Core Topics in General and Emergency Surgery
Third Edition

Take a look at the other great titles in the Companion Series...

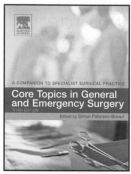

Paterson-Brown
Core Topics in
General and
Emergency Surgery
3rd Edition
0702027332

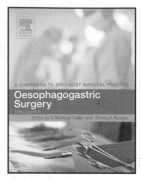

Griffin & Raimes
Oesophagogastric
Surgery
3rd Edition
0702027359

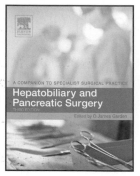

Garden
Hepatobiliary and
Pancreatic Surgery
3rd Edition
0702027367

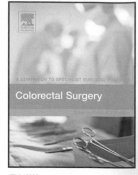

Phillips
Colorectal Surgery
3rd Edition
0702027324

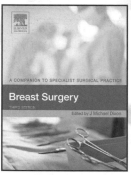

Dixon
Breast Surgery
3rd Edition
0702027383

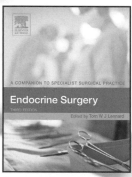

Lennard
Endocrine Surgery
3rd Edition
0702027391

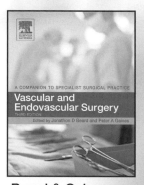

Beard & Gaines
Vascular and
Endovascular
Surgery
3rd Edition
0702027340

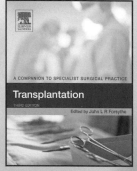

Forsythe
Transplantation
3rd Edition
0702027375

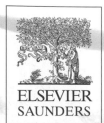

ELSEVIER
SAUNDERS

Order either through your local bookshop, direct from Elsevier
(call customer services on +44 (0)1865 474000) or log on to
http://www.elsevierhealth.com/surgery

A Companion to Specialist Surgical Practice
Third Edition

Series Editors
O. James Garden
Simon Paterson-Brown

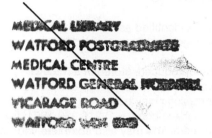
Core Topics in General and Emergency Surgery
Third Edition

Edited by
Simon Paterson-Brown
Honorary Senior Lecturer
Clinical and Surgical Sciences (Surgery)
University of Edinburgh
and
Consultant General and Upper Gastrointestinal Surgeon
Royal Infirmary of Edinburgh

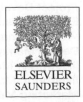

ELSEVIER
SAUNDERS

ELSEVIER
SAUNDERS

An imprint of Elsevier Limited

First edition 1997
Second edition 2001
Third edition 2005
© 2005, Elsevier Limited. All rights reserved.

The right of S. Paterson-Brown to be identified as editor of this work has been asserted by him in accordance with the Copyright, Designs and Patents Act 1988

ISBN 0 7020 2733 2

British Library Cataloguing in Publication Data
A catalogue record for this book is available from the British Library

Library of Congress Cataloging in Publication Data
A catalog record for this book is available from the Library of Congress

Notice
Medical knowledge is constantly changing. Standard safety precautions must be followed, but as new research and clinical experience broaden our knowledge, changes in treatment and drug therapy may become necessary or appropriate. Readers are advised to check the most current product information provided by the manufacturer of each drug to be administered to verify the recommended dose, the method and duration of administration, and contraindications. It is the responsibility of the practitioner, relying on experience and knowledge of the patient, to determine dosages and the best treatment for each individual patient. Neither the Publisher nor the editor assume any liability for any injury and/or damage to persons or property arising from this publication.
The Publisher

Printed in The Netherlands
Last digit is the print number: 9 8 7 6 5 4 3 2 1

Commissioning Editor: Michael Houston
Project Development Manager: Sheila Black
Editorial Assistants: Kathryn Mason, Liz Brown
Project Manager: Cheryl Brant
Design Manager: Jayne Jones
Illustration Manager: Mick Ruddy
Illustrator: Martin Woodward
Marketing Managers: Gaynor Jones (UK), Ethel Cathers (USA)

Contents

Contents

Colour plate section follows p. 116

Contributors

Faisal Abbasakoor MB ChB BAO BA FRCS(Gen Surg)
Clinical Research Fellow
Department of Surgery
Royal Free and University College
Medical School
London, UK

Andrew C. de Beaux MB ChB MD FRCS
Consultant General and Upper
Gastrointestinal Surgeon
Department of Surgery
Royal Infirmary of Edinburgh
Edinburgh, UK

David H. Bennett BSc MB BS DM FRCS
Consultant Surgeon
Department of Surgery
The Royal Bournemouth Hospital
Bournemouth, UK

Kenneth D. Boffard BSc MB BCh FRCS(Gen Surg) FRCS(Ed) FRCPS(Glasg) FCS(SA) FACS
Professor and Clinical Head
Department of Surgery
Johannesburg Hospital and
University of the Witwatersrand
Johannesburg, South Africa

John Broom BSc MB ChB FRCP FRCPath
Consultant in Clinical Biochemistry
and Metabolic Medicine
Grampian University Hospitals
Trust;
Research Professor in Clinical
Biochemistry and Metabolic
Medicine
Robert Gordon University
Aberdeen, UK

Linda de Cossart ChM FRCS
Consultant Vascular and General
Surgeon
Countess of Chester NHS Trust
Chester, UK

Nick Everitt MB ChB MD FRCS
Consultant Surgeon
Chesterfield Royal Hospital
Chesterfield, Derbyshire, UK

David C. Gotley MD FRACS
Professor of Surgery
University of Queensland
Department of Surgery
Princess Alexandra Hospital
Wooloongabba
Queensland, Australia

R. Michael Grounds MD MB BS LRCP MRCS FRCA DA
Reader in Intensive Care
Medicine
St George's Hospital Medical
School;
Consultant in Anaesthesia and
Intensive Care Medicine
St George's Hospital
London, UK

George Hamilton MB ChB MD FRCS
Professor of Vascular Surgery
Royal Free and University College
School of Medicine;
Consultant Vascular Surgeon
Royal Free Hospital
London, UK

Steven D. Heys BMedBiol MD PhD FRCS FRCS(Ed) FRCS(Glasg)
Professor of Surgical Oncology
University of Aberdeen;
Honorary Consultant Surgeon
Grampian University Hospitals
Trust
Aberdeen, UK

Douglas McWhinnie MD FRCS
Consultant Surgeon
Milton Keynes General Hospital
Milton Keynes, UK

B. James Mander BSc MS MB BS FRCS FRCS(Gen Surg)
Consultant Colorectal Surgeon
Edinburgh Colorectal Unit
Western General Hospital
Edinburgh, UK

Jonathan A. Michaels MChir FRCS
Professor of Vascular Surgery
Academic Vascular Unit
Northern General Hospital
Sheffield, UK

Rowan W. Parks MD FRCSI FRCS(Ed)
Senior Lecturer in Surgery
University of Edinburgh;
Honorary Consultant Surgeon
Royal Infirmary of Edinburgh
Edinburgh, UK

Simon Paterson-Brown MB BS MPhil MS FRCS(Ed) FRCS
Honorary Senior Lecturer
Clinical and Surgical Sciences
(Surgery)
University of Edinburgh;
Consultant General and Upper
Gastrointestinal Surgeon
Royal Infirmary of Edinburgh
Edinburgh, UK

James J. Powell BSc MD, FRCS(Ed) FRCS(Gen Surg)
Lecturer in Surgery
Department of Clinical and Surgical
Sciences
University of Edinburgh
Edinburgh, UK

Kathryn A. Rigby MSc MB ChB FRCS
Specialist Registrar in General
Surgery
Sheffield Vascular Institute
Northern General Hospital
Sheffield, UK

Brian J. Rowlands MD FRCS FACS
Professor of Surgery
University of Nottingham;
Head of Section of Surgery
Queen's Medical Centre
University Hospital
Nottingham, UK

Russell Slack BSc MSc
Research Associate
Sheffield Health Economics Group
University of Sheffield
Sheffield, UK

Lewis Spitz MB ChB PhD MD FRCS FRCS(Ed) FRCPCH, FAAP
Nuffield Professor of Paediatric Surgery
Institute of Child Health
University College London
London, UK

Ian D. Sugarman MB ChB FRCS(Paed)
Consultant Paediatric Surgeon
Leeds General Infirmary
Leeds, UK

Carolynne J. Vaizey MD FRCS(Gen Surg) FCS(SA)
Consultant Surgeon
St Mark's Hospital at
Northwick Park
Harrow, UK

Preface

The *Companion to Specialist Surgical Practice* series was designed to meet the needs of surgeons in higher training and the practising consultant who wish up-to-date and evidence-based information on the subspecialist areas relevant to their surgical practice. In trying to meet this aim, we have recognised that the series will never be as all-encompassing as many of the larger reference surgical textbooks. However, by their very size, it is rare that the latter are completely up to date at the time of publication. The first edition of this series was published in 1997, with the second following in 2001. In this third edition, we have been able to bring up to date the relevant specialist information that we and the individual volume editors consider important for the practising subspecialist surgeon. Where possible, all contributors have attempted to identify evidence-based references to support key recommendations within each chapter. These should all be interpreted with the help of the guidance summary 'Evidence-based practice in surgery', which follows this preface.

We are extremely grateful to each volume editor and to their contributors to this third edition. It is thanks to their enthusiasm and hard work that the relatively short time frame between each of the editions has been maintained, thereby providing to the reader the most accurate and up-to-date infor-mation possible. We were all immensely saddened by the sudden and tragic death of Professor John Farndon, who edited the first and second editions of the volumes *Breast Surgery* and *Endocrine Surgery*. While recognising that he was a unique and talented individual, we are pleased to welcome the additional editorial skills of Mike Dixon and Tom Lennard for this third edition.

We are also grateful for the support and encouragement of Elsevier Ltd and hope that our aim – of providing up-to-date and affordable surgical texts – has been met and that all readers, whether in training or in consultant practice, will find this third edition a valuable resource.

O. James Garden BSc, MB, ChB, MD, FRCS(Glasg), FRCS(Ed), FRCP(Ed)
Regius Professor of Clinical Surgery, Clinical and Surgical Sciences (Surgery), University of Edinburgh, and Honorary Consultant Surgeon, Royal Infirmary of Edinburgh

Simon Paterson-Brown MB BS, MPhil, MS, FRCS(Ed), FRCS
Honorary Senior Lecturer, Clinical and Surgical Sciences (Surgery), University of Edinburgh, and Consultant General and Upper Gastrointestinal Surgeon, Royal Infirmary of Edinburgh

EVIDENCE-BASED PRACTICE IN SURGERY

The third edition of the *Companion to Specialist Surgical Practice* series has attempted to incorporate, where appropriate, **evidence-based practice in surgery**, which has been highlighted in the text and relevant references. A detailed chapter on evidence-based practice in surgery, written by Kathryn Rigby and Jonathan Michaels, has been included in this volume *Core Topics in General and Emergency Surgery*, to which the reader is referred for further information on assessing levels of evidence. We are grateful to them for providing this summary for each volume.

Critical appraisal for developing evidence-based practice can be obtained from a number of sources, the most reliable being randomised controlled clinical trials, systematic literature reviews, meta-analyses and observational studies. For practical purposes three grades of evidence can be used, analogous to the levels of 'proof' required in a court of law:

1. **Beyond reasonable doubt** – such evidence is likely to have arisen from high-quality randomised controlled trials, systematic reviews, or high-quality synthesised evidence such as decision analysis, cost-effectiveness analysis or large observational data sets. The studies need to be directly applicable to the population of concern and have clear results. The grade is analogous to burden of proof within a criminal court and may be thought of as corresponding to the usual standard of 'proof' within the medical literature. (i.e. $P<0.05$).

2. **On the balance of probabilities** – in many cases a high-quality review of literature may fail to reach firm conclusions owing to conflicting or inconclusive results, trials of poor methodological quality, or the lack of evidence in the population to which the guidelines apply. In such cases it may still be possible to make a statement as to the best treatment on the 'balance of probabilities'. This is analogous to the decision in a civil court where all the available evidence will be weighed up and the verdict will depend upon the balance of probabilities.

3. **Not proven** – insufficient evidence upon which to base a decision or contradictory evidence.

Depending on the information available three grades of recommendation can be used:

a. strong recommendaton, which should be followed unless there are compelling reasons to act otherwise;

b. a recommendation based on evidence of effectiveness but where there may be other factors to take into account in decision-making, for example the user of the guidelines may be expected to consider patient preferences, local facilities, local audit results or available resources;

c. a recommendation made where there is no adequate evidence regarding the most effective practice, although there may be reasons for making a recommendation in order to minimise cost or reduce the chance of error through a locally agreed protocol.

 The text and references that are considered to be associated with reasonable evidence are highlighted in this volume with a 'scalpel code', leaving the reader to reach his or her own conclusion.

Acknowledgements

I remain eternally grateful for the ongoing support and understanding of my long-suffering wife, Sheila, and our three daughters, without whose support and encouragement I would not have been able to complete this volume. It is likely that this sentiment will be echoed by all the chapter authors for this volume, who have all played their part in helping to put together this book. The additional onerous hours dedicated to academic activities by busy practising surgeons should never be under-estimated, and I am extremely grateful to all of them for their contributions. I would also like to acknowledge the help, enthusiasm and friendship of my co-editor of the *Companion to Specialist Surgical Practice*, James Garden, not only for helping to get this project off the ground way back in 1995 but also for his ongoing support and commitment during these first three editions.

SPB

One

Evidence-based practice in surgery

Kathryn A. Rigby and
Jonathan A. Michaels

INTRODUCTION

Evidence-based medicine is the conscientious, explicit and judicious use of current best evidence in making decisions about the care of individual patients. The practice of evidence-based medicine means integrating individual clinical expertise with the best external clinical evidence from systematic research.[1]

The concept of evidence-based medicine (EBM) was introduced in the 19th century but has only flourished in the last few decades of the 20th century. Historically, its application to surgical practice can be traced back to the likes of John Hunter and the American Ernest Amory Codman, who both recognised the need for research into surgical outcomes in an attempt to improve patient care.

In mid-19th century Paris, Pierre-Charles-Alexander Louis used statistics to measure the effectiveness of bloodletting, the results of which helped put an end to the practice of leeching. Ernest A. Codman began work as a surgeon in 1895 in Massachusetts. His main area of interest was the shoulder and he became a leading expert in this topic as well as being instrumental in the founding of the American College of Surgeons. He developed his 'End Result Idea', a notion that all hospitals should follow up every patient it treats 'long enough to determine whether or not its treatment is successful and if not, why not?' in order to prevent similar failures in the future.[2] Codman also developed the first registry of bone sarcomas.

In the UK, one of the most important advocates of EBM was Archie Cochrane. His experiences in the prisoner of war camps, where he conducted trials in the use of yeast supplements to treat nutritional oedema, influenced his belief in reliable and scientifically proven medical treatment. In 1972 he published his book *Effectiveness and Efficiency*. Cochrane advocated the use of the randomised controlled trial (RCT) as the gold standard in the research of all medical treatment and, where possible, systematic reviews of these trials. One of the first systematic reviews of RCTs was of the use of corticosteroid therapy to improve lung function in threatened premature birth. Although RCTs had been conducted in this area, the message of the results was not clear from the individual studies, until the review overwhelmingly showed that corticosteroids reduced both neonatal morbidity and mortality. Had a systematic review been conducted earlier, then the lives of many babies could have been saved, as the review clearly showed that this inexpensive treatment reduced the chance of these babies dying from complications of immaturity by 30–50%.[3] In 1992, as part of the UK National Health Service (NHS) Research and Development (R&D) Programme, the Cochrane Collaboration was founded.

Subsequently, in 1995, the first centre for EBM in the UK was established at the Nuffield Department of Clinical Medicine, University of Oxford. The driving force behind this was the American David Sackett, who had moved to a new Chair in Clinical Epidemiology in 1994 from McMaster University in Canada, where he had pioneered self-directed teaching for medical students.

From these roots, the interest in EBM has exploded. The Cochrane Collaboration is rapidly expanding, with review groups in many fields of medicine and surgery. EBM is not limited only to hospital-based medicine but is increasingly seen in nursing, general practice and dentistry, and there are many new evidence-based journals appearing.

While clinical experience is invaluable, the rapidly changing world of medicine means that clinicians must keep abreast of new advances and, where appropriate, integrate research findings into everyday clinical practice. Neither research nor clinical experience alone is enough to ensure high-quality patient care; the two must complement each other. Sackett et al. identified five steps that should become part of day-to-day practice and in which a competent practitioner should be proficient:[4]

1. to convert information needs into answerable questions;
2. to be able to track down efficiently the best evidence with which to answer them (be it evidence from clinical examination, the diagnostic laboratory, research evidence or other sources);
3. to be able to appraise that evidence critically for its validity and usefulness;
4. to apply the results of this appraisal in clinical practice;
5. to evaluate performance.

This chapter discusses the steps that are necessary to identify, critically appraise and combine evidence, to incorporate the findings into clinical guidance and to implement and audit any necessary changes in order to move towards EBM in surgery. Many of the organisations and information sources that are relevant to EBM are specific to a particular setting. Therefore, the emphasis in this chapter is on the health services within the UK, although there are comparable arrangements and bodies in many other countries. Links to a number of these are given in the Internet resources described at the end of the chapter.

THE NEED FOR EVIDENCE-BASED MEDICINE

In 1991, there was still a widely held belief that only a small proportion of medical interventions were supported by solid scientific evidence.[5] Jonathan Ellis and colleagues, on behalf of the Nuffield Department of Clinical Medicine, conducted a review of treatments given to 109 patients on a medical ward.[6] The treatments were then examined to assess the degree of evidence supporting their use. The authors concluded that 82% of these treatments were in fact evidence based. However, they did suggest that similar studies should be

conducted in other specialties. The importance of evidence-based health care in the NHS was formally acknowledged in two government papers, *The new NHS*[7] and *A first class service*.[8] These led to the development of the National Service Frameworks and the National Institute of Clinical Excellence (NICE).

In surgery there is a limited body of evidence from high-quality RCTs. For an RCT to be ethical there needs to be a clinical equipoise. That is to say, there needs to be a sufficient level of uncertainty about an intervention before a trial can be considered. For example, it would be unethical to conduct an RCT in the use of burr holes for extradural haematomas, because the observational data alone are so overwhelming as to the high degree of effectiveness that it would be unethical to deny someone a burr hole to prove the point.

Many surgeons feel unhappy with having to explain to a patient that there is clinical uncertainty about a treatment, as patients have historically put their trust in surgeons' hands. This reluctance to perform RCTs and the belief that they would be difficult to carry out has led to practices that are poorly supported by high-quality evidence. For example, there is widespread use of radical prostatectomy to treat localised prostatic carcinoma in the USA, despite a distinct lack of evidence to support this procedure.[9]

New technologies in surgery may be driven into widespread use by market forces, patients' expectations and clinicians' desire to improve treatment options. For example, with laparoscopic surgery, many assumed that it must be 'better' because it made smaller holes, there was less pain involved and therefore patients left hospital sooner. It was only after many hospitals had instituted its use that concerns were raised about its real benefits and the adequacy of training in the new technology. In 1996, a group of surgeons from Sheffield published a randomised, prospective, single-blind study that compared small-incision open cholecystectomy with laparoscopic cholecystectomy.[10] They demonstrated that in their hands the laparosopic technique offered no real benefit over a mini-cholecystectomy in terms of the postoperative recovery period, hospital stay and time off work, but it took longer to perform and was more expensive.[10]

The MRC Laparoscopic Groin and Hernia Trial Group undertook a large multicentre randomised comparison between laparoscopic and open repair of groin hernias.[11] The results demonstrated that the laparoscopic procedure was associated with an earlier return to activities and less groin pain 1 year after surgery but it was also associated with more serious surgical complications, an increased recurrence rate and a higher cost to the health service. They suggested that laparoscopic hernia surgery should be confined to specialist surgical centres. NICE have since published guidelines which state that laparoscopic hernia repairs should only be offered to patients with bilateral or recurrent hernias.

Some would argue that surgery, unlike drug trials, is operator dependent and that operating experience and skill can affect the outcome of an RCT and cite this as a reason for not undertaking surgical trials. Although operator factors can introduce bias into a trial, the North American Symptomatic Carotid Endarterectomy Trial has shown that such problems can largely be overcome through appropriate trial design.[12] Only surgeons who had been fully trained in the procedure, and who already had a proven low complication rate, were accepted as participants in the trial.

These examples illustrate a clear need for high-quality research to be undertaken into any new technology to assess both its efficacy and its cost-effectiveness before it is introduced into the health-care system.

However, concerns have been raised about EBM. Sceptics have suggested that it may undermine clinical experience and instinct and replace it with 'cookbook medicine' or that it may ignore the elements of basic medical training such as history-taking, physical examination, laboratory investi-gations and a sound grounding in pathophysiology. Another fear is that purchasers and managers will use it as a means to cut costs and manage budgets.

Nevertheless, EBM can formalise our everyday procedures and highlight problems. It can provide answers by ensuring that the best use is made of existing evidence or it can identify areas in which new research is needed. Although it has a role in assessing the cost-effectiveness of an intervention, it is not a substitute for rationing and often results in practice that, despite being more cost-effective, has greater overall cost.[13]

THE PROCESS OF EVIDENCE-BASED MEDICINE

EBM requires a structured approach to ensure that clinical interventions are based upon best available evidence. The first stage is always to pose a clinically relevant question for which an answer is required. Such a question should be clear, specific, important and answerable. One way of formulating questions is to think of them as having three key elements:

- the population to whom the question applies;
- the intervention of interest (and any other interventions with which it is to be compared);
- the outcome of interest.

Therefore the question 'What is the best treatment for cholecystitis?' needs to be much more clearly formulated if an adequate, evidence-based approach is to be used. A much better question would be 'For adult patients admitted to hospital with acute cholecystitis (the **population**), does early open cholecystectomy, laparoscopic cholecystectomy or best medical management (the **interventions**) produce the lowest mortality, morbidity and total length of stay in hospital (the **outcomes**)?' Even this may require more refinement to define further the exact interventions and outcomes of interest.

Once such a question has been clearly defined, a number of further stages of the process can follow.

1. Relevant sources of information must be searched to identify all available literature that will help in answering the question.
2. Published trials must be critically appraised to assess whether they possess internal and external validity in answering the question posed (**internal validity** is where the effects within the study are free from bias and confounding; **external validity** is where the effects within the study apply outside the study and the results are therefore generalisable to the population in question).
3. Where relevant, a systematic review and meta-analysis may be required to provide a clear answer from a number of disparate sources.
4. The answers to the question need to be incorporated into clinical practice through the use of guidelines or through other methods of implementation.
5. Adherence to 'best practice' needs to be monitored through audit, and the process needs to be kept under review in order to take account of new evidence or clinical developments.

SOURCES OF EVIDENCE

Once a question has been formulated, the next step in undertaking EBM is the identification of all the relevant evidence. The first line for most prac-titioners is the use of journals. Many clinicians will subscribe to specific journals in their own specialist area and have access to many others through local libraries. However, the vast increase in the number of such publications makes it impossible for an individual to access or read all the relevant papers, even in a highly specialised area.

There has been a huge expansion in the resources that are available for identifying relevant material from other publications, including indexing and abstracting services such as MEDLINE (computerised database compiled by the US National Library of

Medicine) and EMBASE. The rapid technological developments of the past few years have made these widely available through Internet services, electronic publications and online databases.

There is also a rapidly expanding set of journals and other services that provide access to selected, appraised and combined results from primary information sources.

As a result, the information sources that provide the evidence to support EBM are vast and include the following.

- Media: journals, online databases, CD-ROMs and the Internet.
- Independent organisations: research bodies and the pharmaceutical industry.
- Health services: purchasers and providers at local, regional and national level.
- Academic units.

Some of these are described in more detail below and the Appendix to this chapter provides a list of contact details for further information.

Journals

The following are a selection of journals that act as secondary sources, identifying and reviewing other research that is felt to be of key importance to evidence-based practice.

EVIDENCE-BASED MEDICINE

First launched in October 1995, *Evidence-based Medicine* is a collaboration between the American College of Physicians (ACP) and the *British Medical Journal* (BMJ) Publishing Group. The ACP Journal Club, begun in 1991, has a large editorial team who survey a vast array of journals, identifying clinically relevant research articles and summarising the essential information. This consequently allows the reader to keep up with the latest advances in clinical practice. *Evidence-based Medicine* is the UK version of the journal and covers a wide range of specialties and also contains extracts from the American journal, systematic reviews from the Cochrane Collaboration and reports from the York Centre for Reviews and Dissemination.

EVIDENCE-BASED NURSING

Evidence-based Nursing follows similar lines to *Evidence-based Medicine*, but contains articles more relevant to the nursing field. It is edited by the Royal College of Nursing and the BMJ Publishing Group.

EVIDENCE-BASED HEALTH CARE

Evidence-based Health Care is published by Churchill Livingstone (Harcourt). It also contains abstracts and articles about evidence-based issues and results of systematic reviews, etc.

EVIDENCE-BASED PURCHASING

Evidence-based Purchasing is an NHS R&D publication edited by Ben Toth. It summarises evidence about effective health care intended to support the commissioning role.

EVIDENCE-BASED MENTAL HEALTH

The BMJ Publishing Group publishes *Evidence-based Mental Health* in collaboration with the Health Information Research Unit, Department of Clinical Epidemiology and Biostatistics, McMaster University and the NHS R&D programme. It is a quarterly publication that identifies and appraises clinically relevant research.

EVIDENCE-BASED HEALTH POLICY AND MANAGEMENT

Evidence-based Health Policy and Management is also a Churchill Livingstone publication, edited by J.A. Muir and Anna Donaldson.

Internet resources

The Internet is becoming an increasingly useful source of medical information and evidence. Details of Internet addresses for many of the sources referred to below are given in the Appendix to this chapter, although this is a rapidly progressing and changing area. There are many journals and databases that are available either free or through subscription. For example, MEDLINE can be searched free of charge through the National Library of Medicine, PubMed service; the *British Medical Journal* and the *Journal of the American Medical Association* (*JAMA*) are freely available in an electronic form. This medium also provides a number of advantages over printed material, including ease of searching, hyperlinks to other sources, access to additional supporting materials or raw data and the provision of discussion groups. There are, however, potential problems with the Internet in that there is no quality control and much of the available material is of dubious quality or published by those with particular commercial or other interests.

The OMNI (Organising Medical Networked Information) Project is a useful Internet-based resource that provides UK and worldwide coverage of resources in medicine, biosciences and health management. The lead body is the National Institute for Medical Research Library, with contributions from the medical libraries of Nottingham University, Cambridge University, the Royal Free Hospital School of Medicine, the King Edward

Hospital Fund and the Wellcome Centre for Medical Science.

Academic units

COCHRANE COLLABORATION

As described above, the British epidemiologist who inspired this collaboration realised that in order to make informed decisions about health care, reliable evidence must be accessible and kept up to date with any new evidence. It was felt that failure to achieve this might result in important developments in health care being overlooked. This was to be a key aspect in providing the best health care possible for patients. It was also hoped that by making clear the result of an intervention then work would not be duplicated.

The Cochrane library is the electronic publication of the Cochrane Collaboration and it includes several databases.

- The Cochrane Database of Systematic Reviews contains systematic reviews and protocols of reviews in preparation. These are regularly updated and there are facilities for comments and criticisms along with authors' responses.
- The Cochrane Controlled Trials Register is the largest database of RCTs. Information about trials is obtained from several sources including searches of other databases and hand searching of medical journals. It includes many RCTs not currently listed in databases such as MEDLINE or EMBASE.
- The Database of Abstracts of Reviews of Effectiveness (DARE) contains abstracts of reviews that have been critically appraised by peer reviewers at the NHS Centre for Reviews and Dissemination (CRD) and by others.
- The Cochrane Review Methodology Database is a bibliography of articles on the science of research synthesis.
- The Reviewers' Handbook includes information on the science of reviewing research and details of the review groups. It is also available in hard copy.[14]

The Cochrane library is regularly updated and amended as new evidence is acquired. It is distributed on disk, CD-ROM and the Internet.[3] To allow the results of the reviews to be widely used no one contributor has exclusive copyright of the review.

CENTRE FOR EVIDENCE-BASED MEDICINE

The Centre for Evidence-based Medicine is a collaboration between the Health Authority, the NHS R&D programme, medical academia and the hospitals of Oxford. Its chief remit is to promote EBM and the practice of it in health care. It runs workshops and courses in both the practice and teaching of EBM. The members are also involved in RCTs and work closely with the Cochrane Collaboration Methods Working Group.

NHS agencies

NHS CENTRE FOR REVIEWS AND DISSEMINATION

The CRD was established in January 1994 at the University of York; it is funded by the NHS Executive and the health departments of Scotland, Wales and Northern Ireland but is independent of the government. Its sister organisation is the UK Cochrane Centre and they were both set up to support the NHS R&D programme. The CRD concentrates specifically on areas of priority to the NHS. It is designed to raise the standards of reviews within the NHS and to encourage research, by working with health-care professionals. There are two databases that it maintains:

- the NHS Economic Evaluation Database contains mainly abstracts of economic evaluations of health-care interventions and assesses the quality of the studies, stating any practical implications to the NHS;
- DARE (see above).

NHS HEALTH TECHNOLOGY ASSESSMENT PROGRAMME

The Health Technology Assessment (HTA) is the NHS-funded research programme that commissions research into high-priority areas. This includes many systematic reviews and primary research in key areas. The programme publishes details of ongoing HTA projects and monographs of completed research.

CRITICAL APPRAISAL

 This is the process by which we assess the evidence presented to us in a paper. We need to be critical of it in terms of its validity and clinical applicability.

From reading the literature, it is evident that there may be many trials on the same subject, which may all draw different conclusions. Which one should be believed and allowed to influence clinical practice? We owe a duty to our patients to be able to assess accurately all the available information and judge each paper on its own merits before changing our clinical practice accordingly.

Randomised control trials

The RCT is a comparative evaluation in which the interventions being compared are allocated to the units being studied purely by chance. It is the 'gold standard' method of comparing the effectiveness of different interventions.[15] Randomisation is the only way to allow valid inferences of cause and effect,[16] and no other study design can potentially protect as well against bias.

Unfortunately, not all clinical trials are done well, and even fewer are well reported. Their results may therefore be confusing and misleading and it is necessary to consider several elements of a trial's design, conduct and conclusions before accepting the results. The first requirement is that there must be sufficient detail available to make such an assessment.

It has become clear that there is a need for the presentation of clinical trials to be standardised. Two groups published proposals for standardisation in 1994 and the subsequent joint publication became known as the CONSORT statement (**Table 1.1**).[17,18] The statement listed items that should be included in any trial report, along with a flow chart identifying the patient's progress through the trial. Many journals now encourage authors to submit a copy of the CONSORT statement relating to their paper (e.g. *British Medical Journal*, *Journal of the*

Table 1.1 • CONSORT statement regarding the standardisation of presentation of randomised controlled clinical trials

Sections	Content
Title	Identify the study as a randomised trial
Abstract	Use a structured format
Introduction	State prospectively defined hypothesis, clinical objectives and planned subgroup or covariant analyses
Methods Protocol	Planned study population described together with inclusion and exclusion criteria Planned interventions and their timing Primary and secondary outcome measure(s), the minimum important difference(s) and indicate how the target sample size was projected Rationale and methods of statistical analyses Prospectively defined stopping rules
Assignment	Unit of randomisation Method used to generate the allocation schedule Method of allocation concealment Method to separate the generator from the executor of the assignment
Masking (blinding)	Mechanism for masking (e.g. capsules, tablets) Similarity of treatment characteristics Allocation schedule control Evidence for successful blinding among participants, person doing intervention, outcome assessors and data analysts
Results Participant flow	Provide a trial profile, showing patient flow, numbers and follow-up, timing of randomisation assignments, interventions and measurements for each randomised group
Analysis	State estimated effect of intervention on primary and secondary outcome measures including a point estimate and confidence interval State absolute numbers when feasible Present summary data and appropriate statistics in sufficient detail to permit alternative analyses and replication Describe prognostic variables by treatment group and attempt to adjust for them Describe protocol deviations and the reasons why
Discussion	State specific interpretation of study findings, sources of bias and imprecision and discuss internal and external validity State general interpretation of the data in light of the totality of available evidence

American Medical Association, Lancet).[18] The Critical Appraisal Skills Programme (CASP) is a UK-based project designed to develop appraisal skills about effectiveness. It provides half-day workshops and has developed appraisal frameworks based on 10 or 11 questions for RCTs, qualitative research and systematic reviews.

Assuming that the relevant information is available, critical appraisal is required to ensure that the methodology of the trial is such that it will minimise effects on outcome other than true treatment effects, i.e. those owing to **chance**, **bias** and **confounding**.

- Chance: random variation, leading to imprecision.
- Bias: systematic variation leading to inaccuracy.
- Confounding: systematic variation resulting from the existence of extraneous factors that affect the outcome and have distributions that are not taken into account, leading to bias and invalid inferences.

All good study designs will reduce the effects of chance, eliminate bias and take confounding into account. This requires consideration of many aspects of trial design including methods of randomisation, blinding and masking, analysis methods and sample size. It also requires the reviewer to consider aspects such as sponsorship and vested interests that may introduce sources of bias. Discussion of methodology for the critical appraisal of RCTs and other forms of study is readily available elsewhere.[19]

SYSTEMATIC LITERATURE REVIEWS

A systematic review is an overview of primary studies carried out to an exhaustive, defined and repeatable protocol.

There has been an explosion in the published medical literature, with over two million articles a year published in 20 000 journals. The task of keeping up with new advances in medical research has become quite overwhelming. We have also seen that the results of trials in the same subject may be contradictory, and that the underlying message can be masked. Systematic reviews are designed to search out meticulously all relevant studies on a subject, evaluate the quality of each study and assimilate the information to produce a balanced and unbiased conclusion.[20]

One advantage of a systematic review with a meta-analysis over a traditional subjective narrative review is that by synthesising the results of many smaller studies, the original lack of statistical power of each study may be overcome by cumulative size, and any treatment effect is more clearly demonstrated. This, in turn, can lead to a reduction in delay between research advances and clinical implementation. For example, it has been demonstrated that if the original studies done on the use of anticoagulants after myocardial infarction had been reviewed, their benefits would have been apparent much earlier.[21,22] It is essential that the benefit or any harm caused by an intervention becomes apparent as soon as possible.

Unfortunately, as in reported trials, not all reviews are as rigorously researched and synthesised as one would hope and are open to similar pitfalls as RCTs. The Cochrane Collaboration has sought to rectify this and has worked upon refining the methods used for systematic reviews. It has consequently produced some of the most reliable and useful reviews and its methods have been widely adopted by other reviewers. The Cochrane Collaboration advises that each review must be based on an explicit protocol, which sets out the objectives and methods so that a second party could reproduce the review at a later date if required.

Because of the increasing importance of systematic reviews as a method of providing the evidence base for a variety of clinical activities, the methods are discussed in some detail below. There are several key elements in producing a systematic review.

1 Develop a protocol for a clearly defined question

Within a protocol:

- the objectives of the review of the RCTs must be stated;
- eligibility criteria must be included (e.g. relevant patient groups, types of intervention and trial design);
- appropriate outcome measures should be defined.

In the Cochrane Collaboration, each systematic review is preceded by a published protocol that is subjected to a process of peer review. This helps to ensure high quality, avoids duplication of effort and is designed to reduce bias by setting standards for inclusion criteria before the results from identified studies have been assessed.

2 Literature search

All published and unpublished material should be sought. This includes examining studies in non-English journals, grey literature, conference reports, company reports (drug companies can hold a lot of vital information from their own research) and any personal contacts, for personal studies or information. The details of the search methodology and search terms used should be specified in order to make the review reproducible and allow readers to repeat the search to identify further relevant information published after the review. The most frequently used initial source of information is MEDLINE but this does have limitations. It only indexes about one-third of all medical articles that exist in libraries (over 10 million in total),[23] and an average search by a regular user would only yield about one-fifth of the trials that can be identified by more rigorous techniques for literature searching.[24] It also has a bias towards articles published in English. Other electronic and indexed databases should also be searched, but often the only way to ensure that the maximum number of relevant trials are found, wherever published and in whatever language, is to hand search the journals. This is one of the tasks of the Cochrane Collaboration through a database maintained at the Baltimore Cochrane Centre.

One must also be aware, however, that there is a potential for 'publication bias': trials that are more likely to get published are those with a positive result rather than a negative or no-effect result,[25] and these are more likely to be cited in other articles.[26]

3 Evaluating the studies

Each trial should be assessed to see if it meets the inclusion criteria set out in the protocol (eligibility). If it meets the required standards, then the trial is subjected to a critical appraisal, ideally by two independent reviewers to ascertain its validity, relevance and reliability. Any exclusions should be reported and justified; if there is missing information from the published article, it may be necessary to attempt to contact the author of the primary research. Reviewers should also, if possible, be 'blinded' to the authors and journals of publication, etc. in order to minimise any personal bias.

The Cochrane reviewers are assisted in all these tasks by instructions in the Cochrane Handbook[14] and through workshops at the Cochrane Centres.[27]

4 Synthesis of the results

Once the studies have been graded according to quality and relevance, their results may be combined in an interpretative or a statistical fashion. It must be decided if it is appropriate to combine some studies and which comparisons to make. Subgroup or sensitivity analyses may also be appropriate. The statistical analysis is called a meta-analysis and is discussed below.

5 Discussion

The review should be summarised. The aims, methods and reported results should be discussed and the following issues considered:

- quality of the studies;
- possible sources of heterogeneity (reasons for inconsistency between studies, e.g. patient selection, methods of randomisation, duration of follow-up or differences in statistical analysis);
- bias;
- chance;
- applicability of the findings.

As with any study, a review can be done badly, and the reader must critically appraise a review to assess its quality. Systematic errors may be introduced by omitting some relevant studies, by selection bias (such as excluding foreign language journals) or by including inappropriate studies (such as those considering different patient groups or irrelevant outcomes). Despite all precautions, the findings of a systematic review may differ from those of a large-scale high-quality RCT. This will be discussed below in relation to meta-analysis.

META-ANALYSIS

A meta-analysis is a specific statistical strategy for assembling the results of several studies into a single estimate, which may be incorporated into a systematic literature review.[28]

Here we must make the distinction that the term 'meta-analysis' refers to the statistical techniques used to combine the results of several studies and is not synonymous with systematic review, as it is sometimes used.

A common problem in clinical trials is that the results are not clear-cut, either because of size or because of the design of the trial. The systematic review is designed to eliminate some of these problems and give appropriate weightings to the best- and worst-quality studies, regardless of size. Meta-analysis is the statistical tool used to combine the results and give 'power' to the estimates of effect.

Meta-analyses use a variety of statistical techniques according to the type of data being analysed (dichotomous, continuous or individual patient data),[14] and there are two main models used to analyse the results: the fixed-effect model (logistic regression, Mantel–Haenszel test and Peto's method) and the random-effect model. The major concern with fixed-effect methods is that they assume no clinical heterogeneity between the individual trials, and this may be unrealistic.[29] The random-effect method takes into consideration random variation and clinical heterogeneity between trials. In the presentation of meta-analysis, a consistent scale should be chosen for measuring treatment effects and to cope with the possible large scale of difference in proportions, risk ratios or odds ratios that can be used.

Heterogeneity

Trials can have many different components[19] and therefore a meta-analysis is only valid if the trials

that it seeks to summarise are homogeneous: you cannot add apples and oranges.[30] If trials are not comparable and any heterogeneity is ignored, the analysis can produce misleading results.

Figure 1.1 shows an example of this from a meta-analysis of 19 RCTs investigating the use of endoscopic sclerotherapy to reduce mortality from oesophageal varices in the primary treatment of cirrhotic patients.[31] Each trial is represented by a 'point estimate' of the difference between the groups, and a horizontal line showing the 95% confidence interval (CI). If the line does not cross the line of no effect, then there is a 95% chance that there is a real difference between the groups. It can be seen that in this case the trials are not homogeneous as some of the lower limits of the CIs are above the highest limits of CIs in other trials. Such

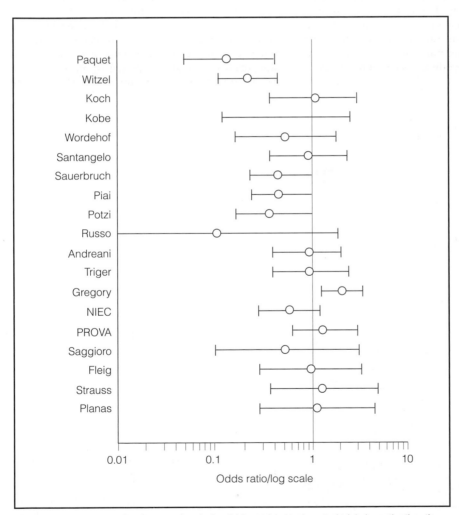

Figure 1.1 • An example of a meta-analysis of 19 randomised control trials investigating the use of endoscopic sclerotherapy to reduce mortality from oesophageal varices in the primary treatment of cirrhotic patients. From Chalmer I, Altman DG. Systematic reviews. London, BMJ Publishing, 1995, p. 119 with permission from Blackwell Publishing Ltd.

a lack of homogeneity may have a variety of causes, relating to clinical heterogeneity (differences in patient mix, setting, etc.) or differences in methods. The degree of statistical heterogeneity can be measured to see if it is greater than is compatible with the play of chance.[32] Such a statistical tool may lack statistical power; consequently results that do not show significant heterogeneity do not necessarily mean that the trials are truly homogeneous and one must look beyond them to assess the degree of heterogeneity.

'Meta-analysis is on the strongest ground when the methods employed in the primary studies are sufficiently similar that any differences in their results are due to the play of chance.'[28]

Views on the usefulness of meta-analyses are divided. On the one hand, they may provide conclusions that could not be reached from other trials because of the small numbers involved. However, on the other hand, they have some limitations and cannot produce a single simple answer to all complex clinical problems. They may give misleading results if used inappropriately where there is a biased body of literature or clinical or methodological heterogeneity. If used with caution, however, they may be a useful tool in providing information to help in decision-making.

Figure 1.2 shows a funnel plot of a meta-analysis relating to the use of magnesium following myocardial infarction.[33] The result of each study in the analysis is represented by a circle plotting the odds ratio (with the vertical line being at 1, the 'line of no effect') against the trial size. The diamond represents the overall results of the meta-analysis with its pooled data from all the smaller studies shown. This study[34] was published in 1993 and showed that it was beneficial and safe to give intravenous magnesium in patients with acute myocardial infarction. The majority of the studies involved show a positive effect of the treatment, as does the meta-analysis. However, the results from this study were contradicted in 1995 by ISIS-4, a very large RCT involving 58 050 patients.[35] It had three arms, in one of which intravenous magnesium was given to patients suspected of an acute myocardial infarction. The results are marked on the

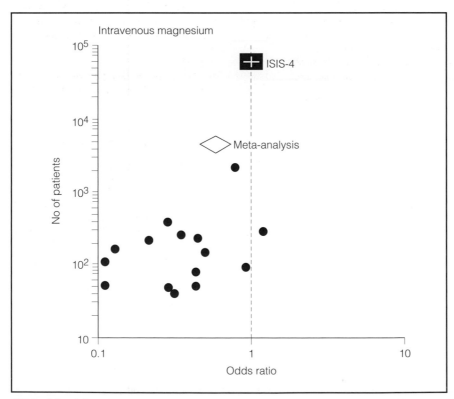

Figure 1.2 • A funnel plot of a meta-analysis relating to the use of magnesium following myocardial infarction. Points indicate values from small and medium-sized trials; the diamond is the combined odds ratio with 95% confidence interval from the meta-analysis of these trials and the square is that for a mega trial. With permission from Egger M, Smith GD. Br Med J 1995; 310:752–4.

funnel plot and show that there is no clear benefit for this treatment, contrary to the results of the earlier meta-analysis.

Some would say that this is one of the major problems with using statistical synthesis. An alternative viewpoint is that it is an example of the importance of ensuring that the material fed into a meta-analysis from a systematic review is researched and critically appraised to the highest possible standard. Explanations for the contradictory findings in this review have been given as:[30,33]

- publication bias, since only trials with positive results were included (see funnel plot);
- methodological weakness in the small trials;
- clinical heterogeneity.

CLINICAL GUIDELINES

Clinical guidelines are systematically developed statements to assist practitioner and patient decisions about appropriate health care for specific clinical circumstances.[36]

EBM is increasingly advocated in health care, and evidence-based guidelines are being developed in many areas of primary health care such as asthma,[37] stable angina[38] and vascular disease.[39] Over 2000 guidelines or protocols have been developed from audit programmes in the UK alone. An observational study in general practice has also shown that recommendations which are evidence based are more widely adopted than those which are not.[40] The UK Department of Health has also endorsed the policy of using evidence-based guidelines.[41]

Guidelines may have a number of different purposes:

- to provide an answer to a specific clinical question using evidence-based methods;
- to aid a clinician in decision-making;
- to standardise aspects of care throughout the country, providing improved equality of access to services and enabling easier comparisons to be made for audit and professional assessment (a reduction in medical practice variation);
- to help to make the most cost-effective use of limited resources;
- to facilitate education of patients and health-care professionals.

For clinical policies to be evidenced based and clinically useful, there must be a balance between the strengths and limitations of relevant research and the practical realities of the health-care and clinical settings.[42]

There are, however, commonly expressed concerns about the use of guidelines.

- There is a worry that the evidence used may be spurious or not relevant, especially in areas where there is a paucity of published evidence.
- Guidelines may not be applicable to every patient and are therefore only useful in treating diseases and not patients.
- Clinicians may feel that they take away their autonomy in decision-making.
- A standardised clinical approach may risk suffocating any clinical flair and innovation.
- There may be geographic or demographic limitations to the applicability of guidelines; for instance a policy developed for use in a city district may not be transferable to a rural area.

The effectiveness of a guideline depends on three areas, as identified by Grimshaw and Russell.[43]

1. How and where the guidelines are produced (development strategy): at a local, regional or national level or by a group internal or external to the area.
2. How the guidelines have been disseminated, e.g. a specific education package, group work, publication in a journal or a mailed leaflet.
3. How the guidelines are implemented (put into use).

In the UK, there are a number of bodies that produce guidelines and summaries of evidence-based advice.

The National Institute for Clinical Excellence

NICE is a special health authority formed on 1 April 1999 by the UK government. The board comprises executive and non-executive members. It is designed to work with the NHS in appraising health-care interventions and offering guidance on the best treatment methods for patients. It assesses all the evidence on the clinical benefit of an intervention, including quality of life, mortality and cost-effectiveness. It will then decide using this information if the intervention should be recommended to the NHS.

Scottish Intercollegiate Guidelines Network

The Scottish Intercollegiate Guidelines Network (SIGN) was formed in 1993. Its objective is to improve the effectiveness and efficiency of clinical care for patients in Scotland by developing, publishing and disseminating guidelines that identify and promote good clinical practice. SIGN is a network of clinicians and health-care professionals including representatives from all the UK Royal Medical Colleges as well as from nursing, pharmacy, dentistry and professions allied to medicine. Patients' views are represented on SIGN through the Scottish Association of Health Councils. SIGN works closely with other national groups and government agencies working in the NHS in Scotland. The SIGN Secretariat is based at the Royal College of Physicians of Edinburgh.

Development and evaluation committees

Development and evaluation committees were set up at a regional level and provide similar information to NICE and are intended as a guide to purchasing decisions. They are due to be phased out and incorporated into NICE.

Royal colleges

The Royal College of Surgeons of England has produced guidelines on topics such as:

- management of head injuries;
- management of groin hernias in adults;
- management of gastroscopy;
- management of ankle fractures.

Effective health-care bulletins

Effective health-care bulletins have been commissioned by the UK Department of Health to provide an overall summary of the clinical and cost effectiveness of health-care interventions.

Effective Practice and Organisation of Care

Effective Practice and Organisation of Care (EPOC) is a subgroup of the Cochrane Collaboration that reviews and summarises research about the use of guidelines.

Guidelines also need to be critically appraised and a framework has been developed by Cluzeau et al. to do this.[44] It uses 37 questions to appraise three different areas of a clinical guideline:

1. rigour of development;
2. content and context;
3. application.

INTEGRATED CARE PATHWAYS

Integrated care pathways (ICPs) are known by a number of names, including integrated care plans, collaborative care plans, critical care pathways and clinical algorithms. ICPs are a development of clinical practice guidelines and have emerged over recent years as a strategy for delivering consistent high-quality care for a range of diagnostic groups or procedures. They are usually multidisciplinary, patient-focused pathways of care that provide a framework for the management of a clinical condition or procedure and are based upon best available evidence.

The advantage of ICPs over most conventional guidelines is that they provide a complete package of protocols relating to the likely events for all health-care personnel involved with the patient during a single episode of care. By covering each possible contingency with advice based upon best evidence, they provide a means of both identifying and implementing optimum practice.

GRADING THE EVIDENCE

There is a traditional hierarchy of evidence, which lists the primary studies in order of perceived scientific merit. This allows one to give an appropriate level of significance to each type of study and is useful when weighing up the evidence in order to make a clinical decision. One version of the hierarchy is given in **Box 1.1**.[19] It must be remembered, however, that this is only a rough guide and that one needs to assess each study on its own merits. Although a meta-analysis comes above an RCT in the hierarchy, a good-quality RCT is far better than a poorly done meta-analysis. Similarly, a seriously flawed RCT may not merit the same degree of importance as a well-designed cohort study. Checklists have been published that may assist in assessing the methodological quality of each type of study.[19]

Similar checklists are available for systematic reviews.[19,45,46] As already discussed, the preparation of a systematic review is a complex process involving a number of steps, each of which is open to bias and inaccuracies that can distort the results. Such lists can be used as a guide when preparing a review as well as in assessing one. One checklist used to assess the validity of a review does so by identifying potential sources of bias in each step (**Table 1.2**).[47]

It is hoped that the results of a systematic review will be precise, valid and statistically powerful in order to provide the highest quality information

Box 1.1 • Hierarchy of evidence

1. Systematic reviews and meta-analyses
2. Randomised controlled trials with definitive results (the results are clinically significant)
3. Randomised controlled trials with non-definitive results (the results have a point estimate that suggests a clinically significant effect)
4. Cohort studies
5. Case–control studies
6. Cross-sectional studies
7. Case reports

From Greenhalgh T. How to read a paper: the basics of evidence based medicine. London: British Medical Journal Publications, 1997; vol xvii, p. 196, with permission.

Table 1.2 • Checklist for assessing sources of bias and methods of protecting against bias

Source	Check
Problem formulation	Is the question clearly focused?
Study identification	Is the search for relevant studies thorough?
Study selection	Are the inclusion criteria appropriate?
Appraisal of the studies	Is the validity of the studies included adequately assessed?
Data collection	Is missing information obtained from investigators?
Data synthesis	How sensitive are the results to changes in the way the review is done?
Interpretation of results	Do the conclusions flow from the evidence that is reviewed? Are recommendations linked to the strength of the evidence? Are judgements about preferences (values) explicit? If there is 'no evidence of effect', is care taken not to interpret this as 'evidence of no effect'? Are subgroup analyses interpreted cautiously?

From Oxman A. Checklists for review articles. Br Med J 1994; 309:648–51, with permission.

on which to base clinical decisions or to produce clinical guidelines. The strength of the evidence provided by a study also needs to be assessed before making any clinical recommendations. A grading system is required to specify the levels of evidence, and several have previously been reported (e.g. those of the Antithrombotic Therapy Consensus Conference[48] or that shown in **Table 1.3**).

The grading of evidence and recommendations within textbooks, clinical guidelines or ICPs should allow users easily to identify those elements of evidence that may be subject to interpretation or modification in the light of new published data or local information. It should identify those aspects of recommendations that are less securely based

Table 1.3 • Agency for Health Care Policy and Research grading system for evidence and recommendations

Category	Description
Evidence	
Ia	Evidence from meta-analysis of randomised controlled trials
Ib	Evidence from at least one randomised controlled trial
IIa	Evidence from at least one controlled study without randomisation
IIb	Evidence from at least one other type of quasi-experimental study
III	Evidence from non-experimental descriptive studies, such as comparative studies and case–control studies
IV	Evidence from expert committee reports or opinions or clinical experience of respected authorities, or both
Recommendation strength	
A	Directly based on category I evidence
B	Directly based on category II evidence or extrapolated recommendation from category I evidence
C	Directly based on category III evidence or extrapolated recommendation from category I or II evidence
D	Directly based on category IV evidence or extrapolated recommendation from category I, II or III evidence

From Hadorn DC, Baker D, Hodges JS, Hicks N. Rating the quality of evidence for clinical practice guidelines. J Clin Epidemiol 1996; 49:749–54, with permission.

upon evidence and therefore may appropriately be modified in the light of patient preferences or local circumstances. This raises different issues to the grading of evidence for critical appraisal and for systematic reviews.

In 1979, the Canadian Task Force on the Periodic Health Examination was one of the first groups to propose grading the strength of recommendations.[49] Since then there have been several published systems for rating the quality of evidence, although most were not designed specifically to be translated into guideline development. The Agency for Health Care Policy and Research has published such a system, although this body considered that its level of classification may be too complex to allow clinical practice guideline development.[50] Nevertheless, the Agency advocated evidence-linked guideline development, requiring the explicit linkage of recommendations to the quality of the supporting evidence. The Centre for Evidence-based Medicine has developed a more comprehensive grading system, which incorporates dimensions such as prognosis, diagnosis and economic analysis.[51]

These systems are complex; for textbooks, care pathways and guidelines, such grading systems need to be clear and easily understood by the relevant audience as well as taking into account all the different forms of evidence that may be appropriate to such documents.

Determining strength of evidence

There are three main factors that need to be taken into account in determining the strength of evidence:

- the type and quality of the reported study;
- the robustness of the findings;
- the applicability of the study to the population or subgroup to which the guidelines are directed.

TYPE AND QUALITY OF STUDY

Meta-analyses, systematic reviews and RCTs are generally considered to be the highest quality evidence that is available. However, in some situations these may not be appropriate or feasible. Recommendations may depend upon evidence from other kinds of study, such as observational studies of epidemiology or natural history, or synthesised evidence, such as decision analyses and cost-effectiveness modelling.

For each type of evidence, there are sets of criteria as to the methodological quality, and descriptions of techniques for critical appraisal are widely available.[19] Inevitably, there is some degree of subjectivity in determining whether particular flaws or a lack of suitable information invalidates an individual study.

ROBUSTNESS OF FINDINGS

The strength of evidence from a published study would depend not only upon the type and quality of a particular study but also upon the magnitude of any differences and the homogeneity of results. High-quality research may report findings with wide confidence intervals, conflicting results or contradictory findings for different outcome measures or patient subgroups. Conversely, sensitivity analysis within a cost-effectiveness or decision analysis may indicate that uncertainty regarding the exact value of a particular parameter does not detract from the strength of the conclusion.

APPLICABILITY

Strong evidence in a set of guidelines must be wholly applicable to the situation in which the guidelines are to be used. For example, a finding from high-quality research based upon a hospital population may provide good evidence for guidelines intended for a similar setting but a lower quality of evidence for guidelines intended for primary care.

Grading system for evidence

The following is a simple pragmatic grading system for the strength of a statement of evidence, which will be used to grade the evidence in this book. Details of the definitions are given in **Table 1.4**. For practical purposes, only the following three grades are required, which are analogous to the levels of proof required in a court of law.

I 'Beyond reasonable doubt'. Analogous to the burden of proof required in a criminal court case and may be thought of as corresponding to the usual standard of 'proof' within the medical literature (i.e. $P <0.05$).

II 'On the balance of probabilities'. In many cases, a high-quality review of literature may fail to reach firm conclusions because of conflicting evidence or inconclusive results, trials of poor methodological quality or the lack of evidence in the population to which the guidelines apply. Where such strong evidence does not exist, it may still be possible to make a statement as to the 'best' treatment on the 'balance of probabilities'. This is analogous to the decision in a civil court where all the available evidence will be weighed up and a verdict will depend upon the balance of probabilities.

III 'Unproven'. Where the above levels of proof do not exist.

Table 1.4 • Grading of evidence and recommendations

Category	Description
Evidence	
I	'Beyond reasonable doubt'. Evidence from high-quality randomised controlled trials, systematic reviews, high-quality synthesised evidence, such as decision analyses, cost-effectiveness analyses or large observational datasets, which is directly applicable to the population of concern and has clear results
II	'On the balance of probabilities'. Evidence of 'best practice' from a high-quality review of literature, which fails to reach the highest standard of 'proof' because of heterogeneity, questionable trial methodology or lack of evidence in a relevant population
III	'Unproven'. Insufficient evidence upon which to base a decision or contradictory evidence
Recommendations	
A	A strong recommendation, which should be followed unless there are compelling reasons against to act otherwise
B	Recommendations based on evidence of effectiveness that may need interpretation in the light of other factors (e.g. patient preferences, local facilities, local audit results or available resources)
C	Recommendation where there is inadequate evidence on effectiveness but pragmatic or financial reasons to institute an agreed policy
Other considerations	
	The evidence should be presented as clear and brief points, with reference to original source material Individual evidence requiring early review should be identified with reference to known sources of work in progress

All evidence-based guidelines require regular review because of the constant stream of new information that becomes available. In some areas, there is more rapid development and the emergence of new evidence; in these instances, relevant reference will be made to ongoing trials or systematic reviews in progress.

Grading of recommendations

Although recommendations should be based upon the evidence presented, it is necessary to grade the strength of recommendation separately from the evidence. For example, the lack of evidence regarding an expensive new technology may lead to a strong recommendation that it should only be undertaken as part of an adequately regulated clinical trial. Conversely, strong evidence for the effectiveness of a treatment may not lead to a strong recommendation for use if the magnitude of the benefit is small and the treatment very costly.

The following grades of recommendations are suggested and details of the definition are given in **Table 1.4**.

A. A strong recommendation, which should be followed.
B. A recommendation using evidence of effectiveness, but where there may be other factors to take into account in the decision-making process.
C. A recommendation where evidence as to the most effective practice is not adequate, but there may be reasons for making the recommendations in order to minimise cost or reduce the chance of error through a locally agreed protocol.

IMPLEMENTATION OF EVIDENCE-BASED MEDICINE

Health-care professionals have always sought evidence on which to base their clinical practice. Unfortunately, the evidence has not always been available, reliable or explicit, and when it was available it has not been implemented immediately. James Lancaster in 1601 showed that lemon juice was effective in the treatment of scurvy, and in 1747 James Lind repeated the experiment. The British Navy did not utilise this information until 1795 and the Merchant Navy not until 1865. When implementation of research findings are delayed, ultimately the people who suffer are the patients.

A number of different groups of people may need to be committed to the changes before they can take place with a degree of success. These include:

- health-care professionals (doctors, nurses, etc.);
- health-care providers and purchasers;
- researchers;
- patients and the public;
- government (local, regional and national).

Each of these groups has a different set of priorities. To ensure that their own requirements are met by the proposal, negotiation is required, which takes time. There are many potential barriers to the implementation of recommendations, and clinicians may become so embroiled in tradition and dogma that they are resistant to change. They may lack knowledge of new developments or the time and resources to keep up to date with the published literature. Lack of training in a new technology, such as laparoscopic surgery or interventional radiology, may thwart their use, even when shown to be effective. Researchers may become detached from the practicalities of clinical practice and the needs of the health service and concentrate on inappropriate questions or produce impractical guidelines. Managers are subject to changes in the political climate and can easily be driven by policies and budgets. The resources available to them may be limited and not allow for the purchase of new technology, and even potentially cost-saving developments may not be introduced because of the difficulties in releasing the savings from elsewhere in the service.

Patients and the general public can also influence the development of the health care offered. They are susceptible to the persuasion of the mass media and may demand the implementation of 'miracle cures' or fashionable investigations or treatments. Such interventions may not be practical or of any proven benefit. They can also determine the success or failure of a particular treatment. For instance, a treatment may be physically or morally unacceptable, or there may be poor compliance, especially with preventative measures such as diets, smoking cessation or exercise. All these aspects can lead to a delay in the implementation of research findings.

Potential ways of improving this situation include the following.

- Provision of easy and convenient access to summaries of the best evidence, electronic databases, systematic reviews and journals in a clinical setting.
- Development of better disease management systems through mechanisms such as clinical guidelines, ICPs and electronic reminders.
- Implementation of computerised decision-support systems.
- Improvement of educational programmes: practitioners must be regularly and actively appraised of new evidence rather than relying on the practitioner seeking it out; passive dissemination of evidence is ineffective.
- More effective systems to encourage patients to adhere to treatment and general health-care advice; the information must be clear, concise, correct and actively distributed.

There is a gap between research and practice, and there is a need for evidence about the effectiveness of different methods of implementing changes in clinical practice. The NHS Central R&D Committee set up an advisory group to look into this problem and identified 20 priorities for evaluation, as shown in **Box 1.2**.[52]

An EPOC review has examined the different methods of implementing evidence-based health-care and classified them into three broad groups.[53]

- Consistently effective: educational visits and interactive meetings.
- Sometimes effective: audit and feedback.
- Little or no effect: printed guideline distribution.

Several groups have looked at implementing evidence-based practice, such as grommet use in glue ear and steroids in preterm delivery:

- PACE (Promoting Action on Clinical Effectiveness);[54]
- PLIP (Purchaser Led Implementation Projects);[55]
- GriPP (Getting Research into Practice and Purchasing).[56]

Successful implementation of research findings into practice appears to be due to a multipronged approach and the UK National Association of Health Authorities and Trusts (NAHAT) has produced an action checklist in order to facilitate this process.[57]

It must be remembered, however, that EBM is not the sole preserve of experts or clinicians. The research, dissemination and implementation of clinical and economic evaluations have wide-reaching repercussions for the health service. Managers are under increasing pressure to be effective both clinically and for costs and are accountable at local, regional and national level. They need to be actively involved and understand the process. As with all interactions between elements in the health service, there must be collaboration, the ultimate goal being an improvement in patient care.

AUDIT

 Audit is the systematic critical analysis of the quality of medical care, including the procedures used for diagnosis and treatment, the use of resources, and the resulting outcome and quality of life for the patient.[58]

The Department of Health has set out policy documents that outline the development and role of audit in today's health-care system.[58,59] Everyone involved in the health-care process has a responsibility to conduct audit and to assess the quality of care that they provide. In 1996, Donabedian categorised three important elements in the delivery of health care.[60]

Box 1.2 • Priority areas for evaluation in the methods of implementation of the findings of research: recommendations of the advisory group to the NHS Central Research and Development Committee

1. Influence of source and presentation of evidence on its uptake by health-care professionals and others

2. Principal sources of information on health-care effectiveness used by clinicians

3. Management of uncertainty and communications of risk by clinicians

4. Roles for health service users in implementing research findings

5. Why some clinicians but not others change their practice in response to research findings

6. Role of commissioning in securing change in clinical practice

7. Professional, managerial, organisational and commercial factors associated with securing change in clinical practice, with particular focus on trusts and primary care providers

8. Interventions directed at clinical and medical directors and directors of nursing trusts to promote evidence-based care

9. Local research implementation and development projects

10. Effectiveness and cost-effectiveness of audit and feedback to promote implementation of research findings

11. Educational strategies for continuing professional development to promote the implementation of research findings

12. Effectiveness and cost-effectiveness of teaching critical appraisal skills to clinicians, patients/users, purchasers and providers to promote uptake of research findings

13. Role of undergraduate training in promoting the uptake of research findings

14. Impact of clinical practice guidelines in disciplines other than medicine

15. Effectiveness and cost-effectiveness of reminder and decision support systems to implement research findings

16. Role of the media in promoting uptake of research findings

17. Impact of professional and managerial change agents (including educational outreach visits and local opinion leaders) in implementing research findings

18. Effect of evidence-based practice on general health policy measures

19. Impact of national guidelines to promote clinical effectiveness

20. Use of research-based evidence by policy-makers

From NHS Central Research and Development Committee. Methods to promote the implementation of research findings in the NHS: priorities for evaluation: report to the NHS Central Research and Development Committee. London: Department of Health, 1995, with permission.

• Structure: this relates to physical resources available, e.g. the number of theatres, hospital beds and nurses, etc.
• Process: this refers to the management of the patient, e.g. procedures carried out, drugs used, care delivered, etc.
• Outcome: this refers to the result of the intervention, e.g. the amount of time off work, incidence of complications, morbidity and length of stay.

Audit is a dynamic cyclical process (an audit loop) in which standards are defined and data are collected against these standards (**Fig. 1.3**). The results are then analysed and if there are any variances, proposals for change are developed to address the needs. These changes are then implemented and the quality of care reassessed. This closes the audit loop

and the procedure begins again. The key to effective audit is that the loop must begin with the development of evidence-based standards. Any success in changing care to meet proposed standards is unlikely to produce more effective clinical care if such standards are set in an arbitrary way. The Royal College of Surgeons of England has published its own guidelines on clinical audit in surgical practice.[61]

One result of the drive to implement audit in the UK was the development in 1993 of a National Confidential Enquiry into Perioperative Deaths (NCEPOD). This is an ongoing national audit and has produced a series of reports and recommendations based upon a peer review process. The process has a high rate of participation and reports and recommendations have resulted in a number of changes in practice. For example, there has been a

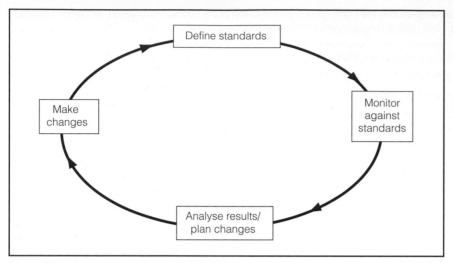

Figure 1.3 • The audit loop.

dramatic reduction in out-of-hours operating following recommendations suggesting that much of this was unsafe and unnecessary.

SUMMARY

This chapter has dealt with some of the issues surrounding the application of EBM in surgery. The key elements of this are:

- the formulation of clear and answerable questions;
- the identification of all the relevant evidence;
- critical appraisal of the evidence;
- the synthesis of information from multiple sources to provide a clear message through systematic review and/or meta-analysis;
- the implementation of findings through mechanisms such as the use of clinical guidelines and ICPs;
- monitoring through audit to ensure continuing adherence to best practice;
- regular review to incorporate new evidence or take account of clinical developments.

Throughout this book and the other volumes in this series, an attempt will be made to take an evidence-based approach. This will include the identification of high-quality evidence from RCTs and systematic reviews, underlining key statements and recommendations relating to clinical practice. All clinicians have a duty to ensure that they act in accordance with current 'best evidence' in order to give patients the highest chance of favourable outcomes and make the best use of limited health-care resources.

REFERENCES

1. Sackett D, Rosenberg WMC, Muirgray JA et al. Evidence based medicine: what it is and what it isn't. Br Med J 1996; 312:71–2.

2. Kaska S, Weinstein JN. Historical perspective. Ernest Amory Codman, 1869–1940. A pioneer of evidence-based medicine: the end result idea. Spine 1998; 23:629–33.

3. Cochrane Collaboration. The Cochrane collaboration: preparing, maintaining and disseminating systematic reviews of the effects of health care. Oxford: Cochrane Centre, 1999.

4. Sackett D, Richardson WS, Rosenberg W. Evidence-based medicine: how to practice and teach EBM. New York: Churchill Livingstone, 1997.

5. Smith R. Where is the wisdom? Br Med J 1991; 303:798–9.

6. Ellis J, Mulligan I, Rowe J et al. Inpatient general medicine is evidence based. Lancet 1995; 346:407–10.

7. Department of Health. The new NHS: modern, dependable. London: Department of Health, 1997.

8. Department of Health. A first class service. London: Department of Health, 1998.

9. Wilt T, Brawer MK. The Prostate Cancer Intervention Versus Observation Trial: a randomized trial comparing radical prostatectomy versus expectant management for the treatment of clinically localized prostate cancer. J Urol 1994; 152:1910–14.

10. Majeed A, Troy G, Nicholl JP et al. Randomised, prospective, single-blind comparison of laparoscopic versus small-incision cholecystectomy. Lancet 1996; 347:989–94.

11. Anon. Laparoscopic versus open repair of groin hernia: a randomised comparison. The MRC

Laparoscopic Groin Hernia Trial Group. Lancet 1999; 354:185–90.

12. Anon. Beneficial effect of carotid endarterectomy in symptomatic patients with high-grade carotid stenosis. North American Symptomatic Carotid Endarterectomy Trial Collaborators. N Engl J Med 1991; 325:445–53.

13. Hunter D. Rationing and evidence-based medicine. J Eval Clin Pract 1996; 2:5–8.

14. Clarke M, Oxman AD (eds). Cochrane Reviewers Handbook 4.1.1 (updated December 2000). Oxford: Cochrane Library, 2000 (Issue 4).

15. Guyatt G, Sackett DL, Sinclair JC, Hayward R, Cook DJ, Cook RG for the Evidence-Based Medicine Working Group. Users' guides to the medical literature. IX. A method for grading health care recommendations. JAMA 1995; 274:1800–4.

16. Altman D. Randomisation. Br Med J 1991; 302:1481–2.

17. Begg C, Cho M, Eastwood S et al. Improving the quality of reports on randomized controlled trials. Recommendations of the CONSORT Study Group. [Not in English] Rev Esp Salvd Publa 1998; 72:5–11.

18. Altman D. Better reporting of randomised controlled trials: the CONSORT statement. Br Med J 1996; 313:570–1.

19. Greenhalgh T. How to read a paper: the basics of evidence based medicine. London: British Medical Journal Publications, 1997; vol xvii, p. 196.

20. Mulrow C. Rationale for systematic reviews. Br Med J 1994; 309:597–9.

21. Lau J, Schmid CH, Chalmers TC. Cumulative meta-analysis of clinical trials builds evidence for exemplary medical care. J Clin Epidemiol 1995; 48:45–57; discussion 59–60.

22. Antman E, Lau J, Kupelnick B, Chalmers TC. A comparison of results of meta-analyses of randomized control trials and recommendations of clinical experts. Treatments for myocardial infarction. JAMA 1992; 268:240–8.

23. Greenhalgh T. How to read a paper. The MEDLINE database. Br Med J 1997; 315:180–3.

24. Adams C, Power A, Fredrick K, Lefebvre C. An investigation of the adequacy of MEDLINE searches for randomized controlled trials (RCTs) of the effects of mental health care. Psychol Med 1994; 24:741–8.

25. Easterbrook P, Berlin JA, Gopalan R, Matthews DR. Publication bias in clinical research. Lancet 1991; 337:867–72.

26. Gotzsche P. Reference bias in reports of drug trials. Br Med J (Clin Res) 1987; 295:654–6.

27. Fullerton-Smith I. How members of the Cochrane Collaboration prepare and maintain systematic reviews of the effects of health care. Evid-Based Med 1995; 1:7–8.

28. Sackett D. Clinical epidemiology: a basic science for clinical medicine, 2nd edn. Boston: Little Brown, 1991; vol xviii, p. 441.

29. Thompson S, Pocock, S. Can meta-analysis be trusted. Lancet 1991; 338:1127–30.

30. Anon. Magnesium, myocardial infarction, meta-analysis and mega-trials. Drug Ther Bull 1995; 33:25–7.

31. Chalmers I, Altman DG. Systematic reviews. London: British Medical Journal Publications, 1995; p. 50.

32. DerSimonian R, Laird N. Meta-analysis in clinical trials. Controlled Clin Trials 1986; 7:177–88.

33. Egger M, Smith GD. Misleading meta-analysis. Br Med J 1995; 310:752–4.

34. Yusuf S, Teo K, Woods K. Intravenous magnesium in acute myocardial infarction. An effective, safe, simple, and inexpensive intervention. Circulation 1993; 87:2043–6.

35. Anon. ISIS-4: a randomised factorial trial assessing early oral captopril, oral mononitrate, and intravenous magnesium sulphate in 58 050 patients with suspected acute myocardial infarction. ISIS-4 (Fourth International Study of Infarct Survival) Collaborative Group. Lancet 1995; 345:669–85.

36. Field MJ, Lohr KN. Clinical practice guidelines: directions for a new program. Washington, DC: National Academy Press, 1990; p. 160.

37. Anon. North of England evidence based guidelines development project: summary version of evidence based guideline for the primary care management in adults. North of England Asthma Guideline Development Group. Br Med J 1996; 312:762–6.

38. Anon. North of England evidence based guidelines development project: summary version of evidence based guideline for the primary care management angina. North of England Stable Angina Guideline Development Group. Br Med J 1996; 312:827–32.

39. Eccles M, Freemantle N, Mason J. North of England evidence based guideline development project: guideline on the use of aspirin as secondary prophylaxis for vascular disease in primary care. North of England Aspirin Guideline Development Group. Br Med J 1998; 316:1303–9.

40. Grol R, Dalhuijsen J, Thomas S. Attributes of clinical guidelines that influence use of guidelines in general practice: observational study. Br Med J 1998; 317:858–61.

41. NHS Executive. Clinical guidelines: using clinical guidelines to improve patient care within the NHS. Leeds: NHS Executive, 1996.

42. Gray J, Haynes RD, Sackett DL et al. Transferring evidence from health care research into medical practice. 3. Developing evidence-based clinical policy. Evid-Based Med 1997; 2:36–8.

43. Grimshaw J, Russell IT. Effect of clinical guidelines on medical practice: a systematic review of rigorous evaluations. Lancet 1993; 342:1317–22.

44. Cluzeau F, Littlejohns P, Grimshaw J, Feder G. Appraisal instrument for clinical guidelines. London: St George's Hospital Medical School, 1997.

45. Oxman A, Guyatt GH. Guidelines for reading literature reviews. Can Med Assoc J 1988; 138:697–703.

46. Oxman A, Cook DJ, Guyatt GH. Users' guides to the medical literature. VI. How to use an overview. Evidence-Based Medicine Working Group. JAMA 1994; 272:1367–71.

47. Oxman A. Checklists for review articles. Br Med J 1994; 309:648–51.

48. Cook D, Guyatt GH, Laupacis A, Sackett DL. Rules of evidence and clinical recommendations on the use of antithrombotic agents. Chest 1992; 102:305S–311S .

49. Canadian Task Force on the Periodic Health Examination. The periodic health examination. Can Med Assoc J 1979; 121:1193–254.

50. Hadorn DC, Baker D, Hodges JS, Hicks N. Rating the quality of evidence for clinical practice guidelines. J Clin Epidemiol 1996; 49:749–54.

51. Centre for Evidence-based Medicine. Levels of evidence and grades of recommendations. Oxford: Centre for Evidence-based Medicine, 1999. http://cebmjr2.ox.ac.uk/docs/levels.html

52. NHS Central Research and Development Committee. Methods to promote the implementation of research findings in the NHS: priorities for evaluation: report to the NHS Central Research and Development Committee. London: Department of Health, 1995.

53. Bero L, Grilli R, Grimshaw J, Harvey E, Oxman A, Thomson MA. Closing the gap between research and practice. In: Haines A, Donald A (eds) Getting research findings into practice. London: BMJ Publications, 1998; pp. 27–35.

54. Dunning M, Abi-aad G, Gilbert G, Gillam S, Livett H. Turning evidence into everyday practice. London: King's Fund, 1999.

55. Evans D, Haines A. Implementing evidence based changes in healthcare. Oxford: Radcliffe Medical Press, 2000.

56. Dunning M, McQuay H, Milne R. Getting a GRiPP. Health Serv J 1994; 104:18–20.

57. Appleby JWK, Ham C. Acting on the evidence: a review of clinical effectiveness: sources of information, dissemination, and implementation. Birmingham: National Association of Health Authorities and Trusts, 1995.

58. Department of Health. Clinical audit: meeting and improving standards in health care. London: Department of Health, 1998; p. 14.

59. Department of Health. The evolution of clinical audit. Heywood: Health Publications Unit, 1994.

60. Donabedian A. Evaluating the quality of care. Millbank Memorial Federation of Quality 1996; 3:166–203.

61. Royal College of Surgeons of England. Clinical audit in surgical practice. London: Royal College of Surgeons of England, 1995.

Appendix: Possible sources of further information, useful Internet sites and contact addresses

The details below provide references to a number of sources of information, particularly those accessible through the Internet. It must be remembered that there are rapid changes in the material available online and Internet addresses are liable to change. Several of these sources provide extensive links to other sites. In particular the ScHARR site 'Netting the Evidence' (see below) provides an extensive and regularly updated list of other useful sites.

Organisations specialising in evidence-based practice, systematic reviews, etc.

Aggressive Research Intelligence Facility (ARIF)
http://www.bham.ac.uk/arif/index.htm

CASP (Critical Appraisal Skills Program)
http://update-software.com/CASP

Centre for Evidence-based Child Health
http://www.gosh.nhs.uk/ich/html/academicunits/paed_epid/cebh/about.htm

Centre for Evidence-based Medicine
University Department of Psychiatry, Warneford Hospital, Headington, Oxford OX3 7JX
Tel. 01865 226485
http://cebm.net

Centre for Evidence-based Mental Health
http://www.cebmh.com

Centre for Evidence-based Nursing
http://www.york.ac.uk/healthsciences/centres/evidence/cebm.htm

Department of Health R&D Strategy Home Page
http://www.doh.gov.uk/research/index.htm

McMaster University
http://hiru.mcmaster.ca

NHS Centre for Reviews and Dissemination
University of York, Heslington, York YO1 5DD
Tel. 01904 433634
email: crd@york.ac.uk
http://www.york.ac.uk/inst/crd/

National Institute for Clinical Excellence
http://www.nice.org.uk/

OMNI (Organising Medical Networked Information) Project
http://www.omni.ac.uk

Resources for Evidence-based Surgery
A site created for all surgeons and the related medical community, hosted by the Royal College of Surgeons of England.
http://www.rcseng.ac.uk/services/library/hi_resources/ebs_html

Sheffield Centre for Health and Related Research (ScHARR)
An introduction to evidence-based practice is available on the Internet called 'Netting the Evidence', produced by Andrew Booth from Sheffield University. This is a comprehensive guide to a range of sources and tools on the web in EBM.
Regent Court, 30 Regent Street, Sheffield S1 4DA
Tel. 0114 2768555
email: mailto:abooth@sheffield.ac.uk
http://www.shef.ac.uk/~scharr/ir/netting/net.html

Unit for Evidence-Based Practice and Policy
Subunit of the Department of Primary Care and Population Sciences at UCL, maintained by Trish Greenhalgh.
http://www.ucl.ac.uk/openlearning/uebpp/uebpp.htm

UK Cochrane Centre
Summertown Pavilion, Middle Way, Oxford OX2 7LG
Tel. 01865 516300
email: general@cochrane.co

Internet access to the Cochrane library and databases:
http://www.update-software.com/cochrane

Home page:
http://hiru.mcmaster.ca/cochrane/default.htm

Controlled Trials Register, listings of ongoing MRC and NRR clinical trials:
http://www.controlled-trials.com/default.asp

Sources of reviews and abstracts relating to evidence-based practice

ACP Journal Club
http://www.acpjc.org

Bandolier (topics in EBM reviewed for the NHS R&D Directorate)
http://www.jr2.ox.ac.uk:/bandolier/

Cochrane Systematic Reviews (abstracts only)
http://www.cochrane.org/cochrane/revabstr/mainindex.htm

Effective Health Care Bulletins
http://www.york.ac.uk/inst/crd/ehcb.htm

Evidence-based Health Care
http://www.harcourt-international.com/journals/ebhc

Evidence-based Medicine
http://www.ebm.bmjjournals.com/

Evidence-based Purchasing
http://www.epi.bris.ac.uk/rd

Journals available on the internet

eBMJ (Electronic version of the *British Medical Journal*)
http://www.bmj.com

Journal of the American Medical Association (*JAMA*)
http://jama.ama-assn.org/

Canadian Medical Association Journal (*CMAJ*)
http://www.cmaj.ca/

Databases, bibliographies and catalogues

University of Hertfordshire Library
Contains up-to-date information on journals and other publications on EBM with access to many EBM internet resources.

Library and Media Services, College Lane, Hatfield, Hertfordshire AL10 9AD
Tel. 01707 284678
email: c.cox@herts.ac.uk
http://www.herts.ac.uk/lis/subjects/health/ebm.htm

PUBMED (the free version of MEDLINE)
http://www.ncbi.nlm.nih.gov/PubMed/

Best Evidence
http://www.acponline.org/catalog/electronic/best_evidence.htm

Clinical Evidence
A formulary along the lines of the British National Formulary summarising the best evidence for clinical interventions.
http://www.evidence.org/index-welcome.htm

Sources of guidelines and integrated care pathways

AHRQ (Agency for Healthcare Research and Quality)
Provides practical health-care information, research findings and data to help consumers.
http://www.ahcpr.gov/

Cedars-Sinai Medical Center, Health Services Research
Home page: http://www.csmc.edu/

HealthCare: Clinical Information Index Page
Clinical information on evidence-based practice, clinical guidelines, medical effectiveness, pharmaceutical therapy, new technology and screening.
http://www.ahcpr.gov/clinic/

Leicester GH guidelines
http://www.le.ac.uk/Li/lgh/library/internet/audit.htm

National Guideline Clearinghouse
Resource for evidence-based clinical practice guidelines and related documents. The site provides guidelines in multiple medical fields.
http://www.guideline.gov/index.asp

National Electronic Library for Health
http://www.nelh.nhs.uk/carepathways

National Pathways Association
http://www.the-npa.org.uk/

Scottish Intercollegiate Guidelines Network (SIGN)
http://www.sign.ac.uk

Useful texts

Cochrane Collaboration Handbook
http://www.cochrane.org/cochrane/hbook.htm

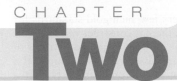

Two

Outcomes and health economic issues in surgery

Jonathan A. Michaels and
Russell Slack

INTRODUCTION

Evidence-based medicine (EBM) demands that all those making decisions regarding clinical management, either on an individual patient basis or at a policy level, consider existing evidence in order to maximise the chance of favourable outcomes and optimise the use of available resources. However, such evidence is rarely clear-cut and there may be conflicting advice because of differences in the way that outcomes are measured, the way in which costs are assessed or the perspective from which an economic evaluation is carried out.

This chapter deals with some of the issues around the measurement of outcomes, the calculation of costs and the methods of economic evaluation. The available outcome measures are considered, drawing the distinctions between disease-specific and generic measures and explaining concepts such as health-related quality of life, quality-adjusted life-years (QALYs) and utilities. The differences between costs, charges and resource use are highlighted, followed by a discussion of issues such as discounting, sensitivity analysis and marginal costing. Finally, a section on economic evaluation describes the different techniques available: cost minimisation, cost-effectiveness, cost–utility and cost–benefit analysis and discusses the use of cost-effectiveness league tables. The intention is not to provide a full reference work on these subjects but to raise awareness of some of the important issues to be considered when evaluating evidence on specific interventions that may rely on differing outcome measurements or methods of economic evaluation.

OUTCOME MEASURES

Clinicians tend routinely to consider health outcomes in terms of clinical or biomedical measures such as blood pressure levels, blood sugar levels or bone mineral density. Process-based outcomes such as readmission rates, reintervention or complications are readily considered alternatives. Data such as these are seen as readily available, easily measured, objective and comparable between differing settings. However, the present environment in medical services makes it necessary for the health-care professional to consider more than just the treatment of the condition. A greater emphasis is now placed upon the consideration by the clinician of the actual status of the patient's quality of life. Now, considerations extend beyond assessing the value of an intervention and the effectiveness, or otherwise, of drug regimens. There should also be an assessment of the patient's physical, mental and social well-being. In line with such interests, there has been considerable research and a greater emphasis upon applying subjective non-biomedical measures and the development of such tools (or 'instruments') has been substantial since the early 1980s.

When considering which instrument of assessment to choose from the plethora now available, the user should carefully consider what parameter is to be measured before making a final selection of an outcome measure. Before applying this measure to a patient population, particular consideration needs to be given to deciding whether it will measure what we are interested in measuring and whether it will answer the questions that we wish to be answered. All too often assessment tools may be applied to patients in the wrong circumstances or used when there is no realistic opportunity to measure what we wish to measure. These are important considerations because the administration and analysis of these measures can be costly, as well as taking up valuable time for both patients and clinicians. In addition, the use of unsuitable measures applied in the wrong context might yield results that are perhaps plausible but wrong, thus leading to erroneous conclusions. The implications of such findings for patients or the health service can be substantial.

Attention must also be given to the psychometric properties of the instruments chosen to measure health, with particular attention given to reliability and validity. Reliability refers to whether the instrument will be reproducible, such that if applied in different settings or circumstances to the same unchanged population then the same results should be achieved. This has particular implications for studies using instruments to derive longitudinal data on a particular sample of patients. In such circumstances, we need to be confident that observed changes over a given time period reflect actual change. Test–retest reliability is an important consideration and is assessed by making repeated assessments under the same circumstances at differing points in time and comparing the results using correlations or differences. Similarly, for instruments that require administration by interviewers, there needs to be a high level of agreement between different raters assessing the same patients but at different periods in time. For example, Collin et al. found a high level of agreement between the patients, a trained nurse and two skilled observers during applications of the Barthel Index to the same group of patients.[1]

Another psychometric criterion for consideration is that of validity, which means that instruments measure precisely what they set out to do. It should be borne in mind that measures can be reliable without being valid, but they cannot be valid without being reliable. Three types of validity are described. First, content validity, which relates to the choice, appropriateness and representativeness of the content of the instrument. Judging content validity involves an assessment of whether all of the relevant concepts are represented. For example, a representative sample of asthmatic patients could be used to develop an asthma questionnaire in order to ensure that it captures all the domains of interest for such a patient population. Second, there is a requirement to consider criterion validity, which is the degree to which the measure obtains results that are comparable to some kind of 'gold standard'. While this is theoretically a simple

concept, there are very few such gold standards for comparison. Finally, there is construct validity. This relates to observation of when expected patterns of given relationships are observed. For example, if a method of valuation of outcomes predicts that a patient prefers option A to option B, then one would expect this to be reflected by their behaviour when faced with genuine clinical choices. This is normally assessed through the use of multitrait–multimethod techniques,[2] which map the correlations between alternative approaches to measuring the same construct and between measures of different constructs.

As can be seen, the choice of an outcome measure is not always as straightforward as it may seem at first. In addition to considerations regarding the patient group, there are also important considerations regarding the psychometric properties of the instruments. Different outcome measures will have uses for differing patient groups. For example, a biomedical measure such as blood pressure alone might be considered suitable for comparing two similar drug regimens to assess 'best' control of blood pressure. However, a study that attempts to compare renal transplant with dialysis might also wish to consider a much broader picture and would be likely to require consideration of quality-of-life issues together with mortality as outcome measures.

It is extremely important to choose the right outcomes for the purpose in question, as different conclusions can be drawn from the application of different outcome measures in the same study. For example, a study of vascular patients compared exercise training with angioplasty for stable claudication with results expressed in terms of ankle brachial pressure indices and walking distance.[3] In the short term, it was found that angioplasty improved the pressure but not the walking distance, while exercise improved the walking distance but not the pressure. This example shows that different outcome measures may not always change in the same direction and used in isolation could lead to opposite conclusions.

The following sections examine some of the issues involved in the evaluation and application of some common specific outcome measures.

Mortality

The mortality rate expresses the incidence of death in a population of interest over a given period of time. It is calculated by dividing the number of fatalities in the given population by the total population.

Mortality is often used as an outcome measure in studies as an indication of the effectiveness, or otherwise, of a treatment. It is often easily derived and as such represents a readily accessible outcome measure. While mortality can indeed provide much useful information, its use in reporting results should always be interpreted with caution. First, procedure- and diagnosis-related mortality rates often refer to inpatient deaths only or perhaps mortality over a given postoperative period, for example 30 days. Variations in short-term survival rates might simply reflect differing discharge practices between differing hospitals or settings. Longer term survival rates are frequently reported for cancer and other chronic conditions. In interpreting these, it must be borne in mind that distortion may occur as a result of the starting point or choice of time frame. For example, survival may be longer in a screened population because there is an earlier starting point[4] and comparisons between surgical and medical treatments may be very sensitive to follow-up periods because of early excess operative mortality in surgical treatments, which may be offset by better long-term survival. For these reasons, it is often necessary to compare survival curves rather than total survival at a specific time point. This may raise further issues regarding the possible need for discounting, to take account of a preference for survival in the earlier years after treatment (see below).

Second, mortality can only be a partial measure of quality, and it is often not the most appropriate outcome measure for use in most situations. Many studies report mortality and tend to ignore other important outcomes such as morbidity and quality of life. These are more complex to quantify and are not routinely collected. Mortality is particularly limited in usefulness for studies investigating low-risk procedures. Accurate assessment of the quality of such procedures requires more sensitive measures.

It is also necessary to highlight the effect that differences in case mix can have on the mortality rate. For example, there is a tendency in studies relating workload to outcome for the results to be reported for the whole sample of patients. It is important to be aware that results reported in this way may be misleading as no account is taken of the diversity of patient characteristics that may be contained in such a sample. Both differences in severity of illness and in risk of adverse outcomes relating to comorbidity can significantly affect any interpretation of mortality rates. This problem is illustrated by Sowden and Sheldon, who discuss examples from coronary artery bypass grafting and intensive care to demonstrate the importance of adjusting for case mix.[5] For coronary artery bypass grafting, they report that the strength of the relationship between low volume and increased mortality is reduced in studies that adjust for differences in risk among patients receiving treatment. With adult intensive care, they cite a study by Jones and

Rowan[6] in which the apparent higher mortality associated with smaller intensive care units ceased to be significant once the data were adjusted to reflect the fact that severity of illness was on average higher among patients admitted to small units. These examples clearly demonstrate that, in order to minimise bias in such studies, account must be taken of any factors (beyond workload) that are likely to affect patient outcomes.

Condition-specific outcome measures

The term 'condition-specific' describes instruments designed to measure health outcomes considered to be of specific interest to patients who incur health problems attributable to a particular disease or as the result of other processes. Such instruments are often referred to as 'disease-specific', but this term is more general as it encompasses more diverse areas such as natural ageing, trauma and pregnancy, which are not diseases.[7]

The measurement of health status is not restricted to broad generic measures. There are many instances when researchers and clinicians are interested in assessing the health status of individuals with a certain condition, or disease. As might be anticipated, many tools have been designed for this purpose and these are primarily aimed at measuring changes that are of importance to clinicians. For example, Spilker et al. identified over 300 such instruments in 1987 and many more are presently available.[8] Examples of such instruments include measures for arthritis, such as the Arthritis Impact Measurement Scales;[9] measures for the heart, such as the Specific Activity Scale;[10] and measures that assess pain, such as the McGill Pain Questionnaire.[11] These instruments have a varying number of dimensions, differing numbers of items and are generally self-completion or interview, though some methods include professional assessment and clinical interview. Such questionnaires are usually scored in a simplistic fashion. Most have simple numeric scaling, such as from 1 to 5, and these scores are usually summed across the items for each dimension, or across all items.

Advantages of condition-specific measures include their relevance and their greater responsiveness to health change.[12] Disadvantages are that they often exclude items relevant to potential complications of treatment and symptoms that do not easily fit the medical model of disease. Generic measures have tended to be used in preference because they can be used to assess benefits for differing treatments or conditions, in a common and exchangeable currency. This enables decisions to be made on allocative efficiency between health-care programmes within the total health-care budget, rather than helping to establish the technical efficiency of producing health benefits for a specific condition.[7]

The measurement of pain

Pain is a common and important symptom of many medical conditions and deserves special consideration. While many generic and condition-specific instruments dedicate specific dimensions to the measurement of pain, there are also a number of instruments designed specifically to assess levels of pain. The measurement of pain cannot be directly assessed through clinical measures (e.g. blood samples) and, in the absence of such objective approaches, it is necessary to assess pain subjectively through the patients' own perceptions.

Subjective measures allow for reproducible results providing that the tools used to assess pain are measured appropriately. While subjective measures for the measurement of pain have many advantages over other instruments, there are problems in assessing subjects for whom communication is difficult. Examples include very young children and patients who are incapable of expressing how they feel. Those patients who are unconscious or who are terminally ill will continue to present particular difficulties for those attempting to assess levels of pain.

As with other outcome measures, options exist to use binary, categorical or visual analogue scales. Within this area, there are both pain-relief scales and pain-intensity scales to be considered. There are often occasions when it will be necessary to measure the state of the pain rather than the effect of a particular intervention or therapy, and in these circumstances pain-intensity scales will be appropriate. In situations where both pain-relief and pain-intensity scales are appropriate, a decision is required regarding which should be used. Pain-relief scales may well encompass more than an intensity scale, as any side effects resulting from an intervention, such as dizziness, might be included in such judgements. Pain-relief scales also require the patient to make judgements about how the current pain now compares with remembered pain, before the intervention. This might make such scales more complicated for patients to grasp compared with intensity scales and this may raise doubts about validity.

Pain can manifest itself in a variety of qualities, and one of the most widely used tools is the McGill Pain Questionnaire.[11] This is a generic instrument, designed primarily for adults, which was developed to specify the qualities and intensities of pain; as such, it is intended to provide a quantifiable profile of pain. The questionnaire can be completed by the patient or administered in an interview. Completion

takes roughly 15–20 minutes but becomes quicker on subsequent applications. The instrument contains 78 pain descriptor words, which are grouped into 20 subclasses, each of which contains two to five words that describe pain on an ordinal scale. These words are arranged to reflect three dimensions of pain: sensory, affective and evaluative. The questionnaire can yield three indices of pain: a pain rating index based on the scale values of the words chosen by the patient; a rank score using the rank values within each subgroup chosen; and the total number of descriptions chosen by the patient.

The McGill Pain Questionnaire has been thoroughly investigated in recent years and the instrument has proved to be the most reliable in applications to patients with moderate-to-severe chronic or acute pain. It has been shown to be particularly useful in disaggregating explained pain from unexplained pain. When the instrument was used in a cohort of cancer patients with lymphoedema, it proved to be more sensitive than categorical or analogue scales.[13]

Health-related quality of life

Recent years have witnessed quite an upsurge in interest in the measurement of health-related quality of life, much of which has no doubt been stimulated by the analytical demands of researchers and the need for outcome information as a basis for policy decisions.

Such health status measures are standardised questionnaires, or instruments, which are used to evaluate patient health across a broad range of areas. These areas include symptoms, physical functioning, mental well-being, work and social activities. Measures can be either generic or condition-specific, and such measures can generate a profile of scores or a single index. These scores can be based upon peoples' preferences (e.g. EQ-5D) or, more usually, arbitrary scoring procedures (e.g. SF-36, assumes equal weighting for most items).[14] Three of the most frequently used instruments are discussed below in further detail.

EQ-5D

Of those instruments that generate a single index, EQ-5D is in regular use, with the use of the instrument reported in over 40 publications.[14] The measure was developed by a group of researchers from seven centres across five countries.[15] The present measure has five dimensions, whereas the original version had six. Patients are classified by the completion of a five-item questionnaire. The Euroqol is a brief, easy-to-use questionnaire of two pages. It can be made even simpler by using the one-page descriptive classification. Self-completion, or interview, usually only takes a matter of minutes, and response rates tend to be extremely high.[14] The five dimensions of the EQ-5D comprise mobility, self-care, usual activities, pain/discomfort and anxiety/depression. Each of the five questions has three levels; therefore combining the five questions defines 243 health states. In addition, the instrument contains a visual analogue scale: a thermometer scale calibrated from zero (representing 'worst possible health state') to 100 (representing 'best imaginable health state').

SF-36

The SF-36 is a self-administered questionnaire composed of 36 items. It measures health across eight multi-item dimensions, covering functional status, well-being and overall evaluation of health. Responses within each of the dimensions are combined in order to generate a score from 0 to 100, where 0 represents 'worst health' and 100 indicates 'best health'. Dimension scores should not be aggregated into a single index score. The questionnaire takes about 5 minutes to complete, attains good response rates and is suitable for completion by the patients themselves or for administration by trained interviewers on a face-to-face or telephone basis.[16]

The questionnaire has been used in a variety of settings, administered on differing populations and exhibits good psychometric properties. Detailed information regarding the scoring process and computation are readily available, as are published data for comparative norms. The question complexity can be a problem in situations where the sample comprises individuals with low education levels, but otherwise the instrument is suitable for administration in a wide range of settings.[16]

NOTTINGHAM HEALTH PROFILE

The Nottingham Health Profile (NHP) measures levels of self-reported distress. The instrument consists of two parts, each of which can be used independent of the other. Part 1, the most frequently used component, comprises 38 statements that are grouped into six sections: physical mobility, pain, sleep, social isolation, emotional reaction, and energy. The number of statements in each of these sections varies from three for the energy dimension to nine for emotional reaction. The second part of the instrument asks respondents to indicate whether or not their state of health influences activity in seven areas of everyday life: work, looking after the home, social life, home life, sex life, interests and hobbies, and holidays. Responses for both parts 1 and 2 are yes/no responses.[17]

Scoring is straightforward, with zero assigned to a 'no' response and 1 to a 'yes' response. Scores for each of the sections range between 0 ('worst health') and 100 ('best health'). The NHP was designed for self-completion and can readily be used in postal surveys, although it can also be administered by an interviewer. Generally, the instrument takes around 5 minutes to complete.

Quality-adjusted life-years

QALYs were developed as an outcome measure to incorporate effects on both the quality and quantity of life. Each year of life is multiplied by a weighting factor reflecting quality of life.[18] An alternative to QALYs is healthy years equivalent (HYE), which is discussed below.

QALYs are estimated by assigning every life-year a weight between 0 and 1, where a weight of 0 reflects a health status that is valued as equal to being dead and a weight of 1 represents full health. For example, a patient receives a surgical intervention and can then be expected to live for an additional number of years. These additional years would be quality-adjusted in some way by comparison with the 0–1 scale. Therefore, if the person who has undergone the surgery is calibrated (scored by raters) to be in a health state of 0.8, then each expected life-year will be assigned a QALY value of 0.8.

The QALY is frequently used by decision-makers or researchers to draw comparisons between differing types of health programme or intervention. The QALY can be used in economic evaluation: the number of additional QALYs that a new surgical intervention might yield can be compared with the costs of the new procedure, thus enabling cost per QALY ratios to be generated.[19] Such ratios have been used in so-called QALY league tables, whereby procedures or interventions are ranked on this basis. These tables might be seen as useful within the decision-making process, but caution should be exercised in making quick decisions regarding the allocation of resources based upon these comparative tables.[20–23]

More recently, HYEs have been developed as an alternative in order to address some of the suggested shortcomings of QALYs.[24] HYEs produce a hypothetical combination of the number of years in full health that equates to the individual's utility of living a number of years at a health state rated at less than full health. In effect, this can be considered as a lifetime profile of health and is often referred to as a stream of health states. In order to produce the values for the HYEs, a two-stage gamble procedure is used. There has, however, been criticism of the use of HYEs and it remains to be seen whether they become an accepted alternative to the QALY.[25,26] For the QALY to be a useful measure of outcome, it should reflect patient or individual preferences, which means that if an individual has a choice between two or more treatments or interventions then they should choose the treatment option that yields the most QALYs.

UTILITIES

Quality weights for use in QALYs can be obtained directly using one of three main methods: visual analogue scales (VAS), standard gamble and time trade-off. Each of these is described in turn below. In addition to these direct methods of measurement, it is possible to obtain utilities through the mapping of health states derived from generic quality-of-life scores onto valuations obtained from members of the general population.[27] The method for obtaining utility weightings is currently the subject of considerable research, and there is evidence that different values are obtained depending on the method of evaluation and framing of questions. In addition, there is considerable controversy as to whether the most appropriate utility values for economic evaluation are those of the general population or of patients with the particular conditions.[28]

Visual analogue scales

With the VAS approach, respondents are required to locate their present health state on a straight line chart, often a thermometer with fixed points, where the bottom of the thermometer is represented by zero, which is a health state equivalent to being dead, and the top of the thermometer is 1, which indicates full health. If thermometers ranging between 0 and 100 are used, these values are equated to 0–1, and the same assumptions regarding the health states hold. If, by way of an example, we wanted to measure the quality weight for being an amputee, and the respondent selects the health state at 55 on the thermometer scale of 0–100, then for that health state their quality weight is equivalent to 0.55. Advantages for VAS scales include their simplicity, but this can be counterbalanced by the fact that there is no choice to be made between health states and therefore it is not possible to observe any trade-offs that the individual might have between health states. Another problem with VAS is that it is uncertain whether the responses lie on a linear interval scale: it is questionable whether moving from 20 to 30 is equivalent to moving from 70 to 80. Given these reservations, it is difficult to use VAS methods to determine quality weights in a way that is consistent with the theoretical basis of utility measurement.[29]

Standard gamble

The second method routinely used to estimate quality weights is standard gamble. Under this approach, the quality weight of a health state can be constructed by comparing a specific number of years in the health state to a gamble with a probability (P) of achieving full health for the same number of years and a complementary probability $(1 - P)$ of immediate death. The probability of full health is varied until the individual is indifferent between the alternatives, and the quality weight of the assessed health state is therefore equal to P. As an example, let us consider that we are comparing 10 years with heart disease with the gamble of full health for 10 years (probability P) or immediate death, with a complementary probability $(1 - P)$. Here, let us assume that the individual is indifferent at a probability of 0.6 of full health. In practical terms, this means that the individual would consider a certainty of living 10 years with the heart disease to be equivalent to taking a gamble that gives a 60% chance of living 10 years in full health and a 40% chance of immediate death. The quality weight here would be 0.6 for the heart disease health state. The advantages of standard gamble include the fact that it is based on expected utility theory;[29] however, one of the major disadvantages is that respondents might find the concept difficult to understand because of the probabilities associated with the method. Another drawback is that the hypothetical choices used in such an approach are not representative of 'real' life, since choices between large improvements in health status and large mortality risks are seldom encountered, especially with the assumption that we will live for a certain number of years for sure.

Time trade-off

A third approach to estimating quality weights is time trade-off.[30] This method compares D years duration in the health state, with X years in full health. The number of years in full health is varied until the individual is indifferent between their options; at this point, the quality weight of the health state is calculated by X/D. As an example, consider that we wish to calculate the quality weight for heart disease and that we assess the measurement for 10 years of heart disease. If the individual considers that 10 years of living with heart disease $(D = 10)$ is equivalent to 6 years of full health $(X = 6)$, then the quality weight is equal to 0.6 (6/10).

COSTS, CHARGES AND RESOURCE USE

From the above discussion, it can be seen that, from a health economists' perspective, there are several methods for assessing the benefits that might be accrued from a health-care intervention within the context of an economic evaluation. Whichever approach is adopted within the economic evaluation, the methods of identifying either the costs or the benefits is essentially the same for each of the approaches. In order to identify the relevant costs, it will be necessary to categorise all items of resource that will be utilised within the health-care programme. Therefore, we need to identify which resources are required and which are not. Measurement requires an estimation of the amount of resources that are used within the programmes, and these should be measured using natural units of measurement. For example, to look specifically at staffing time, one would use units of time (such as hours) that are spent on activities relating to the programme and the specific grades of staff. For other categories of resource use, different units would be appropriate. One might look at drug use in units such as doses of specific drugs. Other examples of resource use and their relevant methods of measurement are outlined in **Table 2.1**.

Many of the items in **Table 2.1** are readily identifiable and straightforward to value. Of these, staffing costs usually have the greatest impact upon health-care costs, and these can be readily costed providing that we are aware of the staffing scale and can use wage rates or salary levels attached to the staff level. For example, to cost consultant time one would multiply the number of hours of consultant time in our study by their hourly pay, with added allowance to cover the costs of leave, sick pay and superannuation, etc. The majority of the other categories of resource use for health services identified in the table (consumables, overheads, capital, etc.) can be readily costed through the use of the market price. Elsewhere, community services, ambulance services and the expenses incurred by patients and their families would usually be costed in the same manner as health service resources.

Within the above, certain components are notoriously difficult to cost. For example, using patient or family leisure time incurs an opportunity cost, which is complex to measure as there are differing types of activity that are forgone in such situations. It is also complex to attach monetary values to activity involving voluntary care or time lost from housework. No accessible market value exists for either of these areas; therefore, it is customary to use a comparable market value from another market. As an example, Gerard used the wage rate for auxiliary nursing staff in order to cost the inputs by volunteers assisting with respite services for mentally handicapped adults.[31] However, there are occasions when comparable proxy market values are not readily accessible. This is often the case for the costing of 'time off usual activities', such as housework, which by its nature is not of routine duration and is often irregular in its occurrence, making comparison with other occupations virtually impossible. One approach that is advocated in such circumstances is to use average female labour costs as a relatively accurate reflection of the opportunity cost of housework.[32]

While costing might appear to be rather simplistic and straightforward, there are a number of considerations that need to be taken into account before embarking upon such an exercise.

Counting costs in base year

First, we should consider whether health-care costs should be counted during the base year. By this, we mean that the costs should be adjusted in order to take account of inflation. If we assume that the

Table 2.1 • Resource use and methods for measurement

Resource	Measurement	Valuation
Health services		
Staff time	Time (e.g. hours/days worked)	Salary levels
General consumables	Units/quantities used	Market price
Capital	Units/quantities used	Market price
Overheads	Units/quantities used	Market price/salary levels
Other services		
Community services	Units/quantities used	Market price
Ambulance services	Units/quantities used	Market price
Voluntary services	Units/quantities used	Estimated values for staff costs
Patients and their families		
Personal time	Hours of input	Salary levels
Expenses	Units/quantities used	Market price or cost of actual expenses
Time off work	Duration of time	Salary levels plus other imputed values

Table 2.2 • Adjusting costs to base year (assuming 5% inflation)

Options	Costs arising (£/person/year)			
	Year 0	Year 1	Year 2	Total
Surgery	3000			
Drug (unadjusted for inflation)	1000	1050	1102.5	3125.5
Drug (adjusted to year 0 prices)	1000	1000	1000	3000

annual inflation rate is running at 6% then £1060 would be required to purchase an item of medical equipment in a year's time that would currently cost £1000. The two values (both now and in 1 year's time) are considered to be equivalent in real terms, although of course they represent two different amounts of money. This problem becomes more acute if we are considering a comparison of two or more health programmes that have their costs spread at differing proportions over a different number of years. To illustrate this point, let us consider the following example taken from Donaldson and Shackley[32] where surgical and drug treatment options are considered for the same hypothetical condition (**Table 2.2**). We assume that each option has the same effect, but the cost streams are different between the two options, and the inflation rate is at 5% per annum. This rate means that a cost of £1050 in a year's time is equivalent to £1000 now (i.e. £1050/1.05), and likewise £1102.5 in 2 years' time is also equivalent to £1000 now (i.e. £102.5/1.05²). If we compare the costs between the different options in this example, we would conclude that surgery is the more efficient option when compared with the unadjusted drug option, since it is the least costly of the two but equally effective. However, it should be noted at this point that the drug therapy option is only greater in terms of cost owing to inflation. Therefore, if the costs are adjusted to take account of inflation, by adjusting costs to year 0 prices, then both therapies cost exactly the same, with the same effectiveness, and neither of the options could be considered superior to the other.

Discounting

Not all costs and benefits of health-care programmes are observed to occur at the same point in time. For example, the costs associated with a vaccination programme are incurred very early in order to provide benefits to the individual, or society, in later life. In general, individuals prefer to reap the benefits sooner rather than later and prefer to incur the costs later rather than sooner. The most common method of allowing for such circumstances is to apply a discount rate to future costs and benefits.[33]

This leads us to consider whether the costs (and benefits) occurring at differing time points should be allocated equal weighting. There is not a consensus amongst health economists over what the appropriate discount rates are, or whether costs and benefits should be discounted at the same rate. Choosing the appropriate discount rate can have significant implications for the results of evaluations; the recommended rates in England and Scotland are 6%. Consequently, sensitivity analysis is essential to assess the implications of varying the discount rate. Recent convention dictates that costs should be discounted at the same rate as benefits,[34,35] though again this should be done in conjunction with sensitivity analysis to assess variations in such assumptions. Issues of discounting of costs and benefit may have a particularly dramatic effect on conclusions if different options have marked differences in the timing of expenditure or outcomes. This is particularly important when considering screening programmes and preventative treatments.

Sensitivity analysis

Evaluations will always be subject to elements of uncertainty, be it in terms of resource use, costs or effectiveness. Sensitivity analysis is essential in such circumstances as it allows us to assess how sensitive the study results are to variations in key parameters or assumptions that have been used in the analysis. This allows us to assess whether changes in key parameters will result in savings or costs.

It is possible to undertake sensitivity analysis using as few or as many variables as desired. Commonly, variables such as production variables or discount rates will be used, or if statistical analysis of the variables has been undertaken one can carry out sensitivity analysis around known confidence intervals. Although sensitivity analysis is advocated for evaluations, Briggs and Sculpher, in a recent literature review,[36] found that only 39% of articles reviewed had taken at least an adequate account of uncertainty, while only 14% were judged to have provided a good account of uncertainty. In addition, 24% had failed to consider uncertainty at all. There are differing methods of sensitivity analysis, which are discussed below.

SIMPLE SENSITIVITY ANALYSIS

Simple sensitivity analysis, in which one or more parameters contained within the evaluation are varied across a plausible range, is the most common method. With one-way analysis, each uncertain component of the evaluation is varied individually in order to assess the separate impact that each component will have upon the results of the analysis. Multiway sensitivity analysis involves varying two or more of the components of the evaluation at the same time and assessing the impact upon the results. It should be noted that multiway sensitivity analysis becomes more difficult to interpret as progressively more variables are varied in the analysis.[36]

THRESHOLD ANALYSIS

Threshold analysis involves the identification of the critical value of a parameter above or below which the conclusion of a study will change from one conclusion to another.[37] Threshold analysis is of greatest use when a particular parameter in the evaluation is indeterminate, for example a new drug with a price that has not yet been determined. A major limitation of threshold analysis is that it deals only with uncertainty in continuous variables, meaning that it is normally only useful for addressing uncertainty in analyses with data inputs.[36]

ANALYSIS OF EXTREMES

In analysis of extremes, a base-case analysis is undertaken that incorporates the best estimates of the inputs and then further analyses consider extreme estimates of the relevant variables. For example, if two alternative treatment strategies are being compared, then both the high and low costs can be considered for both therapies and costs can be assessed for each of the options based upon combinations of these. Analysis of extremes can be particularly effective in situations where a base-case value is known together with a plausible range, but the actual distribution between the outer limits is unknown. However a problem with this approach is that it does not consider how likely it is that the various scenarios will arise.[36]

PROBABILISTIC SENSITIVITY ANALYSIS

A final approach to dealing with uncertainty is through the use of probabilistic sensitivity analysis. This method allows ranges and distributions to be assigned to variables about which we are uncertain, thus allowing for combinations of items that are more likely to take place. For example, it is unlikely that all of the pessimistic factors regarding costs will occur in the evaluation. Techniques such as Monte Carlo simulations allow for the random simultaneous selection of items at designated values and undertake analysis based upon hypothetical patient cohorts. This approach allows the proportion of patients to be estimated for whom one of the options under evaluation is preferred; generally, proportions approaching 100% suggest that the intervention is nearly always preferable under a range of conditions.[36]

Marginal (incremental) costing

The marginal cost is the cost incurred or saved from producing one unit more, or one unit less, of a health-care programme. This is in contrast to the average cost, which is the total cost of a programme divided by the total units produced.

Evaluations should normally measure marginal costs, rather than average costs (and benefits). The costs of treating an extra case, or moving from one programme to another, need to be calculated. For example, if there is currently a breast screening programme for 50–65-year-old women and one wishes to consider whether breast screening is as cost-effective in women aged 40–50 years of age, this should be done by looking at the marginal costs and benefits of reducing the age at which screening is started rather than assessing average costs for the entire programme. The use of marginal rather than average costs has been found to be extremely important in screening programmes, where the marginal cost of screening an additional individual can be significantly lower than the average cost.[38]

Donaldson and Shackley illustrate this point with an example of hospital care.[32] Although it may well cost £25 000 per annum, on average, to care for an elderly person in hospital, it is extremely unlikely that this amount would be saved if one person less were admitted to the hospital. Similarly, this figure is unlikely to equate to an additional expense if one person more were admitted to the hospital. The reasoning behind this is that some costs, such as capital and overhead costs plus some staffing costs, will not differ with small incremental changes in the numbers of patients entering the hospital.

Summary of cost analysis

This section highlights the importance of adhering to the appropriate methods when undertaking the costing component of an evaluation. Failure to do so might well lead to incorrect conclusions and to recommendations based upon flawed analysis. Clearly, not all studies that are published will have fully adopted the principles underlying the methods outlined in this section, and it is important when assessing the results from evaluations to consider whether appropriate analyses have been undertaken.

ECONOMIC EVALUATION

Economic evaluation is widely accepted as the method for assessing health-care programmes.

Within the health-care sector, there will never be enough resources to allow the sufficient provision of health-care resources to satisfy the demands of society. Quite simply, resources are scarce and choices need to be made about how best to distribute such resources. Such problems are further increased by the fact that health care is a mercurial environment with changing technology and population structures. This leads on to the concept of opportunity cost. Because of the scarcity of resources, choices need to be made regarding the best method for their deployment. It is therefore inevitable that choosing to use resources for one activity requires that their use in other activities must be forsaken. The benefits, often referred to as utility, that would have resulted from these forsaken activities are referred to as opportunity costs. In health care, the opportunity costs of the use of resources for a particular health-care programme or intervention are equivalent to the benefits forsaken in the best alternative use of these resources.

It is necessary to identify from whose perspective the economic evaluation is undertaken. The perspective can be that of the individual patient, the NHS, the individual hospital or service provider, the government or society as a whole. If we considered the societal perspective, then we would seek to include all costs and benefits, no matter where they occur. More often than not it is from the societal perspective that economic evaluations are undertaken.

Within health care, economic evaluation is used as a rather general term to describe a range of methods that look at the costs and consequences of different programmes or interventions.[38] Each of the methods involves identifying, measuring and, where necessary, valuing all of the relevant costs and consequences of the programme or intervention under review.

There are four main approaches for undertaking economic evaluation: cost-minimisation analysis, cost-effectiveness analysis, cost–utility analysis and cost–benefit analysis. A summary of the features of these is given in **Table 2.3** and each is discussed below, outlining their appropriate use in health care.

Cost-minimisation analysis

Cost-minimisation analysis is often considered to be a form of cost-effectiveness analysis but is treated here as a separate method of economic evaluation. This particular form of economic evaluation is appropriate in circumstances where, prior to investigation, there is no reason to expect that there will be any therapeutic difference in the outcomes of the procedures under consideration. For example, we might wish to consider two different forms of treatment for varicose veins, such as day case and inpatient treatment. Here, one might assume that there would be no expected differences in outcome between the two forms of treatment, and therefore the preferred option would involve choosing the treatment method that was the least costly of the two. It should be considered, however, that if there is no evidence available to suggest that the outcomes of the options were similar, then ignoring outcomes might well yield misleading results based upon cost differences alone.

Cost-effectiveness analysis

Cost-effectiveness analysis should be used when the outcomes from the different programmes or interventions are anticipated to vary. The outcomes are expressed in natural units, though the appropriate measure to be used in such studies depends ultimately upon the programmes that are being compared. For interventions that would be expected to extend life, natural units such as life-years gained would be an appropriate measure. However, there might be a programme, such as the treatment for hypertension, where other measures might be considered appropriate, in this case unit reductions in blood pressure. Likewise, there might be a comparison of two different preventative treatments for

Table 2.3 • Methods of economic evaluation

Type of economic evaluation	Units of measurement
Cost-minimisation analysis	Outcomes are the same between the different options; evaluation based upon cost
Cost-effectiveness analysis	Benefits are quantity or quality of life, which are measured in natural units (e.g. life-years gained, cases avoided, etc.)
Cost–utility analysis	Benefits are quantity and quality of life, which are measured using QALYs or HYEs
Cost–benefit analysis	Benefits are quantity and quality of life, which are measured in monetary terms such as human capital or willingness to pay

QALY, quality-adjusted life-year; HYE, healthy years equivalent.

coronary heart disease, where heart attacks avoided might be a suitable measure to use.

In order to assess the cost-effectiveness, or otherwise, of the interventions, cost is expressed per unit of outcome (cost-effectiveness ratios). However, this means that the impact upon quantity and quality of life cannot be expressed in a single ratio and this is a substantial limitation to the use of cost-effectiveness analysis. Furthermore, the outcome of interest in the appraisal of two or more interventions must be exactly the same for each of the alternatives that are considered. Therefore the results from cost-effectiveness studies cannot often be generalised in order to assess the impact of interventions for differing conditions. In conclusion, cost-effectiveness analysis is a useful tool for informing choices between alternatives within comparable therapeutic areas but is of little use in comparing alternatives across differing areas.

As an example, one might assess the cost per stroke avoided in comparing the cost-effectiveness of a drug treatment for stroke prevention with that of carotid endarterectomy. However, such figures would be of little help in comparing the value of these treatments with that of a treatment for a different condition, such as joint replacement.

Cost–utility analysis

As has been discussed above, one of the major limitations of cost-effectiveness analysis is that it does not allow for decisions to be made regarding different treatments for differing diseases or conditions. This is because the units of outcome often differ between disease areas.

Cost–utility analysis can be thought of as a special case of cost-effectiveness analysis where the outcomes are expressed in generic units that are able to represent the outcome for different conditions and treatments. Therefore, the units of outcome combine both mortality and morbidity information into a single unit of measurement (such as QALYs or HYEs). This two-dimensional outcome measure allows comparisons to be drawn between treatments for different therapeutic areas. These units of measurement are often expressed in terms of a universal unit, usually cost per QALY gained. Such units have resulted in league tables that compare the outcomes for treatments in different areas, and these will be discussed below.

Cost–benefit analysis

Cost–benefit analysis is a type of evaluation that places a monetary value upon the benefits or outcome from differing programmes of health care, i.e. it determines the absolute benefit. Other methods of economic evaluation do not seek to assess whether the benefits of the intervention actually outweigh their costs. Basically, cost–benefit seeks to allocate monetary values for both the inputs (costs) and outcomes (benefits). This has many difficulties in that there are no simple or widely accepted methods of allocating a monetary value to health outcomes.

Choosing an evaluation method

The appropriate method of economic evaluation depends upon which choices need to be made, and the context within which those choices need to be reached. If outcomes are expected to be similar then the choice is quite straightforward: cost-minimisation analysis should be used. The limitations of cost-effectiveness should be borne in mind, although it is still an extremely popular method of economic evaluation. Cost–utility analysis has increased in popularity in an attempt to overcome some of the limitations that cost-effectiveness analysis possesses. Cost–benefit analysis may offer decision-makers even greater flexibility for assessing alternative health-care programmes.

Cost-effectiveness league tables

Decision-makers face difficult decisions when asked how to allocate resources in health care. Such decisions are increasingly influenced by the relative cost-effectiveness of different treatments and by comparisons between health-care interventions in terms of their cost per life-year or per QALY gained. The first compilation of such league tables was undertaken by Williams, who calculated the cost per QALY of a range of interventions and divided them into strong candidates for expansion and less strong candidates for expansion.[19] Advocates of such analyses argue that if properly constructed, these tables provide comprehensive and valid information to aid decision-makers.

There are, however, problems with the use of such tables and these can make interpretation and comparison between studies problematical.[39] First, the year of origin for the studies varies and, because of technological changes and shifts in relative prices, the ranking might not be truly reflective of the intervention under current practice. Second, differing discount rates have been used in the studies, some appropriately and others inappropriately, which impacts upon the results. Third, there have been a variety of preference values for health states, and currently it is difficult to determine which measure of quality of life has been used to derive the estimates concealed within the statistics presented in the league table. Clearly, if there is a high degree of homogeneity between the methods used to derive such estimates then these statistics might well aid decision-makers. Fourth, there is a wide range of costs used within the studies, and often costs are presented at an insufficient level of detail to allow recalculation to reflect local circumstances. In addition, many studies used in such league tables are often compared with differing programmes from which the incremental cost per QALY has been assessed. For example, some might compare with a 'do nothing' or 'do minimum' alternative, while other programmes would compare with the incremental cost per QALY of expanding services to other groups of patients. Finally, the setting of the study will prove important in drawing comparisons between the statistics in such tables, especially in situations where the studies are undertaken in different countries, requiring adjustments for exchange rates.

There has been a substantial amount of literature on the topic in recent years[20–23] and, while these tables might aid the decision-maker, they also need to be interpreted with extreme caution as there is ample opportunity to mislead the casual observer.

Ethical issues

Any formal method for determining the costs and benefits of different treatments that may be used to allocate resources is likely to raise complex ethical issues. In particular, certain methods may create apparent discrimination against certain groups, such as the elderly or disabled, due to reduced capacity to gain from a particular treatment. Such methods may also fail to take into account other issues that are seen by society as being important in allocating resources, such as preferences relating to the process of care and issues such as equity.[40] It is important that such economic methods should not be used without considering these wider implications of the decisions which stem from such analyses.

SUMMARY

Whether making individual or policy decisions regarding health-care provision, it is becoming increasingly important for clinicians to take into account evidence about both the effectiveness and the cost-effectiveness of the treatment options. This requires that they examine the available evidence with particular attention to the appropriateness of the outcome measures used and of any techniques for economic analysis. In particular, there is a need for both clinicians and researchers to focus upon outcomes that are relevant to patients and truly represent their views about the relative values of the health states and events that they may encounter. Outcome research and economic evaluation are relatively new areas of health-care research but they are progressing rapidly. An understanding of the methods used is a prerequisite for an adequate interpretation of the conclusions drawn from such work.

• Key points

- The choice of outcome measure is important in assessing the results of surgical treatment and needs to be carefully considered.
- The measure used should be clinically relevant and preferably have been validated by previous research.
- Possible measures relevant to surgery include mortality, condition-specific measures, standard pain questionnaires and generic measures of health-related quality of life.
- Quality-adjusted life-years are a commonly used measure of outcome and there are several different ways to produce the weights (utilities) that are required to calculate these.
- The estimation of the cost of treatments should include a detailed analysis of the resources used and their valuation, and may require consideration of the timing of incurring various costs.
- There are several different methods of economic evaluation, including cost-minimisation, cost-effectiveness, cost–utility and cost–benefit analysis.
- The use of cost-effectiveness league tables may allow comparison of health benefits to be gained by expenditure on different treatments but is not without both technical and ethical problems in its application.

REFERENCES

1. Collin C, Wade DT, Davies S, Horne V. The Barthel ADL Index: a reliability study. Int Disabil Stud 1988; 10:61–3.

2. Campbell D, Fisk D. Convergent and discriminant validity by the multi-trait multi-method matrix. Psychol Bull 1959; 56:81–105.

3. Perkins JMT, Collin J, Creasy TS et al. Exercise training versus angioplasty for stable claudication. Long and medium term results of a prospective, randomised trial. Eur J Vasc Endovasc Surg 1996; 11:409–13.

4. Stockton D, Davies T, Day N, McCann J. Retrospective study of reasons for improved survival in patients with breast cancer in East Anglia: earlier diagnosis or better treatment. Br Med J 1997; 314:472–5.

5. Sowden A, Sheldon T. Does volume really affect outcome? Lesson from the evidence. J Health Serv Res Policy 1998; 3:187–90.

6. Jones J, Rowan K. Is there a relationship between the volume of work carried out in intensive care and its outcome. Int J Technol Assess Health Care 1995; 11:762–9.

7. Brazier J, Dixon S. The use of condition specific outcome measures in economic appraisal. Health Econ 1995; 4:255–64.

8. Spilker B, Molihek FR, Johnston KA et al. Quality of life bibliography and indexes. Med Care 1990; 28(suppl. 12):DS1–DS77.

9. Meenan RF, Mason JH, Anderson JJ et al. AIMS2. The content and properties of a revised and expanded Arthritis Impact Measurement Scales Health Status Questionnaire. Arthritis Rheum 1992; 35:1–10.

10. Goldman L, Hashimoto B, Cook EF et al. Comparative reproducibility and validity of systems for assessing cardiovascular functional class: advantages of a new specific activity scale. Circulation 1227; 64:1227–34.

11. Melzack R. The McGill Pain Questionnaire: major properties and scoring methods. Pain 1975; 1:277–99.

12. Guyatt GH, Berman LB, Townsend M et al. A measure of quality of life for clinical trials in chronic lung disease. Thorax 1987; 42:773–8.

13. Carroll D, Rose K. Treatment leads to significant improvement. Effect of conservative treatment on pain in lymphoedema. Prof Nurse 1992; 8:32–3.

14. Brazier J, Deverill M, Green C et al. A review of the use of health status measures in economic evaluation. Health Technol Assess 1999; 3:1–164.

15. Euroqol Group. Euroqol: a facility for the measurement of health related quality of life. Health Policy 1990; 16:199–228.

16. Brazier JE, Harper R, Jones NM et al. Validating the SF-36 health survey questionnaire: new outcome measure for primary care. Br Med J 1992; 305:160–4.

17. Hunt SM, McKenna SP, McEwen J. Measuring health status. London: Croom Helm, 1986.

18. Torrance G. Measurement of health state utilities for economic appraisal: a review. J Health Econ 1976; 10:129–36.

19. Williams A. Economics of coronary artery bypass grafting. Br Med J (Clin Res Ed) 1985; 291:326–9.

20. Drummond M, Torrance G, Mason J. Cost effectiveness league tables: more harm than good? Social Sci Med 1993; 37:33–40.

21. Mason J, Drummond M, Torrance G. Some guidelines on the use of cost effectiveness league tables. Br Med J 1993; 306:570–2.

22. Birch S, Gafni A. Cost-effectiveness ratios: in a league of their own. Health Policy 1994; 28:133–41.

23. Drummond M, Mason J, Torrance G. Cost-effectiveness league tables: think of the fans. Health Policy 1995; 31:231–8.

24. Mehrez A, Gafni A. Healthy-years equivalents versus quality-adjusted life years: in pursuit of progress. Med Decis Making 1993; 13:287–92.

25. Buckingham K. A note on HYE (Healthy Years Equivalent). J Health Econ 1993; 11:301–9.

26. Johannesson M, Jonsson B, Karlsson G. Outcome measurement in economic evaluation. Health Econ 1996; 5:279–96.

27. Brazier J, Roberts J, Deverill M. The estimation of a preference-based measure of health from the SF-36. J Health Econ 2002; 21:271–92.

28. Johannesson M, O'Conor RM. Cost-utility analysis from a societal perspective. Health Policy 1997; 39:241–53.

29. von Neumann J, Morgenstern O. Theory of games and economic behavior. New York: Wiley, 1967.

30. Torrance GW, Thomas WH, Sackett DL. A utility maximization model for evaluation of health care programs. Health Serv Res 1972; 7:118–33.

31. Gerard K. Determining the contribution of residential respite care to the quality of life of children with severe learning difficulties. Child Care Health Dev 1990; 16:177–88.

32. Auld C, Donaldson C, Mitton C, Shackley P. Economic evaluation. In: Detels R, Holland W, McEwan J, Omenn G. (eds) Oxford textbook of public health, 4th edn. Oxford: Oxford University Press, 2001.

33. Drummond MF. Methods for the economic evaluation of health care programmes, 2nd edn. Oxford: Oxford University Press, 1997.

34. Parsonage M, Neuburger H. Discounting and health benefits. Health Econ 1992; 1:71–6.

35. Cairns J. Discounting and health benefits: another perspective. Health Econ 1992; 1:76–9.

36. Briggs A, Sculpher M. Sensitivity analysis in economic evaluation: a review of published studies. Health Econ 1995; 4:355–71.

37. Pauker SG, Kassirer JP. The threshold approach to clinical decision making. N Engl J Med 1980; 302:1109–17.

38. Drummond MF, Maynard AK. Purchasing and providing cost-effective health care. Edinburgh: Churchill Livingstone, 1993.

39. Mason J, Drummond M. Reporting guidelines for economic studies. Health Econ 1995; 4:85–94.

40. Ubel PA, DeKay ML, Baron J, Asch DA. Cost-effectiveness analysis in a setting of budget constraints: is it equitable? N Engl J Med 1996; 334:1174–7.

CHAPTER

Three
Day case surgery

Douglas McWhinnie

INTRODUCTION

The NHS plan, proposed by the Government of the UK in 2001, set the patient firmly at the centre of a framework for modernising the National Health Service (NHS).[1] The idea was to reduce waiting times, implement booking systems and introduce patient choice. However, the Government was faced with capacity constraints and one solution to increase patient throughput was to reduce the length of patients' stay by focusing on a National Day Surgery Programme.

 The day surgery strategy was launched in 2002 with the broad aim of achieving 75% of all elective surgery in the UK to be performed on a day case basis by the year 2005.[2]

Day surgery may be defined as the admission of selected patients to hospital for a planned surgical procedure, returning home on the same day. Patients who have their procedure as an outpatient or as an endoscopy where full operating theatre facilities and/or general anaesthetic is not required are no longer classified as 'true' day surgery.

In North America, day surgery is often defined as any procedure following which the patient is discharged within 24 hours. Several day units in the UK have recently adopted this North American concept but have renamed it 'extended day surgery', '23 hour surgery' or even 'ambulatory surgery'. Consequently it is difficult to compare statistics between countries as definitions vary but at least within the UK it is now possible to record variations in data between hospitals and even individual surgeons.

THE DEVELOPMENT OF DAY SURGERY

The concept of day surgery is not new. In 1909, a surgeon by the name of James Nicholl, working at the Royal Hospital for Sick Children in Glasgow, reported on nearly 9000 children undergoing day surgery for conditions such as hernia and hair lip.[3] Even then, Nicholl stressed the importance of suitable home conditions in the success of day surgery. A decade later, in 1919, Ralph Waters, an anaesthetist in Sioux City, Iowa, reported on the 'downtown anesthesia clinic' where adults underwent minor surgical procedures, returning home within a few hours.[4]

The modern era of day surgery began in the years following World War II with the realisation that prolonged bed rest was associated with high rates of postoperative complications such as deep vein thrombosis.[5] The move towards early ambulation led to earlier discharge and, for the first time, the economic benefits of day surgery were noted.[6] In 1955, Eric Farquharson of Edinburgh described a series of 458 consecutive inguinal hernia repairs performed on a day case basis at a time when the average length of postoperative stay was approximately 2 weeks.[7] The potential impact on surgical waiting lists was also considered.

The development of day surgery in the USA, Canada and Australia was driven by financial gain and progressed at a more rapid pace than in the UK with its state-run NHS. The first hospital-based day case units were opened in Grand Rapids, Michigan in 1951 and Los Angeles in 1952. The first free-standing ambulatory surgical centre, in Phoenix, Arizona, did not open until 1969. The 1970s and 1980s saw a great increase in the number of such units as medical insurance companies attempted to contain rising health costs.

In the UK, day surgery developed at a much slower pace. The first stand-alone day surgery unit was only built at the Hammersmith Hospital in London in 1967. Many more day units were organised in the 1970s but utilisation proved rather variable. Day surgery required consultant surgeons and anaes-thetists to be involved in minor and intermediate procedures, normally delegated in the inpatient setting to the junior trainees. Day surgery was held in low esteem and was therefore unpopular.[8] A culture change was also required to see patients on the morning of operation rather than on the pre-operative visit the day before surgery.

By 1985, there was a sufficient number of pro-active day units reporting good clinical and economic results to encourage the Royal College of Surgeons of England to publish a report (revised in 1992) entitled *Guidelines for day case surgery*.[9] At that time, it was estimated that only 15% of elective surgery was performed on a day case basis and the report suggested 50% as an appropriate target. In 1989, the gathering momentum of day surgery demonstrated a need for a professional body to promote the specialty and set quality standards of care. The result was the British Association of Day Surgery (BADS) encompassing surgeons, anaes-thetists and nurses involved in day surgery. The same year saw the Government's first major initiative to promote day surgery through the NHS Manage-ment Executive's value-for-money unit. They con-cluded that the cost of treating patients as day cases was significantly less than as inpatients and therefore supported the concept of day surgery.[10] By 1990, the Audit Commission had taken over the role of external auditors within the NHS and it introduced the concept of a 'basket' of 20 surgical procedures suitable for day case surgery to allow benchmarking between health authorities.[11] These 20 procedures were essentially minor and inter-mediate procedures (e.g. inguinal hernia repair, varicose vein stripping, arthroscopy, dilatation and curettage) and the audit figures demonstrated wide variation between districts, with the greatest differ-ences noted in carpal tunnel decompression. In some centres, all were performed as day cases while in others all received inpatient care.

The early 1990s saw considerable investment in day surgery infrastructure and practice. In 1991,

Box 3.1 • Audit Commission basket of 25 procedures 2001

Orchidopexy

Circumcision

Inguinal hernia repair

Excision of breast lump

Anal fissure dilatation or excision

Haemorrhoidectomy

Laparoscopic cholecystectomy

Varicose vein stripping or ligation

Transurethral resection of bladder tumour

Excision of Dupuytren's contracture

Carpal tunnel decompression

Excision of ganglion

Arthroscopy

Bunion operations

Removal of metalware

Extraction of cataract with or without implant

Correction of squint

Myringotomy

Tonsillectomy

Submucous resection

Reduction of nasal fracture

Operation for bat ears

Dilatation and curettage/hysteroscopy

Laparoscopy

Termination of pregnancy

the Audit Commission Report *Measuring quality: the patient's view of day surgery* found that 80% of day case patients preferred this mode of treatment to traditional inpatient treatment, adding impetus for the further development of day surgery.[12] In 1993, the national Day Surgery Task Force suggested that 60% of elective surgery should be performed on a day case basis nationally.[13] By 2001 the Audit Commission had produced an updated basket of procedures (**Box 3.1**) to include more major pro-cedures such as laparoscopic cholecystectomy and haemorrhoidectomy and this was incorporated into the Department of Health's *Day surgery: operational guide* published to support the National Day Surgery Programme to achieve a 75% day case rate for elective surgery by 2005.[2]

FACILITIES FOR DAY SURGERY

The organisation of day surgery services differs from inpatient surgery in several ways. The patient arrives at the hospital on the day of surgery, fully assessed with the results of investigations already checked. Following operation, patients recover in the day unit and are discharged home, accompanied by their carer. The entire admission episode is preplanned and the routine nature of the hospital visit ensures quality care. Any error in the system results in an unnecessary overnight admission and it is therefore not surprising that the facilities for day surgery differ from inpatient surgery.

Initially, day surgery was attempted from the inpatient ward, but the patient's procedure was often cancelled on the day of admission as their projected bed had been occupied overnight by an emergency admission. The inpatient ward environment was a mixture of emergency admissions, patients undergoing complex elective surgery and the day surgery patient undergoing a more 'minor' procedure. Quality of care for the day case patient suffered as the busy ward staff naturally concentrated on the acutely ill. Furthermore, there was no incentive to ensure the day patient was able to go home the same evening.

Self-contained day units or dedicated day wards were therefore developed and unplanned overnight admission rates dropped dramatically from 14% on an inpatient ward to 2.4% in a dedicated day unit.[2] These units may be free-standing or integrated within the main hospital where they benefit from the full range of available support services. The self-contained unit should have its own day surgery theatre within the day surgery suite. A less costly option is to provide a dedicated day ward for patient admission and recovery but to use the main theatre complex for the surgery itself. Provided the distance between the day ward and theatres is minimal, a rapid changeover of patients can be facilitated. The arrangement works even better if dedicated theatre lists are adopted. Attempting a day case following a major surgical procedure, especially if delegated to a junior surgeon, does not allow maximum time for recovery and runs the risk of cancellation if the major case overruns. Dedicated lists require appropriate staffing levels to be allocated as there is a greater intensity of work for theatre staff if several day cases are to be treated rather than a single major case.

As part of the NHS Plan, the Government has embarked on an ambitious programme of building a number of free-standing or integrated treatment centres financed by public money or by public/ private finance initiatives. This increased capacity for day surgery and short-stay surgery should ease capacity constraints and allow day surgery rates to increase throughout the country.

THE DAY SURGERY CYCLE

In traditional inpatient surgery, the patient is admitted either from the waiting list or directly from the surgical outpatient clinic if the patient is classified as urgent. In day surgery, referral patterns are different. In many hospitals the patient is seen in the outpatient clinic and then sent directly for pre-assessment. While this has the advantage of a single hospital visit, there is a fear that some patients may become overwhelmed with the amount of information they are given in a short space of time. Indeed, many patients find it convenient to come back to the preassessment clinic at a later date if they already have planned commitments on the day of the outpatient clinic. Many surgeons now hold outreach clinics in general practitioners' surgeries, and often the preassessment is performed by the practice nurse at the time of surgical consultation in the local surgery. More recently, some hospitals have accepted fast tracking by general practitioners, who refer patients direct for preassessment through the day unit's bed manager. In this case, the surgeon does not see the patient until the morning of operation. This is only suitable for the young and fit patient with a straightforward surgical problem (**Fig. 3.1**).

Patient selection

Patient selection addresses the suitability of both patient and procedure for day surgery and assesses the risk of major and minor complications for the individual patient. Factors that influence the selection of patients for day surgery include social conditions, the age of the patient, obesity and medical fitness. For the 23-hour stay patient, selection need not be so rigid. There are no upper limits on age or body mass index (BMI), although each patient is judged on an individual basis. Social factors rarely restrict admission and American Society of Anesthesiologists (ASA) class III patients are accepted. In a district general hospital, over 50% of traditional inpatient procedures can be performed on an extended day case basis.[14]

SOCIAL FACTORS

The effects of general anaesthesia on cerebral function, affecting judgement and coordination, are well recognised. After day surgery, all patients must be accompanied home by a responsible and physically

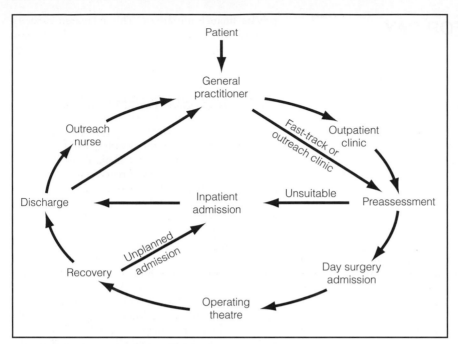

Figure 3.1 • The day surgery cycle.

able adult (over 16 years of age), who should be present for the first 24 hours following operation. Patients themselves must not drive home and the journey preferably should avoid public transport. Greater travelling times are associated with increased discomfort and nausea[15] and patients should reside within an hour's journey from the hospital in case of emergency. The patient's home conditions should be sufficient to allow them to recover in comfort. In general, they should have access to a telephone in case of emergency, there should be adequate toilet facilities and household stairs should be minimal, but each set of circumstances requires individual judgement.

AGE

Biological age is more important than chronological age, although many day units arbitrarily and illogically apply upper limits of 65 or 70 years of age. The older patient is more likely to suffer from respiratory and/or cardiovascular disease and the carer may also be in an elderly age group. However, with careful preoperative evaluation, the elderly patient can benefit from day surgery through a rapid return to familiar home circumstances and less postoperative confusion.

BODY MASS INDEX

Obesity is measured by BMI (in kg/m²) and height–weight charts are used as 'ready reckoners' to cal-

culate it (**Fig. 3.2**). Obesity is defined as a BMI equal to or greater than 30.[16] The prevalence of obesity has doubled in the 1990s, with 35% of adults now fulfilling the definition.[17] The very obese are excluded from day surgery because of delayed recovery related to the absorption of volatile anaesthetic agents into body fat but this is less of a problem with modern total intravenous anaesthetic agents such as propofol.[18] The problems that do occur with the obese patient are related to comorbidity, the surgical procedure and the anaesthetic. Obesity is associated with cardiac disease, diabetes mellitus, hiatus hernia, hypertension and sleep apnoea, and it may be the comorbidity factor that excludes an obese patient from day surgery rather than the obesity itself. Operating on the obese patient is often more technically demanding, and the complication rate is often higher, with increased rates of postoperative haematoma formation and pain as a result of the need for greater surgical access. Anaesthetic problems include problems of venous access, intubation and airway control. Operating on patients early in the day is advisable to ensure that any minor postoperative complications can be corrected and do not prevent the patient from returning home.

The upper safe BMI limit for day surgery remains controversial. While some day units still remain at a restrictive BMI of 30, others have safely increased this upper limit to 35, 37 and even 40.[19]

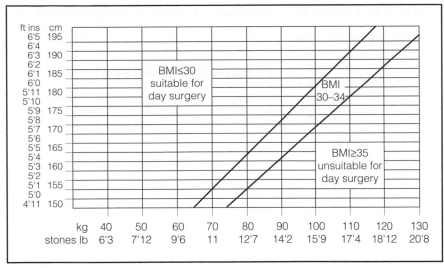

Figure 3.2 • Assessment chart for body mass index (BMI).

SMOKING

Smokers undergoing surgery have increased intra-operative complications such as impaired gas exchange and increased secretions, with postoperative problems consisting of an increased incidence of bronchospasm, chest infection and wound complications.[20] Advice at preassessment regarding cessation of smoking depends on whether the patient would like to stop permanently or else temporarily suspend their habit in the perioperative period. For those attempting permanent cessation, this should commence 6–8 weeks before surgery since this is the minimum time required for lung function to significantly improve.[21] It also allows the effects of physical addiction to nicotine (anxiety, depression and agitation) to subside, these effects being maximal 2–4 days after cessation. The least effective time of smoking cessation is therefore in the week before surgery when the effects of withdrawal are maximal, adding to the stress of hospital admission.[22] For those who intend continuing their habit, temporary cessation 12 hours before surgery confers a reduction in circulating carboxy-haemoglobin, thereby improving perioperative lung function.

MEDICAL FACTORS

 In 1991, the ASA classified surgical patients into five classes of physical fitness (**Box 3.2**), which has provided a framework for patient selection in day surgery.[23]

While ASA class I or class II patients are generally accepted for day surgery, the suitability of patients in the ASA class III group is less clear. While hypertension, chronic lung disease and symptomatic heart

Box 3.2 • Adaptation of the American Society of Anesthesiologists' classification of physical status

Class I	A healthy patient
Class II	Mild-to-moderate systemic disease caused by the surgical condition to be treated or by another disease process, with no functional limitation, controlled hypertension, mild diabetes, mild asthma
Class III	Severe systemic disease with some functional limitation plus diabetes with complications, severe asthma, myocardial infarction >6 months
Class IV	Severe systemic disease that is a constant threat to life plus unstable angina, severe cardiac, pulmonary, renal, hepatic or endocrine insufficiency
Class V	Moribund patient not expected to survive 24 hours even with surgical intervention

disease increase the risk of complications, this is not evident with asthma or insulin-dependent diabetes mellitus.

 Stable ASA class III patients have the same risk of unplanned overnight admissions as lower ASA status patients,[24] and any increase in complications with ASA class III patients is related to the surgical procedure rather than comorbidity.

Diabetes mellitus

Patients with diabetes mellitis can undergo successful day surgery. Type I diabetic patients are more difficult to manage in the perioperative period than type II patients and are more liable to unplanned admission. Stability of the disease in the months before surgery is central to success of the admission, especially in the type I patient. The stability of the diabetic patient can be assessed by blood group profiles in the preceding few months, unplanned hospital admissions, changes in medication, hypoglycaemic attacks and glycosylated haemoglobin (HbA$_{1c}$) levels. An HbA$_{1c}$ result of less than 8% suggests that the patient is suitable for day surgery. Most minor intermediate surgical procedures, such as those in the Audit Commission basket of 25 (**Box 3.1**), can be safely undertaken in adult diabetic patients with the possible exception of laparoscopic cholecystectomy due to the relatively high risk of postoperative nausea and vomiting. Where possible the patient should be managed with local or regional anaesthesia as this may remove the need for the patient to starve preoperatively. However if general anaesthesia is required, diabetic medication is omitted on the morning of surgery, the procedure is scheduled as early as possible on the list and the normal regimen is resumed as soon as possible.[25] Well-controlled non-insulin-dependent diabetics present few problems but insulin-dependent diabetics require intensive monitoring throughout the day surgery process and may in many units be considered unsuitable for inclusion into day surgery practice.

Cardiac disease

The risk of myocardial ischaemia during anaesthesia is increased in the hypertensive patient, and elevated blood pressure is one of the most common reasons for 'on the day' cancellation: the blood pressure has either not been accurately measured at preoperative assessment or it has not been adequately treated. Preoperative sedation can lower a marginally elevated blood pressure but the underlying cause requires further investigation. Many patients with significant cardiovascular disease can still undergo day surgery procedures provided exercise tolerance is good.

The specific blood pressure that is unsafe for the patient undergoing day surgery remains unclear but a systematic review and meta-analysis of 30 observational studies found little evidence for an association between admission arterial pressure and perioperative complications if systolic and diastolic pressures are less than 180 and 110 mmHg respectively.[26]

Asthma

The younger asthmatic using an inhaler and with good exercise tolerance is suitable for day surgery. Only those with steroid-controlled asthma are excluded or require investigation before proceeding. Non-steroidal anti-inflammatory drugs (NSAIDs) can be administered safely for pain relief to 95% of

asthmatics.[27] A history of previous administration without bronchial spasm, usually from over-the-counter preparations, is often available.

Preoperative assessment

The admission, operation and discharge of a patient within a day requires accurate forward planning, with the procedure occurring on a scheduled day at a scheduled time. Unlike traditional inpatient surgery, where planning, assessment and investigations are often performed after admission in the day or days leading up to the operation, day surgery requires day of surgery admission (DOSA) with full preoperative assessment having been performed in advance, up to 6 weeks previously. As a result, nursing, anaesthetic and surgical assessment on the day of admission is both rapid and minimal and accurate preassessment of patients ensures that 'on the day' cancellation for clinical reasons is rare. Cancellations not only waste hospital resources but cause distress to patients and their families and often disrupt work commitments.

While strict assessment criteria ensure patient safety, the assessment process also identifies those patients who could be converted to day surgery provided their exclusion factors can be addressed. The most common remedial factors are treatment of hypertension and identifying an overnight carer for patients living on their own. Assessment also allows the patient a second chance to discuss anxieties that may not have been considered at initial outpatient consultation. Involvement of the patient at this early stage permits flexibility and choice regarding their operating date and improves non-attendance rates.

Day surgery preassessment is best performed by trained assessment nurses in nurse-based preassessment clinics. The use of junior doctors for assessment is inappropriate because of limitations of hours of work and the greater demand on time from more intensive inpatient care.

To maximise day surgery throughput, a cultural change is required from an 'opt in' policy such as 'Is this patient suitable for day surgery?' to an 'opt out' policy such as 'Is there any reason this patient cannot be a day case?' The redesign of preassessment may be accomplished by:

- automatic assessment for day surgery of all patients undergoing a procedure included in the Audit Commission's basket of procedures (**Box 3.1**);
- hospital-wide preassessment for all elective surgical procedures (with procedure-specific exclusions for major surgical procedures such as major bowel resection and aortic aneurysm repair).

Preassessment clinics use a patient questionnaire to screen for social and medical problems. Nurse-based assessment allows the patient adequate consultation time and nursing colleagues are also more adept at the assessment of the patients' social situation. Most questionnaires follow a standard format to rapidly screen and triage the suitability of patients for day surgery. Questionnaires should address the generic status of the health of the patient, but additional questions may be added for specific surgical specialties (e.g. ophthalmology; ear, nose and throat; orthopaedics).

Preassessment is rapid for patients who are either clearly suitable or entirely unsuitable for day surgery and the latter patients are returned to the inpatient waiting list. Most preoperative time and effort is spent on patients who are marginal for day case surgery, and their suitability may only become apparent once the results of further investigations are available. These can be discussed with the appropriate anaesthetist and/or surgeon. Patients may therefore attend the preoperative clinic on more than one occasion, but these extra attendances are still more cost-effective than condemning the patient to inpatient surgery. However, one of the major consequences of a shift to day surgery is that the removal of day surgery patients undergoing mainly intermediate surgery from the inpatient environment leaves a case mix of mainly high dependency and acutely ill patients in the inpatient ward which may require a revaluation of the inpatient ward skill mix.

INVESTIGATIONS

Routine investigations are unnecessary in the asymptomatic day surgery patient[28] and preoperative testing should be limited to circumstances in which the results will affect patient treatment and outcomes. Investigations should not be prescriptive but should be tailored to the individual's needs because most investigations required can be predicted from the history alone. Even when minor abnormalities are found they rarely influence cancellation. A full blood count is only required if there is a risk of anaemia, chronic renal disease, rectal bleeding or menorrhagia. Similarly, analysis for urea and electrolytes is only indicated if the patient has renal disease or is taking diuretics. Urinalysis is often routinely performed as part of the preoperative culture but, again, unsuspected disease is more likely to be picked up on history alone. In Oxford, routine urine testing of more than 30 000 day case admissions resulted in only one cancellation, caused by unsuspected diabetes mellitus.[18]

The incidence of electrocardiographic (ECG) abnormalities increases with age[29] but minor preoperative ECG abnormalities do not predict adverse cardiovascular perioperative events in day surgery.[30]

The only indications for preoperative ECG include chest pain, palpitations and dyspnoea, but these patients have often already been excluded from day surgery by other comorbidity. A chest X-ray examination is also unnecessary. If required, then the patient is probably unsuitable for day surgery in the first place.

Testing for sickle cell disease is more controversial. Patients with sickle cell disease usually present in childhood with chronic haemolytic anaemia. Preoperative screening in adults is unlikely to identify a patient with previously unknown sickle cell disease but will, of course, identify those with sickle cell trait. However, the 'at-risk' population (those of African, Asian and Mediterranean origin) is often difficult to define in Britain today as a result of ethnic mixing. Furthermore, those factors which precipitate sickling (hypotension, hypoxaemia and acidosis) are unlikely to occur during day case surgery.

Day of surgery admission

On arrival at the day unit on the prearranged day of operation, most documentation is complete and bureaucracy is minimised. Any change of circumstance, either social or medical, should be noted since the time of preassessment, and the surgical visit, ideally by the person performing the operation, should consist of verification of the consent and marking the appropriate operation site. The final anaesthetic assessment is performed at this time and **not** in the anaesthetic room where levels of anxiety are already high. Many day surgery units have successfully introduced staggered admission times for patients, which is more convenient for both patient and the day unit. In most centres, the 12-hour fasting ritual has now been replaced by more realistic regimens of no solids within 4–6 hours and up to 300 mL of clear fluid within 2 hours of surgery.

Patient discharge

Discharge after inpatient surgery for those 'basket' procedures suitable for day case surgery usually occurs a minimum of 18–24 hours after the completion of the surgical procedure. By then, there is little concern regarding postoperative complications or the adverse effects of the anaesthetic. In contrast, discharge on the day of surgery must address strict discharge criteria if unacceptable complications are to be avoided. Before returning home, every patient should be seen by a surgeon and anaesthetist involved in their care, but the final decision to discharge is nurse initiated, based on discharge guidelines (**Box 3.3**). Some units adhere to strict scoring systems,[31] which address vital signs, patient activity,

Box 3.3 • Discharge criteria

Vital signs stable for at least 1 hour

Correct orientation as to time, place and person

Adequate pain control and supply of oral analgesia

Understanding the use of oral analgesia supplied, supported by written information

Ability to dress, walk (where appropriate)

Minimal nausea, vomiting or dizziness

Taken oral fluids

Minimal bleeding (or wound drainage)

Has passed urine (if appropriate)

Has a responsible escort for the homeward journey

Has a carer at home for next 24 hours

Written and verbal instructions given about postoperative care

Knows when to return for follow-up (if appropriate)

Emergency contact number supplied

---

postoperative nausea and vomiting (PONV), pain and bleeding, but whether such regimented protocols confirm any advantage over the checklist of criteria outlined in **Box 3.3** is debatable. Generic criteria have their limitations. For example, the criterion of being able to 'walk unaided' from the day unit may be inappropriate following orthopaedic surgery to the foot. Common sense in such situations is clearly required and the individual surgical procedure or type of surgery undertaken may prompt additional specific criteria.[32]

ANAESTHESIA

Day surgery may be performed under four basic anaesthetic techniques: sedation, local, regional or general anaesthesia, with or without premedication.

Premedication

In day surgery, premedication relates to any drugs administered in the day unit before the patient leaves for surgery and they are usually administered orally or rectally. There is a widely held belief that premedication sedatives for anxiety are unnecessary in day surgery and, if given, recovery time may be prolonged. In most cases this is true, but up to 19% of patients suffer significant anxiety and these benefit from sedative premedication.[33] Patients who are young, female and are undergoing their first general anaesthetic, especially if it is for breast

surgery, are at highest risk. Short-acting benzo-diazepines such as temazepam 20 mg orally or midazolam 15 mg orally are both effective but recovery times are prolonged. Standard midazolam tastes bitter and if given orally needs to be given with a sweet drink to hide the bitter taste. Other premedication drugs commonly used in day surgery include oral ranitidine 150 mg for known acid reflux and NSAIDs for postoperative pain if the procedure is of short duration. In addition, the patient's normal drug therapy, including antihypertensive agents, should be given as normal.

SEDATION

Sedation, commonly used in dental and endoscopy practice, may be defined as 'a technique in which the use of a drug or drugs produces a state of depression of the central nervous system enabling treatment to be carried out, but during which verbal contact with the patient is maintained'.[34] Standards of monitoring for sedation in gastro-intestinal endoscopy were published in 1991 and address safety issues such as the availability of resuscitation equipment and the safe use and administration of benzodiazepines.[35] Patient responses to sedative agents vary considerably and they should be titrated to the desired clinical effect to minimise overdose. Ideally, the sedationist should be an experienced anaesthetist, but this is not always practical in the 'real' world. Monitoring during the procedure is mandatory and consists of pulse oximetry to measure oxygen saturation, an assessment of the patient's level of consciousness and ECG and blood pressure monitoring, especially for patients with a history of ischaemic heart disease or cardiac arrhythmias. Oxygen supplementation is provided by oxygen mask or nasal cannulae.

In surgical practice, especially where the sedation is often performed in the procedure, intravenous sedation should be kept simple and consists in adults of midazolam in a titrated dose of 0.07 mg/kg. Dosage is reduced in the elderly patient because hypotension and respiratory depression can occur. It is a much better amnesic drug than diazepam and its solubility has reduced the incidence of pain on injection or phlebitis. As it has a short half-life of 2–4 hours, 'hangover' effects are reduced. If overdose occurs, the competitive benzodiazepine antagonist flumazenil is given, but as its half-life is only approximately 1 hour, it is important to recognise that re-sedation may occur and premature discharge of the patient must be avoided.

Sedo-analgesia is a combination of a benzo-diazepine and an analgesic agent such as pethidine (meperidine) or morphine. It is often used in the more painful endoscopic procedures such as colonoscopy. The longer-acting traditional opioids are often now replaced by the more rapid onset short-acting agents such as fentanyl (50–200 µg i.v.), alfentanil and remifentanil, which act within several minutes.

Local and regional anaesthesia

The application of local anaesthesia creates a temporary loss of sensation from the surgical field, whereas in regional anaesthesia nerves are blocked at a distance from the site of surgery. As with sedation, perioperative monitoring is required and should include pulse oximetry, with ECG and blood pressure monitoring in the elderly or cardiovascularly unfit. Several local anaesthetic agents are available (Table 3.1) but toxic reactions can occur in overdosage. Toxic blood levels lead to circumoral tingling, tinnitus and dizziness. Serious overdosage is reflected in loss of consciousness, convulsions or cardiac dysrhythmia. Dosage levels therefore need to be controlled. Higher dosage can be administered if it is given with adrenaline (epinephrine) (1 in 200 000), which causes vasoconstriction. This assists haemostasis, slow absorption and prolongs anaesthesia. The administration of adrenaline is contraindicated in end-artery procedures such as in the penis or in the digits of the hand or feet.

Local or regional anaesthesia may be used alone, with sedation or with general anaesthesia to prolong pain relief after completion of the procedure. Cocaine, which also has vasoconstrictor properties, may be topically applied to the nasal mucosa prior to nasal surgery. Amethocaine (tetracaine), which is systemically toxic, is mainly used for topical anaesthesia in ophthalmology. Prilocaine is short acting, has less toxic levels in the blood and is useful in intravenous regional anaesthesia such as Bier's block. Field infiltration with local anaesthetic and adrenaline may be used for the removal of minor 'lumps and bumps'. Bupivacaine (and the newer ropivacaine) has a long duration of action, lasting several hours, but can take up to 30 minutes to achieve simple nerve block. It is therefore a useful adjunct for wound infiltration or nerve block in association with general anaesthesia. Commonly performed nerve blocks include digital nerve block, scalene block, wrist block, penile block and blockade of the ileo-inguinal, ileo-hypogastric and genito-femoral nerves in inguinal hernia repair.

Spinal anaesthesia is not currently used routinely in UK day surgery practice in contrast to many other parts of the world. The main advantage of spinal anaesthesia is for operations below the waist such as arthroscopic surgery on the knee, foot surgery, haemorrhoidectomy or other minor rectal surgery, neurological surgery and inguinal hernia repair. The principal reasons for selecting spinal anaesthesia are in the obese or those with cardio-respiratory diesease who would otherwise be excluded from day surgery.[36]

General anaesthesia

General anaesthesia occurs when a drug or combination of drugs produces loss of both sensation and consciousness, with or without relaxation. The techniques and drugs used in general anaesthesia today permit up to 90 minutes of anaesthetic time for day surgery. The use of the laryngeal mask rather than the endotracheal tube has changed anaesthetic practice in day surgery since its introduction in 1988. Muscle relaxants are not required with its insertion, which is quicker and easier, and it is tolerated in light anaesthesia, allowing rapid patient turnaround. The introduction of total intravenous anaesthesia using propofol for induction and maintenance of anaesthesia has major advantages over inhalation agents; these include reduced PONV, early recovery and rapid control of the depth

Table 3.1 • Dosage and application of local anaesthetic agents

Agent	Dose (mg/kg)		Application
	Alone	With adrenaline	
Cocaine	–	–	Topical
Amethocaine (tetracaine)	–	Topical	
Prilocaine	5	7	Intravenous regional anaesthesia
Lignocaine (lidocaine)	3	5	Infiltration nerve blocks
Bupivacaine	1–2	1–2	Infiltration nerve blocks, spinal/epidural
Ropivacaine	1–2	1–2	Infiltration nerve blocks, spinal/epidural

of anaesthesia making it ideal for day case surgery. PONV after surgery is best prevented rather than treated.

 Adequate hydration reduces PONV and intravenous fluid should be administered during longer procedures. Intravenous fluids in a dose of 20 mL/kg significantly reduce the incidence of postoperative drowsiness and dizziness.[37]

While the choice of anaesthetic is considered a major contributing factor in PONV, surgery lasting more than 1 hour or involving laparoscopy, dental procedures, squint surgery or correction of bat ears is associated with an increased incidence. Certain types of patient are also predisposed to PONV. Women are two to three times more likely to suffer PONV than men[38] and it is perhaps greatest during the menstrual period.[39] Patients with a history of PONV or motion sickness have a three times increased incidence than the general population. Therefore, patients with risk factors or who are undergoing surgery associated with a high incidence of PONV should receive intravenous prophylactic antiemetic treatment at induction of anaesthesia. Droperidol (0.5 mg i.v.) is cheap but even in low doses may cause drowsiness, restlessness, anxiety or acute dystonia. Ondansetron (4 mg i.v.), a 5-hydroxytryptamine type 3 (5HT$_3$) receptor antagonist, has fewer side effects but is expensive. Accurate identification of high-risk patients may justify the use of ondansetron. In established PONV, ondansetron 4 mg i.v. is the treatment of choice despite cost when trying to avoid an unplanned admission. If prophylactic ondansetron has already been given, then droperidol administration should be attempted.

Pain management during anaesthesia is based on a concept of multimodal analgesia, which is a combination of two or more analgesic agents or analgesic techniques to minimise side effects. A common strategy is to use an NSAID or opioid in combination with regional or local anaesthesia. In recovery, rescue analgesia may be required if pain is severe, especially if the surgical procedure was more extensive than anticipated. Short-acting opioids such as fentanyl or alfentanil are preferred as PONV side effects are short-lived. The administration of morphine and pethidine at this stage is likely to lead to unplanned overnight admission because of their longer-lasting effects. Administration of analgesia in recovery and on the day ward before discharge should be given before 'breakthrough' pain occurs and is based on the accurate measurement of pain by the patients themselves. It usually takes the form of a visual analogue score from 0 to 10 or a description from 'no pain' through to 'worst possible pain'.

SURGERY

The rapid, safe and effective surgery required for a day case procedure demands the surgical competence of a consultant or an experienced specialist registrar. In the past, the day surgery list of intermediate procedures was often delegated to the most junior surgical trainee to perform without supervision. Not surprisingly, this led to prolonged operating times, patient cancellations, increased complications (such as bleeding or haematoma formation) and an inevitable rise in the unplanned overnight admission rate. Such practice offers poor-quality treatment and should be condemned. It is reassuring to note that the number of units offering suboptimal surgery is on the decrease. Nevertheless, many consultant surgeons' attitudes towards day surgery remain lukewarm, with the surgery itself considered mundane, boring and lacking the technical challenge of complex major procedures. With the introduction of more major minimal access procedures into the field of day surgery, this author would contend that intermediate and major surgery performed on a day case basis is a true surgical challenge if morbidity is to be maintained at near zero levels.

Day surgery rates for specific procedures vary between hospitals and between individual surgeons. The reasons for such variations are complex and remain largely unexplained. Patient preference must always be considered but it is accepted that only 5–10% of patients are actively opposed to day surgery. Patients in rural areas living more than 1 hour's travel from the hospital are also more likely to require overnight admission. Large teaching hospitals tend to attract complex tertiary referrals and therefore day surgery accounts for a smaller percentage of their overall activity. Population demographics might also explain why day case activity can be low in hospitals that serve a large geriatric population. Medical personnel may have strong views for or against day surgery and may therefore influence local day surgery rates.

Procedures suitable for day surgery

The original Audit Commission basket of 20 procedures published in 1990 was updated to a basket of 25 in 2001 (**Box 3.1**). The introduction of newer surgical anaesthetic techniques to the day unit and the loss of others into the outpatient department forced a reassessment of the surgical basket to reflect modern day case activity. Changing practice and fiscal rationing has made several of the surgical procedures on the original list poor comparators of day surgery. Rigid cystoscopy has been largely replaced by flexible cystoscopy, which is a local anaesthetic outpatient procedure. Dilatation and curettage has, in many units, been replaced by outpatient hysteroscopy. Varicose vein surgery has, in many strategic health authorities, been rationed to patients with varicose eczema or venous ulceration. Such patients are often the elderly with comorbidity and often require inpatient or 23-hour surgery.

However, more advanced day units were already performing more complex procedures on a day surgery basis and in 1999, continuing with the supermarket analogy, the British Association of Day Surgery recommended an additional 20 operations to form a 'trolley' of procedures suitable for day surgery in the more experienced day unit (**Box 3.4**). The procedures themselves include more major operations such as laparoscopic cholecystectomy, thoracoscopic sympathectomy, partial thyroidectomy and laser prostatectomy. The concept of the trolley is that a target of 50% of these procedures on a day case basis would be realistic.

Box 3.4 • British Association of Day Surgery 'trolley' of procedures 1999, of which 50% should be suitable for day case surgery

Laparoscopic hernia repair
Thoracoscopic sympathectomy
Submandibular gland excision
Partial thyroidectomy
Superficial parotidectomy
Wide excision of breast lump with axillary clearance
Haemorrhoidectomy
Urethrotomy
Bladder neck incision
Laser prostatectomy
Transcervical resection of endometrium
Eyelid surgery
Arthroscopic meniscectomy
Arthroscopic shoulder decompression
Subcutaneous mastectomy
Rhinoplasty
Dentoalveolar surgery
Tympanoplasty
Laparoscopic cholecystectomy
Bunion operations

Surgical practice: controversies

BREAST SURGERY

Simple excision biopsy or lumpectomy has long been accepted as a day case procedure. Wide local excision with axillary node dissection/sampling is more controversial. The procedure itself is suitable for day surgery, with similar complication rates of haematoma, seroma and infection as with overnight stay.[40] Axillary drainage may not be necessary in all patients.[41] However, the success of such a procedure requires a dedicated breast care team in both the hospital and the community to oversee drain removal and wound management and to offer appropriate psychological support.

HAEMORRHOIDECTOMY

Only 16% of all haemorrhoidectomies in the UK are currently performed as day cases. It is possible to perform the traditional Milligan–Morgan technique on a day case basis but the raw rectal surface created by the procedure often results in unacceptable postoperative pain. The newer haemorrhoid techniques such as Ligasure haemorrhoidectomy,[42] stapled anopexy[43] and haemorrhoidal artery ligation[44] are less invasive and are associated with a reduction in operative pain when compared with the conventional techniques and may therefore be more suitable for day surgery. Spinal or caudal anaesthesia[36] may also confer an advantage for the day surgery patient. Aftercare consists of non-constipatory analgesia, pre-emptive laxatives to avoid unnecessary hospital stay until the bowels open, glyceryl trinitrate ointment for local pain relief and metronidazole antibiotics to reduce incidents of pain and secondary haemorrhage in the days following the procedure.[45]

LAPAROSCOPIC CHOLECYSTECTOMY

The day case rate for laparoscopic cholecystectomy in the UK is 5% and has changed little over the last few years. The reasons for this relate to fears about reactionary haemorrhage, delayed haemorrhage and bile leak. Reactionary haemorrhage occurs within 4–6 hours after surgery and can be addressed within the ordinary working day if the surgery is performed before noon. Delayed haemorrhage usually occurs 3–4 days after cholecystectomy and even if the patient had undergone their operation as an inpatient, they would still have gone home before the secondary haemorrhage was apparent. Bile leaks rarely become apparent before 48 hours after surgery: accessory duct injury is often insidious, diathermy injury to the biliary tree may take days to leak and cystic duct stump leakage likewise. Again, if the patient had undergone inpatient surgery the likelihood is that they would already have been discharged home.

Successful day case laparoscopic cholecystectomy relies on rigorous patient selection, accepting only well-motivated and non-obese patients, and attention to detailed surgical technique. Patients undergoing day case laparoscopic cholecystectomy require approximately 6 hours of recovery time and the procedure is best performed early in the operating day.

 Age greater than 50 and ASA class II and III are poor prognostic indicators.[46,47]

Good operative technique is also relevant when creating the pneumoperitoneum, as carbon dioxide inadvertently placed in the extraperitoneal space can cause considerable discomfort. Shoulder tip pain from diaphragmatic irritation has been related to the size of the gas bubble under the diaphragm[48] and attempts should therefore be made to expel as much gas as possible at the end of the procedure. Blood in the peritoneal cavity is irritant and liver bed haemostasis and peritoneal lavage before exiting the abdomen is worthwhile. While much of the postoperative pain in laparoscopic cholecystectomy is deep in nature, laparoscopy port sites should always be infiltrated with a long-acting local anaesthetic (such as bupivacaine). There appears to be little difference between infiltration at the beginning or the end of the procedure.[49,50] The puncture-site local anaesthesia can be supplemented by NSAIDs administered at the beginning of the operation by either the rectal or sublingual route. It also seems likely, although not proven, that a reduction in the number and size of ports may confer a pain advantage in the postoperative period.

PROSTATECTOMY

Patients requiring prostatectomy tend to be older and less fit and many are excluded from day surgery by comorbidity. Conventional transurethral resection of the prostate (TURP) can be performed as a day case but postoperative haemorrhage remains a problem. Successful laser prostatectomy day case programmes have been reported,[51,52] with the patients discharged with a catheter in situ, returning to the day unit approximately 1 week later for trial without catheter.

THYROIDECTOMY (PARTIAL)

Partial thyroidectomy in non-toxic patients who are not obese may be a suitable day case procedure.[53] The thyroid gland is anatomically accessible via a transverse neck incision below the thyroid notch rather than by the more extensive necklace incision. Meticulous attention to haemostasis is required and

the patient can have the drain (if used) removed in the outpatient clinic, by outreach or community nurse. In the UK the legitimate fear of postoperative haemorrhage leading to tracheal pressure has all but excluded thyroid surgery from the day unit but performing the procedure on a 23-hour basis is gaining popularity.

THORACOSCOPIC SYMPATHECTOMY

Surgical operating time for a unilateral thoracoscopic sympathectomy is commonly under 30 minutes and it may therefore be suitable for day surgery.[54] Access to the thoracic cavity may be obtained through two 5-mm trocars inserted in the region of the third to fifth interspace in the anterior axillary line. Some operators favour a 10-mm telescope with a working channel, but in the small-framed individual, intercostal nerve irritation may preclude day case discharge. A double-lumen endotracheal tube to allow individual lung ventilation is no longer required; a largyngeal mask is safe and the lung is deflated by inserting 600–800 mL carbon dioxide by Veress needle into the thoracic cavity before trocar insertion. After completion of the procedure, the lung is reinflated under direct vision and a postoperative chest radiograph is taken 2–3 hours later before day surgery discharge to check for a pneumothorax. The incidence of significant pneumothorax requiring a chest drain and overnight admission is less than 1%.

TONSILLECTOMY

 In the UK, 6% of tonsillectomies are performed on a day case basis due to worries about reactionary haemorrhage. This risk is small and in a recent series of 668 adults and children undergoing day case tonsillectomy in Salisbury, the reactionary haemorrhage rate was 0.3% occurring within the first 6–8 hours after the operation while the patient was still on the day unit.[55]

Secondary haemorrhage occurs in approximately 1% of post-tonsillectomy patients and occurs several days after discharge but may cause rapid airway obstruction at home with fatal consequences. The Salisbury Unit has a high readmission rate of 6% and reflects their policy of readmitting even minor bleeds for 24 hours in case they herald a more major bleed.

Recovery

Upon completion of anaesthesia at the end of a surgical procedure, the patient is transferred to the operating theatre recovery area known as 'first-stage recovery'. Formerly, the patient remained here for a predetermined period, commonly 30 or 60 minutes. However, the development of short-acting

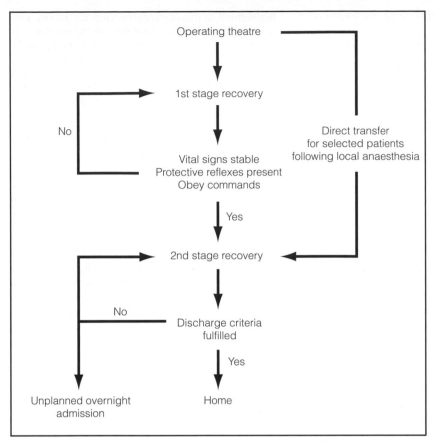

Figure 3.3 • Staged patient recovery.

anaesthetic agents, the introduction of minimally invasive surgical techniques and individual patient variability meant that patients were often ready for transfer to 'second-stage recovery' before their predetermined time. Therefore 'time-based recovery' is no longer necessary and has in many units been superseded by 'criteria-based recovery', where discharge is determined by the observations of stable vital signs, return of protective reflexes and the ability to obey commands. 'Second-stage recovery' occurs in the day unit itself, where patients recover sufficiently to allow safe discharge home. Certain patients may be suitable for direct transfer to second-stage recovery from the operating theatre itself (**Fig. 3.3**) and include patients who have received local or regional anaesthesia with or without minimal sedation.

Postoperative complications

Precise patient selection should ensure that postoperative morbidity is minimised, but complications do occur and can be classified into major and minor problems (**Box 3.5**).[56] Major complications occur less often than anticipated in the day surgery patient population,[57] with an incidence of 1 in 1455, and are independent of ASA status. Mortality is low and varies between 1 in 66 500 and 1 in 11 273.

Minor complications are more common and may precipitate unplanned overnight admission; these range from 0.1 to 5% depending on case mix.[58] Postoperative morbidity is usually related to the procedure undertaken and the anaesthetic used rather than the ASA status, which predicts complications in major inpatient surgery but not in day surgery patients. Surgical causes account for 60–70% of unplanned admissions and are usually the result of the surgeon embarking on a more extensive procedure than planned rather than surgical misadventure. Day surgery lists require careful planning, with the more major surgical procedures performed earlier in the day to allow adequate recovery time. Failure to adhere to this policy often leads to unplanned admissions.[59] Surgical inexperience may prolong a straightforward procedure if consultant supervision is absent. The

Box 3.5 • Postoperative morbidity after day surgery

Major complications
Unrecognised visceral damage
Severe postoperative haemorrhage
Myocardial infarction
Pulmonary embolus
Cerebrovascular accident
Respiratory failure
(Death)

Minor complications
Pain
Postoperative nausea and vomiting
Drowsiness/dizziness
Sore throat/hoarseness
Headache
Minor bleeding
Infection

more lengthy and invasive surgical procedures tend to increase postoperative pain, PONV and drowsiness and preclude safe discharge. Even once the patient has returned home, PONV may return and last up to 5 days in 35% of patients[60] and is often severe. Readmission rates are similar to unplanned admission rates (0.7–3.1%) and again are most often from surgically related causes.

Before leaving the day unit, patients require specific information regarding their medication, wound care and when they are able to bath or shower, arrangements for suture removal or dressing renewal, when they can resume normal activities and arrangements for follow-up (if appropriate). It is also important to offer a contact telephone number for emergency purposes on the night of discharge. In addition, patients must be clearly instructed not to drive a motor vehicle for at least 24 hours. After groin or limb surgery, patients are advised only to drive when they can safely perform an emergency stop, usually 1 week later.

The most common reason for a patient visiting their general practitioner after day surgery is to obtain certification for time off work. The second commonest reason, usually in an unplanned manner, relates to worries about their wound. After discharge, many day surgery units offer outreach or telephone follow-up for their patients 24 hours later. This can be an effective evaluation tool, where any identified actual or potential problems can be

highlighted to the day surgery team for action. This may only be necessary after specialised surgery (e.g. cataract surgery where a change of dressing can be combined with outreach follow-up) or after the introduction of an unfamiliar procedure to the unit. Such follow-up should be voluntary as some patients may object to this intrusion of their privacy.

PAEDIATRIC DAY SURGERY

Children find surgery and hospital visits a daunting and stressful prospect and are therefore treated both separately and differently from adults. In 1991, the National Association for the Welfare of Children in Hospital published quality standards for care of paediatric day cases and suggested that children should be managed by staff trained in their care, in a child-safe and child-friendly environment with open access to the conscious child for the parents.[61] Ideally, paediatric day surgery should be performed in a dedicated paediatric day unit, but this is only achievable in specialised children's hospitals. In non-specialised hospitals where the availability of anaesthetists and surgeons with appropriate paediatric training and registered children's nurses is limited, it is savings efficient to plan 'children's days' in the day unit, for example one day per week. At the very least, on these lists children should have their operation on the first part of the list and in the ward be separated from adults and nursed in a paediatric area with play facilities available.

Most children are fit and healthy ASA class I patients. ASA class II and III patients are not excluded but an anaesthetist with paediatric expertise is recommended. ASA class III children include those with stable asthma, epilepsy or minor corrected congenital heart problems. Procedures for children with respiratory infections should be postponed for 2–4 weeks depending on severity, but after measles or whooping cough this should be extended to 6 weeks because of irritability of the respiratory tract.[62] In many units, children under the age of 6 months are considered unsuitable for day surgery but if specialist facilities are available, full-term neonates are acceptable provided inpatient neonatal care is available. Premature babies are excluded up to 60 weeks after conception because of the risk of postoperative apnoea.[63] Many units also exclude children who are less than 5 kg because of the risk of hypothermia or hypoglycaemia associated with their physical status.

Psychosocial factors also determine a child's fitness for day surgery, and preparation begins with the preadmission visit to the day unit, the anaesthetic room and theatre recovery area, to allay the fears of both child and parents. At these so-called

'Saturday Clubs', routine information is given to the parents about day surgery, the procedure and preoperative fasting: a period of 3 hours is required following clear fluids, 4 hours after breast-feeding and 6 hours after solids or cows' milk. Formal pre-assessment or preoperative investigation is not usually required. Very timid children, especially with overly anxious parents, may find the day surgery episode with all the associated unfamiliarity totally unacceptable and should be excluded. Single parents with many children and little help similarly cannot cope with a child's recovery.

The range of surgical procedures undertaken is more restrictive than in adult day surgery. Any operation with excessive postoperative pain, such as abdominal and invasive orthopaedic procedures, is contraindicated. Therefore, day surgery in children is confined to a restricted list (Box 3.6).

On the day of admission, sedative premedication is required for selected cases only, where the child is very anxious, has a needle phobia or has had a previous traumatic experience with anaesthetic induction. Oral midazolam given 30 minutes before induction in a dose of 0.5 mg/kg up to a maximum of 10 mg is usually effective, provided the standard preparation is mixed with a sweet drink to mask its bitter taste. Alternatively, rapid gas induction with sevoflurane can be used. In the anaesthetic room, venous access is obtained after the application of topical local anaesthetic 1 hour before; parental

presence in the anaesthetic room is useful, especially in the pre-school group. Postoperative pain relief is obtained first through adjunctive local or regional anaesthesia. NSAIDs cannot be given to children under 1 year of age or 10 kg in weight because of their immature kidneys but paracetamol is effective if given in a premedication dose of 20 mg/kg. Before discharge, the parents require clear instructions regarding pain control, wound care, mobilisation and resumption of normal activities.

DAY SURGERY EXPANSION

A target of 75% of all elective activity on a day case basis by 2005 may be an easily achievable goal for some units but a challenge for others, and this will partly be related to the case mix of individual units. There are several strategies that can be adopted for the further expansion of day surgery.

Preassessment Preassessment should be nurse led, and the preassessment team, rather than the surgeon, should make the final decision regarding the suitability of the patient for true day surgery, 23-hour surgery or inpatient stay. The system should implement an 'opt in' rather than an 'opt out' policy (i.e. 'Is there any reason this patient cannot be a day case?'). In many hospitals significant day surgery activity is not captured due to incorrect coding of the length of stay. If funding is dependent on day surgery performance, then the normal 5–10% coding error rate may have to be addressed.

Expand patient selection criteria Accept biological rather than chronological age and abandon formal upper age limits. Consider patients with a BMI up to 37 but with caution in laparoscopic surgery. Evaluate patients with stable ASA class III for day surgery suitability. Liaise with outreach nurses and social workers for patients with difficult social situations.

Consider alternative anaesthetic methods Local and regional anaesthetic methods reduce PONV and uncontrolled pain, which are factors contributing to unplanned overnight admissions. In many patients with major comorbidity, the use of methods other than general anaesthesia can convert the patient to day surgery. By using local and regional anaesthesia in inguinal hernia repair, 80–90% of patients can undergo day surgery.

Adopt new surgical procedures Several of the original Audit Commission 'basket' of procedures are now outpatient or office-based procedures. Varicose vein surgery in many health authorities is effectively rationed and only patients suffering from complications of varicose vein surgery such as eczema and ulceration are accepted for treatment. The introduction of new technology is often a catalyst for converting a traditional inpatient

Box 3.6 • Paediatric day surgery procedures

General surgery

Herniotomy, hydrocele excision, examination under anaesthesia, anal stretch, excision of minor lumps and bumps, ingrowing toenail treatment, endoscopy, biopsy (rectal, skin, lymph node)

Urology

Circumcision and associated procedures, orchidopexy

ENT

Myringotomy/grommets, adenoidectomy, tonsillectomy

Dental

Extractions

Ophthalmology

Correction of squint

Orthopaedic

Change of plaster cast

procedure to day case procedures. Examples include laparoscopic rather than open cholecystectomy, newer and less invasive techniques for haemorrhoidectomy and the introduction of laser technology for prostatectomy.

Organisational redesign Maximising elective surgery on a day case basis requires resolute planning of operating lists for both patients and staffing. Dedicated day lists are best allocated to morning sessions, with the more major day surgery procedures scheduled at the beginning of the list and the intermediate procedures towards the end of the list. If it is an all-day list, then intermediate procedures performed under local anaesthesia or regional block can be scheduled late in the afternoon and the patients can still return home that evening. For mixed inpatient and day surgery lists, it seems obvious to schedule day surgery procedures first on the list before the more major inpatient cases. All too often traditional surgical practice commences with the most major surgery of the day, finishing the list with the day surgery cases and risking an unplanned overnight admission. Reduction in junior doctors' hours and the resultant patterns of shift work indicate that many surgeons will be operating without a surgical trainee. Many hospitals have introduced non-medical practitioners to help with the task of assistance and they now form permanent and valuable members of the surgical team.

Lengthen the day-surgery day Increase the traditional 12-hour day to 14 or even 16 hours. This increases the time available for recovery and maximises use of theatre time even allowing day case procedures to be performed late in the afternoon. Alternatively, consider 'hotel' facilities, where the patient remains overnight but without medical or nursing supervision. This is certainly useful for patients who travel long distances or where the facilities at home are inadequate. Finally, if clinical overnight observation is required, then the day may be extended to 23 hours with the creation of an extended day surgery unit, allowing more surgical procedures to be performed on an ambulatory basis.

• Key points

- The Government has targeted 75% of all elective surgery to be performed on a day case basis by the end of 2005.
- All elective surgical patients should be preassessed by a nurse preassessment team who make the decision to allocate to 12-hour, 23-hour or inpatient surgery.
- Day surgery should be independent and separate from the inpatient infrastructure as successful day surgery depends on day of surgery admission, preassessment and nurse-led discharge.
- Regional and local anaesthetic block techniques are ideal for day surgery but are currently underutilised.
- Major surgical procedures, such as laparoscopic cholecystectomy, TURP, bilateral varicose vein surgery and arthroscopic procedures, can now be performed safely and routinely as day cases.

REFERENCES

1. Department of Health. The NHS plan: a plan for investment, a plan for reform. London: Department of Health, 2000.

2. Department of Health. Day surgery: operational guide. London: Department of Health, 2002.

   Department of Health operational guide for day surgery assists day surgery units achieve 75% elective surgery on a day case basis and covers aspects of patient selection, day surgery activity, day surgery accommodation, management and staffing.

3. Nicholl JH. The surgery of infancy. Br Med J 1909; ii:753–6.

4. Waters RM. The down-town anesthesia clinic. Am J Surg 1919; 33(Suppl.):71–3.

5. Asher RAJ. The dangers of going to bed. Br Med J 1947; ii:967–8.

6. Palumbo LT, Laul RE, Emery FB. Results of primary inguinal hernioplasty. Arch Surg 1952; 64:384–94.

7. Farquharson EL. Early ambulation with special references to herriorrhaphy as an outpatient procedure. Lancet 1955; ii:517–19.

8. Morgan M, Beech R, Reynolds A, Swan AV, Devlin HB. Surgeons' views of day surgery: is there a consensus among providers? J Public Health Med 1992; 14:192–8.

9. Royal College of Surgeons of England. Report of the working party for day case surgery. London: RCS, 1992.

10. NHS Management Executive. A study of the management and utilisation of operating departments. London: HMSO, 1989.

11. Audit Commission. A short cut to better services: day surgery in England and Wales. London: HMSO, 1990.

12. Audit Commission. Measuring quality: the patient's view of day surgery. London: HMSO, 1991.

13. NHS Management Executive. Day surgery: report by the Day Surgery Task Force. London: NHS Health Publications Unit, 1993.

14. Phillips D, Healy J, McWhinnie D et al. Extended day surgery. J One Day Surg 1999; 8:5–6.

15. Fogg KJ, Saunders PRI. Folly! The long distance day surgery patient. Ambul Surg 1995; 3:209–10.

16. National Institute of Health. Clinical guidelines on the identification, evaluation, and treatment of overweight and obesity in adults – evidence report. Obesity Res 1998; 6(Suppl. 2): 515–2095.

17. Garrow J. Gluttony. Br Med J 1996; 313:1595–6.

18. Miller JM. Selection and investigation of adult day cases. In: Miller JM, Rudkin GE, Hitchcock M (eds) Practical anaesthesia and analgesia for day surgery. Oxford: BIOS Scientific, 1997; pp. 5–16.

19. Davies KE, Houghton K, Montgomery J. Obesity and day case surgery. Anaesthesia 2001; 56: 1090–115.

   A prospective review of 258 morbidly obese day patients showed no increase in unplanned admission rates or postoperative complications, indicating that morbid obesity alone should not be an exclusion criterion for day case surgery.

20. Myles PS, Iacono GA, Hunt JO et al. Risks of respiratory complications and wound infection in patients undergoing ambulatory surgery: smokers versus non-smokers. Anesthesiology 2002; 97:842–7.

21. Buist AS, Sexton GJ, Magy JM, Ross BB. The effect of smoking cessation and modification on lung function. Am Rev Respir Dis 1976; 114:115–22.

22. Stechman MJ, Healy J, McMillan R, McWhinnie D. Is current advice on smoking prior to day surgery in the UK appropriate? J One Day Surg 2004; 14:5–8.

23. American Society of Anesthesiology. ASA classification of surgical patients. Chicago: American Society of Anesthesiology, 1991.

   A definitive classification of comorbidity by the American Society of Anesthesiology that has become universally accepted to assess fitness for anaesthesia.

24. Ansel GL, Montgomery J. Outcome of ASA III patients undergoing day case surgery. Br J Anaesth 2004; 92:71–4.

   In a retrospective case–control review of 896 ASA III patients who had undergone day case procedures there were no significant differences in unplanned admission rates, contact with health-care services or postoperative complications 24 hours after discharge between ASA III and ASA I or II patients confirming the safety of operating on ASA III patients as day cases.

25. Watson B, Smith I, Jennings A, Wilson F. Day surgery and the diabetic patient. London: British Association of Day Surgery, 2002.

26. Howell SJ, Sear JW, Foex P. Hypertension, hypertensive heart disease and perioperative cardiac risk. Br J Anaesth 2004; 92:570–83.

   A systematic review and meta-analysis of 30 observational studies demonstrated no association between admission arterial pressure when less than 180 mmHg systolic and 110 mmHg diastolic and perioperative complications. This evidence indicates that patients whose blood pressure is elevated within these limits can undergo routine safe surgery without cancellation.

27. Committee on Safety of Medicines. Avoid all NSAIDs in aspirin sensitive patients. Curr Prob Pharmacovig 1993; 19:8.

28. Carlisle J. Guidelines for pre-operative testing. J One Day Surg 2004; 14:13–16.

29. Goldberger AL, O'Konski M. Utility of routine electrocardiogram before surgery and on general hospital admission. Ann Intern Med 1986; 105:552–7.

30. Gold BS, Young ML, Kinman JL et al. The utility of preoperative electrocardiograms in the ambulatory surgical patient. Arch Intern Med 1992; 152: 301–5.

31. Aldrete BA. The Post-anaesthesia Recovery Score revisited. J Clin Anesth 1995; 7:89–91.

32. Cahill H, Jackson I, McWhinnie D. Ready to go home? London: British Association of Day Surgery, 2000; pp. 1–8.

33. Mackenzie JW. Day case anaesthesia and anxiety. Anaesthesia 1989; 44:437–40.

34. Wylie Report. Report of the Working Party on Training in Dental Anaesthesia. Br Dent J 1981; 151:385–8.

35. Bell GD, McCloy RF, Charlton JE et al. Recommendations for standards of sedation and patient monitoring during gastrointestinal endoscopy. Gut 1991; 32:823–7.

36. Watson B, Allen J, Smith I. Spinal anaesthesia: a practical guide. London: British Association of Day Surgery, 2004.

37. Yogendran S, Asokumar B, Cheng DC, Chung F. A prospective randomised double blinded study of the effect of intravenous fluid therapy on adverse outcomes on outpatient surgery. Anaesth Analg 1995; 80:682–6.

   Two hundred ASA Grade I–III ambulatory surgical patients were prospectively randomised into two groups to receive high (20 mL/kg) or low (2 mL/kg) prospective isotonic infusion over 30 minutes preoperatively. The incidence of thirst, drowsiness and dizziness was significantly lower in the high-infusion group 60 minutes after surgery, confirming an advantage to routine perioperative intravenous fluid administration.

38. Zelcer J, Wells DG. Anaesthetic related recovery room complications. Anaesth Intensive Care 1987; 15:168–74.

39. Honkavaara P, Lehtinen AM, Hovorka J et al. Nausea and vomiting after gynaecological laparoscopy depends upon the phase of the menstrual cycle. Can J Anaesth 1991; 38:876–9.

40. Seltzer MH. Partial mastectomy and limited axillary dissection performed as a same day surgical procedure in the treatment of breast cancer. Int Surg 1995; 80:79–81.

41. Jeffrey SS, Goodson WH III, Ikeda DM et al. Axillary lymphadenectomy for breast cancer without axillary drainage. Arch Surg 1995; 130:909–12.

42. Jayne DG, Botterill I, Ambrose NS et al. Randomised clinical trial of Ligasure versus conventional diathermy for day case haemorrhoidectomy. Br J Surg 2002; 89:428–32.

43. Rowsell M, Bello M, Hemingway DM. Circumferential mucosectomy (stapled haemorrhoidectomy) versus conventional haemorrhoidectomy: randomised controlled trial. Lancet 2000; 355:779–81.

44. Morinaga K, Hasuda K, Ikeda T. A novel therapy for internal haemorrhoids. Am J Gastroenterol 1995; 90:610–13.

45. Carapeti EA, Kamm M, McDonald PJ et al. Double blind randomised controlled trial of effect of metronidazole on pain after day case haemorrhoidectomy. Lancet 1998; 351:169–72.

46. Robinson TN, Biffl WL, Moore EE. Predicting failure of outpatient laparoscopic cholecystectomy. Am J Surg 2002; 184:515–18.

47. Lau H, Brookes DC. Predictive factors for unanticipated admission after ambulatory laparoscopic cholecystectomy. Arch Surg 2001; 136: 1150–3.

   Univariate and multivariate analyses of clinical variables associated with unplanned admission in a retrospective case–control series of 706 patients discharged on the day of operation after a laparoscopic cholecystectomy. Length of operation was the only independent risk factor and operative time greater than 60 minutes incurred a fourfold increased risk for unplanned admission.

48. Jackson SA, Lawrence AS, Hill JC. Does post laparoscopy pain relate to residual carbon dioxide? Anaesthesia 1996; 51:485–7.

49. Rademaker BM, Kalkman CJ, Odoom JA et al. Intraperitoneal local anaesthetics after laparoscopic cholecystectomy. Br J Anaesth 1994; 72:263–6.

50. Mjaland O, Raeder J, Aasboe V, Trondsen E, Buanes T. Outpatient laparoscopic cholecystectomy. Br J Surg 1997; 84:958–61.

51. Keoghane SR, Millar JM, Cranston DW. Is day case prostatectomy feasible? Br J Urol 1995; 76:600–3.

52. Cornford PA. Day case transurethral incision of prostate using holmium YAG laser: initial experience. Br J Urol 1997; 79:383–4.

53. Samson PS, Reyes FR, Saludares WN et al. Outpatient thyroidectomy. Am J Surg 1997; 173: 499–503.

54. Grabham JA, Raitt D, Barrie WW. Early experience with day case trans-thoracic endoscopic sympathectomy. Br J Surg 1998; 85:1266.

55. Dennis S, Georgallow M, Elcock L, Brockbank M. Day case tonsillectomy: the Salisbury experience. J One Day Surg 2004; 14:17–22.

   A prospective audit of 668 patients undergoing day case tonsillectomy indicating primary and secondary haemorrhage rates of 0.3% and 0.9% respectively, confirming the safety of day case tonsillectomy in the UK.

56. Natof HE. Complications. In: Wetcher BV (ed.) Anaesthesia for ambulatory surgery. Philadelphia: Lippincott, 1985; p. 321.

57. Hitchcock M. Postoperative morbidity following day surgery. In: Millar JM, Rudkin GE, Hitchcock M (eds) Practical anaesthesia and analgesia for day surgery. Oxford: BIOS Scientific, 1997; pp. 205–11.

58. Levy ML. Complications: prevention and quality assurance. Anesth Clin North Am 1987; 5:137–66.

59. Twersky RS, Abiona M, Thorne AC et al. Admissions following ambulatory surgery: outcome in seven urban hospitals. Ambul Surg 1995; 3:141–6.

60. Carrol NV, Miederhoff P, Cox FM et al. Postoperative nausea and vomiting after discharge from

outpatient surgery centres. Anesth Analg 1995; 80:903–9.

61. Thornes R. Just for the day. London: National Association for the Welfare of Children in Hospital, March 1991.

62. McEwan AI, Birch M, Bingham R. The pre-operative management of the child with a heart murmur. Paediatr Anaesth 1995; 5:151–5.

63. Steward DJ. Preterm infants are more prone to complications following minor surgery than are term infants. Anesthesiology 1982; 56:304–6.

David H. Bennett

INTRODUCTION

A hernia may be defined as a protrusion of a viscus or part of a viscus through an abnormal opening in the walls of its containing cavity. The anterior abdominal wall can be divided into two structural/functional zones: the upper 'parachute area' aiding respiratory movement and a lower 'belly support' area.[1] Functional failure in the abdomen may lead to epigastric and umbilical hernia in the upper zone and to inguinal and femoral hernia in the lower zone. The external abdominal hernia is the commonest form of hernia, the most frequent varieties being the inguinal (75%), femoral (8.5%) and umbilical (15%).

Hernias may be described as reducible, incarcerated or strangulated. A reducible hernia is one in which the contents of the hernial sac can be manually introduced back into the abdomen while, conversely, an irreducible or incarcerated hernia cannot be manipulated back into the abdomen. A strangulated hernia occurs when the vascular supply to the bowel contained within the hernia is compromised, resulting in ischaemic and gangrenous bowel. Multiple factors contribute to the development of hernias, the commonest of which are shown in **Box 4.1**.

EPIGASTRIC HERNIA

An epigastric hernia may be defined as a fascial defect in the linea alba between the xiphoid process and the umbilicus. The true incidence is unknown but autopsy studies have suggested a prevalence of 0.5–10% in the general population. There is a male preponderance, with a male to female ratio of approximately 4:1. Infant and child epigastric hernias are very rare, the diagnosis usually being made in the third to fifth decades.

Aetiology

The aetiology is related to the functional anatomy of the 'parachute area'. The anterior abdominal wall aponeurosis consists of tendinous fibres that lie obliquely in aponeurotic sheets, allowing for changes in the shape of the abdominal wall, for example during respiration. However, the midline can change only in length and breadth, an increase in one necessitating a decrease in the other. During abdominal distension, the linea alba must increase in both dimensions, the resulting tearing of fibres possibly resulting in the development of an epigastric hernia.

Clinical presentation

The majority of epigastric hernias (75%) are asymptomatic.[2] Typical symptoms, if present, include vague upper abdominal pain and nausea associated with epigastric tenderness. The symptoms tend to be more severe when the patient is lying down, attributed to traction on the hernial contents. Pain on exertion localised to the epigastrium is also a common symptom. Incarceration is common, while strangulation of preperitoneal fat or omentum results in localised pain and tenderness. Incarceration or strangulation of intra-abdominal

From Mensching JJ, Musielewicz AJ. Abdominal wall hernias. Emerg Med Clin North Am 1996; 14:739–56, with permission.

Box 4.1 • Predisposing factors for abdominal wall hernias

Congenital anomalies
Fetal hydrops
Ambiguous genitalia
Hypospadias
Epispadias
Extrophy of the bladder
Cryptorchid testis
Circumstances surrounding birth
Prematurity
Low birth weight
Meconium peritonitis
Hereditary disorders
Mucopolysaccharidoses
Cystic fibrosis
Connective tissue disorders
Hunter–Hurler syndrome
Ehlers–Danlos syndrome
Increased abdominal pressure
Liver disease with ascites
Ventriculoperitoneal shunts
Continuous ambulatory peritoneal dialysis
Chylous ascites

viscera is extremely rare, symptoms depending on the incarcerated organ.

The presence of a midline mass on physical examination usually confirms the diagnosis. In obese patients, palpation of the mass may be difficult and confirmation of the diagnosis by ultrasound or computed tomography may be helpful.[3]

Management

Epigastric hernias are rare in infants and children and there is some evidence that asymptomatic hernias in children under the age of 10 years resolve spontaneously.[4] The decision for surgical intervention depends on the presence and severity of symptoms. An operation offers the only chance of permanent cure of these defects in adults.

Small solitary defects may be approached with either a vertical or transverse incision in the midline, centred over the hernia. For larger hernias, if the defects are multiple or in the emergency setting when a strangulated viscus is suspected, a vertical incision is preferred. The hernia and its contents are dissected free of the surrounding tissues and, if present, the hernial contents examined and dealt with appropriately. If the defect is small (<2 cm), repair by primary suture closure with non-absorbable sutures is sufficient. The orientation of the suture closure remains controversial, some surgeons preferring a vertical closure while others a horizontal orientation. There are very few data to support one technique over the other and probably the direction resulting in the least tension is the most appropriate. If the defect is large (>4 cm), the hernia should be repaired with prosthetic mesh. This technique is described later in the chapter when considering incisional hernias. The technique applied to intermediate-sized hernias is controversial and either technique is currently deemed acceptable. Laparoscopic repair of epigastric hernias[5] was first described in 1992 and the technique has grown in popularity over the last 12 years. Several comparative studies are now available, which support the assertions that the technique offers shorter hospital stays, improved patient outcomes and fewer complications than traditional techniques.[6–10]

Complications

Complication rates are low and most are the usual complications associated with abdominal wall incisions (haematoma, infection). There are very few data on recurrence rates, historical series reporting rates between 7%[11] and 9.4%.[12] In perhaps 50% of patients, however, the recurrence actually represents the persistence of a second hernia or area of weakness overlooked at the initial procedure. The laparoscopic technique avoids this problem because all fascial defects are visible laparoscopically.

UMBILICAL AND PARAUMBILICAL HERNIAS

There are several distinct types of hernia that occur around the umbilicus: congenital (omphalocele), infantile, paraumbilical and adult umbilical hernias.

Congenital umbilical hernias

A congenital umbilical hernia occurs when the abdominal viscera herniate into the tissue of the umbilical cord. Normally, the gut returns to the abdominal cavity at 10 weeks of gestation. If this fails to occur, normal rotation and fixation of the intestine is prevented, the umbilicus is absent and a funnel-shaped defect in the abdominal wall is present through which viscera protrude into the umbilical cord. The abdominal wall defect may vary in size from no larger than an umbilical stump to a defect that appears to involve the entire abdominal wall. Defects less than 5 cm usually contain gut only, whereas defects greater than 5 cm usually contain liver and other viscera. Congenital umbilical hernia occurs in 1 in 5000 births and is associated with other serious congenital anomalies.

CLINICAL PRESENTATION

Clinically, congenital umbilical hernia may be diagnosed in utero or at birth. On ultrasound examination, fetal abdominal wall defects are not subtle and may be visualized as early as 15 weeks of gestation, appearing as fluid-filled loops of intestine contained in a smooth sac anterior to the normal fetal abdominal wall. The management is surgical correction and one of the most important contributors to the morbidity and mortality of isolated abdominal wall defects is the delay between delivery and appropriate surgical repair. Antenatal knowledge of the existence of a congenital hernia can allow for the birth of the child at a tertiary care institution with the appropriate neonatal and paediatric surgical expertise.[13] The method of birth is still contentious. In giant omphaloceles, in which dystocia or rupture may occur at the time of vaginal delivery, caesarean section may be advantageous. The superiority of the routine use of caesarean section in smaller defects has not been proven.[14]

MANAGEMENT

Surgical correction should only be undertaken in specialised centres. If the diagnosis is made prenatally, the mother should be transferred to such a centre for delivery. If the diagnosis only becomes apparent at birth, the baby should be kept warm and hydrated, and the sac handled with care to avoid rupture or twisting of the sac. The sac should be wrapped in moist sterile gauze and covered with impervious plastic sheeting or aluminium foil. Mother and baby should then be transferred as soon as feasible to a tertiary centre for further management.

Infantile umbilical hernias

Infantile umbilical hernias occur when the umbilical vessels fail to fuse with the urachal remnant and umbilical ring. It presents with a protrusion of the umbilicus, usually at the superior margin of the ring. The infantile hernia, as opposed to the congenital type, is always covered by skin. It is the third most common surgical disorder in children, occurring in approximately one in five live births. The incidence in black and Asian infants is up to eight times higher than in Caucasian infants and there is a 9–12% familial predisposition, although no genetic pattern of inheritance has been identified.

CLINICAL PRESENTATION

Clinically, the commonest presenting 'symptom' is the cosmetic appearance, the hernia resulting in a cone-like protrusion of the umbilicus that bulges every time the child cries or strains. Infantile umbilical hernias rarely enlarge over time and 90% disappear by the time the child is 2 years of age. Several authors have reported failure of hernias to close spontaneously if they persist to the age of 5 years.[15-17] Spontaneous resolution of umbilical hernias appears to be directly influenced by the size of the umbilical ring. If, at the age of 3 months, the hernia has a fascial ring of <0.5 cm, 96% heal spontaneously within 2 years. Defects that have a fascial diameter >1.5 cm are unlikely to heal spontaneously. Complications of umbilical hernias are rare, occurring in approximately 5–7%,[18,19] and include strangulation of the omentum, strangulation of the intestine and evisceration.

MANAGEMENT

Management of the infant with an umbilical hernia is expectant. The majority will resolve spontaneously without surgical correction. The indications for surgery in children less than 2 years of age are the development of complications or tenderness over the site of the hernia. There is no consensus on the appropriate timing of herniorrhaphy in older children. In the USA, most paediatric surgeons delay repair until the age of 4 years,[20] while in the UK the British Association of Paediatric Surgeons has no set protocol. Generally repair is performed before school/nursery to avoid the child becoming self-conscious of the umbilical protrusion.

Elective repair of infantile umbilical hernia is performed on an outpatient basis under general anaesthesia. A curvilinear incision is made within a skin fold on the inferior aspect of the hernia. The sac is then encircled by blunt dissection. If there is any concern regarding the contents of the sac, the sac should be opened on its caudal aspect, as abdominal contents usually adhere to the fundus of the sac, and the contents inspected. Once dealt with appropriately, the contents should be reduced and the incision continued to the cephalic aspect of the sac. If the sac is empty, the fundus may simply be disconnected from the umbilicus and reduced intact. Repair is by simple fascial apposition using horizontal mattress sutures of absorbable material. While the Mayo ('vest-over-pants') technique of umbilical hernioplasty is frequently taught, there is no evidence that the results are any better than simple apposition of the fascial edges. The umbilicus is refashioned by leaving a small button of the fundus of the sac attached to the inner surface of the cicatrix and tacking it down to the area of fascial repair. Haemostasis must be meticulous. Skin closure is by subcuticular absorbable suture.

COMPLICATIONS

Complications of umbilical hernioplasty are rare, but include seroma or haematoma formation and infection. Recurrence is possible if large defects are closed under tension or if an associated paraumbilical hernia is overlooked.

Paraumbilical hernias

Paraumbilical hernias are acquired hernias and occur in all age groups. They occur secondary to disruption of the linea alba and generally occur above the umbilical cicatrix. Aetiological factors (see **Box 4.1**) include stretching of the abdominal wall by obesity, multiple pregnancy and ascites. Paraumbilical hernias are more common in patients over the age of 35 years and are five times more common in females.

CLINICAL PRESENTATION

Clinically, paraumbilical hernias are frequently symptomatic. Patients complain of intermittent abdominal pain (possibly caused by dragging on the fat and peritoneum of the falciform ligament) and, when the hernial sac contains bowel, colic resulting from intermittent intestinal obstruction. The hernia tends to progress over time and intertrigo and necrosis of the skin may occur in patients with large dependent hernias.

It is important to distinguish paraumbilical hernias from umbilical defects as the latter may resolve spontaneously in the young, whereas the former require surgical correction. Umbilical hernias classically produce a symmetric bulge with the protrusion directly under the umbilicus. This is in contrast to paraumbilical hernias where about half the fundus of the sac is covered by the umbilicus and the remainder is covered by the skin of the abdomen directly above or below the umbilicus. Paraumbilical hernias do not resolve spontaneously and have a high incidence of incarceration and strangulation; therefore, surgical repair is always indicated.

MANAGEMENT

For solitary hernias separated from the umbilicus, a transverse incision over the hernia produces the best exposure. In patients with a paraumbilical and umbilical hernia, a midline incision may provide better access. Similarly, if multiple fascial defects are present or there is concern about the integrity of

visceral contents of the sac, a vertical incision may be better employed. If the defect simply contains preperitoneal fat, this may be reduced. In patients with strangulated or infected preperitoneal fat, it is best excised. If there is a sac present, it should be dissected free from the fascial edges, opened and the contents examined. Once the contents have been dealt with appropriately, they may be reduced and redundant sac excised. There is no requirement to close the peritoneum but some authors recommend transfixing the neck of the sac once the contents have been reduced. Repair is performed by fascial apposition either transversely or longitudinally, depending on the defect and the direction of least tension. As this is an acquired defect, non-absorbable sutures or sutures with a long half-life, such as PDS, are recommended.

Adult umbilical hernias

Umbilical hernias in adults represent a spectrum of conditions from the partially unfolded cicatrix to huge dependent sacs. The umbilicus may become partially unfolded in patients with acute abdominal distension. Persistent elevation of intra-abdominal pressure eventually results in the umbilical cicatrix giving way and the development of an umbilical hernia. Although uncommon, causes include ascites from cirrhosis, congestive cardiac failure or nephrosis. Patients undergoing peritoneal dialysis also have a high incidence of these hernias. Management should be conservative, as the majority of these patients have serious underlying pathology. Operative repair is not indicated unless the hernia incarcerates or becomes extremely large and the overlying skin is thinned down to such an extent that spontaneous rupture is possible.

Umbilical hernias in adults do not represent persistence of infantile hernias but are indirect herniations through an umbilical canal, which is bordered by umbilical fascia posteriorly, the linea alba anteriorly and the medial edges of the two rectus sheaths on each side. They have a tendency to incarcerate and strangulate and do not resolve spontaneously. Umbilical hernias in adults have a high morbidity and mortality. Over 90% occur in females and almost all patients are obese and multiparous.

CLINICAL PRESENTATION

Clinically, the diagnosis is usually obvious. The hernias are usually large and complete reduction is not possible because of the adherence of omentum to the fundus of the sac. The hernia is usually painful because, as it enlarges, it has a tendency to sag downwards, causing traction on the stomach and transverse colon. Attacks of intermittent colicky pain may be caused by episodes of incomplete intestinal obstruction. Treatment should be conservative for as long as possible, but these patients often have incarcerated hernias and surgical intervention inevitably becomes necessary.

MANAGEMENT

Umbilical hernias in high-risk adult patients are generally operated on using regional or local anaesthesia. In smaller umbilical hernias, a subumbilical incision may be used, but with large hernias, and particularly incarcerated hernias, a large midline incision may be necessary. The sac is isolated and the entire mass of fat and sac elevated while the neck of the sac is incised. The incarcerated contents must be evaluated and treated as required. The sac is frequently loculated and Richter-type hernias may occur within one or more of the loculi. After the contents are dealt with, the peritoneal sac is repaired and an edge-to-edge fascial closure performed in the direction of least tension, which may be either transverse or vertical. For small hernias (<2 cm in diameter), primary edge-to-edge apposition with non-absorbable sutures of appropriate size is sufficient. The classic Mayo approach[21] was to overlap the edges, but it has been demonstrated that the bursting strength of the wound was not improved by imbrication and was actually impaired to a degree proportional to the amount of overlapping and tension.[22] In larger hernias (>4 cm diameter), it is important to obtain closure without tension. If the fascial edges can be brought together with ease, the repair is reinforced with prosthetic mesh placed extraperitoneally and retromuscularly, behind the rectus muscle (anterior to the posterior rectus sheath). If the fascial edges cannot be apposed easily, mobilisation of the lateral abdominal muscles and skin flaps will be required before placement of mesh in the extraperitoneal retromuscular space. Only rarely, when the defect cannot be closed, should a mesh be placed to bridge the defect in the extraperitoneal space, with an overlap of the fascial edges of at least 5 cm. The mesh should be secured with interrupted non-absorbable sutures.

The overlying umbilical skin need not be excised unless it is macerated or infected, although the cosmetic appearance is often enhanced by judicious removal of excess skin and subcutaneous fat. All patients should be warned that it might be necessary to excise the umbilicus. If a new umbilicus is to be created, care should be taken, as recurrences may occur at the point on the linea alba where the new umbilicus is fixed to the fascia.

COMPLICATIONS

Complications include the development of seromas, haematomas and infection. Sealed suction drains may be employed in the retromuscular and subcutaneous planes to avoid the development of large seromas. In addition to local problems, these patients often have respiratory and cardiovascular complications and may require prolonged hospitalisation.

INGUINAL HERNIAS

Anatomy

The anatomy of the inguinal region is complex. The inguinal canal is approximately 4 cm in length and is located just above the inguinal ligament between the internal and external rings. The inguinal canal allows passage of the spermatic cord into the scrotum, along with the testicular, deferential and cremasteric vessels. The superficial ring is a triangular aperture in the aponeurosis of the external oblique and lies 1.25 cm above the pubic tubercle. The ring is bounded by a superomedial and an inferolateral crus joined by the criss-cross intercrural fibres. Normally, the ring will not admit the tip of the little finger. The deep ring is a U-shaped condensation of the transversalis fascia and it lies 1.25 cm above the inguinal (Poupart's) ligament, midway between the pubic tubercle and the anterior superior iliac spine. The transversalis fascia is the fascial envelope of the abdomen and the competency of the deep inguinal ring depends on the integrity of this fascia.

The anterior boundary of the inguinal canal comprises mainly the external oblique aponeurosis with the conjoined muscle laterally. The posterior boundary is formed by the fascia transversalis and the conjoined tendon (internal oblique and transversus abdominus medially). The inferior epigastric vessels lie posteriorly and medially to the deep inguinal ring. The superior boundary is formed by the conjoined muscles (internal oblique and transversus) and the inferior boundary by the inguinal ligament.

Definition

An indirect hernia travels down the canal on the outer (lateral and anterior) side of the spermatic cord. A direct inguinal hernia comes out directly forwards through the posterior wall of the inguinal canal. While the neck of an indirect hernia is lateral to the epigastric vessels, the direct hernia usually emerges medial to these vessels, except in the saddle-bag or pantaloon type, which has both a lateral and a medial component.

Inguinal hernia in infants and children (see also Chapter 12)

Repair of congenital inguinal hernia is the most frequently performed operation in the paediatric age group. Although inguinal hernias can present at any age, the peak incidence is during infancy and childhood. About 3–5% of full-term infants may be born with a clinical inguinal hernia.[23,24] Between 80 and 90% of paediatric hernias occur in boys, about one-third of the hernias presenting in the first 6 months of life. Congenital inguinal hernias present more commonly on the right side (55–60%), while 15% have a bilateral presentation.

CLINICAL PRESENTATION

Examination of the inguinal area for a hernia may show an obvious bulge at the site of the external ring or within the scrotum. This bulge can often be gently reduced. However, the bulge may only be seen during severe straining, such as with crying or defecation. If the infant is old enough to stand, he or she should be examined in both the supine and standing positions. If not, the parent can hold the infant upright so that the surgeon can closely observe the inguinoscrotal area.

Before an examination for an inguinal hernia, it is essential to make sure that the testis is within the scrotal sac to avoid mistaking a retractile testis for a hernial bulge. The presence of an empty scrotum should alert the examining surgeon to a possible undescended or ectopic testis, which is associated with an inguinal hernia more than 90% of the time. Although routine orchidopexy is usually delayed until the child is 1 year of age, a coexisting symptomatic hernia should be promptly repaired and orchidopexy accomplished at the same time.

Inguinal hernias are prone to incarcerate, the overall rate being 12%.[25] Incarceration is most common in the first 6 months of life, when more than half of instances are observed. The incidence of incarceration is higher in females as is the frequency of emergency operation. An incarcerated hernia usually presents as an acute tender mass in the inguinal canal. The mass may protrude beyond the external inguinal ring or into the scrotum. The skin over the mass may be discoloured, oedematous, erythematous or blue. Inability to reduce the mass may result in strangulation, characterised by abdominal distension, vomiting, failure to pass faecal material, tachycardia and radiological evidence of small bowel obstruction. These findings all suggest emergency operative intervention for relief of obstruction, intestinal salvage and hernia repair.

MANAGEMENT

In most instances (80%), incarcerated hernias in children may be managed initially by conservative measures. In patients with incarceration of short duration and no evidence of toxicity, conservative measures may be employed. These include sedation, using a cold pack and, when the baby is quiet,

gentle manipulation of the involved hernia. Exploration may be safely delayed for about 4–6 hours; however, if the hernia remains irreducible at this stage, emergency repair is indicated. The complication rate is approximately 20 times greater after emergency repair for incarcerated hernia than after elective procedures.[25] It is therefore worthwhile to reduce the hernia whenever possible and perform an elective procedure within 24–48 hours of the reduction.

The high risk of incarceration in the paediatric age group makes the presence of an inguinal hernia an indication for surgical repair. The procedure is performed as a day case, reducing the child's psychological trauma by avoiding hospitalisation, limiting family separation and reducing the incidence of cross-infection. In addition to the standard surgical preparation, special precautions should be made for young infants, including the wrapping of the extremities in bubble-wrap or Webril, positioning the child on a warming pad and the use of an overhead heater. Surgical access is achieved through a short (3 cm) transverse incision in the lowest inguinal skin crease. The superficial fascia (Scarpa's fascia) is incised and the external oblique fascia identified. The aponeurosis is traced laterally to identify the inguinal ligament and the exact location of the external inguinal ring identified. Although some surgeons advocate repair through the external ring (Mitchell Banks technique[26]), an alternative approach is to incise the external oblique fascia in the long axis of its fibres, perpendicular to the external inguinal ring. This exposes the cremasteric muscle and fascia, which envelop the cord structures.

The hernial sac is always located in an anteromedial position in relation to the cord and gentle blunt dissection of the cremasteric fibres usually brings the sac into view. The sac is elevated with a haemostat and the cremasteric fibres carefully freed from the anterior and lateral aspects. Retraction of the sac medially allows identification of the spermatic vessels and vas deferens and these structures may be carefully teased away from the sac in a posterolateral direction. If the layers are adherent, injection of 1–2 mL of saline into the cord may help to define the planes of separation. The vas itself should not be grasped and the floor of the canal not disturbed. Once the end of the sac has been freed, the dissection of the sac is carried superiorly to the level of the deep inguinal ring. If the sac extends down into the scrotum, it may be divided once the cord structures are identified and protected. The base of the sac may then be gently twisted to reduce any fluid or viscera into the peritoneal cavity.

The base of the sac should be suture ligated with 3–0 or 4–0 absorbable suture and, once the suture is cut, the peritoneal stump should retract proximally through the deep inguinal ring. Free ties should not be used because of the risk of them becoming dislodged if abdominal distension occurs. If it is excessively large, the deep inguinal ring should be 'snugged' with an interrupted 3–0 vicryl suture that approximates the transversalis fascia inferior to the cord structures. Closing the ring too tightly, however, may result in vascular compression of the cord and severe swelling. Absolute haemostasis is essential to prevent postoperative haematoma formation. The position of the testis within the scrotum should be confirmed to avoid iatrogenic entrapment within the inguinal canal. Wound closure is accomplished in layers.

There is no role for laparoscopic hernia repair in infants and young children. It may have a role to play in adolescents with recurrent hernia in whom a preperitoneal procedure requiring mesh insertion is anticipated. It also enables examination of the contralateral side.

An emergency operation is required for patients with an incarcerated hernia, with toxicity and obvious intestinal obstruction or after failed attempts at reduction. Infants and children with incarcerated hernias should be given antibiotics preoperatively. A nasogastric tube is inserted and intravenous volume replacement initiated with 20 mL/kg Hartmann's solution. The operation begins with preparation of the whole abdomen in case laparotomy is required. An inguinal incision is utilized and the incarcerated intestine must be carefully inspected for viability once the obstruction at the internal ring is relieved. A rapid return of pink colour, sheen, peristalsis and palpable or visible pulsations at the mesenteric border should be observed. If there is any question regarding intestinal viability, resection and anastomosis should be carried out and hernial repair accomplished.

In certain circumstances, the incarcerated intestine may reduce during surgical manipulation, before the intestine has been visualized. The incarcerated segment of bowel should be retrieved and inspected. If this is not possible, a counter-incision should be made and a formal laparotomy performed to assess intestinal viability more accurately. An operation for incarcerated hernia may be difficult because of oedema, tissue friability and the presence of the mass, which may obscure the anatomy. The gonad should be carefully inspected because it may become infarcted by vascular compression caused by the incarcerated intestine. The undescended testis is more vulnerable to this complication in the presence of incarcerated intestine.

COMPLICATIONS

Complications may be divided into intraoperative and postoperative categories. Intraoperative complications include division of the ilioinguinal nerve, which can be avoided if the external oblique fascia is elevated before incision; division of the vas deferens, which should be repaired with interrupted 7–0 monofilament sutures; and bleeding, which is usually secondary to needle-hole injury and can usually be controlled with withdrawal of the suture and the application of pressure.

Postoperative complications include wound infection, scrotal haematoma, postoperative hydroceles and recurrence. The wound infection rate is low (1–2%) and recurrence rates of less than 1% are reported;[27] 80% of recurrences are noted within the first postoperative year. The major causes of recurrence in infants and children include (i) a missed hernial sac or an unrecognised tear in the peritoneum; (ii) a broken suture ligature at the neck of the sac; (iii) failure to repair a large internal inguinal ring; (iv) injury to the floor of the inguinal canal, resulting in the development of a direct inguinal hernia; (v) severe infection in the inguinal canal; and (vi) increased intra-abdominal pressure, as is noted in patients with ascites after ventriculoperitoneal shunts, in children with cystic fibrosis, after previous operation for incarceration and in patients with connective tissue disorders. Reoperations for recurrent inguinal hernia may be a technical challenge and a preperitoneal approach is an extremely useful alternative for recurrent hernias.

Adult inguinal hernias

Inguinal hernias are more frequent in males, with a male to female ratio of 10 or 12:1. The peak incidence is in the sixth decade and 65% are indirect in type. Right-sided inguinal hernias are slightly more common than left-sided, 55% occurring on the right. Bilateral hernias are four times more common in direct than indirect forms.

AETIOLOGY

The pathogenesis of groin hernias is multifactorial. It was initially believed that persistence of a patent processus vaginalis into adult life was the predisposing factor for inguinal hernia formation. However, postmortem studies have shown that 15–30% of adult males without a clinically apparent inguinal hernia have a patent processus vaginalis.[28] Similarly, review of the contralateral side in infantile inguinal hernias reveals a patent processus vaginalis in 60% of neonates and a contralateral hernia in 10–20%. During 20 years of follow-up after infantile hernia repair, only 22% of men will develop a contralateral hernia.

It is therefore apparent that the problem of indirect inguinal hernia is not simply one of a congenital defect. The high frequency of indirect inguinal hernia in middle-aged and older people suggests a pathological change in connective tissue of the abdominal wall to be a contributory factor.

There is now extensive experimental evidence to support collagen derangement as an aetiological factor in inguinal hernia development.[29–31]

MANAGEMENT

The essential goal of hernia repair is to restore the functional integrity of the laminar musculo-aponeurotic structure of the groin region and the musculo-aponeurotic fenestration, which allows the vessels to the genitalia to penetrate this structure. It is beyond the scope of this chapter to review the history of the various repair techniques that have been previously employed and are now mainly historical. **Figure 4.1** illustrates how the popularity of the various techniques has changed and only the latest techniques (i.e. prosthetic repairs) will be considered here.

Tension-free prosthetic mesh repair

Lichtenstein first described the technique of tension-free repair of groin hernia, which now bears his name.[32] Tension-free repair of primary groin hernias may be performed as an outpatient procedure under local anaesthesia. Field-block injections are unnecessary, while epidural anaesthesia is only required in exceptional circumstances, such as extreme obesity, simultaneous bilateral hernioplasty and large irreducible scrotal hernias. General anaesthesia may be reserved for hernias with suspected bowel incarceration and when it is decided, at the time of operation, to revert to an open preperitoneal approach.

Operative details Once the local anaesthesia has been administered, a groin-crease incision is made and a window established through the subcutaneous tissues at the lateral end of the wound, exposing the external oblique aponeurosis. The window is increased in size to expose the medial end of the external oblique aponeurosis, the inguinal ligament and the superficial ring. A small incision is made in the external oblique along the line of the fibres, approximately 1 cm above the inguinal ligament. The edges are carefully lifted with haemostats to avoid damage to the ilioinguinal nerve. The external oblique aponeurosis is then opened along a line from the incision to the superficial ring and the contents of the inguinal canal gently separated from it. The spermatic cord is mobilised utilising the avascular space between the pubic tubercle and the cord itself to avoid damage to the floor of the canal, injury to the testicular blood flow and crushing of the genital nerve, which always lies in juxtaposition to the external spermatic vessels.

In order to thin out the spermatic cord and remove any lipoma present (**Fig. 4.2**), the cremaster fibres are incised longitudinally at the level of the deep ring. Complete excision of the cremaster fibres from the spermatic cord is unnecessary and may result in damage to the vas deferens, increasing the likelihood of postoperative neuralgia and ischaemic orchitis. Indirect hernial sacs are opened and digital exploration performed to detect any other defects or the presence of a femoral hernia. Lichtenstein states that the sac may be simply inverted into the abdomen without excision, suture or ligation, which he feels is unnecessary and may contribute to postoperative discomfort.[32] However, it is the author's practice to suture ligate any but the smallest hernial sacs at the level of the deep ring and excise any redundant peritoneum. To prevent postoperative hydrocele formation, complete scrotal sacs are transected at the midpoint of the canal, with the distal section left in place.

In the event of a large direct hernia, the sac is invaginated with an imbricating suture to achieve a flat surface over which to lay the prosthetic mesh.

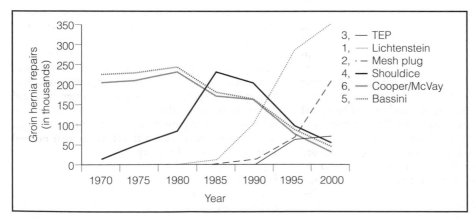

Figure 4.1 • Popularity of techniques of herniorrhaphy since the 1970s. 1, Lichtenstein; 2, mesh plug; 3, transoesophageal procedure (TEP); 4, Shouldice; 5, Bassini; 6, Cooper/McVay. With permission from Rutkow IM. Epidemiologic, economic, and sociologic aspects of hernia surgery in the United States in the 1990s. Surg Clin North Am 1998; 78:941.

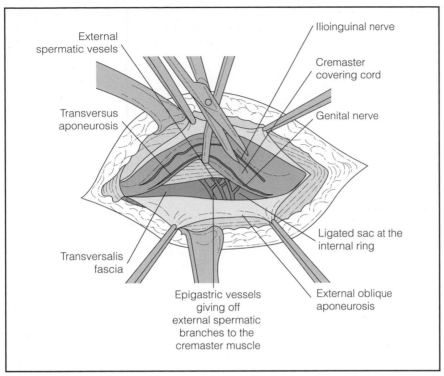

External
spermatic vessels

Ilioinguinal nerve

Cremaster
covering cord

Transversus
aponeurosis

Genital nerve

Transversalis
fascia

Ligated sac at the
internal ring

Epigastric vessels
giving off
external spermatic
branches to the
cremaster muscle

External oblique
aponeurosis

Figure 4.2 • Elevation of cord. With permission from Lichtenstein IL, Shulman AG, Amid PK. The tension-free repair of groin hernias. In: Nyhus LM, Condon RE (eds) Hernia. Philadelphia: JB Lippincott, 1995; 237–49.

The external oblique aponeurosis is separated from the underlying internal oblique muscle at a point high enough to accommodate a mesh measuring 15 × 10 cm.

A sheet of polypropylene mesh is trimmed as appropriate so that the patch overlaps the internal oblique muscle and aponeurosis by at least 2 cm above the border of the Hesselbach triangle. The medial portion of the mesh is rounded to the shape of the medial corner of the inguinal canal. The mesh is sutured to the aponeurotic tissue over the pubic bone, overlapping the bone to prevent any tension or weakness at this critical point, but ensuring the periosteum is not caught in the suture. The same suture is continued along the lower edge, attaching the mesh to the shelving portion of the inguinal ligament to a point just lateral to the deep ring with a continuous suture (**Fig. 4.3a**).

A slit is made at the lateral end of the mesh, creating a wider tail above the cord and a narrower one below the cord. This manoeuvre positions the cord between the two tails of the mesh and avoids the keyhole opening, which is less effective and results in an occasional reported recurrence. The upper edge of the patch is sutured to the internal oblique aponeurosis using a few interrupted sutures. Sharp retraction of the upper leaf of the external

oblique aponeurosis from the internal oblique muscle is important because it provides the appropriate amount of laxity for the patch. When the retraction is released, a true tension-free repair is taken up when the patient strains on command during the operation or resumes an upright position afterwards. Using a single non-absorbable monofilament suture, the lower edges of the two tails are fixed to the shelving margin of the inguinal ligament just lateral to the completion knot of the lower continuous suture. This creates a new deep ring of mesh (**Fig. 4.3b**).

The excess patch is trimmed on the lateral side, leaving 3–4 cm beyond the deep ring. This is tucked underneath the external oblique aponeurosis and the external oblique aponeurosis closed with a continuous suture. Unrestricted activity is encouraged and patients are expected to return to their normal activity 2–7 days after surgery.

Laparoscopic repair

The alternative to an open operation is a laparoscopic approach. Ger is credited with the first laparoscopic approach to hernia, repairing indirect hernias with a stapling instrument developed for this purpose.[33,34] In parallel, Gazayerli described a suture repair technique through a transabdominal

(a)

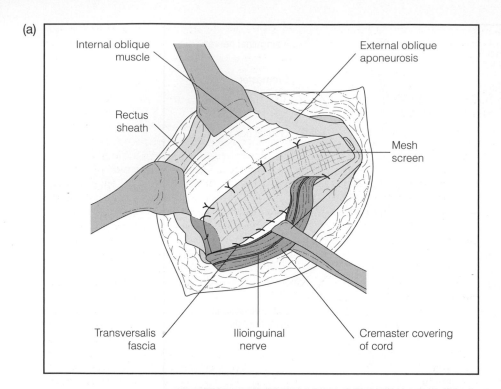

Internal oblique muscle

External oblique aponeurosis

Rectus sheath

Mesh screen

Transversalis fascia

Ilioinguinal nerve

Cremaster covering of cord

(b)

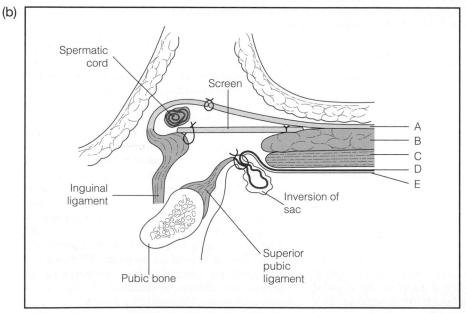

Spermatic cord

Screen

A
B
C
D
E

Inguinal ligament

Inversion of sac

Pubic bone

Superior pubic ligament

Figure 4.3 • Use of a prosthetic mesh. **(a)** The mesh sutured in place. **(b)** The implanted mesh in parasagittal section: A, external oblique aponeurosis; B, internal oblique muscle; C, transverse muscle and aponeurosis; D, transversalis fascia; E, peritoneum. With permission from Lichtenstein IL, Shulman AG, Amid PK. The tension-free repair of groin hernias. In: Nyhus LM, Condon RE (eds) Hernia. Philadelphia: JB Lippincott, 1995; 237–49.

approach, approximating the transversus abdominis aponeurotic arch and the iliopubic tract.[35] After the repair is completed, the peritoneum is reapproximated. Since the early 1990s, laparoscopic hernia repair has evolved from simple closure of a small indirect hernia, through the placement of mesh plugs and a small mesh patch over the internal ring, to the current use of large pieces of prosthetic mesh to reinforce the lower abdominal wall.

The rationale for the use of large mesh sheets placed into the preperitoneal space was based on the surgical experience of the open preperitoneal hernia repair, especially in the treatment of recurrent hernias[36,37] Although a variety of laparoscopic repairs have been described, they can be categorized in general according to the approach used to expose the defect. Three exposures are used: the intraperitoneal approach, in which the prosthesis is placed as an onlay graft over the peritoneum; the transabdominal preperitoneal prosthetic (TAPP) repair; and the totally extraperitoneal prosthetic (TEP) repair.

Intraperitoneal repair In the intraperitoneal repair with an onlay graft, the prosthesis is placed within the peritoneal cavity. The technique is well described by Toy and Smoot.[38] Compared to the TAPP and TEP approaches, it has the advantages of being less time-consuming to perform and requires less dissection of the preperitoneal space. It has the disadvantage of leaving the prosthetic material exposed within the peritoneal cavity and has a higher recurrence rate (**Table 4.1**).

Transabdominal preperitoneal prosthetic repair The TAPP repair is one of the most popular approaches used for laparoscopic herniorrhaphy, particularly in Europe. The abdomen is insufflated with carbon dioxide and the laparoscope introduced through an umbilical incision. Two accessory trocars are used to provide access for the dissecting instruments and the stapler. After both groins have been inspected, making a second incision in the pelvic peritoneum several centimetres above the hernia defect and peeling the peritoneum away exposes the hernia defect. The peritoneum is dissected bluntly away from the abdominal wall, allowing the hernia sac to be inverted and dissected free of adherent tissue. Preperitoneal fat is removed to allow identification of the transversus abdominis arch, the pubic tubercle, the iliopubic tract and the Cooper ligament. A prosthetic mesh of approximately 10 × 12 cm is inserted and fixed in place with staples or sutures so that it covers the entire myopectineal orifice. The peritoneum is closed over the mesh with staples or sutures. This approach has the advantage of permitting inspection of the abdomen in general, and of the opposite side in particular, enabling bilateral repairs to be performed if necessary. In addition, exposure is usually excellent. The disadvantage is that a wider dissection is required to accommodate the mesh than is used in the intraperitoneal onlay procedure. In addition, the intra-abdominal incision presents the possibility of injury to intraperitoneal structures and a second peritoneal incision in the groin increases the potential for adhesion formation and late bowel obstruction.

Totally extraperitoneal prosthetic repair The TEP is a laparoscopic adaptation of the open posterior preperitoneal approach first described by Annandale.[39] The laparoscope is introduced into the preperitoneal space through a paraumbilical incision. The preperitoneal space is dissected toward the symphysis pubis, the Cooper ligament and the iliac vessels with a blunt probe or balloon. Carbon dioxide is insufflated into the preperitoneal space to maintain exposure. Care must be taken to avoid entering the peritoneum; if this occurs, loss of pressure in the preperitoneal space results and exposure is lost. If an indirect hernia is present, the hernia sac is reduced. A polypropylene mesh is used to reconstruct the inguinal floor and is fixed to the Cooper ligament, along the iliopubic tract and to the edges of the rectus sheath using staples or sutures. Typically, the mesh is split so that it can be placed around the cord in the preperitoneal space. The TEP approach avoids the risks of entering the peritoneal cavity and subsequent intraperitoneal adhesion formation. However, the operating space is more limited than in transabdominal procedures and the approach can be more tedious and time-consuming. The learning curve is also longer for this approach.

Table 4.1 • Recurrence rates of laparoscopic herniorrhaphy

Laparoscopic technique	No. of patients/hernias	Recurrence (%)
Intraperitoneal	182/186	3.2
TAPP	328/359	0.8
TEP	53/90	0

TAPP, transabdominal preperitoneal prosthetic repair;
TEP, totally extraperitoneal prosthetic repair.
From MacFadyen BV Jr, Arregui ME, Corbitt JD Jr et al.
Complications of laparoscopic herniorrhaphy. Surg Endosc
1993; 7:155–9, with permission of Springer-Verlag ©.

The TEP approach is currently the technique recommended by the National Institute for Clinical Excellence (NICE) for recurrent inguinal hernias and bilateral primary inguinal hernias.[40]

COMPLICATIONS

Complications of herniorrhaphy include recurrence, urinary retention, ischaemic orchitis and testicular atrophy, wound infection and nerve injuries (neuromas of the ilioinguinal or genitofemoral nerves). A wide variation in recurrence rates is reported in the literature, depending on both the surgical technique employed and the method and length of follow-up (questionnaire, physical examination, etc.). There is no doubt that the Bassini technique has a high rate of recurrence (>10%)[41] and is now of historical interest only.

The Shouldice technique, which remains very popular in Europe (accounting for 50% of primary hernia repairs in Germany), has numerous publications reporting recurrence rates of 1–2%.[42] To date, the Lichtenstein tension-free repair has the largest number of published repairs with the lowest recurrence rates. Lichtenstein and colleagues published a multicentre series of 22 300 hernioplasties performed by this technique with a recurrence rate of 0.77%.[43]

The recurrence rates for laparoscopic herniorrhaphy are still in their infancy as the technique is less than 10 years old and up to 15% recurrences may occur after this time. However, the preliminary results for primary hernia are promising.

There are now more than 20 randomised trials comparing laparoscopic with open herniorrhaphy, summarised by Goh.[44] The results show that while laparoscopic herniorrhaphy takes longer, postoperative analgesic requirement, time to return to work and recurrence rates are generally superior in the laparoscopic group. Recurrence rates in large reported series are <1%,[45] with the TEP having the lowest recurrence rate of the various laparoscopic approaches: intraperitoneal 3.2%, TAPP 0.8% and TEP 0%.[46]

Recurrent inguinal hernias

Tables **4.2** and **4.3** present an overview of the re-recurrence rates for the open procedures. **Table 4.2** illustrates a re-recurrence rate of 27.5–35% for the Bassini technique and there is now no indication to use this procedure in the repair of recurrent inguinal hernias.

The McVay procedure and transversalis repair are not commonly employed and the results are probably of historic interest only.

The use of the Shouldice technique to treat recurrent groin hernias has been carefully evaluated in numerous studies with high numbers of patients. A few well-known investigators with up to 2500 participating patients and an observation period of

Table 4.2 • Sutured procedures for recurrent inguinal hernias

Procedure	Reference	No. of cases	Re-recurrences (%)
Bassini	Kux et al.[47]	–	13.5
	Herzog[48]	295	30.0
	Guthy and Boom[49]	70	35.3
	Witte[50]	160	27.5
McVay	Alexandre[51]	142	0
	Barbier et al.[52]	95	9.5
	Rutledge[53]	127	2.4
	Horn and Paetz[54]	35	14.0
	Halverson and McVay[55]	580	5.5
Transversalis repair	Kuttel[56]	124	5.9
	Chevally et al.[57]	394	7.5
	Berliner[58]	171	4.3
Shouldice	Schippers et al.[59]	197	3.1
	e-Silva et al.[60]	102	4.9
	Jan[61]	22	4.5
	Wantz[62]	639	7.2
	Berliner[58]	272	5.9
	Obney[63]	1057	3.9
	Glasgow[64]	2524	2.5

From Tons C. Suture repair of recurrent inguinal hernia – a review of the literature. In: Schumpelick V, Kingsnorth AN (eds) Incisional hernia. Berlin: Springer-Verlag, 1999; 367–73, with permission.

Table 4.3 • Open approach using prosthetic augmentation

Procedure	Reference	No. of cases	Re-recurrences (%)
Lichtenstein	Fuchsjager[65]	55	3.6
	Gilbert[66]	412	0.24
	Rutkow and Robbins[67]	1313	0
	Law and Ellis[68]	52	10.0
Mesh plug	Lichtenstein et al.[69]	1500	1.6
	Amid et al.[70]	1400	1.0
	Shulman et al.[71]	1402	2.0
TIPP/Rives	Schumpelick et al.[72]	54	0
	Munegato et al.[73]	121	5.7
	Bendavid[74]	280	3.2
	Flament[75]	586	1.7
Wantz	Hoffman and Traverso[76]	52	0.5
	Fong and Wantz[77]	827	0.5
	Schaap et al.[78]	98	25.0
	Mozingo et al.[79]	100	3.0
Stoppa	Beets et al.[80]	126	1.0
	Langer et al.[81]	58	12.0
	Wantz[82]	108	8.3
	Baeten[83]	150	0.75
	Stoppa and Verhaeghe[84]	270	1.1

TIPP, transinguinal preperitoneal prosthesis.
From Tons C. Suture repair of recurrent inguinal hernia – a review of the literature. In: Schumpelick V, Kingsnorth AN (eds) Incisional Hernia. Berlin: Springer-Verlag, 1999; 367–73.

10–18 years report a re-recurrence rate ranging between 2.5 and 7%. Relevant studies performed in non-specialized hospitals also report a low re-recurrence rate, no higher than 7.6%. In centres where alloplastic material is unavailable or too expensive for routine use, the Shouldice technique is probably the technique of choice.

PROSTHETIC MESH REPAIR OF RECURRENT INGUINAL HERNIAS

 The use of prosthetic mesh to repair recurrent hernias varies throughout Europe and the USA, although it is probably now the technique of choice.

If the mesh is used with the onlay technique using the inguinal approach, the recurrence rate varies between almost 0%[67] and 10%,[68] a difference that may be explained both by the short follow-up times and the methods of follow-up. Since its introduction, excellent results have been reported when the mesh-plug method has been used in specialized centres.[69–71] The transinguinal preperitoneal prosthetic (TIPP) repair/Rives procedure tends to be reserved for selected cases and is not indicated for the majority of recurrent inguinal hernias. Even so, it is highly successful when employed, with a reported re-recurrence rate of less than 6% after a 10-year observation period. When a preperitoneal approach is used with preperitoneal mesh implantation, the re-recurrence rate ranges between 0.5 and 5.3% after an observation period of up to 10 years.[76,77,79] However, one series reported a re-recurrence rate of 25%, suggesting that this technique may require a degree of surgical experience for success. Divergent results are also reported for the Stoppa technique, with re-recurrence rates varying between 1 and 12% (**Table 4.3**). The most likely explanation for this wide variation is that the size and type of recurrence probably varied between the centres reporting.

LAPAROSCOPIC REPAIR OF RECURRENT INGUINAL HERNIAS

During the 1990s, the laparoscopists have challenged the open approach to recurrent hernia repair. **Table 4.4** lists the reported re-recurrence rates for laparoscopic repair of recurrent inguinal hernias. Although the reported follow-up times are relatively

Table 4.4 • Laparoscopic repair of recurrent inguinal hernias

Reference	No. of repairs	Type of repair	Recurrence rate (%)	Follow-up (months)
Felix[85]	124 49	TAPP TEP	0.8 0	24 24
Liebel[86]	210	TAPP	0.95	6–36
Sandbichler[87]	200	TAPP	0.5	9–31
Birth[88]	117	TAPP	0	3–36
Stancanelli[89]	51	TAPP	0	1–31
Gadacz[90]	45	TEP	0	Not reported

TAPP, transabdominal preperitoneal prosthetic repair; TEP, totally extraperitoneal prosthetic repair.

short, the preliminary results are very encouraging. The advantages of the laparoscopic approach include elimination of one of the commonest causes of recurrence, the missed hernia; allowing the surgeon to identify those patients with complex hernias; and covering the entire myopectineal orifice, buttressing the intrinsic collagen deficit, thereby overcoming one of the causes of late recurrence. The complication rate is low (<2%),[91] the main cause of failure being technical error.

FEMORAL HERNIA

Femoral hernia represents the third commonest type of primary hernia. It accounts for 20% of hernias in women and 5% in men, strangulation being the initial presentation in 40%.

Anatomy

The femoral canal occupies the most medial compartment of the femoral sheath, extending from the femoral ring above to the saphenous opening below. It contains fat, lymphatic vessels and the lymph node of Cloquet. It is closed above by the septum crurale, a condensation of extraperitoneal tissue pierced by lymphatic vessels, and below by the cribriform fascia. The femoral ring is bounded anteriorly by the inguinal ligament and posteriorly by the iliopectineal (Cooper) ligament, the pubic bone and the fascia over the pectineus muscle. Medially, the boundary is the edge of the lacunar ligament, while laterally it is separated from the femoral vein by a thin septum.

Aetiology

Femoral hernias are considered to be acquired, possibly as a result of increased abdominal pressure. A postulated mechanism is the insinuation of

fat into the femoral ring secondary to raised intra-abdominal pressure. This bolus of fat drags along pelvic peritoneum to develop a peritoneal sac. Once the peritoneal sac has moved the short distance down the canal and out of the femoral orifice, the sac becomes apparent. The hernia not only becomes visible and palpable, but the contents of the sac become at risk of incarceration and strangulation. The incidence of femoral herniation increases with age, and a potential mechanism for this involves the muscle bulk adjacent to the distal femoral canal. Normally, the iliopsoas and pectineus muscle bundles encroach on the canal and thus act as a barrier to the development of a femoral hernia. With the natural atrophy of muscle tissue that occurs with senescence, the actual volume of muscle within the canal decreases, allowing positive intra-abdominal pressure to push the peritoneum into the canal. This would explain the high rate of femoral hernia among elderly women as well as men. In women of all ages, the muscle mass is not as great as in men. Consequently, women are predisposed to femoral hernias with any condition that increases intra-abdominal pressure, such as pregnancy or obesity.

Management

The treatment of femoral hernia is surgical repair. Several operative approaches have been described: the low approach (Lockwood), the high approach (McEvedy) and the inguinal approach (Lothiessen). To these can now be added the laparoscopic approach.

LOW APPROACH (LOCKWOOD)

The low approach is based on a groin-crease incision and dissection of the femoral hernia sac below the inguinal ligament. The anatomical layers covering the sac should be peeled away and the sac opened to inspect its contents. Once empty, the neck of the sac is pulled down, ligated as high as possible and redundant sac excised. The neck then retracts through the femoral canal and the canal is closed with a plug or cylinder of polypropylene mesh, anchored to the inguinal ligament and iliopectineal ligament with non-absorbable sutures. Suturing of the iliopectineal ligament to the inguinal ligament may result in tension due to the rigidity of these structures and may predispose to recurrence.

TRANSINGUINAL APPROACH (LOTHIESSEN)

Techniques of femoral repair that open the posterior inguinal wall for exposure and repair (the inguinal approaches of Lothiessen, Bassini, Shouldice, McVay–Cooper, Halsted and Andrews) should rarely be used. It is unnecessary to incise this natural fascial barrier in Hesselbach's triangle for exposure; the low or high approach leaves the inguinal floor intact.

HIGH APPROACH (MCEVEDY)

The high approach was classically based on a vertical incision made over the femoral canal and continued upwards above the inguinal ligament. This has now been replaced with a transverse 'unilateral' Pfannenstiel incision, which can be extended to form a complete Pfannenstiel incision if a formal laparotomy is required. The dissection is continued through the subcutaneous tissue and anterior rectus sheath. The rectus muscle is retracted medially and the transverse incision is extended laterally a few centimetres through the full thickness of the musculo-aponeurotic layers formed by the external oblique aponeurosis and the internal oblique and transversus abdominis muscles. The transversalis fascia is now exposed, which is opened transversely, and the preperitoneal space entered. The femoral hernia sac is identified medial to the iliac vessels and reduced by traction. If the hernia is incarcerated, the sac may be released by incising the insertion of the iliopubic tract into the Cooper ligament at the medial margin of the femoral ring. The sac is then opened, the contents dealt with appropriately and the sac ligated at its neck. The hernioplasty may then be completed by either suturing the iliopubic tract to the posterior margin of the Cooper ligament or by insertion of a prosthetic mesh, either as a sheet covering the whole of the myopectineal opening or as a mesh plug. The wound is closed in layers with apposition of the anterior sheath and lateral muscle aponeurosis.

LAPAROSCOPIC APPROACH

The laparoscopic approach is the same as for inguinal hernias and may employ the TAPP or TEP technique. The femoral ring is easily seen during either of these approaches and, indeed, visualisation of the whole of the myopectineal opening is fre-

quently quoted as one of the advantages of laparoscopic herniorrhaphy. There are no data yet published on laparoscopic series of femoral herniorrhaphy, the current data being extrapolated from femoral hernias detected during surgery for inguinal hernias. However, none of the series reported in **Table 4.4** described the subsequent development of a femoral hernia.

INCISIONAL HERNIA

Aetiology

Incisional hernias are unique in that they are the only hernia to be considered iatrogenic. The cause of wound complications after laparotomy is multifactorial, conditioned by local and systemic factors and by preoperative, perioperative and postoperative factors. Several factors such as advanced age, pulmonary disease, morbid obesity, malignancy and intra-abdominal infection are associated with impaired wound healing and predispose patients to serious wound complications such as wound dehiscence, wound infection and incisional herniation. Prospective trials in the 1990s show burst abdomen rates of 1–3%, wound infection rates of 10–15% and incisional hernia rates of 4–21%.[92] Technical factors influencing wound complications include surgical technique and suture material.

The results of prospective randomised trials comparing absorbable versus non-absorbable sutures are shown in **Table 4.5**. No difference was demonstrated in wound dehiscence rate when absorbable sutures were compared with non-absorbable sutures.

A higher incidence of incisional hernia rate was reported when absorbable sutures were employed in three trials.[93,97,99] Several trials of continuous versus interrupted suture closure have failed to show any difference in the rate of wound dehiscence or incisional hernia.[93,101]

The continuous method has the advantages of being quicker, cheaper and adjusts to some degree the tension in the tissues along the line of closure, so that tissues are less ischaemic than when they are approximated comparably with multiple interrupted sutures.

There is also a difference in wound complication rates when the skill of the surgeon is taken into account. Gislason[92] compared the results of experienced surgeons performing the same type of procedures and found wound failure rates ranging from 3.9 to 20%. When surgeons expressing an interest in the field of abdominal wall closure performed similar procedures, much lower complication rates were reported (wound dehiscence <0.5%, incisional hernia 3%, wound infection 3–4%).

Table 4.5 • Results of prospective randomised trials comparing absorbable versus non-absorbable suture

Location	No. of patients	Sutures	Dehiscence (%)	Hernia (%)
Netherlands[93]	1156	Vicryl	1.9	18.8
		PDS	3.5	13.2
		Nylon	2.1	10.4
Montreal[94]	200	Dexon	0.0	4.2
		Prolene	1.0	10.5
Aberdeen[95]	757	PDS	0.3	3.5
		Prolene	0.3	4.7
London[96]	347	Dexon	0.6	6.1
		Prolene	0.6	5.2
London[97]	210	Dexon	1.0	11.5
		Nylon	1.0	3.8
Burlington[98]	161	Vicryl	0	0
		Nurolon	0	8.9
		Prolene	1.9	4.4
New Brunswick[99]	229	PDS	0	10
		Ethibond	1.8	18
Milwaukee[100]	225	Maxon	0	8.7
		Nylon	2.7	4.4

PDS, polydioxanone

The final technical consideration is the ratio of suture length to wound length (SL:WL). This ratio depends on the stitch interval, the amount of tissue included in the stitches and the tension on the suture. A strong correlation between the SL:WL ratio and the development of incisional hernia has been found. With an SL:WL ratio of at least 4, the wound tension seems to be distributed in such a way that the suture-holding capacity of the tissues is not exceeded.

The incisional hernia rate is lower if the SL:WL ratio is 4 or more, and suturing with a lower ratio is associated with a threefold increase in the rate of incisional hernia.[96]

However, the SL:WL ratio should not be higher than 5 since this has been associated with a higher rate of both wound infection and incisional hernia, probably because a large amount of tissue other than fascia is then included in the suture. An SW:LW ratio of 4 equates to 1-cm bites of tissue on each side of the incision taken at 1-cm intervals along the length of the incision.

Management

The large number of surgical procedures described in the literature to repair incisional hernias illustrates that no single technique has stood out as

being effective. While 50% of incisional hernias occur within 1 year after primary operation, 10–18% are diagnosed more than 5 years after laparotomy. Any study reporting re-recurrence rates following incisional hernia repair should therefore ideally have at least 5 years of follow-up data for analysis. Unfortunately, prospective randomised trials comparing different types of incisional hernia repair are lacking and the majority of studies are retrospective. However, recurrence rates ranging from 6 to 46% for primary closure are documented.[102] The results for the Mayo ('vest-over-pants') procedure are no better (overall recurrence rate 33.1%).[102]

As a consequence of the disappointing data on mesh-free repair of incisional hernias, meshes were introduced to strengthen the abdominal wall repair. Several different techniques were developed: inlay, onlay and sublay (**Fig. 4.4**). Implantation as an inlay did not achieve any strengthening of the abdominal wall, and recurrence rates of up to 50% have been reported.

MESH REPAIR

The onlay technique is relatively popular in the USA and preliminary reports suggest relatively low recurrence rates (0–20%). The technique is dependent on adequate fixation of the mesh to the fascia and an overlap of 5–8 cm is recommended. If the

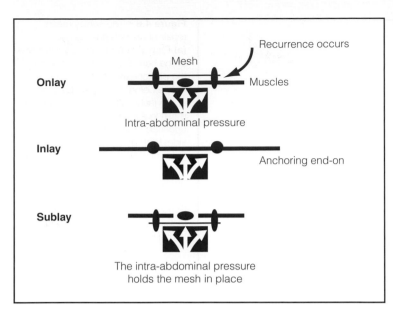

Figure 4.4 • Cross-sectional appearance of techniques of incisional hernia repair. With permission from Schumpelick V, Klinge V. Immediate follow-up results of sublay polypropylene repair in primary or recurrent incisional hernias. In: Schumpelick V, Kingsnorth AN (eds) Incisional hernia. Berlin: Springer-Verlag ©, 1999; pp. 312–26.

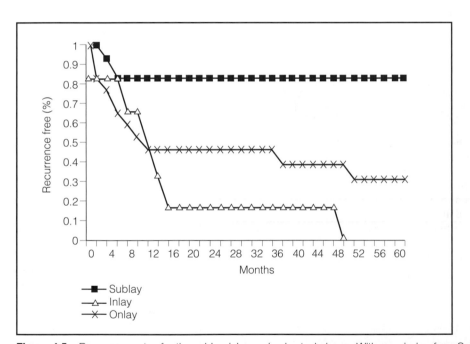

Figure 4.5 • Recurrence rates for the sublay, inlay and onlay techniques. With permission from Schumpelick V, Klinge V. Immediate follow-up results of sublay polypropylene repair in primary or recurrent incisional hernias. In: Schumpelick V, Kingsnorth AN (eds) Incisional hernia. Berlin: Springer-Verlag ©, 1999; pp. 312–26.

connection between the mesh and the fascia is lost, a buttonhole hernia develops at the edge of the mesh.

The sublay technique is the procedure favoured by the author. A mesh in the sublay position is not only sutured into position but is also held in place by the intra-abdominal pressure. Polypropylene mesh in this position is therefore able to strengthen the abdominal wall both by mechanical sealing and by the induction of strong scar tissue. **Figure 4.5** compares the recurrence rate in a single institution where all three techniques have been used and illustrates the favourable results achieved by the sublay technique. **Figure 4.6** illustrates pictorially the steps in a sublay mesh repair of an incisional

(a)

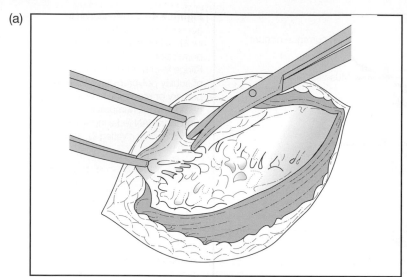

Figure 4.6 • The sublay mesh repair of an incisional hernia. **(a)** Preparation of the fascial borders of the hernia gap with separation of the peritoneum. **(b)** Preparing the hernia before the repair. **(c)** Closure of the fascia after placement of the mesh in a sublay position with an underlap of at least 5–8 cm on each side. With permission from Schumpelick V, Klinge V. Immediate follow-up results of sublay polypropylene repair in primary or recurrent incisional hernias. In: Schumpelick V, Kingsnorth AN (eds) Incisional hernia. Berlin: Springer-Verlag ©, 1999; pp. 312–26.

(b)

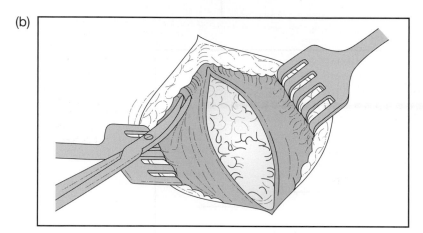

(c)

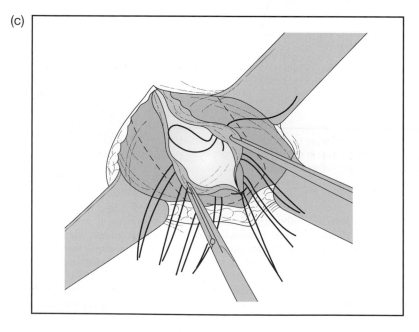

hernia, while the cross-sectional appearance is illustrated in **Fig. 4.7**.

The laparoscopic approach has also been applied to incisional hernias, the approach guaranteeing the same safety as the use of a prosthetic mesh placed at open surgery but avoiding the extensive dissection and wide surgical wounds required for open insertion. **Table 4.6** summarises comparative series that have been published, suggesting that the outcome for laparoscopic incisional hernia repair is at least equivalent to open surgery.

The laparoscopic approach has the advantages of shorter hospital stay, lower analgesic requirements, fewer wound complications and an earlier return to normal activities.

The mesh employed in laparoscopic incisional hernia repair is frequently a composite mesh with a smooth microporous surface on one side and a corrugated (rough) surface on the other. The smooth side faces the intestine and serves as an adhesion barrier, while the rough side is applied against the abdominal wall and promotes mesh fixation via collagen and cellular ingrowth.

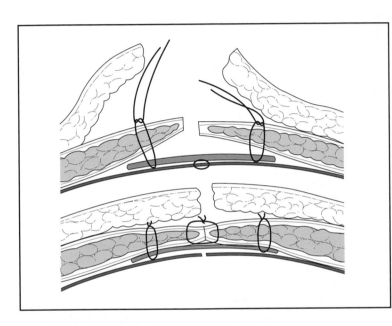

Figure 4.7 • Cross-sectional appearance of peritoneum closure showing the sublay position of the mesh, which is fixed either to the muscle or (better) only to the posterior sheath of the rectus muscle. The fascia is closed continuously with a non-absorbable end-to-end suture. With permission from Schumpelick V, Klinge V. Immediate follow-up results of sublay polypropylene repair in primary or recurrent incisional hernias. In: Schumpelick V, Kingsnorth AN (eds) Incisional hernia. Berlin: Springer-Verlag ©, 1999; pp. 312–26.

Table 4.6 • Comparison of laparoscopic and open hernia repair

Reference	No. of patients		Prosthesis		Follow-up (months)		Recurrences (%)	
	Open	Lap.	Open	Lap.	Open	Lap.	Open	Lap.
Holzman et al.[10]	16	21	PP	PP	19	20	1 (12)	2 (9)
Park et al.[6]	49	56	PTFE/PP	PTFE/PP	53	24	17 (34)	6 (10)
Ramshaw et al.[7]	174	79	PP	PTFE	21	21	36 (21)	2 (2)
Carbajo et al.[8]	30	30	PTFE/PP	PTFE	27	27	2 (6)	0 (0)
DeMaria et al.[9]	18	21	PP	PTFE	24	24	0 (0)	1 (4)
Chari et al.[103]	14	14	PP	PTFE	6–27	6–27	0 (0)	0 (0)
Zanghi et al.[104]	15	11	PTFE/PP	PTFE	40	18	0 (0)	0 (0)
Wright et al.[105]	119	90	None	PP	24	32	11 (9)	5 (6)
Bencini et al.[106]	49	42	PP	PTFE	18	17	3 (6)	0 (0)

PP, polypropylene; PTFE, expanded polytetrafluoroethylene.

Key points

- Herniorrhaphy is one of the commonest operations performed.
- Techniques have advanced considerably during the 1990s.
- The use of prosthetic mesh should now be considered for the repair of all hernias.
- The laparoscopic approach may be more appropriate than a traditional open approach.
- Recurrent hernias may be best managed in specialist centres or by surgeons with a specialist interest in hernia surgery who are technically competent to perform both open and laparoscopic procedures.
- A multidisciplinary approach, including plastic surgeons, may be appropriate for complex, multiply recurrent hernias.

REFERENCES

1. Devlin B. Functional anatomy. In: Schumpelick V, Kingsnorth AN (eds) Incisional hernia. Berlin: Springer-Verlag, 1999; pp. 32–44.

2. Robin AP. Epigastric hernia. In: Nyhus LM, Condon RE (eds) Hernia. Philadelphia: Lippincott, 1995; pp. 372–80.

3. Truong SN, Muller M. Diagnosis of abdominal wall defects. In: Schumpelick V, Kingsnorth AN (eds) Incisional hernia. Berlin: Springer-Verlag, 1999; pp. 117–35.

4. Pentney BH. Small ventral hernias in children. Practitioner 1960; 184:779–84.

5. LeBlanc KA, Booth WV. Laparoscopic repair of incisional abdominal hernias using expanded polytetrafluoroethylene: preliminary findings. Surg Laparosc Endosc 1993; 3:39–41.

6. Park A, Birch DW, Lovrics P. Laparoscopic and open incisional hernia repair: a comparison study. Surgery 1998; 124:816–21.

7. Ramshaw BJ, Esartia P, Schwab J et al. Comparison of laparoscopic and open ventral herniorrhaphy. Ann Surg 1999; 65:827–31.

8. Carbajo MA, Martin del Olmo JC, Blanco JI et al. Laparoscopic treatment vs open surgery in the solution of major incisional and abdominal wall hernias with mesh. Surg Endosc 1999; 13:250–52.

9. DeMaria EJ, Moss JM, Sugarman HJ. Laparoscopic intraperitoneal polytetrafluoroethylene (PTFE) prosthetic patch repair of ventral hernia. Prospective comparison to open prefascial polypropylene mesh repair. Surg Endosc 2000; 14:326–9.

10. Holzman MD, Purut CM, Reintgen K et al. Laparoscopic ventral and incisional hernioplasty. Surg Endosc 1997; 11:32–5.

11. Askar OM. Aponeurotic hernias: recent observations upon paraumbilical and epigastric hernias. Surg Clin North Am 1984; 64:315–29.

12. McCaughan JJ. Epigastric hernia. Results obtained by surgery. AMA Arch Surg 1956; 73:972–9.

13. Nakayama DK, Harrison MR, Gross BH et al. Management of the fetus with an abdominal wall defect. J Pediatr Surg 1984; 19:408–11.

14. Sipes SI, Weiner CP, Sipes DR, Grant SS, Williamson RA. Gastroschisis and omphalocele: does either antenatal diagnosis or route of delivery make a difference in perinatal outcome? Obstet Gynecol 1990; 76:195–9.

15. Woods GE. Some observations on umbilical hernia in infants. Arch Dis Child 1953; 28:450–5.

16. Sibley WL III, Lynn HB, Harris LE. A 25-year study of infantile umbilical hernias. Surgery 1964; 55:462–70.

17. Walker SH. The natural history of umbilical hernia. A six-year follow-up of 314 negro children with this defect. Clin Pediatr 1967; 6:29–32.

18. Morgan WW, White JJ, Stumbaugh S, Haller JA Jr. Prophylactic umbilical hernia repair in childhood to prevent adult incarceration. Surg Clin North Am 1970; 50:839–43.

19. Lassaletta L, Fonkalsrud EW, Tovar JA, Dudgeon D, Asch MJ. The management of umbilical hernias in infancy and childhood. J Pediatr Surg 1975; 10:405–8.

20. Skinner MA, Grosfield JL. Inguinal and umbilical hernia repair in infants and children. Surg Clin North Am 1993; 73:439–51.

21. Mayo WJ. An operation for the radical cure of umbilical hernia. Ann Surg 1901; 34:276–8.

22. Farris JM, Smith GK, Beattie AS. Umbilical hernia: an inquiry into the principle of imbrication and a note on the preservation of the umbilical dimple. Am J Surg 1959; 98:236–9.

23. Gray SW, Skandalakis JE. Embryology for surgeons. Philadelphia: WB Saunders, 1972; pp. 417–22.

24. Holder TM, Ashcroft KW. Groin hernias and hydroceles. In: Holder TM, Ashcroft KW (eds) Pediatric surgery. Philadelphia: WB Saunders, 1980; pp. 594–608.

25. Rowe MI, Clatworthy HW Jr. Incarcerated and strangulated hernias in children. Arch Surg 1970; 101:136–43.

26. Kurlan MZ, Web PB, Piedad OH. Inguinal herniorrhaphy by the Mitchell Banks technique. J Pediatr Surg 1972; 7:427–31.

27. Grosfeld JL, Minnick K, Shedd F et al. Inguinal hernia in children: factors affecting recurrence in 62 cases. J Pediatr Surg 1991; 26:159–64.

28. Hughson W. The persistence or performed sac in relation to oblique inguinal hernia. Surg Gynecol Obstet 1925; 41:610–14.

29. Read RC. Attenuation of the rectus sheath in inguinal herniation. Am J Surg 1970; 120:610–14.

   Excellent description of abdominal wall anatomy.

30. Peacock EE, Madden JW. Studies on the biology and treatment of recurrent inguinal hernia. II. Morphological changes. Ann Surg 1974; 179: 567–71.

31. Cannon DJ, Casteel L, Read RC. Abdominal aortic aneurysm, Leriche's syndrome, inguinal herniation and smoking. Arch Surg 1984; 119:387–9.

   A good summary of the aetiological factors in hernia development.

32. Lichtenstein IL, Shulman AG, Amid PK, Montilier MM. The tension-free hernioplasty. Am J Surg 1989; 157:188–93.

33. Ger R. The management of certain abdominal hernias by intra-abdominal closure of the neck. Ann R Coll Surg Engl 1982; 64:342–5.

34. Ger R, Monroe K, Duvivier R, Mishrock A. Management of indirect inguinal hernias by laparoscopic closure of the neck of the sac. Am J Surg 1990; 159:370–6.

35. Gazayerli MM. Anatomical laparoscopic hernia repair of direct or indirect inguinal hernias using the transversalis fascia and iliopubic tract. Surg Laparosc Endosc 1992; 2:49–52.

36. Nyhus LM, Pollak R, Bombeck CT, Donahue PE. The preperitoneal approach and prosthetic buttress repair for recurrent hernia. Ann Surg 1988; 203:733–8.

37. Rignault DP. Properitoneal prosthetic inguinal hernioplasty through a Pfannenstiel approach. Surg Gynecol Obstet 1986; 163:465.

38. Toy FK, Smoot RT Jr. Laparoscopic herniorrhaphy update. Laparoendosc Surg 1992; 2:197–9.

39. Annandale T. Case in which a reducible oblique and direct inguinal and femoral hernia existed on the same side and were successfully treated by operation. Edinb Med J 1876; 27:1087–9.

40. National Institute for Clinical Excellence. Laparoscopic surgery for inguinal hernia repair. Technology Appraisal Guidance 83. London: NICE, 2004. Available at www.nice.org.uk/TA083guidance

41. Bendavid R. The Shouldice repair. In: Nyhus LM, Condon RE (eds) Hernia. Philadelphia: Lippincott, 1995; pp. 217–36.

   Original description of the Shouldice technique.

42. Treutner KH, Arlt G, Schumpelick V. Shouldice repair for recurrent inguinal hernia: a ten-year follow-up. In: Schumpelick V, Kingsnorth AN (eds) Incisional hernia. Berlin: Springer-Verlag, 1999; pp. 359–66.

43. Shulman AG, Amid PK, Lichtenstein IL. The safety of mesh repair for primary inguinal hernias. Am Surg 1992; 58:255–9.

44. Goh PM. Overview of randomised trials of laparoscopic hernia repair. Semin Laparosc Surg 1998; 5:238–41.

   An excellent summary of randomised trials in laparoscopic inguinal hernia surgery.

45. Klaiber C, Banz M, Metzger A. Endoscopic repair: totally endoscopic preperitoneal prosthesis in recurrent inguinal hernia. In: Schumpelick V, Kingsnorth AN (eds) Incisional hernia. Berlin: Springer-Verlag, 1999; pp. 424–30.

   Reviews the TEP technique for recurrent inguinal hernia repair.

46. MacFadyen BV Jr, Arregui ME, Corbitt JD Jr et al. Complications of laparoscopic herniorrhaphy. Surg Endosc 1993; 7:155–9.

47. Kux M, Fuchsjager N, Hirbawi A. Verstarkung des Peritonealsacks mittels groser Prothese (Operation nach Stoppa). Chirurg 1993; 64:329–3.

48. Herzog U. Das Leistenhernienrezidiv. Schweiz Rundsch Med Prax 1990; 79:1166–9.

49. Guthy E, Boom H. Das Mehrfachrezidiv beim Leistbruch. 01 XV 088. Langenbecks Arch Chir 1983; 361:315–18.

50. Witte J. Die Rezidivleistenhernie im Erwachsenenalter; Operationsindikation, Verfahrenswahl, Ergebnisse. 01 XV 361. Langenbecks Arch Chir 1983; 361:309–13.

51. Alexandre JH. Recurrent inguinal hernia: surgical repair with a sheet of Dacron mesh by the inguinal route. Eur J Surg 1996; 162:29–33.

52. Barbier J, Carretier M, Richer JP. Cooper ligament repair: an update. World J Surg 1989; 13:499–505.

53. Rutledge RH. The Cooper ligament repair. Surg Clin North Am 1993; 73:471–84.

54. Horn J, Paetz B. Rezidiveingriffe nach Leisten- und Schenkelbrucheingriffen. Chirurg 1984; 55: 558–63.

55. Halverson K, McVay CB. Inguinal and femoral hernioplasty. Arch Surg 1970; 101:127–35.

56. Kuttel JC. Recurrent inguinal hernias: surgery with transversalis fascia repair. [In German] Helv Chir Acta 1992; 58:847–50.

57. Chevally JP, Rothenbuhler JM, Harder F. Erste Erfahrungen mit der Transversalisplastik in der Behandlung der Leistenhernie. Helv Chir Acta 1989; 56:221–4.

58. Berliner SD. An approach of groin hernia. Surg Clin North Am 1984; 64:197–213.

59. Schippers E, Peiper C, Schumpelick V. Pro-Shouldice: primary tension-free hernia repair. Conditio sine qua non? [In German] Swiss Surg 1996; Suppl. 4:33–6.

60. e-Silva NC, Reis MC, Candido Lima AP, de Carvalho Canuto R. Inguinal hernia repair with

the Shouldice technique. [In Portuguese] Rev Hosp Clin Fac Med Sao Paulo 1995; 50:314–16.

61. Jan SE, Wu CW, Lui WY. Shouldice inguinal hernioplasty. Zhonghua Yi Xue Za Zhi (Taipei) 1992; 50:26–8.

62. Wantz GE. The Canadian repair: personal observations. World J Surg 1989; 13:516–21.

63. Obney N. Application of Shouldice technique in large scrotal hernias and sliding hernias. Contemp Surg 1984; 25:11–16.

64. Glassow F. Inguinal hernia repair using local anaesthesia. Ann R Coll Surg Engl 1984; 66:382–7.

65. Fuchsjager N. Lichtenstein patch versus Shouldice technique in primary inguinal hernia with a high risk of recurrence. [In German] Chirurg 1994; 65: 59–62.

66. Gilbert AI. Sutureless repair of inguinal hernia. Am J Surg 1992; 163:331–5.

67. Rutkow IM, Robbins AW. 'Tension-free' inguinal herniorrhaphy: a preliminary report on the 'mesh-plug' technique. Surgery 1993; 114:3–8.

68. Law NW, Ellis H. Preliminary results for the repair of difficult recurrent inguinal hernias using expanded PTFE patch. Acta Chir Scand 1990; 156:609–12.

69. Lichtenstein IL, Shulman AG, Amid PK. The cause, prevention and treatment of recurrent groin hernia. Surg Clin North Am 1993; 73:529–44.

70. Amid PK, Shulman AG, Lichtenstein IL. Critical scrutiny of the open 'tension-free' hernioplasty. Am J Surg 1993; 165:369–71.

71. Shulman AG, Amid PK, Lichtenstein IL. The plug repair of 1402 recurrent inguinal hernias: 20-year experience. Arch Surg 1990; 125:265–7.

72. Schumpelick V, Treutner KH, Arlt G. Inguinal hernia repair in adults. Lancet 1994; 344:375–9.

73. Munegato G, Da Dalt GF, Godina M et al. The surgical treatment of preperitoneal inguinal hernia: a comparison between the methods of Rines and Stoppe. [In Italian] Minerva Chir 1992; 47:919–23.

74. Bendavid R. The rational use of mesh in hernias: a perspective. Int Surg 1992; 77:229–31.

75. Flament JB. Use of prostheses in emergency surgery. Retrospective study of 204 strangulated inguinal hernias. [In French] Chirurgie 1996; 12:48–50.

76. Hoffman HC, Traverso ALV. Preperitoneal prosthetic herniorrhaphy. Arch Surg 1993; 128:964–9.

77. Fong Y, Wantz GE. Prevention of ischaemic orchitis during inguinal hernioplasty. Surg Gynecol Obstet 1992; 174:399–402.

78. Schaap HM, van de Pavoordt H, Bast TJ. The preperitoneal approach in the repair of recurrent inguinal hernias. Surg Gynecol Obstet 1992; 174:460–4.

79. Mozingo D, Walters J, Otchy D, Rosenthal D. Preperitoneal synthetic mesh repair of recurrent inguinal hernias. Surg Gynecol Obstet 1992; 174:33–5.

80. Beets GL, Dirkoen CD, Go PM et al. Open or laparoscopic mesh repair for recurrent inguinal hernia. A randomised controlled trial. Surg Endosc 1999; 13:323–7.

81. Langer I, Herjog U, Schuppisser JP et al. Preperitoneal prosthesis implantation in surgical management of recurrent inguinal hernia. Retrospective evaluation of our results 1989–1994. [In German] Chirurg 1996; 67:394–402.

82. Wantz GE. The technique of giant prosthetic reinforcement of the visceral sac performed through an anterior groin incision. Surg Gynecol Obstet 1995; 176:497–500.

83. Baeten CGMI, Beets GL, Van Geldere D, Go PMNYH. Long term results of giant prosthetic reinforcement of the visceral sac for complex recurrent inguinal hernia. Br J Surg 1996; 83:203–6.

84. Stoppa RE, Verhaeghe P. Results after Stoppa procedure. In: Schumpelick V, Wantz GE (eds) Inguinal hernia repair. Basel: Karger, 1995; pp. 399–402.

85. Felix EL. Laparoscopic repair of recurrent hernia. Am J Surg 1996; 172:580–4.

86. Liebel B. Endoscopic hernia surgery (TAPP): gold standard in the management of recurrent hernias? Chirurg 1996; 67:1226–30.

87. Sandbichler P, Draxl H, Gstir H. Laparoscopic repair of recurrent inguinal hernias. Am J Surg 1996; 171:366–8.

88. Birth M. Laparoscopic transabdominal preperitoneal hernioplasty: results of 1000 consecutive cases. J Laparosc Surg 1996; 6:293–300.

89. Stancanelli V. Laparoscopic repair of bilateral and/or recurrent hernia. G Chir 1994; 15:519–23.

90. Gadacz T. Totally preperitoneal laparoscopic inguinal herniorrhaphy using balloon dissection. Surg Rounds 1995; March:107–12.

91. Klaiber C, Banz M, Metzger A. Endoscopic repair: totally endoscopic preperitoneal prosthesis in recurrent inguinal hernia. In: Schumpelick V, Kingsnorth AN (eds) Incisional hernia. Berlin: Springer-Verlag, 1999; pp. 424–30.

92. Gislason H. Closure of the abdomen in acute wound failure. In: Schumpelick V, Kingsnorth AN (eds) Incisional hernia. Berlin: Springer-Verlag, 1999; pp. 253–7.

93. Wissing J, van Vroonhoven TJMV, Schattenkerk ME et al. Fascia closure after midline laparotomy: results of a randomised trial. Br J Surg 1987; 74:738–45.

94. Lewis RT, Wiegand FM. Natural history of vertical abdominal parietal closure: Prolene versus Dexon. Can J Surg 1989; 32:196–9.

95. Krukowski ZH, Cusick EL, Engeset J et al. Polydioxanone or polypropylene for closure of midline abdominal incisions: a prospective comparative clinical trial. Br J Surg 1987; 74:828–32.

96. Cameron AEP, Gray RCF, Talbot RW et al. Abdominal wound closure: a trial of Prolene and Dexon. Br J Surg 1980; 67:487–91.

97. Bucknall TE, Ellis H. Abdominal wound closure: a comparison of monofilament nylon and polyglycolic acid. Surgery 1981; 89:672–5.

98. Corman ML, Veidenheimer MC, Clooer JA. Controlled clinical trial of three suture materials for abdominal wall closure after bowel operations. Am J Surg 1981; 141:510–14.

99. Brolin RE. Prospective, randomised evaluation of midline fascial closure in gastric bariatric operations. Am J Surg 1996; 172:328–31.

100. Carlson MA, Condon RE. Polyglyconate (Maxon) versus nylon suture in midline abdominal incision closure: a prospective randomised trial. Am J Surg 1995; 61:980–7.

101. Sahlin S, Ahlberg J, Granstrom L, Ljungstrom KG. Monofilament versus multifilament absorbable sutures for abdominal closure. Br J Surg 1993; 80:322–4.

A good summary of the evidence for type of suture used in abdominal wall closure.

102. Decurtins M. Significance of fascia doubling in the management of incisional hernia. In: Schumpelick V, Kingsnorth AN (eds) Incisional hernia. Berlin: Springer-Verlag, 1999; pp. 287–93.

103. Chari R, Chari V, Eisenstat M, Chung R. A case controlled study of laparoscopic incisional hernia repair. Surg Endosc 2000; 14:117–19.

104. Zanghi A, Di Vita M, Lomenzo E, De Luca A, Cappellani A. Laparoscopic repair vs open surgery for incisional hernias: a comparison study. Ann Ital Chir 2000; 71:663–7.

105. Wright BE, Niskanen BD, Peterson DJ et al. Laparoscopic ventral hernia repair: are there comparative advantages over traditional methods of repair? Am Surg 2002; 68:291–6.

106. Bencini L, Sanchez LJ, Buffi B et al. Incisional hernia repair: retrospective comparison of laparoscopic and open techniques. Surg Endosc 2003; 17:1546–51.

An excellent study highlighting the benefits and complications of laparoscopic compared with open incisional hernia repair.

Five

Early assessment and investigation in the acute abdomen

Simon Paterson-Brown

INTRODUCTION

The care of emergency surgical admissions remains one of the most important aspects of general surgical practice[1] and, with the current trend of increasing emergency admissions throughout the UK in all medical specialties,[2] this responsibility will undoubtedly increase. It has been estimated that at least 50% of all general surgical admissions are emergencies,[3] and as approximately half of these are due to acute abdominal pain the workload for the general surgeon remains substantial. The Confidential Enquiry into Post-operative Deaths (CEPOD) has repeatedly demonstrated that the outcome for patients requiring emergency surgery is improved when senior surgical staff are involved not only in preoperative decision-making but also in the surgery and postoperative care.[4]

Attempts to improve preoperative diagnosis and early management of patients with acute abdominal pain are continuously being sought and this chapter discusses all the current available techniques and the evidence for their incorporation into emergency surgical practice. For the purposes of most studies looking at acute abdominal pain, the broad definition is taken as 'abdominal pain of less than one week's duration requiring admission to hospital, which has not been previously treated or investigated'. However, this must be accepted as a fairly loose definition.

OVERALL MANAGEMENT OF EMERGENCY SURGICAL ADMISSIONS

On-call surgical team

Of all the changes that have occurred in general surgery over the last decade, undoubtedly the reduction in junior doctors' hours,[5] associated with the European Working Time Directive (EWTD),[6] has had the strongest influence, followed closely by the reduced overall period of training as recommended in the Calman report.[7] These two factors together have been estimated to have halved the overall experience available for surgical trainees.[8] Where continuity of care was maintained by the 'middle grade' surgical team in the past, the new rotas currently being put into place are increasingly of a shift pattern where the maximum time worked per week is 48 hours and consultants rarely work with the same trainees.[9] One solution to this problem is the establishment of the 'emergency team' where the whole surgical team (consultant and supporting junior staff) have no elective commitments and are on-call for a more extended period of time. Although there will have to be some change of juniors because of the EWTD, these can be kept to a minimum by allocating juniors to emergency activities for a defined period of time, perhaps a week, perhaps longer. Their subsequent attachment to elective activity then no longer suffers from the disruption associated with on-call shifts, a state of affairs which enhances both emergency and elective training opportunities. This 'emergency team' system, with many adaptations according to local requirements, has now been adopted in many units throughout the UK since it was first reported in Edinburgh in 1999.[10]

The emergency team undoubtedly improves the ability of the consultant general surgeon, as well as the middle grade team, to provide safe and effective emergency care, but requires other conditions to be met if this is to be both efficient and cost-effective, not only in terms of lost elective activity for the consultant but also training opportunities for the surgical trainees. These include easy access to radiological imaging, a dedicated emergency operating theatre with full (and senior) anaesthetic support available 24 hours each day, enough surgical admissions to make the system worthwhile, and a distinct and dedicated admission area for emergency patients to be assessed.

Many of these patients have equivocal signs and symptoms of acute appendicitis and the value of 'active observation' with reassessment after 2–3 hours by the same surgeon, repeated thereafter as necessary, is well established[11] and should be routine in all units. This is only really possible if all acute admissions remain in a single identifiable area.

Emergency theatre availability

It is now well established that most emergency surgical procedures do not need to be carried out overnight, but reducing operations during these inappropriate hours requires availability to theatre during the day. It also goes without saying that there is no point having an on-call surgical team available and free of elective commitments during the day if it does not have ready access to theatre. Indeed, as could be anticipated, establishment of an emergency theatre during the day substantially reduces the amount of out-of-hours operating.[10,12]

Early investigation of patients with emergency surgical problems

For an emergency team system to work efficiently the surgical team must have rapid access to diagnostic blood tests and appropriate imaging, which should include plain and contrast radiology, diagnostic and interventional (percutaneous drainage

and biopsy) ultrasound and computed tomography (CT). Furthermore, plain radiography evaluated by senior radiologists substantially enhances senior surgical assessment of patients with acute abdominal pain, resulting in reduced surgical admissions.[13] All these modalities are discussed below.

CONDITIONS ASSOCIATED WITH ABDOMINAL PAIN

Many studies have looked at the spectrum of patients admitted to hospital with acute abdominal pain and the approximate percentage represented by each condition is now well understood. Figures from one study[14] appear to be fairly representative (**Box 5.1**). In this study the 30-day mortality in 1190 emergency admissions was 4%, with a perioperative mortality of 8%. Not surprisingly, the mortality rate was age related, with perioperative mortality in patients below 60 years being 2%, rising to 12% in those 60–69 years and reaching 20% in patients over the age of 80 years. Laparotomy for

Box 5.1 • Conditions that may present with acute abdominal pain

Non-specific abdominal pain (NSAP) (35%)
Acute appendicitis (17%)
Intestinal obstruction (15%)
Urological causes (6%)
Gallstone disease (5%)
Colonic diverticular disease (4%)
Abdominal trauma (3%)
Abdominal malignancy (3%)
Perforated peptic ulcer (3%)
Pancreatitis (2%)
Conditions contributing 1% or less
Exacerbation of peptic ulcer
Ruptured abdominal aortic aneurysm
Gynaecological causes (these may go unnoticed as NSAP)
Inflammatory bowel disease
Medical conditions
Mesenteric ischaemia
Gastroenteritis
Miscellaneous

After Irvin TT. Abdominal pain: a surgical audit of 1190 emergency admissions. Br J Surg 1989; 76:1121–5.

irresectable disease was the most common cause of perioperative mortality (28%), with ruptured abdominal aortic aneurysm (23%), perforated peptic ulcer (16%) and colonic resections (14%) all being associated with significant perioperative mortality.

What stands out from all the studies on acute abdominal pain published over the last three decades is the high incidence of non-specific abdominal pain (NSAP), with published figures of 40% or more.[15] NSAP usually reflects a failure of diagnosis as many of these patients do have a cause for the pain and it has been shown that further investigations, such as laparoscopy, can reduce the overall incidence of NSAP to around 27%.[16]

Some authors have examined this diagnosis of NSAP further and describe a certain number of alternative conditions that could be related (**Box 5.2**),[15] including abdominal wall pain[17] and rectus nerve entrapment.[18] In some cases of NSAP, detection of abdominal wall tenderness (increased abdominal pain on tensing the abdominal wall muscles) may be a useful diagnostic test.[19] Possible causes of abdominal wall pain are also given in **Box 5.2**. The major problem with making a diagnosis of NSAP is in missing serious underlying disease, and the late Tim de Dombal estimated that 10% of patients over the age of 50 years who were admitted to hospital with acute abdominal pain were subsequently found to have intra-abdominal malignancy.[20] Half of these patients had colonic carcinoma and the major concern was that 50% of the patients who were subsequently proved to have intra-abdominal cancer were discharged from hospital with a diagnosis of NSAP.

Box 5.2 • Causes of non-specific abdominal pain

Viral infections

Bacterial gastroenteritis

Worm infestation

Irritable bowel syndrome

Gynaecological causes

Psychosomatic pain

Abdominal wall pain[17]
  Iatrogenic peripheral nerve injuries
  Hernias
  Myofascial pain syndromes
  Rib tip syndrome
  Nerve root pain
  Rectus sheath haematoma

From Gray DWR, Collin J. Non-specific abdominal pain as a cause of acute admission to hospital. Br J Surg 1987; 74:239–42, with permission.

Acute gynaecological conditions such as pelvic inflammatory disease and ovarian cyst accidents are another group of diagnoses that may often be included under the umbrella of NSAP, simply because of failure to take a good history or examination or even perform a thorough pelvic examination, whether digitally, ultrasonographically or at operation. In one study from a general surgical unit, gynaecological causes represented 13% of all diagnoses in a consecutive series of all emergency admissions (both male and female) initially presumed to be 'surgical' in origin.[21] As many of these patients present with 'query appendicitis', accurate assessment is essential if unnecessary operations are to be avoided, and even then the diagnosis may remain hidden unless the surgeon examines the pelvic organs once a normal appendix has been found. However, with the increased use of diagnostic laparoscopy, discussed later in this chapter, these conditions are now being recognised by the emergency surgeon with much greater frequency. Early recognition and appropriate treatment of pelvic inflammatory disease may help to avoid potentially serious long-term sequelae and must be encouraged.[22] Indeed the condition of Curtis–Fitz-Hugh syndrome, when transperitoneal spread of pelvic inflammatory disease produces right upper quadrant pain due to perihepatic adhesions, is now well recognised and care must be taken to differentiate this from acute biliary conditions.[23] Although much is made of possible 'medical' causes of acute abdominal pain in surgical textbooks, the incidence of conditions such as myocardial infarction, lobar pneumonia and some metabolic disorders is extremely small though many still masquerade as NSAP. However, the possibility of such conditions must still be borne in mind during the clinical assessment of all patients with acute abdominal pain: one study has shown that 19 of 1168 children (1.6%) admitted to hospital with acute abdominal pain had pneumonia as the sole cause of symptoms.[24] It is therefore still extremely important to recognise these medical conditions when they do present, before exploratory surgery, as the mortality can be significantly increased.[25]

HISTORY AND EXAMINATION (INCLUDING COMPUTER-AIDED DIAGNOSIS)

In the early 1970s, de Dombal[26] in Leeds and Gunn[27] in Edinburgh developed a computer program based on Bayesian reasoning that produced a list of probable diagnoses for individual patients with acute abdominal pain. They demonstrated that the accuracy of clinical diagnosis could be improved by around 20%, and since then many other studies have confirmed this finding.[28–30] Furthermore, these studies have shown that there is a reduction in the unnecessary laparotomy rate and in bad management errors (patients whose surgery is incorrectly delayed); when used in the accident and emergency department, there is an associated reduction in 'inappropriate' admissions.[27] When the reasons for the improvement in diagnostic accuracy associated with the use of computer-aided diagnosis (CAD) are examined, there appear to be three main factors involved: (i) peer review and audit, which is invariably associated with improved results in most aspects of medical management;[31,32] (ii) an educational factor related to feedback;[33] and (iii) probably of greatest significance, the use of structured data sheets onto which the history and examination findings are documented before being entered into the computer program. One study demonstrated that the diagnostic accuracy of junior doctors improved by nearly 20% when they used structured data sheets alone, without going on to use the CAD program.[34] The same study also demonstrated that medical students assessing patients with the structured data sheets and then using the CAD program reached similar levels of diagnostic accuracy. Other studies have since confirmed similar improvements in clinical decision-making following the introduction of these data sheets.[35]

The message is clear: a good history and examination remain essential for both diagnostic accuracy and good clinical decision-making, and the use of a structured data sheet helps the clinician to achieve this objective.

A more recent study that examined the role of structured data collection in patients with suspected appendicitis again showed improvement in diagnostic accuracy, but only in female patients between the ages of 13 and 40 years.[36] This is of course the group that continually poses the greatest challenge to the admitting surgeon.

The aim of both the history and examination is to determine a diagnosis and clinical decision. There are undoubtedly specific features associated with all acute abdominal conditions that are well established; however, it remains the ability to identify the presence or absence of peritoneal inflammation that probably has the greatest influence on the final surgical decision. In other words, the presence or absence of guarding and rebound tenderness, and a history of pain on coughing, correlates well with the presence of peritonitis.[37] The differential diagnosis of acute appendicitis from NSAP is always difficult, particularly in children, and both guarding and rebound tenderness are significantly more likely to be present in acute appendicitis.[38] There has

always been great store taken from tenderness elicited on rectal examination during the assessment of patients with suspected acute appendicitis. However, when rebound tenderness is detected in the lower abdomen, as evident by pain on gentle percussion, further examination by rectal examination has been shown to provide no new information.[39] Rectal examination can therefore be avoided in such cases and reserved for those patients without rebound tenderness or where specific pelvic disease needs to be excluded. Measurement of temperature has also been shown to be relatively non-discriminatory in the early assessment of the acute abdomen.[40] Urgent urinary microscopy should be carried out on anyone with any symptoms that could relate to the urinary tract and it is a good principle to dip test the urine on admission of every patient with acute abdominal pain. A recent study has reported a reliable urine dip test for acute pancreatitis that detects trypsinogen-2.[41]

INITIAL INVESTIGATIONS AND MANAGEMENT

After the initial assessment (history and examination) of patients with acute abdominal pain, steps should be taken towards resuscitation, pain relief and further diagnostic tests as required.

There is now good evidence to support the early administration of opiate analgesia in patients with acute abdominal pain.[42] This has been clearly shown to have no detrimental effect on subsequent clinical assessment;[43] on the contrary, because the patient becomes more comfortable, further assessment may actually be facilitated. The cruel practice of withholding analgesia until the emergency surgeon has examined the patient with acute abdominal pain must be condemned.

Once the initial assessment has been completed, the surgeon will reach a differential diagnosis and, perhaps more importantly, a clinical decision: early operation definitely required, early operation definitely not required or need for early operation uncertain. Clearly, further investigations in the first category are unlikely to influence management, with the exception of a serum amylase level, which may reveal acute pancreatitis.[44] Further investigations in the group in which the surgeon considers early operation is not required can be organised on a more leisurely basis, and it is not surprising that it is in the group in which the surgeon is uncertain as to whether early operation is required that most difficulty exists.[45] Most of the uncertainty relates to 'query appendicitis', particularly in the young female, but also involves patients with intestinal obstruction and the elderly patient, in whom the diagnosis of mesenteric ischaemia must always be considered.[46]

This is particularly important in those with venous thrombosis and arterial embolic disease, whose survival after surgery is much better than those with arterial thrombosis.[47]

In the assessment of the role of subsequent investigations in the acute abdomen, it is important to identify their potential influence on clinical decision-making rather than evaluating them purely on diagnostic potential.

BLOOD TESTS

Although blood tests are often useful as a baseline, their influence on the diagnosis of acute abdominal pain remains unclear, with the exception of serum amylase for acute pancreatitis.[44] As already mentioned, a quick and reliable dip test has recently been developed to confirm acute pancreatitis[41] and may complement testing of serum amylase levels, particularly if they are equivocal. Studies examining the influence of white cell concentration,[48] C-reactive protein[49] and skin temperature in the right iliac fossa[50] in patients with 'query appendicitis' have concluded that serial white cell counts are useful (compared with a single measurement), while measurement of skin temperature over the right iliac fossa is of little value. Although isolated C-reactive protein levels may also be fairly non-discriminatory, when they are interpreted with white cell count and both are normal, acute appendicitis is unlikely.[51]

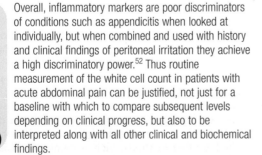

Overall, inflammatory markers are poor discriminators of conditions such as appendicitis when looked at individually, but when combined and used with history and clinical findings of peritoneal irritation they achieve a high discriminatory power.[52] Thus routine measurement of the white cell count in patients with acute abdominal pain can be justified, not just for a baseline with which to compare subsequent levels depending on clinical progress, but also to be interpreted along with all other clinical and biochemical findings.

Liver function tests are increasingly becoming available during the early assessment of the acute abdomen, and are extremely useful in confirming or refuting acute biliary disease.[53,54]

The other area that has attracted great interest in the role of blood tests for aiding diagnosis in the acute abdomen is intestinal ischaemia, whether from strangulated obstruction or mesenteric ischaemia

and infarction. Estimation of acid–base status to assess the degree of metabolic acidosis is often a late change and measurement of serum phosphate, lactate, kinase, creatine, lactate dehydrogenase, alkaline phosphatase, diamine oxidase and porcine ileal peptide have all been shown to be unreliable.[46]

RADIOLOGICAL INVESTIGATIONS

With advances in technology and improved radiological techniques, the radiologist is playing an ever-important role in the diagnosis of patients with acute abdominal pain. Furthermore abdominal ultrasonography and plain radiography evaluated by senior radiologists substantially enhances senior surgical assessment of patients with acute abdominal pain, resulting in reduced surgical admissions.[55]

Plain radiology

The role of plain radiology in the investigation of the acute abdomen has been extensively examined. Until recently there was general consensus that the erect chest radiograph was the most appropriate investigation for the detection of free intraperitoneal gas,[56] with use of the lateral decubitus film if either the erect chest film could not be taken (due to the patient's condition) or was equivocal. This no longer seems to be true following a report from Taiwan where ultrasonography was shown to be superior to the erect chest radiograph, with a sensitivity of 92% in the detection of pneumoperitoneum compared with only 78% for plain radiology.[57] Undoubtedly there will be operator dependence and for now the erect chest radiograph should still be the initial test for suspected perforation. The routine use of the supine abdominal radiograph has also been questioned. In the past some surgeons have felt that the supine abdominal radiograph provided valuable information in patients with an acute abdomen, which contributed to management.[58] However, this view is not supported by other reports. One study, performed by radiologists and surgeons,[59] demonstrated that across the spectrum of the 'acute abdomen' the plain abdominal radiograph altered the clinical diagnosis in only 7% of patients and actually only influenced management in 4%. This, of course, does not suggest that its use should be abandoned but that it should not be 'routine',[60] and perhaps merely limited to circumstances when diagnostic or management uncertainty exists, such as intestinal obstruction, suspected perforation, renal colic and trauma.[61–63] If requests for plain abdominal radiography were based on these criteria, its use could be reduced by 50%.[60]

Similar controversy exists in the use of erect abdominal radiographs for the assessment of patients with suspected intestinal obstruction. The majority of radiologists consider that the supine abdominal film is sufficient,[64,65] but most surgeons still prefer both views on the basis that in those patients in whom the supine radiograph is normal or equivocal the erect film may be helpful.[66] As most radiographs taken in patients with suspected obstruction are assessed by junior surgeons, it is not unreasonable to request both the supine and erect view, unless an experienced radiologist is available to perform immediate reporting.

Contrast radiology

Although contrast radiology has been available for many years, its role in the acute abdomen has, until relatively recently, been poorly understood. As a result, its use has been erratic and ill-defined, with the exception of intravenous urography for the assessment of patients with ureteric colic. It has been recognised for many years that gastrointestinal contrast studies can be used to differentiate between intestinal obstruction and postoperative ileus,[67,68] and their ability to evaluate other acute gastrointestinal conditions is now generally well accepted.[69]

PERFORATED PEPTIC ULCER

Although the erect chest radiograph is recognized as the most appropriate first-line investigation for a suspected perforated peptic ulcer,[56] in approximately 50% of patients no free gas can be identified on the radiograph.[70] This leaves the emergency surgeon with three options: (i) to review the diagnosis, such as reconsidering acute pancreatitis; (ii) to proceed to laparotomy based on the clinical findings alone; or (iii) particularly if there are reasonable grounds for uncertainty, to arrange a water-soluble contrast study.[71] This test will confirm or refute the presence of perforation (**Fig. 5.1**) but will not differentiate between the patient without a perforation and one in whom the perforation has sealed.[70] The addition of ultrasonography,[57] as already discussed, and even CT in this scenario may help by revealing free abdominal air and fluid in the patient whose perforation has sealed spontaneously. As has been well understood for quite some time now, many patients with perforated peptic ulcers can be managed non-operatively;[72,73] with this knowledge, the assessing surgeon has plenty of time to resuscitate the patient and make efforts to confirm or refute the diagnosis before rushing to emergency surgery. Patients who might be considered for non-operative treatment of their perforation should have a contrast meal to confirm spontaneous sealing of

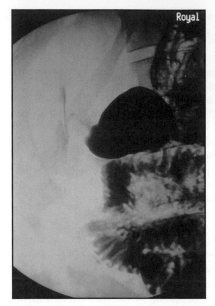

Figure 5.1 • Supine abdominal radiograph taken 20 minutes after the oral administration of 50 mL of water-soluble contrast material in a patient with a suspected perforated peptic ulcer in whom the erect chest radiograph was normal. Note the small trickle of contrast through the perforation. These findings were confirmed at laparotomy. From Hamilton Bailey's Emergency Surgery, 13th edn, reproduced by permission of Hodder Murray.

the perforation. This topic is discussed in more detail in Chapter 6.

SMALL BOWEL OBSTRUCTION

Surgery for small bowel obstruction is performed for one of two reasons: first, there has been failure of non-operative management or, second, there is clinical suspicion of impending strangulation. Although plain abdominal radiographs are useful in establishing the diagnosis of small bowel obstruction, they cannot differentiate between strangulated and non-strangulated gut. The criteria on which strangulated intestine must be suspected are well established: peritonism, fever, tachycardia and leucocytosis.[74] However, even when the diagnosis is suspected, the changes at operation are often irreversible and resection required. Some workers have looked at other methods, such as computer-assisted prediction[75] and serum markers such as phosphate and lactate concentrations,[44] to help identify patients with possible strangulation in order to allow earlier surgery but unfortunately none are reliable. As in other areas of acute abdominal imaging ultrasonography also appears to be able to contribute to the diagnosis of intestinal obstruction,[76,77] but the problem of detecting early ischaemic changes in small bowel obstruction remains largely unsolved.

Many centres have assessed the influence of water-soluble contrast studies in patients with small bowel obstruction, hypothesising that if those patients whose obstruction will not settle with non-operative treatment can be identified early, then these patients can undergo surgery without waiting for a 'trial' of non-operative treatment. This would reduce the number who may develop strangulation. Although small bowel contrast studies do appear to improve the diagnostic accuracy of small bowel obstruction[78] and can provide useful clinical information in more than three-quarters of patients,[79] their influence on clinical decision-making remains to be established. What can probably be agreed is that failure of contrast to reach the caecum within 4 hours,[80,81] and certainly by 12 hours,[82] strongly suggests that surgical intervention is likely to be required, and better sooner than later (**Fig. 5.2**). Suffice to say that in selected patients contrast studies can be of value in helping the surgeon reach a decision as to whether to proceed on a course of non-operative management or abandon it in favour of laparotomy,[83] particularly when the underlying cause is likely to be adhesions.[84]

More detailed information on the surgical management of small bowel obstruction is provided in Chapter 9.

LARGE BOWEL OBSTRUCTION

The management algorithm for large bowel obstruction has now become well established following the more widesdpread recognition that colonic pseudo-obstruction could not be distinguished from mechanical obstruction on plain radiographs alone (**Fig. 5.3a,b**).[85,86] The decision that all patients with suspected large bowel obstruction should now undergo a contrast enema (**Fig. 5.3c,d**) before laparotomy has probably been the most important factor in reducing not only the unnecessary operation rate for pseudo-obstruction but also the associated mortality. As long ago as 1896 this functional obstruction was recognised and termed 'spastic ileus',[87] later refined to 'pseudo-obstruction',[88] which is the term recognised today. Patients with acute colonic pseudo-obstruction present with similar history and clinical signs to the patient with a mechanical obstruction. Although factors recognised as precipitating pseudo-obstruction, such as dehydration, electrolyte abnormalities, pelvic and spinal surgery, acid–base imbalance, and so on,[88] may alert the clinician as to the possible cause, it cannot be confirmed without further investigation. As the treatment for one is non-operative and for the other is usually operative, accurate assessment is essential.

 The data to support the routine use of water-soluble contrast enemas in all patients who present with a clinical and radiological diagnosis of large bowel obstruction have been available for many years.[85,86]

In one study,[85] 35 of 99 patients thought to have a mechanical large bowel obstruction had other diagnoses following a contrast enema, of whom 11 had pseudo-obstruction. Of the 18 patients thought

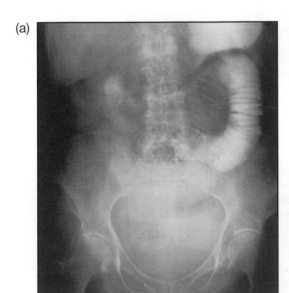
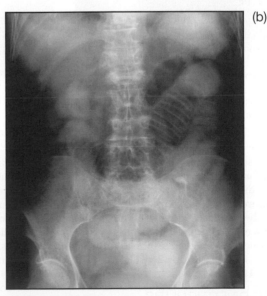

Figure 5.2 • Supine abdominal radiograph taken **(a)** 90 minutes and **(b)** 4 hours after oral administration of 50 mL of water-soluble contrast material. Note failure of contrast to reach the caecum and the obvious small bowel obstruction. These findings were not obvious on plain radiographs. Laparotomy confirmed small bowel obstruction due to adhesions.

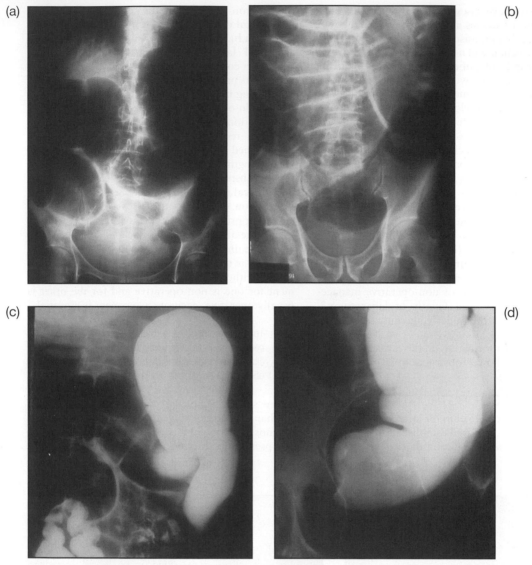

Figure 5.3 • Supine abdominal radiographs in two patients with large bowel obstruction. **(a)** Patient A has pseudo-obstruction; **(b)** patient B has mechanical obstruction. Water-soluble contrast enema confirmed pseudo-obstruction in patient A **(c)** and an obstructing carcinoma of the sigmoid colon in patient B **(d)**.

to have pseudo-obstruction, two were discovered to have a mechanical cause. Although colonoscopy can also differentiate the two conditions and can be therapeutic in the case of pseudo-obstruction,[89] it is less easily arranged in the emergency setting and experienced personnel are required. The surgical management of both large bowel obstruction and the next topic, acute diverticulitis, is covered in Chapter 10.

ACUTE DIVERTICULITIS

The majority of patients who present with symptoms and signs of acute diverticulitis can be managed non-operatively, with the exception of those patients who have overt peritonitis from perforation. Although ultrasonography in experienced hands might identify a thickened segment of colon, perhaps with an associated paracolic collection of fluid, invariably there is too much gas for adequate assessment and quite significant collections can go unnoticed. For this reason clinicians have attempted to evaluate other modalities, such as water-soluble contrast radiology and CT.[90] The former has the ability to identify a 'leak', the latter a collection. Both of these pieces of information may be of use to the surgeon in reaching a decision to operate, even though the ultimate decision must be based on clinical rather than radiological criteria. Overall, CT is no more specific than a contrast enema but does allow guided percutaneous drainage to be carried out if a collection is identified.[91]

Ultrasonography

Over the last two decades, high resolution real-time ultrasonography has become firmly established in the investigative algorithm for many patients with acute abdominal pain. Accurate detection of small amounts of intraperitoneal fluid associated with conditions such as perforated peptic ulcer, acute cholecystitis, acute appendicitis, strangulated bowel and ruptured ovarian cysts can be very helpful in alerting the clinician to the possible severity of the patient's symptoms. Furthermore, reports on the accuracy of ultrasonography in the detection of specific conditions such as acute cholecystitis and appendicitis are impressive. The presence of free fluid, gallstones, a thickened gallbladder wall and a positive ultrasonographic Murphy's sign are all good indicators of acute cholecystitis.[92] This has allowed ultrasound to replace all other investigations, such as radioisotope scanning (HIDA scanning), as the first-line investigation for acute biliary disease, with a sensitivity greater than 95% for the detection of acute cholecystitis.[93] As approximately 25% of patients admitted to hospital with suspected acute cholecystitis are subsequently shown to have another, non-biliary diagnosis,[94] an accurate early diagnosis is essential if current trends in early cholecystectomy for acute cholecystitis, established in the era of open surgery,[95] are to continue in the laparoscopic era.[96] Suspicion of acute biliary disease usually follows clinical assessment, although abnormal liver function tests are additional useful markers of underlying biliary disease.[53] Discriminant analysis of patients admitted with suspected acute biliary disease has shown that abnormal liver function tests and a fever are the only reliable features;[54] consequently, in the majority of patients, if not all, ultrasonography should be performed.

The role of ultrasonography in the detection of acute appendicitis is less well defined than for acute biliary disease. One of the seminal studies on ultrasonography and acute appendicitis came from a group of radiologists and surgeons from the Netherlands, who demonstrated that an acutely inflamed non-perforated appendix can be identified by ultrasonography with a sensitivity of 81% and specificity of 100%.[97] Because the technique relies on visualising a non-compressible swollen appendix, the sensitivity for perforated appendicitis was much lower (29%). Since then other studies have con-

firmed the high sensitivity and specificity of ultrasound in the diagnosis of acute appendicitis[98] and there is little doubt that its use has risen as a result over the last few years. When a scoring system is used for both clinical diagnosis and ultrasonographic findings, the addition of the latter increases the diagnostic accuracy for acute appendicitis.[99,100] Clearly, it would be inappropriate to scan everyone with suspected appendicitis, but where the diagnosis is uncertain, particularly in women, the case for ultrasound scanning is strong, as many alternative diagnoses can be detected.[101]

As surgeons began to achieve a better understanding of ultrasonography, it was only a matter of time before they started performing the ultrasound examination in the acute setting themselves.[102] Early reports were mixed, with some centres demonstrating little value for immediate scanning in all patients,[103] whereas others found it valuable.[104] However, there does appear to be agreement that surgical trainees can reach similar levels of accuracy to radiological trainees, and the main question remaining to be answered is whether immediate bedside ultrasonography in all patients admitted with acute abdominal pain, whether performed by trainees in surgery or radiology, is better than a more selective policy performed by an experienced radiologist after a period of observation. Until this question is answered, the current practice of selective ultrasonography performed by senior personnel based on clinical grounds is likely to continue.

Other areas where ultrasonography is specifically used to assess the acute abdomen are abdominal aortic aneurysms, renal tract disease and acute gynaecological emergencies. The preliminary report suggesting that ultrasonography may also have a role to play in the diagnosis of strangulated small bowel obstruction, by detecting dilated non-peristaltic loops of bowel in association with free intraperitoneal fluid,[76] has been further substantiated by a prospective study from the same unit.[77] Ultrasound can, of course, be useful in detecting acute abdominal wall problems, such as rectus sheath haematoma, and differentiating them from intra-abdominal pathology.[105] Although covered in detail in Chapter 13, ultrasonography also has a role in the early assessment of patients with blunt abdominal trauma.[106]

Computed tomography

The place of CT in the early assessment of the acute abdomen is difficult to evaluate. Its role in the investigation of severity of acute diverticulitis has already been discussed,[90,91] and it can also be used to identify miscellaneous intra-abdominal collections resulting from other conditions. Attempts to improve the diagnostic accuracy of acute appendicitis using CT have been impressive, with a 98% accuracy in 100 consecutive patients with suspected appendicitis, of whom 53 had acute appendicitis.[107] However, irrespective of the cost and availability issue, care must be taken to ensure that such techniques of investigation are used to complement rather than to replace the clinical assessment.[108] A randomised study from Cambridge that examined the effect of early CT (within 24 hours of admission) on patients with acute abdominal pain demonstrated a significant reduction in missed serious diagnoses.[109]

Certainly at present, few if any units would advocate routine use of CT as a first-line diagnostic test for the acute non-traumatic abdomen, perhaps with the exception of acute pancreatitis, where contrast-enhanced CT has an important role in demonstrating the presence of pancreatic necrosis (see Chapter 8).

PERITONEAL INVESTIGATIONS

Ultimately, the surgeon assessing the acute abdomen wishes to determine exactly what is going on within the peritoneal cavity. Needle paracentesis has been successfully used for many years to detect conditions such as intestinal perforation, infarction and peritonitis, by demonstrating foul-smelling fluid in the aspirate.[110] Subsequently, surgeons attempted to quantify these results in a more meaningful fashion using both peritoneal lavage[111] and fine catheter aspiration cytology.[112]

Peritoneal lavage

A standard peritoneal lavage is carried out using the 'open' technique and the effluent evaluated for white cell concentration, amylase, bacteria and bile. A review of the literature[111] demonstrated impressive results, with a mean accuracy of 93%, false-positive rate of 1.6% and false-negative rate of 1%.

Fine catheter peritoneal cytology

Fine catheter peritoneal cytology was first introduced by Richard Stewart from Wellington, New Zealand,[112] and is more simple than lavage but equally accurate. It involves the insertion of a venous cannula into the peritoneal cavity under local anaesthesia through which a fine umbilical catheter is inserted. Peritoneal fluid is aspirated back, placed on a slide, stained and examined under a light microscope for percentage of polymorphonuclear cells. A value greater than 50% suggests a significant underlying inflammatory process but obviously cannot identify the exact cause. This procedure can be carried out at the bedside or even in the accident and emergency department and has been shown to significantly improve surgical decision-making, whether it is used in all patents with acute abdominal pain[113] or just those with suspected acute appendicitis,[114] when the sensitivity and specificity have been reported as 91% and 94% respectively.[115]

Laparoscopy

The first reported use of laparoscopy to evaluate acute abdominal pain was in 1978 when Sugarbaker and colleagues performed laparoscopy before laparotomy in a group of patients in whom the decision to operate was uncertain.[116] They showed that following laparoscopy 18 patients were spared an unnecessary laparotomy, whereas 6 of 27 patients going straight to laparotomy did not require surgery. Following on from this, other surgeons became interested in laparoscopy, which until then had previously been left to the gynaecologists since its introduction in 1902 and early use by surgical gastroenterologists to investigate liver disorders, intra-abdominal masses and malignancies.

Many studies have now demonstrated that laparoscopy significantly improves surgical decision-making in patients with acute abdominal pain,[117] particularly when the need for operation is uncertain.[45] If one specifically looks at suspected appendicitis, then the argument for laparoscopy increases. In a study from St Mary's Hospital in London[118] of 90 patients with suspected appendicitis, 50 were thought definitely to require appendicectomy and in 40 the decision was uncertain, but the surgeon had elected to 'look and see' rather than 'wait and see'. The error rate in the 50 patients going straight to appendicectomy was 22% but was only 8% in the uncertain group, who all underwent laparoscopy first and those with a normal appendix had no further surgery. In a hypothetical situation without laparoscopy, the overall unnecessary appendicectomy rate in the whole series would have been 25/90, with the error rate in women (19/49, 39%) being more than twice that in men (6/41, 15%). Thus there is a strong argument in support of the view that all women with suspected appendicitis should undergo laparoscopy before appendicectomy. A recent randomised trial comparing early laparoscopy versus observation in patients admitted to hospital with suspected NSAP[119] has clearly supported the use of early laparoscopy because of its higher diagnostic accuracy and subsequent improved quality of life (assessed 6 weeks after discharge from hospital).

As mentioned earlier, more than 13% of all women admitted to a surgical ward with acute abdominal pain have a gynaecological cause,[21] which may only come to light at laparoscopy. With the recognised complication rate associated with the removal of a normal appendix lying somewhere between 17 and 21%, depending on whether other conditions have been found,[120] continuing to accept an unnecessary appendicectomy rate of around 20% or higher[121] is no longer defensible. There is, of course, the question of what to do if at laparoscopy a normal appendix is seen but no other condition can be identified which could account for the patient's symptoms. Some surgeons might argue that in this case the appendix should be removed, either by formal open appendicectomy or by using the laparoscopic approach, because a normal-looking appendix can be found to have histological evidence of mucosal inflammation.[122] However, there have been other studies which have shown that even histologically normal appendices can subsequently be shown to contain inflammatory changes if more advanced analyses are used.[123] A study attempting to evaluate accurately the ability of laparoscopy to discriminate between a normal and an inflamed appendix demonstrated a sensitivity of 100% and a specificity of 85% only if an appendix with isolated mucosal inflammation was considered as normal. If an appendix with mucosal inflammation was considered to be inflamed, the sensitivity fell to 92% while the specificity remained at 85%.[124] As the significance of isolated mucosal inflammation in an otherwise normal-looking appendix is highly debatable, a pragmatic approach would be to remove the appendix when it looks inflamed at laparoscopy but do nothing further if it looks normal. The decision may differ in each patient and the final course of action has to be left to the operating surgeon. The author has always taken this pragmatic view and has never knowingly had reason for regret. This area remains controversial and is discussed further in Chapter 9.

 What remains clear is the overwhelming evidence in support of the use of diagnostic laparoscopy in the management of patients with acute abdominal pain in whom the need for surgery is uncertain and in women with suspected appendicitis.

As laparoscopes have reduced in size with optical quality maintained, so it has become possible to carry out 'minilaparoscopy' (**Fig. 5.4**) under local anaesthesia for acute abdominal pain,[125] with results comparable to those already reported using larger laparoscopes and general anaesthesia. This is certainly an area which is likely to receive increasing attention over the next few years.

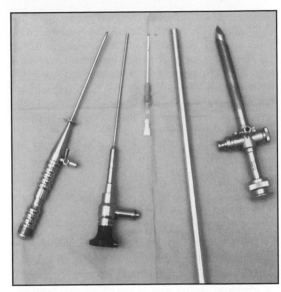

Figure 5.4 • A 2.7-mm 'minilaparoscope' (second from the left). From left to right: trocar and port, minilaparoscope, size 14G venous cannula, 10-mm laparoscope and its trocar and port.

SURGICAL SUBSPECIALISATION

All general surgeons treating emergencies must keep up to date in all the subspecialties and be aware of new developments in both diagnosis and early management in order to provide the best care for their patients. However, the increasing trend towards subspecialisation in elective general surgery has, not surprisingly, resulted in some consultants becoming increasingly uncomfortable with the broader knowledge and skills required for emergency surgery when their elective practice is in an unrelated field, such as breast and endocrine surgery. Although separate on-call rotas for vascular emergencies are now extremely common in the UK, there is an increasing number of hospitals where subspecialty inter-unit referrals for complex emergency oesophago-gastric, hepatobiliary–pancreatic and colorectal problems are undertaken.[126] This is yet another on-call commitment for the increasingly pressurised consultant with a subspecialist interest. However, there appears to be no doubt that, even within abdominal surgery, emergency subspecialisation influences outcome. Patients undergoing emergency colorectal surgery are less likely to have a stoma fashioned if the surgeons operating have a specialist interest in colorectal surgery;[127] likewise, patients with acute biliary disease are more likely to undergo laparoscopic cholecystectomy during their index admission when a subspecialist upper gastrointestinal surgical service is available.[128] If implemented throughout the UK, this policy of emergency subspecialisation would have widespread and far-reaching effects, not only on the surgical rotas within larger hospitals but on the very existence of emergency surgical services in smaller hospitals. Early results from Edinburgh, where upper and lower gastrointestinal surgery, both elective and emergency, was divided in 2002, have been encouraging,[129,130] although different solutions will need to be tailored to local requirements.

• **Key points**

- The art of good management of patients with acute abdominal pain lies in an accurate history, careful examination and logical decision-making, taking into account results from all appropriate and available investigations.
- Regular reassessment of patients is an essential part of this process and emergency surgeons who do not make use of the investigative options discussed in this chapter are in danger of falling short of providing the standards of care which patients with acute abdominal pain now have a right to expect.
- The ability to provide adequate emergency surgical care, with careful observation and reassessment, is increasingly likely to be provided in the future by dedicated emergency surgical teams without elective commitments.
- Swift access to investigations and an emergency theatre must also be made available.
- Although emergency subspecialisation has great attractions for the overall care of the emergency patient with complex problems, this area of development will depend very much on local resources, requirements and workload.

REFERENCES

1. Senate of the Royal Surgical Colleges of Great Britain and Ireland. Consultant practice and surgical training in the UK. London: Royal Surgical Colleges, 1994.

2. Hobbs R Rising emergency admissions. Br Med J 1995; 310:207–8.

3. Ellis BW, Rivett RC, Dudley HAF. Extending the use of clinical audit data: a resource planning model. Br Med J 1990; 301:159–62.

4. Campling EA, Devlin HB, Hoile RW, Lunne JN. Report of the National Confidential Enquiry into Peri-operative Deaths 1990. London: HMSO, 1992.

5. NHS Management Executive. Junior doctors, the New Deal. Working arrangements for hospital doctors and dentists in training. London: Department of Health, 1991.

6. European Working Time Directive 93/104/EC.

7. Calman K. Hospital doctors: training for the future. The report of the working group on specialist medical training. London: HMSO, 1993.

8. Beecham L. New Scottish CMO criticises training reforms. Br Med J 1996; 313:947.

9. Hilton JR, Shiralkar SP, Samsudin A et al. Disruption of the on-call surgical team. Ann R Coll Surg Engl 2002; 84(Suppl.):50–3.

10. Addison PDR, Getgood A, Paterson-Brown S. Separating elective and emergency surgical care (the emergency team). Scot Med J 2001; 46:48–50.

 11. Thomson HJ, Jones PF. Active observation in acute abdominal pain. Am J Surg 1986; 152:522–5.

12. Calder FR, Jadhav V, Hale JE. The effect of a dedicated emergency theatre facility on emergency operating patterns. J R Coll Surg Edinb 1998; 43:17–19.

13. Cochrane RA, Edwards AT, Crosby DL et al. Senior surgeons and radiologists should assess emergency patients on presentation: a prospective randomised controlled trial. J R Coll Surg Edinb 1998; 43:324–7.

14. Irvin TT. Abdominal pain: a surgical audit of 1190 emergency admissions. Br J Surg 1989; 76:1121–5.

15. Gray DWR, Collin J. Non-specific abdominal pain as a cause of acute admission to hospital. Br J Surg 1987; 74:239–42.

16. Paterson-Brown S. The acute abdomen: the role of laparoscopy. In: Williamson RCN, Thompson JN (eds) Baillières clinical gastroenterology: gastrointestinal emergencies, Part 1. London: Baillière Tindall, 1991; pp. 691–703.

17. Gallegos NC, Hobsley M. Abdominal wall pain: an alternative diagnosis. Br J Surg 1990; 77:1167–70.

18. Hall PN, Lee APB. Rectus nerve entrapment causing abdominal pain. Br J Surg 1988; 75:917.

19. Gray DWR, Seabrook G, Dixon JM, Collin J. Is abdominal wall tenderness a useful sign in the diagnosis of non-specific abdominal pain? Ann R Coll Surg Engl 1988; 70:233–4.

20. de Dombal FT, Matharu SS, Staniland JR et al. Presentation of cancer to hospital as 'acute abdominal pain'. Br J Surg 1980; 67:413–16.

21. Paterson-Brown S, Eckersley JRT, Dudley HAF. The gynaecological profile of acute general surgery. J R Coll Surg Edinb 1988; 33:13–15.

22. Pearce JM. Pelvic inflammatory disease. Br Med J 1990; 300:1090–1.

23. Shanahan D, Lord PH, Grogono J, Wastell C. Clinical acute cholecystitis and the Curtis–Fitz-Hugh syndrome. Ann R Coll Surg Engl 1988; 70:45–7.

24. Ravichandran D, Burge DM. Pneumonia presenting with acute abdominal pain in children. Br J Surg 1996; 83:1706–8.

25. Blidaru P, Blidaru A, Popa G. False acute abdomen in emergency surgery. Br J Surg 1996; 83(Suppl. 2): 61–2.

26. de Dombal FT, Leaper DJ, Staniland JR, McCann AI, Horrocks JC. Computer-aided diagnosis of acute abdominal pain. Br Med J 1972; 2:9–13.

27. Gunn AA. The diagnosis of acute abdominal pain with computer analysis. J R Coll Surg Edinb 1976; 21:170–2.

28. Adams ID, Chan M, Clifford PC et al. Computer aided diagnosis of acute abdominal pain: a multi-centre study. Br Med J 1986; 293:800–4.

29. Clifford PC, Chan M, Hewett DJ. The acute abdomen: management with microcomputer aid. Ann R Coll Surg Engl 1986; 6:182–4.

30. Scarlett P, Cooke WM, Clarke D, Bates C, Chan M. Computer aided diagnosis of acute abdominal pain at Middlesbrough General Hospital. Ann R Coll Surg Engl 1986; 68:179–81.

31. Batstone GF. Educational aspects of medical audit. Br Med J 1990; 301:326–8.

32. Gruer R, Gunn AA, Gordon DS, Ruckley CV. Hospital practice: audit of surgical audit. Lancet 1986; ii:23–5.

33. Marteau TM, Wynne G, Kaye W, Evans TR. Resuscitation: experience without feedback increases confidence but not skill. Br Med J 1990; 300:849–50.

34. Lawrence PC, Clifford PC, Taylor IF. Acute abdominal pain: computer aided diagnosis by non-medically qualified staff. Ann R Coll Surg Engl 1987; 69:233–4.

This paper demonstrates that medical students assessing patients with acute abdominal pain using a structured proforma and then CAD have the same diagnostic accuracy as medical staff who use the proforma but not CAD.

35. Paterson-Brown S, Vipond MN, Simms K, Gatzen C, Thompson JN, Dudley HAF. Clinical decision-making and laparoscopy versus computer prediction in the management of the acute abdomen. Br J Surg 1989; 76:1011–13.

The addition of structured patient proformas without CAD significantly improved clinical decision-making and laparoscopy.

36. Korner H, Sondenaa K, Soreide JA, Andersen E, Nysted A, Lende TH. Structured data collection improves the diagnosis of acute appendicitis. Br J Surg 1998; 85:341–4.

37. Bennett DH, Tambeur LJMT, Campbell WB. Use of coughing test to diagnose peritonitis. Br Med J 1994; 308:1336–7.

38. Williams NMA, Johnstone JM, Everson NW The diagnostic value of symptoms and signs in child-hood abdominal pain. J R Coll Surg Edinb 1998; 43:390–2.

39. Dixon JM, Elton RA, Rainey JB, McLeod DAD. Rectal examination in patients with pain in the right lower quadrant of the abdomen. Br Med J 1991; 302:386–8.

40. Howie CR, Gunn AA. Temperature: a poor diag-nostic indicator in abdominal pain. J R Coll Surg Edinb 1984; 29:249–51.

41. Kylanpaa-Back M-L, Kemppainen E, Puolakkainen P et al. Reliable screening for acute pancreatitis with rapid urine trypsinogen-2 test strip. Br J Surg 2000; 87:49–52.

42. 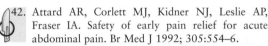 Attard AR, Corlett MJ, Kidner NJ, Leslie AP, Fraser IA. Safety of early pain relief for acute abdominal pain. Br Med J 1992; 305:554–6.

Assessment of patients with acute abdominal pain is not affected adversely by early analgesia.

43. Thomas SH, Cheema F, Reisner A et al. Effects of morphine analgesia on diagnostic accuracy in emergency department patients with abdominal pain: a prospective randomized trial. J Am Coll Surg 2003; 196:18–31.

This was a randomised study of 74 patients who received either morphine or placebo. The diagnostic accuracy was not affected by morphine.

44. Clavien PA, Burgan S, Moossa AR. Serum enzymes and other laboratory tests in acute pancreatitis. Br J Surg 1989; 76:1234–43.

45. Paterson-Brown S, Eckersley JRT, Sim AJW, Dudley HAF. Laparoscopy as an adjunct to decision-making in the acute abdomen. Br J Surg 1986; 73:1022–4.

46. Bradbury AW, Brittenden J, McBride K, Ruckley CV. Mesenteric ischaemia: a multi-disciplinary approach. Br J Surg 1995; 82:1446–59.

47. Schoots IG, Koffeman DA, Levi M, van Gulik TM. Systematic review of survival after acute mesenteric ischaemia according to diease aetiology. Br J Surg 2004; 91:17–27.

Data from 45 observational studies including 3692 patients were reviewed. Prognosis after acute mesenteric venous thrombosis is better than for arterial ischaemia; and that for arterial embolism is better than that for arterial thrombosis.

48. Thompson MM, Underwood MJ, Dookeran KA, Lloyd DM, Bell PRF. Role of sequential leucocyte counts and C-reactive protein measurements in acute appendicitis. Br J Surg 1992; 79:822–4.

49. Davies AH, Bernau F, Salisbury A, Souter RG. C-reactive protein in right iliac fossa pain. J R Coll Surg Edinb 1991; 36:242–4.

50. Middleton SB, Whitbread T, Morgans BT, Mason PF. Combination of skin temperature and a single white cell count does not improve diagnostic accuracy in acute appendicitis. Br J Surg 1996; 83:499.

51. Gronroos JM, Gronroos P. Leucocyte and C-reactive protein in the diagnosis of acute appendicitis. Br J Surg 1999; 86:501–4.

52. Andersson REB. Meta-analysis of the clinical and laboratory diagnosis of appendicitis. Br J Surg 2004; 91:28–37.

    Systematic Medline search of 28 diagnostic variables in 24 studies.

53. Dunlop MG, King PM, Gunn AA. Acute abdominal pain: the value of liver function tests in suspected cholelithiasis. J R Coll Surg Edinb 1989; 34:124–7.

54. Stower MJ, Hardcastle JD. Is it acute cholecystitis? Ann R Coll Surg Engl 1986; 68:234.

55. Cochrane RA, Edwards AT, Crosby DL et al. Senior surgeons and radiologists should assess emergency patients on presentation: a prospective randomised controlled trial. J R Coll Surg Edinb 1998; 43:324–7.

56. Miller RE, Nelson SW. The roentgenologic demonstration of tiny amounts of free intra-peritoneal gas: experimental and clinical studies. Am J Roentgenol 1971; 112:574–85.

57. Chen S-C, Yen Z-S, Wang H-P, Lin F-Y, Hsu C-Y, Chen W-J. Ultrasonography is superior to plain radiology in the diagnosis of pneumoperitoneum. Br J Surg 2002; 89:351–4.

58. Lee IWR. The plain X-ray in the acute abdomen: a surgeon's evaluation. Br J Surg 1976; 63:763–6.

59. Stower ML, Amar SS, Mikulin T, Kean DM, Hardcastle JD. Evaluation of the plain abdominal X-ray in the acute abdomen. J R Soc Med 1985; 78:630–3.

60. Anyanwu AC, Moalypour SM. Are abdominal radiographs still overutilized in the assessment of acute abdominal pain? A district general audit. J R Coll Surg Edinb 1998; 43:267–70.

61. de Lacey GJ, Wignall BK, Bradbrooke S, Reidy J, Hussain S, Cramer B. Rationalising abdominal radiography in the accident and emergency department. Clin Radiol 1980; 31:453–5.

62. Eissenberg RL, Heineken P, Hedgcock MW, Federle M, Goldberg HI. Evaluation of plain abdominal radiographs in the diagnosis of abdominal pain. Ann Intern Med 1982; 97:257–61.

63. Campbell JPM, Gunn AA. Plain abdominal radiographs and acute abdominal pain. Br J Surg 1988; 75:554–6.

64. Field S, Guy PJ, Upsdell SM, Scourfield AE. The erect abdominal radiograph in the acute abdomen: should its routine use be abandoned? Br Med J 1985; 290:1934–6.

65. Simpson A, Sandeman D, Nixon SJ, Goulbourne IA, Grieve DC, Macintyre IMC. The value of an erect abdominal radiograph in the diagnosis of intestinal obstruction. Clin Radiol 1985; 36:41–2.

66. Traill ZC, Nolan DJ. Imaging of intestinal obstruction. Br J Hosp Med. 1996; 55:267–71.

67. Matheson NA, Dudley HAF. Contrast radiography: an aid to postoperative management. Lancet 1963; i:914–17.

68. Zer M, Kaznelson D, Feigenberg Z, Dintsman M. The value of gastrografin in the differential diagnosis of paralytic ileus versus mechanical intestinal obstruction: a critical review and report of two cases. Dis Colon Rectum 1977; 20:573–9.

69. Ott DJ, Gelfand DW. Gastrointestinal contrast agents: indications, uses and risks. JAMA 1983; 249:2380–4.

70. Wellwood JM, Wilson AN, Hopkinson BR. Gastrografin as an aid to the diagnosis of perforated peptic ulcer. Br J Surg 1971; 58:245–9.

71. Fraser GM, Fraser ID. Gastrografin in perforated duodenal ulcer and acute pancreatitis. Clin Radiol 1974; 25:397–402.

72. Donovan AJ, Vinson TL, Maulsby GO, Gewin JR. Selective treatment of duodenal ulcer with perforation. Ann Surg 1979; 189:627–36.

73. Crofts TJ, Park KGM, Steele RJC, Chung SS, Li AKC. A randomized trial of non-operative treatment for perforated peptic ulcer. N Engl J Med 1989; 320:970–3.

74. Stewardson RH, Bombeck CT, Nyhus LM. Critical operative management of small bowel obstruction. Ann Surg 1978; 187:189–93.

75. Pain JA, Collier D St J, Hanka R. Small bowel obstruction: computer-assisted prediction of strangulation at presentation. Br J Surg 1987; 74:981–3.

76. Ogata M, Imai S, Hosotani R, Aoyama H, Hayaashi M, Ishikawa T. Abdominal ultrasonography for the diagnosis of strangulation in small bowel obstruction. Br J Surg 1994; 81:421–4.

77. Ogata M, Mateer JR, Condon RE. Prospective evaluation of abdominal sonography for the diagnosis of bowel obstruction. Ann Surg 1996; 223:237–41.

78. Dunn JT, Halls JM, Berne TV. Roentenographic contrast studies in acute small bowel obstruction. Arch Surg 1984; 119:1305–8.

79. Riveron FA, Obeid FN, Horst HM, Sorensen VJ, Bivins BA. The role of contrast radiography in presumed bowel obstruction. Surgery 1989; 106:496–501.

80. Chung CC, Meng WC, Yu SC, Leung KL, Lau WY, Li AK. A prospective study on the use of water-soluble contrast follow-through radiology in the management of small bowel obstruction. Aust N Z J Surg 1996; 66:598–601.

81. Brochwocz MJ, Paterson-Brown S, Murchison JT. Small bowel obstruction: the water-soluble follow-through revisited. Clin Radiol 2003; 58:393–7.

82. Chen S-C, Lin F-Y, Lee P-H, Yu S-C, Wang S-M, Chang J-J. Water soluble contrast study predicts the need for early surgery in adhesive small bowel obstruction. Br J Surg 1999; 86:1692–8.

83. Joyce WP, Delaney PV, Gorey TF, Fitzpatrick JM. The value of water-soluble contrast radiology in the management of acute small bowel obstruction. Ann R Coll Surg Engl 1992; 74:422–5.

84. Caroline DF, Herlinger H, Laufer I, Kressel HY, Levine MS. Small-bowel enema in the diagnosis of adhesive obstructions. Am J Roentgenol 1984; 142:1133–9.

85. Stewart J, Finan BJ, Courtney DF, Brennan TG. Does a water soluble contrast enema assist in the management of acute large bowel obstruction: a prospective study of 117 cases. Br J Surg 1984; 71:799–801.

Clinicians cannot differentiate on plain abdominal films and clinical assessment alone between mechanical large bowel obstruction and pseudo-obstruction.

86. Koruth NM, Koruth A, Matheson NA. The place of contrast enema in the management of large bowel obstruction. J R Coll Surg Edinb 1985; 30:258–60.

Should be routine in all patients who present with large bowel obstruction.

87. Murphy JB. Ileus. JAMA 1896; 26:15–22.

88. Dudley HAF, Paterson-Brown S. Pseudo-obstruction. Br Med J 1986; 292:1157–8.

89. Munro A, Youngson GG. Colonoscopy in the diagnosis and treatment of colonic pseudoobstruction. J R Coll Surg Edinb 1983; 28:391–3.

90. Shrier D, Skucas J, Weiss S. Diverticulitis: an evaluation by computer tomography and contrast enema. Am Coll Gastroenterol 1991; 86:1466–71.

91. McKee RF, Deignan RW, Krukowski ZH. Radiological investigation in acute diverticulitis. Br J Surg 1993; 80:560–5.

92. Laing FC, Federie MP, Jeffrey RB, Brown TW. Ultrasonic evaluation of patients with acute right upper quadrant pain. Radiology 1981; 140:449–55.

93. Samuels BL, Freitas JE, Bree RL, Schwab RE, Heller ST. A comparison of radionuclide hepatobiliary imaging and real-time ultrasound for the detection of acute cholecystitis. Radiology 1983; 47:207–10.

94. Schofield PF, Hulton NR, Baildam AD. Is it acute cholecystitis? Ann R Coll Surg Engl 1986; 6:14–16.

95. Addison NY, Finan PJ. Urgent and early cholecystectomy for acute gallbladder disease. Br J Surg 1988; 75:141–3.

96. Lo CM, Liu CL, Tan ST, Lai ECS, Wong J. Prospective randomised study of early versus delayed laparoscopic cholecystectomy for acute cholecystitis. Ann Surg 1998; 227:461–7.

97. Puylaert IBCM, Rutgers PF, Lalisang RI et al. A prospective study of ultrasonography in the diagnosis of appendicitis. N Engl J Med 1987; 317:666–9.

98. Schwerk WB, Ruschoff BWJ, Rothmund M. Acute and perforated appendicitis: current experience with ultrasound-aided diagnosis. World J Surg 1990; 14:271–6.

99. Gallego MG, Fadrique B, Nieto MA et al. Evaluation of ultrasonography and clinical diagnostic scoring in suspected appendicitis. Br J Surg 1998; 85:37–40.

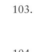

100. Douglas CD, Macpherson NE, Davidson PM, Gani JS. Randomised controlled trial of ultrasonography in diagnosis of acute appendicitis, incorporating the Alvarado score. Br Med J 2000; 321:919–22.

Data from 302 patients randomised to Alvarado scoring then ultrasonography or control. Patients in ultrasonography group who had a therapeutic operation had a significantly shorter time to operation than control group (7 vs. 10 hours) but no difference in hospital stay, nontherapeutic operation rate or delayed treatment in relation to perforation.

101. McGrath FP, Keeling F. The role of early sonography in the management of the acute abdomen. Clin Radiol 1991; 44:172–4.

102. Parys BT, Barr H, Chantarasak ND, Eyes BE, Wu AVO. Use of ultrasound scan as a bedside diagnostic aid. Br J Surg 1987; 74:611–22.

103. Davies AH, Mastorakou I, Cobb R, Rogers C, Lindsell D, Mortensen NJ. Ultrasonography in the acute abdomen. Br J Surg 1991; 78:1178–80.

104. Williams RJLI, Windsor ACJ, Rosin RD, Mann DV, Crofton M. Ultrasound scanning of the acute abdomen by surgeons in training. Ann R Coll Surg Engl 1994; 76:228–33.

105. Klingler PJ, Wetscher G, Glaser K, Tschmelitsch J, Schmid T, Hinder RA. The use of ultrasound to differentiate rectus sheath hematoma from other acute abdominal disorders. Surg Endosc 1999; 13:1129–34.

106. Stengel D, Bauwens K, Sehouli J et al. Systematic review and meta-analysis of emergency ultrasonography for blunt abdominal trauma. Br J Surg 2001; 88:901–12.

107. Rao PM, Rhea JT, Novelline RA, Mostafavi AA, McCabe CJ. Effect of computed tomography of the appendix on treatment of patients and use of hospital resources. N Engl J Med 1998; 338:141–6.

108. McColl I. More precision in diagnosing appendicitis. New Engl J Med. 1998; 338:190–1

109. Ng CS, Watson CJE, Palmer CR et al. Evaluation of early abdominopelvic computer tomography in patients with acute abdominal pain of unknown cause: prospective randomised study. Br Med J 2002; 325:1387–9.

In this study 120 patients were randomised. There was no significant reduction in hospital stay but improved diagnostic accuracy and less missed serious conditions in the group undergoing CT.

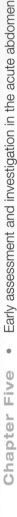

110. Baker WNW, Mackie DB, Newcombe IF. Diagnostic paracentesis in the acute abdomen. Br Med J 1967; 3:146–9.

111. Hoffmann J. Peritoneal lavage in the diagnosis of the acute abdomen of non-traumatic origin. Acta Chir Scand 1987; 153:561–5.

112. Stewart RJ, Gupta RK, Purdie GL, Isbister WH. Fine catheter aspiration cytology of peritoneal cavity improves decision-making about difficult cases of acute abdominal pain. Lancet 1986; ii:1414–15.

113. Baigrie RJ, Saidan Z, Scott-Coombes D et al. Role of fine catheter peritoneal cytology and laparoscopy in the management of acute abdominal pain. Br J Surg 1991; 78:167–70.

114. Baigrie RJ, Scott-Coombes D, Saidan Z, Vipond MN, Paterson-Brown S, Thompson JN. The selective use of fine catheter peritoneal cytology and laparoscopy reduces the unnecessary appendicectomy rate. Br J Clin Pract 1992; 46:173–6.

115. Caldwell MTP, Watson RGK. Peritoneal aspiration cytology as a diagnostic aid in acute appendicitis. Br J Surg 1994; 81:276–8.

116. Sugarbaker PH, Bloom BS, Sanders IH, Wilson RE. Pre-operative laparoscopy in diagnosis of acute abdominal pain. Lancet 1975; i:442–5.

117. Paterson-Brown S. Emergency laparoscopic surgery. Br J Surg 1993; 80:279–83.

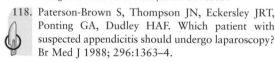

Review article showing the overwhelming evidence in support of diagnostic laparoscopy in the assessment of patients with acute abdominal pain, particularly when the diagnosis and decision to operate is in doubt.

118. Paterson-Brown S, Thompson JN, Eckersley JRT, Ponting GA, Dudley HAF. Which patient with suspected appendicitis should undergo laparoscopy? Br Med J 1988; 296:1363–4.

A prospective evaluation of the accuracy of decision-making in patients with suspected appendicitis, using laparoscopy when the decision is in doubt. Significantly improved results using laparoscopy, especially in women.

119. Decadt B, Sussman L, Lewis MPN et al. Randomised clinical trial of early laparoscopy in the management of acute non-specific abdominal pain. Br J Surg 1999; 86:1383–6.

Only reported randomised trial which has demonstrated the improvements in diagnostic accuracy and subsequent quality of life in the group undergoing laparoscopy.

120. Chang FC, Hogle HH, Welling DR. The fate of the negative appendix. Am J Surg 1973; 126:752–4.

121. Baigrie RJ, Dehn TCB, Fowler SM, Dunn DC. Analysis of 8651 appendicectomies in England and Wales during 1992. Br J Surg 1995; 2:933.

122. Lau WY, Fan ST, Yiu TF, Chu KW, Suen HC, Wong KK. The clinical significance of routine histo-pathological study of the resected appendix and safety of appendiceal inversion. Surg Gynecol Obstet 1986; 162:256–8.

123. Wang Y, Reen DJ, Puri P. Is a histologically normal appendix following emergency appendicectomy always normal? Lancet 1996; 347:1076–9.

124. Champault G, Taffinder N, Ziol M, Rizk N, Catheline JM. Recognition of a pathological appendix during laparoscopy: a prospective study of 81 cases. Br J Surg 1997; 84:671.

125. Pursnani KG, Salman AA. Diagnostic mini-laparoscopy under local anaesthesia in the management of acute abdominal pain. Br J Surg 1997; 84:1583.

126. Dawson EJ, Paterson-Brown S. Emergency general surgery and the implications for specialisation. The Surgeon 2004; 2:165–70.

127. Darby CR, Berry AR, Mortensen N. Management variability in surgery for colorectal emergencies. Br J Surg 1992; 79:206–10.

128. Mercer SJ, Knight JS, Toh SKC, Walters AM, Sadek SA, Somers SS. Implementation of a specialist-led service for the management of acute gallstone disease. Br J Surg 2004; 91:504–8.

129. Elson DW, Sa'adedin F, Partridge R et al. The separation of upper and lower emergency surgery: implications for emergency specialisation. Br J Surg 2004; 91(Suppl. 1):62.

130. Anakwe REB, Collie MHS, Bradnock T, Zorcolo L, Bartolo DCCB. A study to assess the impact of a new specialist colorectal unit. Br J Surg 2004; 91(Suppl. 1):iv–v.

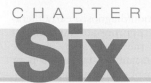

CHAPTER

Six

Perforations of the upper gastrointestinal tract

David C. Gotley

INTRODUCTION

Perforations of the upper gastrointestinal tract can be broadly divided into iatrogenic and 'spontaneous' (**Box 6.1**). Such a classification is helpful in evaluating the published literature for treatment and outcomes since, as a general rule, iatrogenic perforations tend to be recognised earlier than spontaneous perforations, which occur out of hospital, are more difficult to treat and have a worse outcome. This chapter focuses on the more common events in clinical practice, on areas of particular controversy and those subject to recent innovations. Unfortunately, reliable high-level data in this subject are scarce, and hence critical appraisal is difficult. Most authors report results from retrospective clinical experience in small heterogeneous patient groups.

OESOPHAGEAL PERFORATION

Oesophageal perforation has been described as 'the most rapidly fatal and serious perforation of the gastrointestinal tract'.[1] It can occur in the cervical, body or lower oesophagus. Most oesophageal perforations are iatrogenic, caused during instrumentation. Hence measures aimed at prevention, prompt recognition and treatment when the injury occurs all seem to be vital goals for minimising the incidence and impact of iatrogenic oesophageal perforation. Disturbingly, a sizable proportion of these injuries are still diagnosed late.[2]

Box 6.1 • Classification of perforations of the upper gastrointestinal tract

IATROGENIC
Oesophagus
Instrument perforation
Post-irradiation for tumour
Perforation during balloon dilatation for achalasia
Intraoperative
Stomach
Intraoperative
Duodenum
During endoscopic retrograde cholangiopancreatography
SPONTANEOUS
Oesophagus
Boerhaave syndrome
Caustic injury
Stomach
Perforated gastric ulcer
Perforated gastric cancer
Duodenum
Perforated duodenal ulcer

Instrumental perforation

Oesophageal instrumental perforation is a potentially devastating complication. Prompt recognition and treatment of the injury is the key to avoiding death of the patient due to rapid development of overwhelming sepsis, or a protracted and complicated illness and recovery.

Most perforations of the oesophagus are the result of therapeutic endoscopy[3] and the most common follows dilatation of a benign or malignant stricture,[3,4] with the risk higher for malignant strictures.[3] Although modern video/fibreoptic wire-guided dilatation techniques are safer than those employing rigid oesophagoscopes and blind techniques of oesophageal dilatation,[5,6] the increasing frequency of oesophageal instrumentation is probably responsible for the steadily rising rate of iatrogenic oesophageal perforations reported to the UK Thoracic Registry during 1992–96.[2] Perforation rates during dilatation for stricture ranged from 0.5 to 1.6% in recent studies,[4,7] while perforation rates varied from 2 to 6%[3,5] during balloon dilatation for achalasia (Table 6.1).

The principles that underpin low morbidity and mortality rates in managing perforation of the oesophagus are risk minimisation during instrumentation; early recognition/diagnosis; early therapeutic intervention and appropriate tailoring of therapy to the patient, the perforation and the pathology. The most significant risk factors for poor outcome are age, presence of persisting oesophageal obstruction, malignancy and treatment delay.[17–19]

PATHOPHYSIOLOGY

During diagnostic endoscopy, instrumental perforation of the oesophagus tends to occur at anatomical areas of narrowing: the cricopharyngeus–oesophageal junction,[20] the indentation of the aortic arch, the diaphragmatic hiatus and, in obstructive pathology, immediately proximal to a lesion.[21] During dilatation, perforation may occur either just proximal to the stenosis (when non-wire-guided blind dilatation is used)[10] or at the stenosis itself.

Cervical perforation is usually not associated with cervical pathology but is more often related to difficult forceful attempts at oesophageal intubation. The risk, and potential trauma, is amplified by use of the rigid oesophagoscope, and by the presence of kyphosis, pharyngeal diverticulum or a poorly sedated, agitated patient.[21] The posterior wall of the proximal oesophagus is at greatest risk because there is no longitudinal muscle layer (Laimer's triangle) and there is rigid bony confinement by the vertebral bodies (C7/8), which may possess anterior-projecting osteophytes.[22] Because of anatomical attachments in the neck, lateral cervical perforations rarely track into the mediastinum, and this has implications for management. However, posterior perforations of the pharynx and cervical oesophagus may track into the mediastinum because of the relatively loose posterior sagittal connections of the oesophagus to the prevertebral fascia.[23]

Oesophageal body perforations are usually associated with pathology such as a benign or malignant stricture, diverticulum or radiation damage. The pathology consists of either direct instrumental perforation or a longitudinal split through a stricture or tumour owing to shearing or bursting forces. Malignant, radiation and caustic strictures tend to be long, transmural and lack compliance, making them especially susceptible to perforation during dilatation, which results in a crack or rupture of unpredictable length and depth.

Foreign bodies with sharp points or edges may perforate the oesophagus, especially at points of narrowing, or they may pierce the oesophageal wall during retrieval. Perforation can also occur by slow pressure necrosis of the object against the oesophageal wall.

The risk of oesophageal perforation/rupture during balloon dilatation of the lower oesophageal sphincter for achalasia is higher than that for conventional dilatation of the oesophagus (see below). The process results in an uncontrolled tear of the

Table 6.1 • Causes of instrumental oesophageal perforations

Technique	Perforation rate (%)	Reference
Diagnostic endoscopy		
Rigid	0.2–1.9	Wesdorp et al.[8]
Flexible	0.0003–0.01	Dawson and Cockel[9]
Dilatation		
Wire guided	0.5	Adamek et al.[7]
Blind	1.6	Wichern[10]
Achalasia balloon	2–6	Reynolds and Parkman[11]
Stent insertion		
Preformed	7–15	Tytgat[12]
Expandable	1.8	Bartelsman et al.[13]
Laser recanalisation	5	Jensen et al.[14]
Balloon compression of varices	Rare	McGrath[15]
Sclerotherapy for varices	1–3	Lee and Lieberman[16]

Other causes: foreign body removal, argon plasma coagulation, endoscopic mucosal resection, overtube placement, transoesophageal echocardiography, nasogastric tube placement.

oesophagus. The rent is usually (but not always) in the left lateral position, may involve the pleura directly, and is usually longitudinal and at least several centimetres long as a result of the mechanics of the balloon within the oesophagus.

Disruption of the oesophageal wall permits exposure of the mediastinum to a mixture of oropharyngeal secretions, food and bacteria, in addition to gastric contents. Occasionally, the leak is confined to a small local area; this is more likely if there has been previous surgery or pathology in the mediastinum that has resulted in local fibrosis. More often, however, the loose areolar space allows rapid dispersal of this material, with infection, necrosis and systemic toxicity.[10] Most cultures from the mediastinum are polymicrobial, aerobic and anaerobic, with Gram-negative rods (including *Pseudomonas*), streptococci, staphylococci and *Bacteroides* the predominant species.[24] The initiating event may also damage the thin mediastinal pleura, resulting in pleural soiling, fluid extravasation and shock. Early, contained infection may later erode the mediastinal pleura, with similar consequences. Unchecked, these processes will rapidly result in death.

CLINICAL PRESENTATION

The classical clinical features of oesophageal perforation include pain, fever and surgical emphysema, although the condition is notorious for its ability to produce symptoms that mimic a variety of other serious conditions. These include myocardial infarction, aortic dissection, pulmonary embolism, perforated peptic ulcer and pancreatitis. Clearly, if the symptoms follow instrumentation of the oesophagus, the possibility of perforation is increased. Increased levels of suspicion are warranted by a technically 'difficult' procedure, bleeding or otherwise unexplained onset of agitation and restlessness in the patient. Presenting symptoms will obviously depend on the anatomical position of the perforation. Cervical perforation is manifest by cervical pain exacerbated by neck movement and swallowing. There may be tenderness to palpation. Later, the neck may become tense and indurated. Oesophageal body perforation causes retrosternal pain that may radiate to the back, while lower oesophageal perforations may cause acute epigastric pain. Fever invariably accompanies clinically significant perforation of the oesophagus, usually within the first 24 hours. Likewise, surgical emphysema may be detectable during the initial few hours, but it may be a delayed clinical manifestation. It may be palpated in the neck as crepitus or heard on auscultation in synchrony with the heartbeat (Hamman's sign). Cervical perforations result in clinically detectable surgical emphysema more frequently than do thoracic perforations (60% vs. 30%).[25] A pleural effusion may be clinically evident. Dysphagia

or odynophagia can also be a feature. As mediastinal infection spreads, systemic sepsis and shock supervene. Despite these clinical features and an association with recent oesophageal instrumentation, delay in diagnosis is still seen in more than one-third of patients.[2]

In foreign body ingestion/retrieval, sclerotherapy, laser or argon plasma coagulation, a perforation may not manifest for 5–7 days after the procedure.[16,26]

DIAGNOSIS

Since the key element in successful management of oesophageal perforation is early recognition, a high index of suspicion should be maintained in all patients who have undergone therapeutic endoscopy. In the circumstance of persisting pain following oesophageal instrumentation, immediate investigation is warranted. Before the patient has left the endoscopy suite, it may be possible to visualise the rent on re-endoscopy; although this approach is controversial, it can be immediately diagnostic and expedite treatment.[27] A plain chest radiograph will reveal radiological signs in 60% of cases of intrathoracic perforation, such as subcutaneous emphysema, air in prevertebral tissue plains, mediastinal widening and hydropneumothorax.[28] However, it may take at least an hour or more before some of these signs become apparent. The site of perforation can sometimes be deduced on the plain film: mid-oesophageal rupture tends to produce a right-sided pleural effusion, while lower oesophageal perforations produce a left-sided effusion.[29] Although routine chest radiography has been recommended after dilatation of peptic strictures,[30] the cost-effectiveness of this approach has not been established. Contrast radiography using a water-soluble medium will locate 90% of perforations in the thoracic oesophagus[25] but only 60% of cervical perforations because of relatively rapid transit at this level. Hence, a negative result with this technique would not exclude perforation. Although barium sulphate contrast radiology is more accurate, especially with small tears, intramediastinal barium is said to result in an intense granulomatous response, with subsequent severe mediastinal fibrosis. However, when communication with the airway is suspected, soluble hypertonic contrast agents are contraindicated because of the potential for acute pulmonary oedema. Modern low-osmolar non-ionic contrast media, not barium sulphate, are used in the first instance in suspected oesophageal perforation.[31]

Computed tomography (CT) can be a valuable aid in the diagnosis of oesophageal perforation, especially for small subclinical tears. CT-detectable abnormalities include extraluminal air, perioesophageal fluid or abscesses, oesophageal thickening and extraluminal contrast.[32]

PREVENTION

The risk of oesophageal perforation during instrumentation can be minimised with careful technique, including the use of fluoroscopy and appropriate patient selection.[5,33,34] A number of techniques have contributed to prevention.

- *Use of flexible video/fibreoptic endoscopy.* This has substantially reduced the risk of traumatic perforation of the oesophagus compared with rigid oesophagoscopy and should, wherever possible, be the preferred method for routine diagnostic endoscopy. Perforation rates of 0.0003–0.01% have been reported for flexible endoscopy compared with 0.2–1.9% for rigid endoscopy (**Table 6.1**).[8,9] Rigid endoscopy is rarely indicated, except perhaps for removal of large foreign bodies, and it should then only be employed by individuals with appropriate training and experience.
- *Insertion technique.* Gentle introduction of the instrument under vision in a cooperative patient under instruction to swallow (or anaesthetised patient), rather than blind insertion under force through a closed sphincter, will minimise the risk of cervical perforation.
- *Recognition of potential hazards.* The presence of a pharyngo-oesophageal diverticulum, osteoarthropathy of the cervical spine, eccentricity of the cricopharyngeus or oesophagus (indicating external compression and distortion by tumour) and a history of previous surgery in the area are all potential hazards during routine endoscopy. Attempts should be made to recognise the presence of these features before commencing the procedure.
- *Avoidance of force.* Intubation of strictures (benign or malignant) should not be forced.
- *Use of guidewire-directed dilators.* Endoscopically placed guidewires reduce the risk of oesophageal perforation during dilatation.[35] In situations where the endoscope will not pass a tight stricture, trans-stricture placement of a flexible-tipped wire can be confirmed by fluoroscopy.
- *Use of contrast radiology before dilatation.* Tight, long or complex strictures can be delineated with contrast radiology prior to dilatation. In such cases, it may be easier to place a 'floppy' wire radiologically rather than endoscopically. Alternatively, placing the wire through difficult-to-negotiate strictures may be facilitated endoscopically by instillation of water-soluble radiocontrast via the biopsy channel of the instrument.
- *Avoidance of excessive dilatation at the first session.* Graded dilatation should cease beyond one or two size graduations after meeting with resistance, with further sessions of dilatation forming part of a planned programme.[34] Through-the-endoscope balloon dilatation of strictures under direct vision may reduce the risk of perforation because it exerts radial pressure only and the longitudinal shear force exerted by rigid dilators is eliminated.
- *Use of expandable metal/mesh stents for malignant strictures.* These obviate the need for excessive preliminary dilatation of oesophageal tumours, which is required for preformed stents.
- *Awareness of pathology.* Different pathologies produce different stricture characteristics, with different risks of perforation. For example, anastomotic strictures, being surrounded by fibrosis, are more resilient during dilatation than carcinomas or acute inflammatory strictures (such as those from radiation or caustic damage), which are more prone to rupture during dilatation.
- *Use of a sheath or overtube for endoscopic retrieval of sharp foreign bodies.* Sharp foreign bodies in the oesophagus may lacerate the oesophageal wall and cause further trauma on removal. Drawing the foreign body into an overtube reduces this risk.

Achalasia: a case for special consideration

The risk of oesophageal perforation is higher during blind balloon dilatation of the oesophagus than during wire-guided bouginage of benign or malignant strictures, reaching as high as 12% in some series.[36] There are few studies that address the risk factors for perforation in achalasia; the numbers of patients in any individual report are small and the studies retrospective.[37,38] However, it would appear that the risk factors include the presence of a fibrotic stricture, the use of a compliant rather than non-compliant balloon, previous pneumatic dilatation, inflation pressure >69 kPa and high-amplitude oesophageal contractions. Postdilatation indicators of patients with an increased risk of perforation are blood on the balloon, tachycardia and prolonged chest pain lasting longer than 4 hours after dilatation (all patients experience some chest pain or discomfort after balloon dilatation). One group recommends the passage of a 56 Fr oesophageal dilator prior to forceful balloon dilatation to check for easy passage into the stomach; this would exclude the presence of a fibrous or malignant stricture.[5] A safe approach is graduated balloon dilatation. A 30-mm balloon is used in the first instance, with larger balloons (35/40 mm) being reserved for later sessions in those with persisting symptoms.[39]

Routine postdilatation contrast oesophagography is advocated by some because of the relatively high rate of perforation.[40]

MANAGEMENT

The management of oesophageal perforation from any cause remains controversial. Variables attracting debate include conservative versus operative treatment, simple closure/drainage versus resection, oesophageal exclusion, method of closure, early versus late intervention and treatment of cervical versus thoracic oesophageal perforation. More recently, minimally invasive techniques have been introduced. Analysis of published data in this area is difficult because patient numbers are small and different pathologies and methods of treatment have been grouped together. Some studies include spontaneous ruptures, which are known to have a worse outcome compared with ruptures caused by instrumental perforation,[41] and there are too many variables in these cohorts to allow any attempt at meta-analysis. It is clear, however, that delay in treatment increases the risk of morbidity, prolonged hospitalisation and death.[42,43] Since many patients with oesophageal pathology are elderly with clinically significant comorbidity, treatment choice in particular circumstances should be tailored to the individual patient.[44]

Strategies in managing oesophageal instrumental perforations

The principal aims in management of instrumental perforations are to minimise mediastinal or cervical contamination and to treat sepsis.[43] The secondary aim is to restore peroral alimentation. Sometimes this will require an immediate, or staged, procedure to treat the primary pathology. Important variables include site and size of perforation, extent of contamination, presence of systemic sepsis, presence of associated oesophageal disease and the preoperative condition of the patient. As always, resuscitation will be important in some patients but the duration needs to be balanced with the need to avoid undue delay if operation is planned. Treatment with intravenous volume expansion and broad-spectrum antibiotics should be immediate, together with appropriate methods of monitoring such as hourly urine output and central venous pressure measurements. Where a pleural effusion is evident, drainage by basal intercostal catheter should be undertaken. Consideration should be given early to medium-term alimentation, either by parenteral or enteral (jejunal) routes.

The case for non-operative therapy

Non-operative versus operative therapy for oesophageal perforation is contentious, principally because surgical intervention implies the need for thoracotomy, a major procedure with a potentially long recovery time and high risk of morbidity. A case can be made for non-operative treatment of oesophageal perforations for patients in either of two general categories: those with advanced malignant disease and in selected patients with small well-contained perforations. For the latter group, the anatomical position of the perforation is important.

The cervical oesophagus Cervical perforations are often not associated with cervical or oesophageal pathology. Limited local and systemic symptoms and signs of sepsis, lack of surgical emphysema in the mediastinum on chest radiograph, together with radiological demonstration of cervical confinement of the leak have been used to justify a non-operative approach.[45,46] Early instigation of broad-spectrum antibiotics, parenteral nutrition and close observation are the key elements of management, but clinical progression of sepsis, increasing neck pain and induration indicate a need for surgical intervention. Using the above criteria, non-operative management of such perforations has yielded survival rates that compare favourably with surgical management.

The thoracic oesophagus Non-operative treatment of perforations of the thoracic oesophagus is somewhat more difficult and controversial. They are more often associated with underlying pathology in the oesophagus and are less likely to remain localised and contained. Delay in instigation of surgical treatment has resulted in poorer outcomes compared with early surgical intervention,[47] although modern supportive care has tended to reduce mortality rates in these patients, even in those with delayed treatment.

Only a minority of authors have advocated a non-operative approach to perforations of the thoracic oesophagus. An early report by Mengoli and Klassen[48] described the use of nasogastric suction, antibiotics and selective use of intercostal drainage and achieved a survival rate of 14 from 15 patients. To this regimen, others have added the placement of an oesophageal stent to seal the perforation.[8,49] In patients who present late (e.g. >3 days) with oesophageal perforations that are contained and who are without systemic signs of sepsis, non-operative therapy has been successfully employed.[50] Such patients have obviously already undergone a selection process of sorts, since for most the general course of the illness is rapid progression.

There is general agreement that in the conservative management of instrumental oesophageal perforations, selection criteria should include small localised leaks, with ready drainage back into the oesophagus (after contrast radiography), absence of pleural contamination (none or minimal effusion), and low-grade symptoms, with an absence of signs of systemic sepsis.[7,45]

Other variables, including age and level of comorbidity, and extent of the underlying disease (e.g. cancer) will also be important to the decision-making process. Aggressive broad-spectrum antibiotic treatment, parenteral nutrition and nasogastric suction with gastric acid suppression form part of most regimens. Meaningful assessment of outcomes in published reports is difficult, as already mentioned, and there are no randomised studies comparing conservative and operative management in equivalent patients, although, in general, overall survival rates vary from 60 to 90%.[7,8,50-54] The addition of an expandable oesophageal stent to non-operative management presents the potential for improvement in these figures, although no substantial data in support of this technique are yet available.[49,55] The compact nature of the prosthesis obviates the need for dilatation to the extent previously required, and hence has the potential to reduce the risk of complications associated with insertion of preformed stents (**Fig. 6.1**). Use of these stents has been limited to treating those with malignant disease (since they are difficult to remove and may erode into adjacent structures over time). A newly released stent (Polyflex; Rusch, Kernen, Germany) made from silicone has proved useful in treating oesophageal rupture/perforation in benign disease by temporarily occluding the perforation while healing takes place, following which it can

then can easily be removed endoscopically 6–8 weeks later (**Fig. 6.2**). However, stent migration remains a potential problem and needs to be kept in mind during the management of these patients. There are insufficient data as yet to be able to conclude that survival rates are improved; however, the prompt placement of a stent will generally reduce or eliminate gross mediastinal contamination. The timing would seem important not only in early prevention of contamination but also to avoid the risk that late stent placement may prevent drainage of an established cavity back into the oesophagus. Duration of hospitalisation in these patients is an important issue; the length of hospital stay in 20 non-operative patients was no different to that in 66 operatively treated patients (20 vs. 15 days).[50]

If during non-operative management the patient shows signs of clinical deterioration, worsening sepsis or spreading radiographic leakage, then an emergency operation is indicated.[56] The dilemma with this form of treatment is that if the patient deteriorates with spreading sepsis, the optimal timing for surgical intervention is lost (i.e. operation within the first 24 or, perhaps, the first 12 hours[57]) and this remains a potent argument against conservative management for perforation of the thoracic oesophagus.

Endoscopic clipping of an oesophageal rent has also been used successfully as an adjunct to conservative

(a)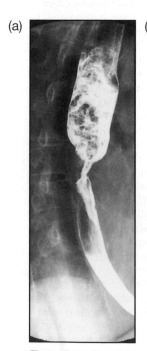

(b)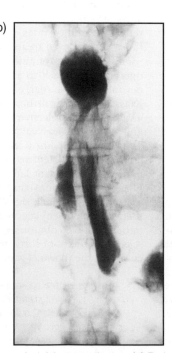

(c)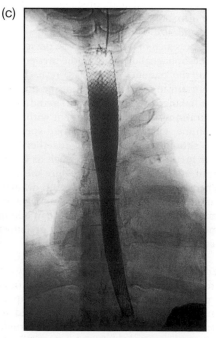

Figure 6.1 • Contrast radiography of the oesophagus. **(a)** Barium swallow demonstrating a tight malignant stricture. **(b)** Water-soluble contrast swallow after dilatation demonstrating a perforation. **(c)** Water-soluble contrast study in the same patient following insertion of an expandable metal stent, demonstrating no further leak.

(a)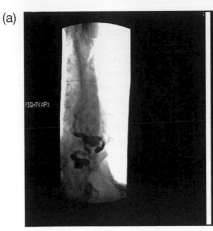

(b)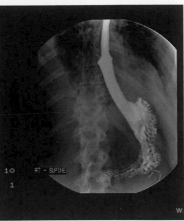

Figure 6.2 • A patient with a ruptured oesophagus which occurred during balloon dilatation for achalasia. The leak was confirmed using oral non-ionic contrast radiography **(a)**. The patient was immediately treated by insertion of a silicone stent **(b)**, which sealed the rent and which was removed endoscopically 8 weeks later when the oesophagus had healed.

management.[58] A conservative non-operative approach has also been advocated for those patients in whom the diagnosis is very delayed or where the patient is very ill or infirm.[59] The justification is on the grounds that thoracotomy only compounds the physical insult. Perhaps minimally invasive techniques through either the chest[60] or abdomen,[61] although not yet widely evaluated, may reduce the added morbidity resulting from thoracotomy.

The case for surgical treatment

The cervical oesophagus Because operations for debridement and drainage of cervical oesophageal perforations carry low morbidity and mortality rates, it could be argued that all perforations in this site should undergo early operation.[62] Historically, surgical exploration and drainage has resulted in lower mortality rates than non-operative methods,[25,63] and most deaths have been related to uncontrolled sepsis.

 As most cervical perforations are not based on local pathology, establishment of adequate drainage for cervical secretions (with or without primary repair) would seem to be the key to these improved results.

The thoracic oesophagus Instrumental perforation of the thoracic oesophagus is an inherently serious complication because it allows oesophageal contents access to the extensive loose tissue plains of the mediastinum, where longitudinal and lateral extension (into the pleura) is common. In these injuries, delay in obtaining control of this process is critical in patient survival,[42,64,65] and effective surgical treatment is early operation. Hence, a decision favouring non-operative management that fails may squander an opportunity for effective surgical salvage and ultimately increase the chances of

death. Late intervention poses increased technical demands because of friability and oedema of the infected tissues, in addition to the undoubted suboptimal physical condition of the patient as a result of established sepsis – both increasing the morbidity and mortality.[65]

 The case for early surgical intervention in perforation of the thoracic oesophagus is therefore compelling on current evidence.

Surgical management of early instrumental perforations

The surgical options available for early perforations include primary repair and drainage, resection, oesophageal exclusion/drainage or bypass. The first two options are currently the most widely used methods. The choice of procedure is based on the time delay since perforation, the general condition of the patient and the type of lesion, i.e. whether it is in otherwise salvageable ('normal') or in diseased oesophagus (e.g. with distal obstruction owing to benign or malignant stricture).

Where the oesophagus is relatively normal without distal obstruction, a promptly diagnosed perforation repaired primarily gives results at least as good or better than those achieved with early resection,[57] and this includes patients with rupture following forced balloon dilatation for achalasia.[27]

Primary repair and drainage A transthoracic approach has been the preferred option over time and has the advantages of excellent exposure, the ability to debride and drain widely and to deal with pleural contamination. The full length of the tear should be clearly exposed, sometimes necessitating vertical oesophago-myotomy above and below the rent.[57] Submucosal and mucosal tissues are debrided to healthy edges and closed with suture or with a stapling device applied vertically to the apposed edges, with an intra-oesophageal bougie (40–46 Fr) for size graduation purposes.[57] The muscle layer can then be closed over the suture line and the area is routinely drained. Some reports have described the addition of buttressing techniques to primary repair, including pleural flap (vascularised), intercostal pedicle and diaphragmatic pedicle.[66] One group has reported reinforcement with absorbable mesh and fibrin glue in four patients with early primary repair, with no leak.[67] However, it is not possible to deduce from published reports whether buttressing improves the results of primary repair in this group with a relatively good prognosis.

Early localised leaks may also be approached using thoracoscopy,[60] which is facilitated by using the prone position. This removes the need for lung retraction and minimises interference from blood and secretions, which drain anteriorly through gravity. The right thorax approach is used for right-sided oesophageal perforations, the left thorax for left-sided oesophageal perforations. Both debridement and suture repair can be readily undertaken using this approach, which has the advantage of avoiding a thoracotomy.

A transabdominal approach to lower oesophageal perforations has been successful too but necessitates that the pleura is intact. A laparoscopic approach is also an option for tears from balloon dilatation for achalasia; this has the potential advantage of reducing postoperative pain and facilitating mobilisation by avoiding a laparotomy.[61]

Following repair, the appropriate timing for removal of the drain is important. In both early and late primary repair, suture line breakdown is common and in this situation controlled external fistulation is essential. A leak will usually manifest from 2 to 8 days or more. Contrast radiography with water-soluble agents should be performed prior to removal of the drain and commencement of alimentation; however, a test swallow of food dye or methylene blue in water can be a sensitive marker of a residual fistula.

Resection Resection of a salvageable oesophagus after early recognition of instrumental perforation is generally regarded as unnecessary.[27]

Diseased oesophagus: primary perforation above a stenosing lesion In the case of benign strictures (caustic or peptic), the extent of oesophageal disease may preclude satisfactory primary repair, and early resection will be indicated. Where dilatation has ruptured the oesophagus immediately above the obstruction, primary repair is likely to break down if the functional distal obstruction is not relieved.[27] Either oesophagoplasty or further stricture dilatation is required, and neither may be realistic in acute

oesophageal perforation. Nevertheless, intraoperative dilatation, primary repair and fundoplication have been employed successfully in the management of perforations above a benign stricture.

In cases of malignant obstruction, primary repair is inappropriate. Stenting with or without drainage may be used as either a temporising or a definitive treatment, especially in frail or very ill patients. However, for those who are fit, resection is the best choice. For those patients with a diseased non-salvageable oesophagus, primary resection can result in early survival rates of 82–100%.[27,64,68] Obviously, longer-term survival will depend on the stage of the tumour.

For perforations of an extensively damaged oesophagus, such as with caustic stricture, long-standing peptic stricture with shortened oesophagus, end-stage achalasia, scleroderma or malignant tumour without dissemination, resection may be the only alternative. In the fit patient, this might be by transthoracic or transhiatal resection.[42,65,69] Alternatively, thoracoscopic mobilisation can be used.[70] Most authors recommend anastomosis outside the field of contamination, but in early perforations this may be less important than achieving an anastomosis with healthy proximal oesophagus, even if this is in the neck. The interposition conduit will usually be the stomach, since in the emergency situation the colon will be unprepared and use of a long jejunal limb is technically demanding and therefore probably inappropriate in the emergency setting. The mortality rate for immediate resection remains around 12–18%.[65]

For the unfit patient, immediate resection poses significant perioperative risks, and attempts to reduce these include resection with a defunctioning oesophagostomy[46] and ongoing alimentation using gastrostomy or jejunostomy. Later reconstruction is necessary to preserve quality of life, but this may be done after a period of recuperation to maximise fitness, with reconstruction through the substernal or subcutaneous route to minimise the technical difficulties and perioperative impact of a repeat transthoracic approach. Alternatively, emergency preliminary stenting may be an appropriate first step to a staged resection of the oesophagus at a later date.

Oesophageal isolation (exclusion), decompression and drainage Oesophageal isolation and drainage has been used in the setting of early-recognised perforations in unfit patients but has been more favoured in the care of the desperately ill with the repair delayed (see below).

Surgical management of delayed perforation
Somewhat more debate surrounds the optimal surgical treatment for patients with delayed perforation

of the thoracic oesophagus. The options include primary closure and drainage,[57,71] immediate resection and reconstruction, staged reconstruction, or oesophageal diversion procedures.[72] In the patient with delayed perforation, primary repair is necessarily undertaken in oedematous, friable and infected tissues and a technically sound closure can be difficult to achieve. Advocates of primary closure, whatever the delay, achieve survival rates of 83–96%, but anastomotic breakdown occurs in 33–83% of patients (after a delay of 24 hours), resulting in a controlled fistula. These generally heal in time and do not appear to affect the mortality rates.[18,57] However, not surprisingly, hospitalisation is often prolonged in these patients (up to 68 days) and, as a result, some surgeons argue for resection. Conversely, prolonged tube drainage associated with jejunostomy feeding need not require long-term hospitalisation.

Uncontrolled sepsis in these situations, requiring further surgical intervention, appears to be uncommon. Buttressing of the suture line with tissue is commonly used but has apparently not improved the results,[43,57] and long-term functional outcome in patients with a normal oesophagus is satisfactory.

It is important to note that localised mediastinal collections may develop in these situations and can sometimes be drained percutaneously under CT guidance. Generally, more extensive drainage (with a large-bore drain) and debridement using an operative approach is needed. For some lower mediastinal collections, drainage can be achieved using either laparotomy or laparoscopy. However, inadequate drainage of a mediastinal abscess is disastrous, with the possible risk of catastrophic secondary haemorrhage.

Resection Proponents of resection for delayed perforation demonstrate survival rates as high as 85%,[64] although in high-risk patients following previous surgical attempts at control of the leak the survival rate can be somewhat lower (44%).[73] The surgical approach is generally transthoracic because wide debridement of necrotic tissue is necessary. However, transhiatal oesophagectomy has also been employed successfully in this setting.[64]

Oesophageal isolation/exclusion and drainage In an attempt to control leakage and preserve the oesophagus in desperate situations, various forms of oesophageal isolation have been used.[72] These techniques generally involve cervical oesophagostomy, oesophageal tube decompression, mediastinal drainage and feeding gastrostomy or jejunostomy. Reflecting the usually desperate circumstances in which these techniques are used, the mortality rates are high (35–80%).[43]

Spontaneous oesophageal rupture (Boerhaave syndrome)

Spontaneous oesophageal rupture is dealt with separately from instrumental oesophageal perforation because the mediastinal/pleural contamination is gross (often being induced following vomiting of a large meal) and at initial presentation the diagnosis is often missed.[74] As a result, the overall survival rates are worse than following instrumental perforation in a fasted patient.

Boerhaave syndrome as 'spontaneous' oesophageal perforation is somewhat of a misnomer, since it is a subset of barotrauma induced by uncoordinated vomiting against a closed cricopharyngeus. Other events that have caused oesophageal rupture in this group include lifting a heavy weight, asthma, childbirth and prolonged coughing. The rent can be small or large and is usually found in the lower oesophagus, just above the lower oesophageal sphincter on the left lateral aspect. Although rupture can take place on the right side of the oesophagus, the left is much more common, perhaps due to thinning of the muscle coat in this area, anterior angulation of the oesophagus and absence of supporting structures at this site.[75] The left pleura is in close proximity at this point and is usually also ruptured.

The clinical presentation is classically with vomiting, lower chest pain and subcutaneous emphysema. The pain is usually excruciating and is exaggerated by swallowing. Dyspnoea is common, perhaps through a combination of pain, splinting and hydropneumothorax. Variations on this presentation account for the frequent misdiagnoses, as high as 50% in one series.[76] Vomiting, however, may be absent, and the patient may present with pneumothorax or pleural effusion. Sometimes the symptoms are predominantly abdominal and a negative laparotomy may have been carried out.

The diagnosis can be made on plain chest radiograph where 88% of patients will have abnormal findings (Fig. 6.3).[29] In fact, the most common error in diagnostic evaluation is failure to obtain a plain chest radiograph when a patient presents with acute upper abdominal symptoms.[77] Pneumothorax, pleural effusion and subcutaneous emphysema are the most common findings. Mediastinal air in fascial plains can be a subtle, but early, sign. Contrast studies are an important adjunct (Fig. 6.4) but, as with oesophageal instrumental perforations, may not reveal the perforation. Tube drainage of an effusion may be diagnostic if it contains food particles, bile, acid or amylase. Oral administration of methylene blue can also be used to confirm a perforation if an intercostal catheter is in place. CT can also be helpful in confirming the diagnosis and visualising any intramediastinal abscesses. Finally,

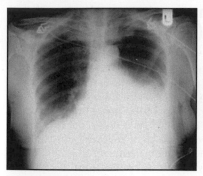

Figure 6.3 • Plain chest radiograph in a patient with Boerhaave syndrome. Note the left-sided pleural effusion.

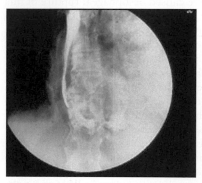

Figure 6.4 • Contrast study in the same patient with Boerhaave syndrome shown in Fig. 6.3, demonstrating a leak into the left pleural cavity.

endoscopic examination can be used to reveal the site, side (right or left) and extent of perforation.

Risk factors for poor outcome are similar to those for instrumental perforation of the oesophagus. They include delay in treatment, size of perforation, underlying disease in the oesophagus, extent of soiling, and age and general condition of the patient.[78] Non-operative treatment is rarely feasible because of the extent of local contamination. The surgical options include drainage alone, drainage and primary repair (with or without buttressing), resection, diversion/exclusion and placement of an intra-oesophageal stent. Extensive debridement of devitalised tissues, pleural cleansing/decortication, elimination of obstruction and both mediastinal and pleural tube drainage are the mainstays of treatment, usually carried out through a left thoracotomy (or right if the perforation is draining into the right pleural cavity). An oesophageal myotomy is necessary to obtain adequate visualisation of the oesophageal mucosal rent (which is usually larger than the muscle tear) and repair can usually be accomplished in two layers. Buttressing is often recommended but there is no firm evidence to support its use. Some surgeons also insert a large

T-tube or even a split chest drain in order to establish a controlled fistula in those patients with gross contamination. Ongoing therapy will include antibiotics, enteric nutrition through a jejunostomy tube and a period of ventilation followed by intensive physiotherapy.

Although reports in the 1980s consistently reflected a high mortality rate from this condition (in the order of 30–60%), a recent report on 21 patients, 12 of whom were referred 24 hours after rupture, described primary oesophageal repair, debridement and drainage with a hospital stay of 14 days and a 14.3% mortality rate.[79] Similar results have been reported following primary repair and fundal wrap.[80] Low mortality rates have also been achieved with oesophagectomy and reconstruction.[17,81]

A single case report describes the successful use of an expandable covered metal stent together with drainage for a small rent.[82] If a Rusch stent is used, it is possible to endoscopically retrieve the stent at a later time, when swelling and oedema have resolved. Expandable metal mesh stents are not removable over time and long-term problems may follow, such as granulation tissue overgrowth and extra-oesophageal erosion. As such they are not recommended.

Caustic injury to the oesophagus

Oesophageal corrosive injury is a major cause of oesophageal perforation and stricture in children. The most common offending agent is sodium hydroxide (caustic soda, lye),[83] but button batteries also cause substantial morbidity when swallowed.[84] Button batteries are constructed of a metal anode and cathode separated by a disc of strong alkali. The battery case is usually not biologically sealed and leakage of the alkali produces rapid localised liquefaction necrosis within a few hours of ingestion. A stored electric charge may facilitate damage, perhaps by aiding leakage. In view of the potential for perforation, all swallowed button batteries should be endoscopically removed, with observation for up to 48 hours to detect delayed perforation.

In adults, oesophageal perforation is a relatively uncommon complication of acute caustic injury (gastric perforation being more common), and the usual scenario is complete recovery for superficial burns but with oesophageal stricture from deep burns. All instances of ingestion of caustic substances, whether accidental or deliberate, need to be taken seriously. Deep oesophageal burns might be evidenced by a history of sodium hydroxide ingestion (particularly the large amount that can occur in deliberate events), bloody emesis and the presence of severe mediastinal pain (although absence of pain cannot be interpreted as indicating a minor burn). Leucocytosis, acidosis, intravascular disseminated coagulopathy and systemic toxicity all indicate extensive necrosis and the likelihood of perforation. Early endoscopy for grading of lesions is mandatory. The presence of grade 3 lesions (mucosal necrosis) on endoscopy places the patient at high risk of perforation. Emergency surgery, when transmural necrosis of the oesophagus or stomach is suspected or manifest, consists of excision of the organ, exteriorisation of the cervical oesophagus and staged reconstruction at a later time, probably using colon because the stomach is often also affected.

Iatrogenic intraoperative oesophageal perforations

Inadvertent intraoperative injury to the oesophagus usually occurs in relation to surgery for reflux, cardiomyotomy for achalasia or excision of oesophageal leiomyoma. It is of critical importance that these injuries are recognised at the time of operation, since delayed recognition carries similar consequences to the intraluminal instrumental injuries described above. In fundoplication, especially when performed laparoscopically, oesophageal injury most commonly occurs while dissecting posterior to the oesophagus and, in this position, can be missed unless specifically sought.[85] In cardiomyotomy and leiomyoma enucleation, careful bloodless dissection is the key to avoid oesophageal perforation. If a tiny perforation is suspected but not obvious, the cavity (abdomen, thorax) can be instilled with warmed normal saline to cover the operative area, and air instilled intraluminally through a nasogastric tube. This method is sensitive for even 'pin-hole' perforations. Alternatively, a coloured tracer in water, such as methylene blue, can be instilled into the oesophagus using a nasogastric tube.

When a mucosal defect is recognised, it should be well defined, even if an extended myotomy is required to do so. The edges can be primarily repaired with interrupted sutures, and the muscle closed over the mucosa in one layer. In fundoplication, the wrap is completed and has the additional effect of bolstering the repair. Likewise, a fundoplication or anterior fundoplasty has the same effect after cardiomyotomy for achalasia. A radiological contrast swallow is a wise precaution in the postoperative period before commencement of oral intake in these patients.

PERFORATED PEPTIC ULCER

Perforated peptic ulcer accounts for the majority of deaths from peptic ulcer disease,[86] with a mortality rate of 5–10%, and up to 40% in the elderly with perforated gastric ulcer. Longitudinal population studies show that, in recent decades, more operations are performed for perforated peptic ulcer than are performed electively for peptic ulcer disease and there is a higher operative mortality rate for perforated peptic ulcer. These findings are thought to be a consequence of the decline in elective surgery for chronic peptic ulcer disease[87] and an ageing population of patients with perforated peptic ulcer disease.[88] Approximately half of patients with perforated peptic ulcer do not report a history of ulcer dyspepsia.[86]

Two factors are associated with most perforated peptic ulcers: chronic use of non-steroidal anti-inflammatory drugs (NSAIDs) and *Helicobacter pylori* infection.[89,90]

The classic presentation is one of sudden onset of severe epigastric pain and upper abdominal peritonitis, although 'silent' perforations can occur in elderly patients or in patients with severe illness. The diagnosis is aided by the detection of free gas under the diaphragm on erect chest radiograph but this may be absent in up to 50% (see also Chapter 5). Water-soluble radiological contrast media administered orally or through a nasogastric tube can be a helpful diagnostic adjunct to detect an intraperitoneal leak (see also Chapter 5). In 50% of patients, the perforation has sealed at presentation, and for those who favour a non-operative approach in this setting, contrast radiology is routine in the management of these patients.[91]

Conservative non-operative management of perforated peptic ulcer has been compared with surgery in a randomised trial, and although mortality was similar there was a higher incidence of sepsis and intra-abdominal abscess for the non-operative approach, which was less successful in patients over 70 years.[92]

General management of perforated peptic ulcer includes resuscitation, nasogastric tube decompression, pain relief and administration of broad-spectrum antibiotics.

Surgical management

Surgical treatment of perforated peptic ulcer is now over 100 years old.[93] The development of an appropriate operation for perforated gastric ulcer has been influenced by the generally older demographics of the disease, the more severe nature of the illness,[94] the technical difficulties in surgically closing the perforation, the high rate of non-healing or recurrence[95] and the potential for underlying malignancy.[96] Surgical mortality after distal gastric resection for perforated gastric ulcer is frequently lower than after simple closure,[97] but this probably reflects selection bias. However, it is clear that the mortality rate rises sharply in the elderly (from 4.3 to 29% in those over 65 years).[97,98] The published literature reports simple closure of perforated gastric ulcers as more commonly performed than gastric resection.

Definitive surgery or not?

The debate about the advisability of definitive ulcer surgery at the time of operation for acute peptic ulcer perforation continued for over 50 years. Until relatively recently, the gold standard surgical treatment included definitive operation for the ulcer[86] in order to reduce the likelihood of recurrence, but the association of H. pylori with peptic ulcer disease and the use of laparoscopic surgery have redefined this paradigm. To this a third factor might be added: the development of a new generation of non-ulcerogenic anti-inflammatory analgesics.

H. pylori and peptic ulcer perforation

There is a strong association between chronic peptic ulceration and H. pylori,[99–101] which can be found in the gastric antral mucosa in over 90% of patients with duodenal ulcers and 60% of those with gastric ulcers. Although ulcer healing by acid suppression can be achieved in over 90% of patients, ulcer recurrence will occur in the majority on cessation of therapy. Eradication of H. pylori, together with ulcer healing, reduces this rate to <10%. Moreover, there is a high prevalence of H. pylori infection found in those with ulcer recurrence.[101]

Perforated peptic ulcer disease as a result of H. pylori infection has been a more elusive hypothesis to substantiate, and currently the evidence is strong but circumstantial.

Guilt by association

Reinbach et al.[102] did not find H. pylori to be any more prevalent in patients with perforated peptic ulcers than in the general population and concluded that the pathogenesis of perforated peptic ulcer therefore differed from that of the non-perforated variety. In their study, 47% of the patients were positive for H. pylori; however, there was a large proportion of NSAID users among the group, which was generally older than most published cohorts. Others have since shown a substantially higher prevalence of H. pylori infection in patients with perforated ulcer, up to 95% when chronic NSAID users are excluded.[103–105] In 36% of patients with perforated duodenal ulcers, a high density of H. pylori organisms was seen histologically throughout the walls of the duodenum.[106] However, there is no doubt that the demographics of patients with H. pylori and perforated peptic ulcer are different. Patients with H. pylori infection and a perforated peptic ulcer tend to be younger, with a male preponderance and a more prolonged period of dyspepsia compared with those with NSAID consumption and perforated ulcer.[105]

Despite the association of H. pylori with perforated peptic ulcer, it is of greater clinical importance to know whether H. pylori is associated with a higher risk of ulcer recurrence after simple closure of the perforation.

H. pylori and postoperative ulcer recurrence

In a small series, Sebastian et al. reported that all patients with persisting duodenal ulceration after simple closure for perforation were positive for H. pylori infection.[104] Chu et al. examined this question in 163 patients with perforated peptic ulceration who were not NSAID users.[107] After a mean of 75 months postoperatively, the prevalence of H. pylori infection was 47%. Recurrent epigastric pain was experienced by 83% of those positive for H. pylori but only by 3.5% of those without H. pylori infection. Almost all patients with recurrent pain had positive endoscopic findings (ulcer, gastritis, duodenitis). The majority of operations were simple omental patch closure (83%), and the ulcer recurrence rate was 17.8%, all of whom were positive for H. pylori. In this study, male gender and H. pylori were independent risk factors associated with recurrent duodenal ulcer.

In randomised controlled trials, although the prevalence of H. pylori infection is no different between those with perforated and non-perforated peptic ulcer, the H. pylori infection rate is significantly higher in patients who had recurrent (or persisting) ulcers.[108,109] These studies have potentially major implications for the acute surgical management of perforated duodenal ulcer. Simple closure with H. pylori eradication from the stomach will substantially reduce both the symptom and ulcer recurrence rates after perforation, thus making definitive ulcer surgery unnecessary. Indeed, a recent survey suggests that the majority of surgeons in the UK no longer perform vagotomy for perforated duodenal ulcer.[110]

Minimally invasive surgery and peptic ulcer perforation

The laparoscopic approach to surgery for perforated peptic ulcer has offered the potential to reduce operative morbidity and mortality and to hasten recovery. Not only is simple omental patch closure possible, but definitive ulcer operations such as posterior truncal vagotomy/anterior seromyotomy,[111] proximal gastric vagotomy[112,113] and even distal gastrectomy[114] are also possible laparoscopically; however, as discussed above, these techniques are now rarely, if ever, required.

Does the laparoscopic approach improve outcomes for patients with perforated peptic ulcer?

Several prospective non-randomised studies have examined key perioperative variables in comparing a laparoscopic and an open approach.[115–118] Consistently, the laparoscopic approach takes longer and is associated with a reduced requirement for postoperative analgesia. Operative mortality, morbidity, hospital stay and overall recovery time are unchanged.

Prospective, randomised, controlled trials published to date are contradictory.[119,120] In one trial, nasogastric aspirate and time to tolerating oral intake was no different between laparoscopic and open approaches, indicating that in this disease, perioperative variables not influenced by the operative wound are important.

However, in 121 patients with perforated peptic ulcer randomised to open or laparoscopic approaches, there were less analgesic requirements, lower pain scores, shorter operative time, similar postoperative stay, fewer chest complications and earlier return to normal activities in the laparoscopically treated group.[120]

Laparoscopic technique

Several techniques of laparoscopic simple closure are now available. These include the traditional Roscoe Graham omental patch repair, 'sutureless' repair with fibrin glue[119] and a pedicled ligamentum teres repair.[121–123] In the randomised controlled study of Lau et al.[119] fibrin glue repair had equivalent results to sutured repair but took significantly less time to perform. An abdominal drain is not necessary following operation.[124]

A new generation of non-steroidal anti-inflammatory drugs

NSAIDs work through their inhibition of the key enzyme of prostaglandin synthesis, cyclooxygenase (COX). Recently, two isoforms have been described: COX-1, which exists in the stomach, intestine, kidneys and platelets; and COX-2, the inducible form, which is present during inflammation. The therapeutic effects of NSAIDs are largely mediated through inhibition of COX-2, whereas the side effects are mediated through COX-1. Newly developed drugs with COX-2 selectivity (meloxicam, celecoxib) have been found to be as effective as traditional NSAIDs but have a much reduced side-effect profile, including reduced gastric complication rates.[125] These drugs appear to have a beneficial impact on peptic ulcer disease, with an eightfold reduction in ulcer complication risk, including perforation,[126] and may influence the type of long-term therapy offered for patients with arthritis.

Risk factors for adverse outcome in perforated peptic ulcer

A number of factors have been associated with adverse outcome in perforated peptic ulcer disease. These include hospitalisation at the time of admission, delay in diagnosis, coexistent medical illness, shock on admission and leucocytosis.[86] The most important factors, determined by multivariate analysis, are delay in diagnosis (12 hours), shock, presence of comorbidity and age over 75 years.[127–129] A delay greater than 24 hours in commencing treatment can increase mortality rates sevenfold, morbidity rates threefold and hospital stay twofold,[130] stressing the need for prompt diagnosis and treatment of this condition. The elderly are at particular risk if treatment is delayed. Older patients may have poorly localised symptoms and signs and tend to have less prevalence of prior symptomatic peptic ulcer disease.[131]

Peptic ulcer: summary

With the current state of knowledge on the role of *H. pylori* in peptic ulcer disease, there are those who feel confident that the era of definitive ulcer surgery for perforated peptic ulceration is well and truly over.[132] Further evaluation of the impact of laparoscopic surgery in these patients requires stratification of data for age/fitness, delay in treatment and ulcer location and size. This will help to identify those for whom this approach might be most appropriate.

PERFORATED GASTRIC TUMOURS

Gastric adenocarcinoma, lymphoma, sarcoma and metastatic tumours such as melanoma may spontaneously perforate. Perforated gastric cancer is the most common of these, although perforation generally is an uncommon complication of gastric malignancy. Patients will usually present with symptoms and signs of perforated peptic ulcer, but there may be antecedent symptoms of weight loss, pain or bleeding. At operation it may be difficult to determine whether a perforated gastric ulcer is in fact a malignancy because of the degree of inflammation and oedema of the stomach and surrounding tissues. If patch repair is to be carried out, biopsy of the ulcer edge is a wise precaution. When malignancy is apparent or diagnosed by frozen section, formal gastric resection, if possible, is indicated. If, following patch repair, subsequent biopsy results confirm malignancy in the absence of evidence of metastatic disease, gastric resection should be considered in otherwise fit patients after full staging investigations. In the case of gastric lymphoma it is now clear that combination chemotherapy is not only as good as surgical resection in relation to cure but is also associated with extremely small perforation rates;[133] it is is therefore the preferred choice of treatment in the majority of patients, permitting gastric preservation. As such biopsy and patch repair of any perforated gastric tumour is probably the best treatment, definitive surgical resection can be left until the results of histology are available.

In those with perforated gastric cancer, long-term prognosis is poor, in keeping with this type of tumour, and perhaps exacerbated by malignant cell seeding of the peritoneum. However, long-term survival does occur in some patients.

Key points

- The risk of iatrogenic perforation of the upper gastrointestinal tract can be minimised by careful technique.
- Early recognition and treatment of iatrogenic perforation minimises morbidity and mortality.
- Primary surgical repair gives best results in an otherwise normal oesophagus, and can be done with low mortality even in cases of delayed intervention.
- Modern oesophageal stents may be successfully used to treat perforations in the diseased oesophagus, with removable ones best for benign conditions.
- Definitive ulcer surgery at the time of operation for perforated peptic ulcer is no longer indicated in the majority of patients.
- Perforated peptic ulcer is best treated by operative closure of the perforation (at open or laparoscopic operation) and subsequent eradication of *H. pylori* and/or substitution of ulcerogenic NSAIDs with COX-2 inhibitor drugs.

REFERENCES

1. Sealy WC. Rupture of the esophagus. Am J Surg 1963; 105:505–10.

2. Lawrence DR, Moxon RE, Fountain SW, Ohri SK, Townsend ER. Iatrogenic oesophageal perforations: a clinical review. Ann R Coll Surg Engl 1998; 80:115–18.

3. Quine MA, Bell GD, McCloy RF, Matthews HR. Prospective audit of perforation rates following upper gastrointestinal endoscopy in two regions of England. Br J Surg 1995; 82:530–3.

   An audit of 14 149 upper gastrointestinal endoscopies detected an overall perforation rate of 0.05%, and 2.6% after dilatation/intubation; these rates are unchanged over 10 years.

4. Muhldorfer SM, Kekos G, Hahn EG, Ell C. Complications of therapeutic gastrointestinal endoscopy. Endoscopy 1992; 24:276–83.

5. Tulman AB, Boyce HWJ. Complications of esophageal dilation and guidelines for their prevention. Gastrointest Endosc 1981; 27:229–34.

6. Katz D. Morbidity and mortality in standard and flexible standard endoscopy. Gastrointest Endosc 1967; 14:134–7.

7. Adamek HE, Jakobs R, Dorlars D, Martin WR, Kromer MU, Riemann JF. Management of esophageal perforations after therapeutic upper gastrointestinal endoscopy. Scand J Gastroenterol 1997; 32:411–14.

   An single-unit audit of upper gastrointestinal endoscopic dilatation revealed a perforation rate of 1.7%.

8. Wesdorp IC, Bartelsman JF, Huibregtse K, Hartog-Jager FC, Tytgat GN. Treatment of instrumental oesophageal perforation. Gut 1984; 25:398–404.

9. Dawson J, Cockel R. Oesophageal perforation at fibreoptic gastroscopy. Br Med J (Clin Res Ed) 1981; 283:583.

10. Wichern WA Jr. Perforation of the esophagus. Am J Surg 1970; 119:534–6.

11. Reynolds JC, Parkman HP. Achalasia. Gastroenterol Clin North Am 1989; 18:223–55.

12. Tytgat GN. Endoscopic therapy of esophageal cancer: possibilities and limitations. Endoscopy 1990; 22:263–7.

13. Bartelsman JF, Bruno MJ, Jensema AJ, Haringsma J, Reeders JW, Tytgat GN. Palliation of patients with esophagogastric neoplasms by insertion of a covered expandable modified Gianturco–Z endoprosthesis: experiences in 153 patients. Gastrointest Endosc 2000; 51:134–8.

14. Jensen DM, Machicado G, Randall G, Tung LA, English-Zych S. Comparison of low-power YAG laser and BICAP tumor probe for palliation of esophageal cancer strictures. Gastroenterology 1988; 94:1263–70.

15. McGrath RB. Inadvertent gastric balloon inflation within the chest in the management of esophageal varices. Crit Care Med 1986; 14:580–2.

16. Lee JG, Lieberman DA. Complications related to endoscopic hemostasis techniques. Gastrointest Endosc Clin North Am 1996; 6:305–21.

17. Reeder LB, DeFilippi VJ, Ferguson MK. Current results of therapy for esophageal perforation. Am J Surg 1995; 169:615–17.

18. Wang N, Razzouk AJ, Safavi A et al. Delayed primary repair of intrathoracic esophageal perforation: is it safe? J Thorac Cardiovasc Surg 1996; 111:114–21.

19. Muir AD, White J, McGuigan JA, McManus KG, Graham AN. Treatment and outcomes of oesophageal perforation in a tertiary referral centre. Eur J Cardiothoracic Surg 2003; 23:799–804; discussion 804.

20. Bavastro P, Schweigert R. Asymptomatic perforation of the esophagus after C6/C7 plate osteosynthesis. [In German] Med Klin 1993; 88:670–5.

21. DeMeester TR. Perforation of the esophagus. Ann Thorac Surg 1986; 42:231–2.

22. Wright RA. Upper-esophageal perforation with a flexible endoscope secondary to cervical osteophytes. Dig Dis Sci 1980; 25:66–8.

23. Barrett N. Report of a case of spontaneous perforation of the oesophagus successfully treated by operation. Br J Surg 1947; 35:216–18.

24. Ajalat GM, Mulder DG. Esophageal perforations. The need for an individualized approach. Arch Surg 1984; 119:1318–20.

25. Sarr MG, Pemberton JH, Payne WS. Management of instrumental perforations of the esophagus. J Thorac Cardiovasc Surg 1982; 84:211–18.

26. Ell C, Riemann JF, Lux G, Demling L. Palliative laser treatment of malignant stenoses in the upper gastrointestinal tract. Endoscopy 1986; 18(Suppl. 1): 21–6.

27. Moghissi K, Pender D. Instrumental perforations of the oesophagus and their management. Thorax 1988; 43:642–6.

28. Parkin GJ. The radiology of perforated oesophagus. Clin Radiol 1973; 24:324–32.

29. Han SY, McElvein RB, Aldrete JS, Tishler JM. Perforation of the esophagus: correlation of site and cause with plain film findings. Am J Roentgenol 1985; 145:537–40.

30. Foster DR. Routine chest radiography following endoscopic oesophageal dilatation for benign peptic oesophageal strictures. Australas Radiol 1998; 42:33.

31. Goh GJ, Pilbrow WJ, Youngs GR. The use of gastrografin for esophageal perforation. Gastroenterology 1995; 108:618.

32. Lee S, Mergo PJ, Ros PR. The leaking esophagus: CT patterns of esophageal rupture, perforation, and fistulization. Crit Rev Diagn Imaging 1996; 37:461–90.

> A review of the salient CT scan findings in cases of oesophageal perforation, including those seen in the early stages after perforation has occurred.

33. Pasricha PJ, Fleischer DE, Kalloo AN. Endoscopic perforations of the upper digestive tract: a review of their pathogenesis, prevention, and management. Gastroenterology 1994; 106:787–802.

34. Graham DY. Treatment of benign and malignant strictures of the esophagus. In: Silvis SE (ed.) Therapeutic gastrointestinal endoscopy. New York: Igaku-Shoin, 1990; pp. 172–6.

35. Boyce HWJ. Peroral esophageal dilatation over a guide wire: fluoroscopy, endoscopy or 'blind' passage. Am J Gastroenterol 1989; 84:358.

36. Sauer L, Pellegrini CA, Way LW. The treatment of achalasia. A current perspective. Arch Surg 1989; 124:929–31.

37. Borotto E, Gaudric M, Danel B et al. Risk factors of oesophageal perforation during pneumatic dilatation for achalasia. Gut 1996; 39:9–12.

38. Nair LA, Reynolds JC, Parkman HP et al. Complications during pneumatic dilation for achalasia or diffuse esophageal spasm. Analysis of risk factors, early clinical characteristics, and outcome. Dig Dis Sci 1993; 38:1893–904.

39. Kadakia SC, Wong RK. Graded pneumatic dilation using Rigiflex achalasia dilators in patients with primary esophageal achalasia. Am J Gastroenterol 1993; 88:34–8.

40. Flynn AE, Verrier ED, Way LW, Thomas AN, Pellegrini CA. Esophageal perforation. Arch Surg 1989; 124:1211–14.

41. Larsen K, Skov JB, Axelsen F. Perforation and rupture of the esophagus. Scand J Thorac Cardiovasc Surg 1983; 17:311–16.

42. Skinner DB, Little AG, DeMeester TR. Management of esophageal perforation. Am J Surg 1980; 139:760–4.

43. Salo JA, Isolauri JO, Heikkila LJ et al. Management of delayed esophageal perforation with mediastinal sepsis. Esophagectomy or primary repair? J Thorac Cardiovasc Surg 1993; 106:1088–91.

44. Kotsis L, Kostic S, Zubovits K. Multimodality treatment of esophageal disruptions. Chest 1997; 112:1304–9.

45. Cameron JL, Kieffer RF, Hendrix TR, Mehigan DG, Baker RR. Selective nonoperative management of contained intrathoracic esophageal disruptions. Ann Thorac Surg 1979; 27:404–8.

46. Shaffer HA Jr, Valenzuela G, Mittal RK. Esophageal perforation. A reassessment of the criteria for choosing medical or surgical therapy. Arch Intern Med 1992; 152:757–61.

47. Schwartz HM, Cahow CE, Traube M. Outcome after perforation sustained during pneumatic dilatation for achalasia. Dig Dis Sci 1993; 38:1409–13.

48. Mengoli L, Klassen K. Conservative management of esophageal perforation. Arch Surg 1965; 91:238–40.

49. Bethge N, Kleist DV, Vakil N. Treatment of esophageal perforation with a covered expandable metal stent. Gastrointest Endosc 1996; 43:161–3.

50. Altorjay A, Kiss J, Voros A, Bohak A. Nonoperative management of esophageal perforations. Is it justified? Ann Surg 1997; 225:415–21.

51. Hine KR, Atkinson M. Instrumental perforation of the oesophagus. [Letter] Lancet 1984; ii:52.

52. Swedlund A, Traube M, Siskind BN, McCallum RW. Nonsurgical management of esophageal perforation from pneumatic dilatation in achalasia. Dig Dis Sci 1989; 34:379–84.

53. Tyrrell MR, Trotter GA, Adam A, Mason RC. Incidence and management of laser-associated oesophageal perforation. Br J Surg 1995; 82:1257–8.

54. Molina EG, Stollman N, Grauer L, Reiner DK, Barkin JS. Conservative management of esophageal nontransmural tears after pneumatic dilation for achalasia. Am J Gastroenterol 1996; 91:15–18.

55. Watkinson A, Ellul J, Entwisle K, Farrugia M, Mason R, Adam A. Plastic-covered metallic endoprostheses in the management of oesophageal perforation in patients with oesophageal carcinoma. Clin Radiol 1995; 50:304–9.

56. Kim-Deobald J, Kozarek RA. Esophageal perforation: an 8-year review of a multispecialty clinic's experience. Am J Gastroenterol 1992; 87:1112–19.

57. Whyte RI, Iannettoni MD, Orringer MB. Intrathoracic esophageal perforation. The merit of primary repair. J Thorac Cardiovasc Surg 1995; 109:140–4.

58. Wewalka FW, Clodi PH, Haidinger D. Endoscopic clipping of esophageal perforation after pneumatic dilation for achalasia. Endoscopy 1995; 27:608–11.

59. Lyons WS, Seremetis MG, deGuzman VC, Peabody JW Jr. Ruptures and perforations of the esophagus: the case for conservative supportive management. Ann Thorac Surg 1978; 25:346–50.

60. Nathanson LK, Gotley D, Smithers M, Branicki F. Videothoracoscopic primary repair of early distal oesophageal perforation. Aust NZ J Surg 1993; 63:399–403.

61. Bell RC. Laparoscopic closure of esophageal perforation following pneumatic dilatation for achalasia. Report of two cases. Surg Endosc 1997; 11:476–8.

62. Trastek VF. Esophageal perforation. A reassessment of the criteria for choosing medical or surgical therapy. Arch Intern Med 1992; 152:693.

63. Michel L, Grillo HC, Malt RA. Operative and non-operative management of esophageal perforations. Ann Surg 1981; 194:57–63.

64. Orringer MB, Stirling MC. Esophagectomy for esophageal disruption. Ann Thorac Surg 1990; 49:35–42.

65. Gupta NM. Emergency transhiatal oesophagectomy for instrumental perforation of an obstructed thoracic oesophagus. Br J Surg 1996; 83:1007–9.

66. Grillo HC, Wilkins EW Jr. Esophageal repair following late diagnosis of intrathoracic perforation. Ann Thorac Surg 1975; 20:387–99.

67. Bardaxoglou E, Campion JP, Landen S et al. Oesophageal perforation: primary suture repair reinforced with absorbable mesh and fibrin glue. Br J Surg 1994; 81:399.

68. Luostarinen M, Isolauri J. Esophageal perforation and caustic injury: approach to instrumental perforations of the esophagus. Dis Esophagus 1997; 10:86–9.

69. Orringer MB, Marshall B, Stirling MC. Transhiatal esophagectomy for benign and malignant disease. J Thorac Cardiovasc Surg 1993; 105:265–76.

70. Smithers BM, Gotley DC, McEwan D, Martin I, Bessell J, Doyle L. Thoracoscopic mobilization of the esophagus. A 6 year experience. Surg Endosc 2001; 15:176–82.

71. Port JL, Kent MS, Korst RJ, Bacchetta M, Altorki NK. Thoracic oesophageal perforations: a decade of experience. Ann Thorac Surg 2003; 75:1071–4.

72. Urschel HC Jr, Razzuk MA, Wood RE, Galbraith N, Pockey M, Paulson DL. Improved management of esophageal perforation: exclusion and diversion in continuity. Ann Surg 1974; 179:587–91.

73. Bladergroen MR, Lowe JE, Postlethwait RW. Diagnosis and recommended management of esophageal perforation and rupture. Ann Thorac Surg 1986; 42:235–9.

74. Henderson JA, Peloquin AJ. Boerhaave revisited: spontaneous esophageal perforation as a diagnostic masquerader. Am J Med 1989; 86:559–67.

75. Bennett DJ, Deveridge RJ, Wright JS. Spontaneous rupture of the esophagus: a review with reports of six cases. Surgery 1970; 68:766–70.

76. Keighley MR, Girdwood RW, Ionescu MI, Wooler GH. Spontaneous rupture of the oesophagus. Avoidance of postoperative morbidity. Br J Surg 1972; 59:649–52.

77. Curci JJ, Horman MJ. Boerhaave's syndrome: the importance of early diagnosis and treatment. Ann Surg 1976; 183:401–8.

78. Janjua KJ. Boerhaave's syndrome. Postgrad Med J 1997; 73:265–70.

79. Lawrence DR, Ohri SK, Moxon RE, Townsend ER, Fountain SW. Primary esophageal repair for Boerhaave's syndrome. Ann Thorac Surg 1999; 67:818–20.

80. Safavi A, Wang N, Razzouk A et al. One-stage primary repair of distal esophageal perforation using fundic wrap. Am Surg 1995; 61:919–24.

81. Altorjay A, Kiss J, Voros A, Sziranyi E. The role of esophagectomy in the management of esophageal perforations. Ann Thorac Surg 1998; 65:1433–6.

82. Davies AP, Vaughan R. Expanding mesh stent in the emergency treatment of Boerhaave's syndrome. Ann Thorac Surg 1999; 67:1482–3.

83. Panieri E, Rode H, Millar AJ, Cywes S. Oesophageal replacement in the management of corrosive strictures: when is surgery indicated? Pediatr Surg Int 1998; 13:336–40.

84. Gordon AC, Gough MH. Oesophageal perforation after button battery ingestion. Ann R Coll Surg Engl 1993; 75:362–4.

85. Watson DI, Jamieson GG. Antireflux surgery in the laparoscopic era. Br J Surg 1998; 85:1173–84.

86. Branicki FJ. Risk factors, *Helicobacter pylori* and a role for laparoscopic treatment of perforated peptic ulcer? J Gastroenterol Hepatol 1996; 11:93–6.

87. Svanes C. Trends in perforated peptic ulcer: incidence, etiology, treatment, and prognosis. World J Surg 2000; 24:277–83.

A detailed review of the epidemiology of perforated peptic ulcer and its treatment, and changing trends over time, which is attributed to a cohort phenomenon. One in four gastric ulcer perforations can be attributed to NSAIDs, and mortality has changed little in recent decades.

88. Higham J, Kang JY, Majeed A. Recent trends in admissions and mortality due to peptic ulcer in England: increasing frequency of haemorrhge among older subjects. Gut 2002; 50:460–4.

A review of the trends in hospital admissions for peptic ulcer from 1989 to 1999. Perforations from gastric ulcer declined but for duodenal ulcer increased for older men.

89. Sontag SJ. Guilty as charged: bugs and drugs in gastric ulcer. Am J Gastroenterol 1997; 92:1255–61.

90. Witte CL. Is vagotomy and gastrectomy still justified for gastroduodenal ulcer? [Editorial] J Clin Gastroenterol 1995; 20:2–3.

91. Donovan AJ, Berne TV, Donovan JA. Perforated duodenal ulcer: an alternative therapeutic plan. Arch Surg 1998; 133:1166–71.

92. Crofts TJ, Park KG, Steele RJ, Chung SS, Li AK. A randomized trial of nonoperative treatment for perforated peptic ulcer. N Engl J Med 1989; 320:970–3.

Randomised study from Hong Kong of 83 patients. No difference in mortality or morbidity but 6 of the 9 patients over 70 years of age randomised to non-surgical treatment required emergency surgery. Conclusion: initial period of non-operative treatment acceptable with close observation in patients under 70 years of age.

93. Lau WY, Leow CK. History of perforated duodenal and gastric ulcers. World J Surg 1997; 21:890–6.

94. de Bakey M. Acute perforated gastroduodenal and gastric ulceration: statistical analysis and review of the literature. Surgery 1940; 8:852.

95. Hodnett RM, Gonzalez F, Lee WC, Nance FC, Deboisblanc R. The need for definitive therapy in the management of perforated gastric ulcers. Review of 202 cases. Ann Surg 1989; 209:36–9.

96. Wilson-Macdonald J, Mortensen NJ, Williamson RC. Perforated gastric ulcer. Postgrad Med J 1985; 61:217–20.

97. Hewitt PM, Krige J, Bornman PC. Perforated gastric ulcers: resection compared with simple closure. Am Surg 1993; 59:669–73.

98. Blomgren LG. Perforated peptic ulcer: long-term results after simple closure in the elderly. World J Surg 1997; 21:412–14.

99. Tepes B, Kavcic B, Gubina M, Krizman I. A four-year follow-up of duodenal ulcer patients after Helicobacter pylori eradication. Hepatogastroenterology 1999; 46:1746–50.

100. Neil GA, Suchower LJ, Johnson E, Ronca PD, Skoglund ML. Helicobacter pylori eradication as a surrogate marker for the reduction of duodenal ulcer recurrence. Aliment Pharmacol Ther 1998; 12:619–33.

101. Laine L, Hopkins RJ, Girardi LS. Has the impact of Helicobacter pylori therapy on ulcer recurrence in the United States been overstated? A meta-analysis of rigorously designed trials. Am J Gastroenterol 1998; 93:1409–15.

102. Reinbach DH, Cruickshank G, McColl KE. Acute perforated duodenal ulcer is not associated with Helicobacter pylori infection. Gut 1993; 34:1344–7.

103. Matsukura N, Onda M, Tokunga A et al. Role of Helicobacter pylori infection in perforation of peptic ulcer: an age- and gender-matched case–control study. J Clin Gastroenterol 1997; 25(Suppl. 1): S235–S239.

104. Sebastian M, Chandran VP, Elashaal YI, Sim AJ. Helicobacter pylori infection in perforated peptic ulcer disease. Br J Surg 1995; 82:360–2.

105. Ng EK, Chung SC, Sung JJ et al. High prevalence of Helicobacter pylori infection in duodenal ulcer perforations not caused by non-steroidal anti-inflammatory drugs. Br J Surg 1996; 83:1779–81.

106. Mihmanli M, Isgor A, Kabukcuoglu F, Turkay B, Cikla B, Baykan A. The effect of H. pylori in perforation of duodenal ulcer. Hepatogastroenterology 1998; 45:1610–12.

107. Chu KM, Kwok KF, Law SY et al. Helicobacter pylori status and endoscopy follow-up of patients having a history of perforated duodenal ulcer. Gastrointest Endosc 1999; 50:58–62.

108. Kate V, Ananthakrishnan N, Badrinath S. Effect of Helicobacter pylori eradication on the ulcer recurrence rate after simple closure of perforated duodenal ulcer: retrospective and prospective randomized controlled studies. Br J Surg 2001; 88:1054–8.

Long-term ulcer prevalence after simple closure of a perforation was correlated with H. pylori status. Hence eradication of H. pylori after simple operative closure of a duodenal ulcer perforation should reduce the chances of ulcer recurrence.

109. Ng EK, Lam YH, Sung JJ et al. Eradication of Helicobacter pylori prevents recurrence of ulcer after simple closure of duodenal ulcer perforation: randomized controlled trial. Ann Surg 2000; 231:153–8.

A randomised controlled trial in which omeprazole alone was compared with H. pylori eradication in patients who had simple closure of duodenal ulcer perforation. Patients with H. pylori eradication had significantly less likelihood of ulcer relapse (4.8% vs. 38.1%), demonstrating the benefits of H. pylori eradication after perforated duodenal ulcer repair, and obviating the need for immediate definitive ulcer surgery in patients with uncomplicated perforated duodenal ulcer.

110. Gilliam AD, Speake WJ, Lobo DN, Beckingham IJ. Current practice of emergency vagotomy and Helicobacter pylori eradication for complicated peptic ulcer in the United Kingdom. Br J Surg 2003; 90:88–90.

111. Katkhouda N, Heimbucher J, Mouiel J. Laparoscopic proximal vagotomy and anterior seromyotomy. Endosc Surg Allied Technol 1994; 2:95–9.

112. Cadiere GB, Himpens J, Bruyns J. Laparoscopic proximal gastric vagotomy. Endosc Surg Allied Technol 1994; 2:105–8.

113. Weerts JM, Dallemagne B, Jehaes C, Markiewicz S. Laparoscopic gastric vagotomies. Ann Chir Gynaecol 1994; 83:118–23.

114. Goh P. Laparoscopic Billroth II gastrectomy. Semin Laparosc Surg 1994; 1:171–81.

115. Bergamaschi R, Marvik R, Johnsen G, Thoresen JE, Ystgaard B, Myrvold HE. Open vs. laparoscopic repair of perforated peptic ulcer. Surg Endosc 1999; 13:679–82.

116. So JB, Kum CK, Fernandes ML, Goh P. Comparison between laparoscopic and conventional omental patch repair for perforated duodenal ulcer. Surg Endosc 1996; 10:1060–3.

117. Naesgaard JM, Edwin B, Reiertsen O, Trondsen E, Faerden AE, Rosseland AR. Laparoscopic and open operation in patients with perforated peptic ulcer. Eur J Surg 1999; 165:209–14.

118. Katkhouda N, Mavor E, Mason RJ, Campos GM, Soroushyan A, Berne TV. Laparoscopic repair of perforated duodenal ulcers: outcome and efficacy in 30 consecutive patients. Arch Surg 1999; 134:845–8.

119. Lau WY, Leung KL, Kwong KH et al. A randomized study comparing laparoscopic versus open repair of perforated peptic ulcer using suture or sutureless technique. Ann Surg 1996; 224:131–8.

120. Siu WT, Leong HT, Law BK et al. Laparoscopic repair for perforated peptic ulcer: a randomized controlled trial. Ann Surg 2002; 235:313–19.

Randomised study from Hong Kong demonstrating a small advantage for the laparoscopic approach, although hospital stay was similar.

121. Costalat G, Alquier Y. Combined laparoscopic and endoscopic treatment of perforated gastroduodenal ulcer using the ligamentum teres hepatis (LTH). Surg Endosc 1995; 9:677–9.

122. Simon IB. Minimally invasive approach to perforated ulcer – is it? Surg Endosc 1995; 9:674–6.

123. Lewis WI. Ligamentum teres not the ideal ulcer patch. [Letter] Surg Endosc 1996; 10:697.

124. Pai D, Sharma A, Kanungo R, Jagdish S, Gupta A. Role of abdominal drains in perforated duodenal ulcer patients: a prospective controlled study. Aust NZ J Surg 1999; 69:210–13.

125. Schachna L, Ryan PF. COX-2 inhibitors: the next generation of non-steroidal anti-inflammatory drugs. [Editorial] Med J Aust 1999; 171:175–6.

126. Goldstein JL, Silverstein FE, Agrawal NM et al. Reduced risk of upper gastrointestinal ulcer complications with celecoxib, a novel COX-2 inhibitor. Am J Gastroenterol 2000; 95:1681–90.

127. Hermansson M, Stael VH, Zilling T. Surgical approach and prognostic factors after peptic ulcer perforation. Eur J Surg 1999; 165:566–72.

128. Suter M. Surgical treatment of perforated peptic ulcer. Is there a need for a change? Acta Chir Belg 1993; 93:83–7.

129. Hamby LS, Zweng TN, Strodel WE. Perforated gastric and duodenal ulcer: an analysis of prognostic factors. Am Surg 1993; 59:319–23.

130. Svanes C, Lie RT, Svanes K, Lie SA, Soreide O. Adverse effects of delayed treatment for perforated peptic ulcer. Ann Surg 1994; 220:168–75.

131. Kum CK, Chong YS, Koo CC, Rauff A. Elderly patients with perforated peptic ulcers: factors affecting morbidity and mortality. J R Coll Surg Edinb 1993; 38:344–7.

132. de Boer WA. Perforated duodenal ulcer. N Engl J Med 1997; 337:1013.

133. Al-Akwaa AM, Siddiqui N, Al-Mofleh IA. Primary gastric lymphoma. World J Gastroenterol 2004; 10:5–11.

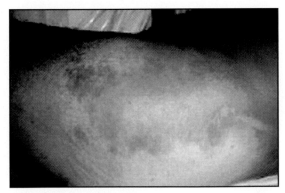

Plate 1 • Grey Turner's sign in severe acute pancreatitis.
Reproduced from Hospital Medicine 2003; 64:150–5.

Seven

Acute non-variceal gastrointestinal bleeding

Andrew C. de Beaux

INTRODUCTION

Non-variceal upper gastrointestinal bleeding remains a significant problem in the Western world. A population-based audit of upper gastrointestinal bleeding (the first in 25 years) gave the incidence of acute bleeding as 103 cases per 100 000 adults per year.[1] Of this, variceal bleeding accounted for only 4% of the total. Overall mortality was 14% (11% in emergency admissions and 33% among inpatients who began bleeding).

It is interesting to compare these figures with those from two previous studies from the 1960s,[2,3] where mortality was 10% and 14% respectively. It is important to note, however, that 27% of patients from the recent audit were over the age of 80 years, compared with less than 10% in the earlier studies, and that both incidence and mortality increased markedly with age.

Consequently, although there has been little improvement in mortality over the years, this observation must be set against a dramatic shift in the age of the population at risk. There is no room for complacency, however, and there is little doubt that the formation of specialist units to deal with gastrointestinal bleeding can minimise the morbidity and mortality of this problem.[4] Many of the therapeutic advances described in this chapter have been shown to have a significant effect, but it must be stressed that they can only be useful when employed by enthusiastic, dedicated and properly trained personnel.

AETIOLOGY

Peptic ulcer is by far the most common cause of upper gastrointestinal haemorrhage in the Western world. Other less common but appreciably frequent causes of non-variceal upper gastrointestinal bleeding include erosions, oesophagitis, Mallory–Weiss tears and malignancy.

Peptic ulcer

The UK audit reported by Rockall et al.[1] found that peptic ulcer accounted for 35% of cases of upper gastrointestinal bleeding (Fig. 7.1), and the rest of this chapter is therefore largely devoted to the management of this problem. Peptic ulcers bleed because of erosion of blood vessels, the severity of the bleed depending on the size of the vessel affected. Simple oozing is caused by damage to small submucosal vessels less than 0.1 mm in diameter, but the more important arterial bleeding indicates that a large vessel (0.1–2 mm in diameter) in the base of the ulcer has been eroded by the inflammatory process.

In arterial bleeding, the vessel tends to loop up to the base of the ulcer (Fig. 7.2), and haemorrhage occurs when the apex of this loop becomes eroded. This defect in the artery may become plugged by a sentinel clot or thrombus, and it is this that is usually interpreted as a visible vessel by the endoscopist. In ulcers on the posterior wall of the duodenum or the lesser curve of the stomach,

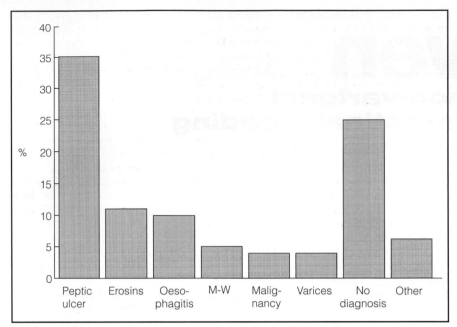

Figure 7.1 • Frequency of causes for upper gastrointestinal bleeding in the United Kingdom. M-W, Mallory–Weiss. With permission from Rockall TA, Logan RFA, Devlin HB, Northfield TC. Incidence of and mortality from acute upper gastrointestinal haemorrhage in the United Kingdom. Br Med J 1995; 311:222–6.

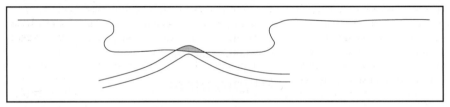

Figure 7.2 • Vessel looping up to the ulcer base.

the gastroduodenal or left gastric arteries can be involved, and these lesions are particularly prone to massive haemorrhage and rebleeding after initial stabilisation.[5]

Erosions

Acute erosive gastritis must be distinguished from the chronic forms of gastritis as the latter do not bleed. Haemorrhagic gastritis is often caused by stressful stimuli such as head injury, burns, shock or hepatic failure and is probably related to impaired mucosal blood flow. Drugs may also be responsible; the agents that are commonly implicated include steroids, non-steroidal anti-inflammatory drugs (NSAIDs) and alcohol.

Oesophagitis

Oesophagitis is a form of peptic ulcer disease but usually only causes minor acute bleeding. Occasion-

ally, however, a significant vessel may be involved, with consequent massive arterial haemorrhage that must be distinguished from variceal bleeding.

Mallory–Weiss tear

The Mallory–Weiss tear occurs in the region of the gastro-oesophageal junction as a result of severe vomiting or retching, often after excessive alcohol intake. The tear is mostly in the gastric mucosa but may extend into the oesophagus. Although bleeding can be profuse, it usually stops spontaneously. Very occasionally, repeated vomiting may result in a full-thickness tear (Boerhaave syndrome; see Chapter 6), and this is typically associated with sudden onset of severe pain in the upper abdomen or chest.

Malignancy

Carcinoma and lymphoma of the stomach, when at an advanced ulcerated stage, commonly bleed.

This usually results in occult blood loss but will occasionally present with acute haemorrhage.

Other diagnoses

There are several other conditions that may present as upper gastrointestinal haemorrhage and these are listed in **Table 7.1**.

PRESENTATION AND ASSESSMENT

Patients with acute gastrointestinal haemorrhage present with haematemesis, melaena or frank rectal bleeding, plus the signs and symptoms of hypovolaemia in varying degrees. Haematemesis implies vomiting of blood, either in a recognisable form or as dark-brown grainy material ('coffee grounds') if the blood has been in the stomach long enough for acid to convert the haemoglobin into methaemoglobin.

Melaena is the passage of altered blood per rectum. This is recognised as jet black liquid stool, sometimes tinged red when very fresh, which has a characteristic pungent smell. It results from the oxidation of haem by intestinal and bacterial enzymes and indicates that the site of bleeding is probably from the upper gastrointestinal tract, and almost certainly proximal to the ileocaecal junction. It is important to appreciate that melaena can persist for several days after the cessation of active bleeding, and its continued appearance may be misleading. It is also very important to distinguish between melaena and oral iron, which results in a sticky but relatively solid grey-black motion.

Fresh rectal bleeding immediately suggests a site within the colon, rectum or anal canal, but it must be remembered that brisk bleeding from the upper gastrointestinal tract can easily present in this way. Therefore, in the patient with massive fresh rectal bleeding, particularly when there are signs of hypovolaemia, urgent steps must be taken to exclude bleeding from the stomach or duodenum. In a patient who has previously undergone aortic surgery involving a prosthetic graft, the possibility of an aorto-enteric fistula must be considered early and advice sought from a vascular surgeon.

When the patient with acute gastrointestinal bleeding has been identified from one of the above symptoms, the following assessment and management plan should be instituted.

1. Assess the patient rapidly to ascertain airway patency, conscious level and external signs of blood loss.
2. Measure pulse and blood pressure.
3. Establish large-bore peripheral venous access, crossmatch blood and check coagulation status.
4. If the patient is haemodynamically stable, obtain a full history, carry out a full examination and proceed with investigations promptly but within normal working hours.
5. If the patient is haemodynamically unstable, fluid resuscitation must start immediately. If an adequate pulse and blood pressure are achieved rapidly and can be maintained without aggressive fluid replacement, then it is possible to proceed as for the stable patient. However, if any difficulty is encountered in stabilisation, it is necessary to investigate the patient rapidly, often with simultaneous resuscitation.

Table 7.1 • Causes of upper gastrointestinal bleeding

	Oesophagus	**Stomach**	**Duodenum**	**Small bowel**
Inflammation	Oesophagitis Barrett's ulcer	Peptic ulcer Gastritis Dieulafoy lesion	Peptic ulcer	Peptic ulcer at stoma or Meckel's diverticulum Crohn's disease
Vascular abnormalities	Varices Aortic aneurysm	Varices Vascular malformation	Aortoduodenal fistula	Vascular malformation
Neoplasia	Carcinoma	Carcinoma Leiomyoma Lymphoma Polyp	Carcinoma of ampulla Carcinoma of pancreas	Tumour
Other	Mallory–Weiss tear		Haemobilia Pancreatitis Post ERCP	Diverticulum

ERCP, endoscopic retrograde cholangiopancreatography.

INVESTIGATION

The mainstay of the investigation of acute upper gastrointestinal bleeding is flexible endoscopy. Accordingly, this section concentrates mostly on endoscopy and is divided into descriptions of endoscopy equipment, technique in acute bleeding, endoscopic appearances in acute bleeding, and other diagnostic techniques.

Endoscopy

EQUIPMENT

Most modern endoscopy units have video-endoscopy equipment, and this has major advantages. First, it affords an excellent view to all the members of the team, which is of great importance for endoscopic intervention where the assistant has to coordinate with the endoscopist, and it greatly facilitates teaching. Second, the head of the endoscope is held away from the endoscopist's face, which reduces the risk of blood or secretions splashing into the eyes.

Earlier generations of video-endoscopy equipment were not ideal for examining the bleeding patient as the image became very dark and fuzzy owing to saturation of the 'red channel' of the chip camera by blood. However, the latest video systems have overcome this problem and the direct viewing fibreoptic instrument is rarely required, except when endoscopy has to be carried out away from the endoscopy unit (e.g. in an intensive care unit). The endoscope itself must be chosen with some care for the particular circumstances. The slim or 'paediatric' instrument is very manoeuvrable, but its 2.8-mm working or biopsy channel limits the use of therapeutic accessories and does not allow good suction. The big double-channel endoscope allows good suction and washing through the unoccupied channel when an accessory is in use, but it is uncomfortable for the patient and cumbersome when trying to reach relatively inaccessible lesions. The best compromise is an endoscope with a single wide (3.7 mm) working channel and a separate forward washing channel, which allows good suction and the passage of a wide range of therapeutic instruments.

Other pieces of equipment that are important in the acute bleeding situation include a lavage tube, a pharyngeal overtube, washing devices and therapeutic accessories. The lavage tube is occasionally required when the stomach is full of clot, and the most useful device is a wide-bore (40 Fr if possible) soft tube with an open end as well as side holes. The pharyngeal overtube is a 30-cm tube with a flange at one end to prevent it slipping into the mouth. This can be passed over the endoscope when lavage is needed; it both facilitates repeated changes between the endoscope and the lavage tube and, at the same time, protects the airway. The simplest washing method is to insert the nozzle of a 20-mL syringe filled with water directly into the working or washing channel of the endoscope and to empty its contents in one rapid action. Finally, it is important to have all the therapeutic accessories that might be required immediately to hand; these are described in a later section.

TECHNIQUE IN ACUTE BLEEDING

Even when not urgent as a life-saving procedure, endoscopy should take place within 24 hours of admission, as this will increase the chance of making a diagnosis and improve the overall outcome.[6] Usually, the endoscopy will take place in the endoscopy room under benzodiazepine sedation, but in the patient who is vomiting copious quantities of blood, general anaesthesia with cuffed endotracheal intubation should be considered. When sedation is considered adequate, careful monitoring is still required, and the patient's pulse and blood pressure should be measured regularly, preferably using an automatic device. Pulse oximetry should also be regarded as mandatory, as arterial desaturation is a particular risk during a prolonged procedure with a large-diameter endoscope. For this reason, it is also wise to administer oxygen throughout the procedure, either nasally or by means of a specially designed mouth guard.

The endoscopy should take place on a bed or trolley that can tip into either the head-up or head-down position. The examination should start with the patient in the strict left lateral position, as this encourages blood to pool in the fundus of the stomach where ulcers are uncommon (**Fig. 7.3**). If it becomes necessary to view the fundus, this can be done by turning the patient on to the right side and tipping the trolley head-up so that the blood falls into the antrum. When the endoscope has been passed beyond the gastro-oesophageal junction, it is not uncommon to encounter a seeming impenetrable mass of blood and clot. However, as long as the stomach is given long enough to distend and the above guidelines are followed, a moderate amount of blood in the stomach rarely prevents adequate visualisation of the responsible lesion. Often clot will be seen overlying an ulcer, and it is important to try to wash this off in order to ascertain whether it is adherent; this has implications for prognosis and treatment, and gentle washing will rarely precipitate haemorrhage.

Occasionally, however, there will be too much blood in the stomach to allow an adequate examination, and lavage will be necessary. The 40 Fr lavage tube, ideally with a pharyngeal overtube in place, is passed into the stomach and direct suction is applied. This will often clear enough blood and

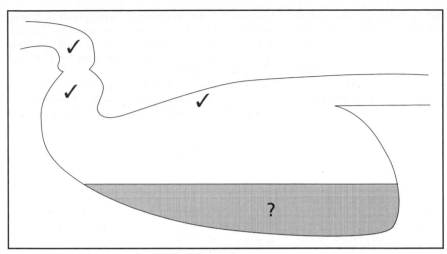

Figure 7.3 • Pooling of blood in the stomach in the left lateral position. This leaves the lesser curve, antrum and duodenum clear of blood. ✓, areas visible; ?, area of uncertainty.

clot to allow the examination to proceed. If not, it then becomes necessary to carry out a formal lavage by rapidly pouring in a litre of water via a funnel. This will break up the clot, which can then be siphoned out by placing the tube in a dependent position.

ENDOSCOPIC APPEARANCE OF THE BLEEDING ULCER

The endoscopic appearance of a peptic ulcer that has bled or is still bleeding provides valuable prognostic information, which can be used to predict outcome and risk of rebleeding.[7–10]

Unfortunately, however, there is considerable interobserver variation in the interpretation of these appearances,[11–13] indicating that the descriptive terms commonly employed lack sufficient precision. It is nonetheless important to have some means of describing the 'stigmata of recent haemorrhage', and the categories given below are widely recognised.

- *Active arterial bleeding*. This indicates erosion of an artery or arteriole. Although studies have indicated that this type of bleeding may stop in up to 40% of patients,[14] it is regarded as a clear indication for intervention.
- *Active non-pulsatile bleeding or oozing from the base of an ulcer*. This implies ongoing bleeding from a partially occluded vessel and is associated with a 20–30% chance of continued bleeding. It must be distinguished from contact bleeding from the edge of an ulcer, which is of no significance.

- *A visible vessel*. This is best defined as a raised lesion in the base of an ulcer. It may represent either an exposed vessel or an organised thrombus plugging a hole in the underlying vessel. This lesion is important as it carries a significant risk of rebleeding if untreated. The precise risk is difficult to ascertain because there is considerable disagreement among endoscopists as to what constitutes a visible vessel, but it is probably in the region of 30–50%.
- *Adherent blood clot*. It may be difficult to distinguish this from a visible vessel but as the underlying pathology is usually identical, the distinction is not absolutely necessary.
- *Flat red or black spots*. These indicate dried blood in the slough of the ulcer base and are of little significance, with a rebleeding rate of less than 5%.

These stigmata change fairly rapidly, and a study from China has indicated that visible vessels disappear in a mean of 4 days.[15]

Other diagnostic techniques

When upper gastrointestinal endoscopy by an experienced endoscopist fails to provide the diagnosis, other approaches are required. If blood is not seen in the stomach and the patient is haemodynamically unstable with continuing signs of bleeding, it is usually best to move immediately to mesenteric angiography.[16] With fresh melaena or rectal bleeding, colonoscopy is usually fruitless, and if the blood loss is more than 0.5 mL/min, on angiography the bleeding site will be seen as contrast entering the bowel lumen.

If the bleeding site is in the colon, its anatomical position will be obvious. However, when it is in the small bowel, localisation can be a problem, and it is helpful for the radiologist to leave a superselective angiogram catheter as close as possible to the lesion so that at laparotomy the affected segment of bowel can be identified by injection of methylene blue.

When the patient is bleeding intermittently, angiography may not be able to detect the blood loss, and in this case labelled red cell scanning may provide useful information.[17] A blood sample is taken, the red cells labelled with an isotope such as ^{99m}Tc-methyl bisphosphonate or ^{111}indium and the blood is reinjected into the patient. When the bleeding occurs, a proportion of the cells will enter the gut and be seen as a distinct 'blush' on the gamma-camera image. Unfortunately, once blood has entered the intestine it rapidly moves along, making localisation of the lesion imprecise. For this reason, it is important for the patient to have regular frequent scans over a prolonged period, and this is often not feasible.

Occasionally, it will be impossible to localise the site of bleeding, and the surgeon will be forced into an exploratory operation. At laparotomy, it is usually possible to determine whether the bleeding is originating from the small or large bowel, and appropriate intraoperative endoscopy can be performed to pinpoint the lesion.[18,19] This is done either per anum after antegrade lavage of the colon with warm saline or through a small bowel enterotomy at the most convenient site. An algorithm for the investigation of massive melaena or rectal bleeding is given in **Fig. 7.4**.

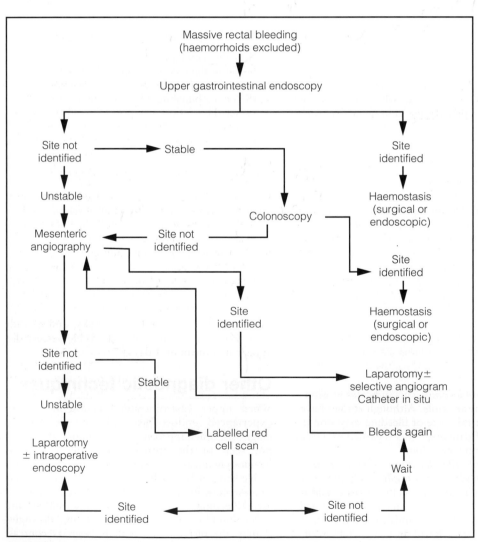

Figure 7.4 • Algorithm for the investigation of massive rectal bleeding.

MEDICAL TREATMENT

The majority of cases of upper gastrointestinal bleeding will resolve spontaneously and supportive care will be all that is necessary. There is, however, increasing evidence that aggressive acid suppression with proton pump inhibitors may influence the outcome in peptic ulcer bleeding. Theoretically, reduction of gastric acid secretion might be expected to help, as an acid environment impairs platelet function and destabilises clot. A meta-analysis of trials of histamine H_2 receptor antagonists has suggested that such therapy might reduce mortality, especially for gastric ulcer bleeding.[20] A more recent trial randomised over 1000 patients with bleeding peptic ulcers to famotidine or placebo.[21] The famotidine and placebo groups had similar rates of death (6% vs. 5%), surgery (16% vs. 17%) and rebleeding (24% vs. 26%).

The evidence for proton pump inhibitors is more compelling. A number of randomised studies[22–26] have suggested that proton pump inhibitors given after endoscopic therapy improve some of the outcomes in peptic ulcer bleeding, such as rebleeding rates, need for surgery, blood transfusion requirements and hospital stay.

To date, however, there is little convincing evidence that the use of proton pump inhibitors influences mortality in peptic ulcer bleeding. Furthermore, the optimal dose of proton pump inhibitor and the route of administration (oral vs. intravenous) to prevent rebleeding is unclear.

Inhibition of fibrinolysis has also been explored, and in one large trial of tranexamic acid a significant 50% reduction in mortality was seen.[27] However, there were no differences in rebleeding or operation rates, and for this reason the study has been criticised. All the trials of tranexamic acid have been put together in a meta-analysis that suggests that patients do benefit,[28] but as this conclusion was greatly influenced by the one positive study, the use of fibrinolysis therapy cannot be firmly recommended.

Somatostatin has also been tested in non-variceal upper gastrointestinal bleeding on the basis of its ability to reduce both acid secretion and splanchnic blood flow.

To date, there have been 14 randomised trials, and a recent meta-analysis has indicated that somatostatin may reduce the risk of continued bleeding from peptic ulcer disease.[29]

The prostaglandin analogue misoprostol appears to be promising, and there is one small trial which indicates that it may reduce the need for emergency surgery in peptic ulcer bleeding.[30]

It would seem that both omeprazole and somatostatin may be of value in reducing risk in bleeding peptic ulcer, but neither is a panacea. They should be seen either as adjuncts to endoscopic therapy or as alternatives only when endoscopic treatment is impossible or not available.

ENDOSCOPIC TREATMENT

Endoscopic haemostasis for peptic ulcer bleeding is now well established, and many randomised trials testify to the ability of several treatment modalities in reducing rebleeding and the need for emergency surgery. In this section, the various available methods are described and evidence relating to their efficacy is reviewed.

Techniques of endoscopic haemostasis

Currently, the main endoscopic techniques available for controlling peptic ulcer bleeding are laser photocoagulation, bipolar diathermy, heater probe, injection sclerotherapy and adrenaline (epinephrine) injection. Each of these will now be considered in turn, in addition to newer techniques.

LASER PHOTOCOAGULATION

Laser photocoagulation is essentially a method of delivering energy that is converted into heat on contact with tissue. The laser that is used almost exclusively for peptic ulcer bleeding is the neodymium–yttrium aluminium garnet (Nd-YAG), as this appears to achieve sufficient tissue penetration to coagulate vessels of reasonable size. A suitable laser unit has to be capable of delivering 60–100 W and is best used with a double-channel endoscope. This allows adequate venting, which prevents over-distension of the stomach and permits escape of the smoke generated by vaporisation of tissue.

When an ulcer is to be treated by laser therapy, it is washed clear of blood and loose clot so that the bleeding point can be clearly seen. A red helium–neon aiming beam is then activated, and a test 0.5-second 70-W pulse of the invisible Nd-YAG laser delivered to the edge of the ulcer. If the settings are correct, this should cause blanching of the mucosa but no ulceration. Ideally, the fibre should be 1 cm from the ulcer when the laser is activated.

The aim is then to coagulate the feeding vessel, but it is impossible to be sure of the course of this vessel from the external appearance of the ulcer (**Fig. 7.5**). For this reason, it is necessary to surround the bleeding point or visible vessel with a tight ring of

124

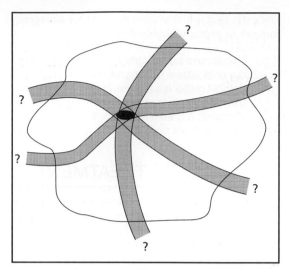

Figure 7.5 • The unpredictability of the course of a vessel that becomes visible in an ulcer base.

pulses. This will maximise the chances of delivering heat both upstream and downstream of the exposed portion of the vessel.

The main reported dangers of laser therapy are perforation of the stomach or duodenum and exacerbation of the bleeding, but these can be minimised by good technique. The laser is also hazardous for staff, and it is important for everyone involved to wear specific filter goggles to prevent possible retinal damage; the room used also has to be specifically modified. These problems, together with the cost of the laser unit, its relative immobility and the rather indifferent results achieved in randomised trials, have resulted in laser therapy being superseded by the simpler methods described below.

BIPOLAR DIATHERMY

Diathermy also relies on the generation of heat, this time by electrical current flowing through tissue near an electrode. This can be achieved by a monopolar or a bipolar system, but the former causes an

unpredictably deep thermal injury and adherence of coagulated tissue to the probe can be a problem. Bipolar diathermy avoids these disadvantages to a greater extent and has now superseded monopolar equipment.

All contact probes, including bipolar diathermy and heat probes, rely on coaptive coagulation to achieve optimum results (**Fig. 7.6**). This implies that the walls of the vessel to be treated are brought into close apposition by external pressure while heat is applied. This has two advantages. First, if the pressure stops active bleeding, it means that the probe must be correctly positioned. Second, the dissipation of heat by the flow of blood ('heat sink') is minimised so that the heat has maximum effect.

The bipolar device that is now most widely used is the BICAP probe, which consists of three pairs of bipolar electrodes arranged radially around the tip. This allows current to pass into the tissue regardless of the angle of the probe tip relative to the surface of the ulcer. The current delivered to tissue is dependent on electrical resistance, and as this increases with desiccation, the current flow is decreased as the tissue heats up and dries out, thus limiting damage. The probes come in various sizes, but the best results have been reported with the largest (3.2 mm).

As for laser therapy, the ulcer must be washed to obtain a good view of the bleeding point. If there is active bleeding, the site should be compressed firmly in order to obtain as much control as possible. The power and pulse length can be varied considerably, and there is some debate as to the ideal settings. Conventionally, a 2-second pulse at 50 W is delivered two or three times, but it has recently been suggested that using a lower power for a longer time produces better results by allowing deeper energy penetration of the tissue.

When there is a non-bleeding visible vessel, tamponade of haemorrhage is not available to provide the clue as to where to place the probe, and it is then necessary to produce a ring of coagulation around the vessel as for laser treatment. When this has been done, it is usual to treat the vessel itself in order to flatten any protruding lesion.

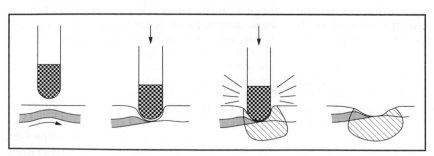

Figure 7.6 • Coaptive coagulation.

HEAT PROBE

The principles of using the heat probe are very similar to that of the BICAP device, but there are two theoretical advantages. First, because no electrical energy has to pass into the tissue, the probe can be coated with non-stick material, which prevents adherence to coagulated tissue. Second, because the temperature developed is independent of tissue desiccation, the delivery of energy is not impeded by coagulum and tissue bonding may therefore be greater.

The heat probe consists of a coated hollow metal tip containing an inner heater coil that can rapidly generate a temperature of 150°C. This temperature is effective for coagulation but avoids excessive vaporisation. The probe also incorporates channels for washing, which allows better visualisation during coaptation and coagulation. As with BICAP, the largest available probe (3.2 mm) is preferable.

The technique for using the heat probe is almost identical to that for the BICAP device, with the exception that the energy settings are graded as joules rather than watts and duration. The probe is positioned with firm pressure, and three to four pulses of around 30 J are delivered.

Both heat probe and bipolar diathermy are relatively safe, but both have been reported as causing perforations and reactivation of bleeding. It is therefore important to exercise great care in their use.

ADRENALINE INJECTION

Adrenaline injection probably achieves immediate haemostasis by virtue of the tamponade effect of the injected fluid, but the permanent effect depends on vasospasm and platelet activation, encouraging the formation of platelet and fibrin thrombus within the vessel lumen.[31] A solution of 1 in 10 000 is most often used, delivered by means of an endoscopic injection needle of the type used for sclerotherapy for oesophageal varices.

When an active bleeding point is identified, the ulcer is washed and the needle assembly, already flushed through with the adrenaline solution, is passed through the working channel of the endoscope with the point withdrawn into the sheath. As soon as the needle is seen emerging from the endoscope, the assistant is asked to push out the needle point. The needle is then advanced into the base of the bleeding point, and the assistant injects 0.5 mL of the adrenaline solution. A fair degree of force is required, and if the injection is very easy, the needle is probably not in the tissue. If the bleeding does not stop immediately, a further 0.5 mL should be injected at the same site and the needle moved to a slightly different site to repeat the process. When the bleeding has stopped, more adrenaline should be injected around the bleeding point in four to six 0.5-mL portions. The non-bleeding visible vessel can be treated in the same manner.

One situation where injection therapy is particularly useful is where adherent clot obscures the bleeding point. This makes thermal coagulation difficult, but it is quite easy to pass a needle through the clot to allow injection of the ulcer base. Exacerbation of the bleeding is not a significant problem, presumably because of the combined tamponade and vasoconstriction.

Adrenaline injection appears to be very safe, with no recorded instances of perforation. Tachycardia and hypertension can occur, however, and although fatal arrhythmias have not been reported, it is a sensible precaution to use electrocardiographic monitoring in addition to pulse and blood pressure recording during the procedure.

INJECTION SCLEROTHERAPY

The sclerosants that have been used in non-variceal haemorrhage include absolute alcohol, 1% polidocanol, 5% ethanolamine (monoethanolamine oleate) and 3% sodium tetradecyl sulphate (STD). Alcohol acts by dehydration and fixation of tissue whereas the others are detergents that cause endothelial damage; the intended end result is obliteration or thrombosis of the feeding vessel.

If there is active bleeding, it is usual to control this with adrenaline injection as above, and then to surround the bleeding point with sclerosant: 0.1-mL portions for alcohol or 0.5 mL for the other sclerosants. Sclerotherapy of a non-bleeding vessel will not require adrenaline injection unless the injection precipitates active bleeding. As for adrenaline, sclerotherapy appears to be safe, although there have been a few cases of extensive necrosis of the stomach wall after injection of the left gastric artery.[32]

NEW TECHNIQUES

The two other techniques that have attracted recent attention are fibrin glue injection and the application of microclips on to visible vessels. Fibrin glue injection involves the simultaneous injection of thrombin and fibrinogen using a specially designed double-syringe needle device. Microclips (sometimes called haemoclips or endoclips) are placed on to visible vessels by means of an applicator that can be passed down the working channel of the endoscope.

Results of endoscopic treatment

Because most upper gastrointestinal bleeding stops without intervention, it is important for techniques of endoscopic therapy to be subjected to randomised trials before they are accepted as effective. Before drawing conclusions from these trials, however, it is important to be clear about the endpoints that are being studied.

Mortality is obviously the most important, but as this is likely to be around 5% in interested centres, it would take a very large trial to demonstrate a convincing improvement in death rate.[33] The next most important is probably need for emergency surgery; this can be associated with a mortality of up to 24%,[34] and any intervention that can reduce urgent operation rates is likely to be translated into a reduction in morbidity and mortality. Rebleeding is less reliable as an endpoint as it does not necessarily represent a clinically significant outcome if it does not result in surgery or death. In many trials, however, rebleeding is the only endpoint measured.

The available trials can be divided into those that have compared a specific form of endoscopic haemostasis with no endoscopic therapy, and those that have compared different techniques. In the remainder of this section, the trials that have examined the efficacy of each of the commonly used methods against conventional treatment are considered, and this is followed by an appraisal of the comparative trials.

LASER PHOTOCOAGULATION

Laser photocoagulation was first used for bleeding peptic ulcer in the 1970s, and since then there have been at least 12 randomised controlled trials comparing it with no endoscopic therapy.[35,36] Both the Nd-YAG and the argon laser have been used, but the former has superseded the latter owing to its superior tissue penetration qualities.

Of the nine trials of the Nd-YAG laser, four were poorly designed or were not based on sufficiently accurate definitions of the lesions being treated. Of the five remaining studies, four produced favourable results.[36–39]

In the first trial, from Rutgeerts and colleagues, significant reduction in clinical rebleeding was seen among those who had active bleeding, but there were no differences in mortality or need for surgery.[37] Two studies have shown a reduction in the need for emergency surgery,[38,39] and one of these showed a reduction in mortality in a high-risk subgroup.[39] In both of these studies, however, relatively large numbers of patients were excluded prior to randomisation, usually because of difficulties in aiming the laser beam. In another study, no benefit whatsoever was seen from laser therapy,[40] but this may have been related to selection of low-risk patients and relative lack of experience among the endoscopists.

BIPOLAR DIATHERMY

Of six controlled trials of bipolar diathermy, three have been unable to demonstrate any benefit.[41–43] One showed a reduction in clinical rebleeding but no difference in the need for emergency surgery.[44]

The most impressive studies, however, were carried out by Loren Laine, who performed one trial in patients with active bleeding[45] and one in patients whose ulcers exhibited non-bleeding visible vessels;[46] in both studies a reduction in the need for emergency surgery was seen.

It is significant that in both of these studies the large 10 Fr probe was used and, perhaps more importantly, all the therapy was delivered by Laine himself.

HEAT PROBE

In heat probe therapy, there have been four randomised controlled trials with 'no endoscopic treatment' arms. Two of these showed no benefit[36,47] and one demonstrated a reduction in rebleeding but no effect on surgery rates.[48] In the CURE study, however, Jensen's group demonstrated significant reduction in both rebleeding and the need for emergency surgery in high-risk patients with arterial bleeding or visible vessels.[49] In this report, the need for the large (3.2 mm) probe, firm tamponade of the vessel and the use of four 30-J pulses was stressed.

ADRENALINE INJECTION

Adrenaline injection of actively bleeding ulcers has been widely used in conjunction with other forms of treatment including laser, heat probe and injection sclerotherapy.[50–53] The rationale has been twofold: first, to facilitate the delivery of the main therapeutic modality by stopping any active bleeding and, second, to reduce the heat sink effect (see above). It is now clear, however, that adrenaline injection can be effective on its own.

There has been one randomised trial of 1 in 10 000 adrenaline versus no endoscopic treatment in actively bleeding ulcers that showed reductions in the need for emergency surgery, blood transfusion and hospital stay in the treated group.[54] Furthermore, there have been several studies comparing adrenaline alone with adrenaline plus another form of treatment, and few of these have shown the supplementary therapy to have been of any value (**Table 7.2**).

INJECTION SCLEROTHERAPY

Although the use of absolute alcohol has been very popular, especially in Japan,[76] there have been no true trials comparing it with no treatment. However, there has been one comparative study which has suggested that it can reduce emergency surgery

Table 7.2 • Comparative trials of different techniques for endoscopic haemostasis in non-variceal haemorrhage. A best result is only indicated where there was a statistically significant difference

Study	Methods compared	Best result
Johnston et al. (1985)[55]	Laser vs. heat probe	Heat probe
Goff (1986)[56]	Laser vs. BICAP	No difference
Rutgeerts et al. (1987)[57]	Laser vs. BICAP	No difference
Rutgeerts et al. (1989)[58]	Laser vs. adrenaline vs. adrenaline + sclerosant	Adrenaline + sclerosant
Chiezzini et al. (1989)[59]	Ethanol vs. adrenaline	No difference
Matthewson et al. (1990)[36]	Laser vs. heat probe	No difference
Loizou and Bown (1991)[60]	Laser vs. adrenaline	No difference
Hui et al. (1991)[61]	Laser vs. heat probe vs. BICAP	No difference
Lin et al. (1990)[62]	Heat probe vs. alcohol	Heat probe
Jensen (1990)[49]	Heat probe vs. BICAP	Heat probe
Laine (1990)[63]	BICAP vs. alcohol	No difference
Chung et al. (1991)[64]	Heat probe vs. adrenaline	No difference
Waring et al. (1991)[65]	BICAP vs. alcohol	No difference
Choudari et al. (1992)[66]	Heat probe vs. adrenaline	No difference
Chung et al. (1993)[67]	Adrenaline vs. adrenaline + sclerosant	No difference
Lin et al. (1993)[68]	Alcohol vs. glucose vs. saline	No difference
Choudari and Palmer (1994)[69]	Adrenaline vs. adrenaline + sclerosant	No difference
Jensen et al. (1994)[70]	Heat probe vs. adrenaline + heat probe	No difference
Chung et al. (1994)[52]	Adrenaline vs. adrenaline + heat probe	No difference
Chung et al. (1996)[53]	Adrenaline vs. adrenaline + alcohol	No difference
Rutgeerts et al. (1997)[71]	Fibrin glue vs. sclerosant	Fibrin glue
Chung et al. (1999)[72]	Adrenaline vs. microclips	Endoclip
Cipolletta et al. (2001)[73]	Endoclip vs. heat probe	Endoclip
Pescatore et al. (2002)[74]	Adrenaline vs. fibrin glue + adrenaline	No difference
Lin et al. (2002)[75]	Fibrin glue vs. adrenaline	Fibrin glue

rates,[77] and a trial which indicated that it produces better results than spraying with adrenaline and thrombin in gastric ulcers with non-bleeding visible vessels.[78]

The sclerosant polidocanol has also been widely used, and it has been tested in two randomised trials, both utilising pre-injection with adrenaline. One showed a reduction in the need for emergency surgery;[79] the other was only able to show an effect on rebleeding.[80] In addition, there have been two trials of adrenaline followed by 5% ethanolamine, which showed reductions in rebleeding and non-significant trends towards less emergency surgery.[81,82]

NEW TECHNIQUES

Fibrin glue injection and endoclip application have recently been subjected to comparative randomised trials, and these are worth considering.

In a study comparing injection of polidocanol and use of fibrin glue in patients with active bleeding or visible vessels, the glue was given either as a single application or repeated daily until the vessel had disappeared.[71] All patients were pretreated with adrenaline injection. Treatment failure was significantly less frequent in the group treated with repeat fibrin glue injection, but only when compared with the polidocanol-treated group. In a more recent study, fibrin glue does not appear to augment the role of adrenaline,[74] while another study found that fibrin glue was more likely to prevent rebleeding compared with adrenaline.[75]

Another study randomly assigned patients with actively bleeding or visible vessels to adrenaline injection, endoclip application or a combination of both techniques.[72] Rebleeding and the need for surgery was less frequent when the endoclip was used. The combination treatment did not appear to confer any added benefit. A more recent study has found the endoclip to be superior to the heater probe in preventing rebleeding.[73]

Comparison between different methods

There is now little doubt that endoscopic haemostasis should be employed. It is effective in producing initial control of active bleeding, reducing clinical rebleeding and reducing the need for emergency or urgent surgical intervention. Whether it saves lives is more contentious, but a meta-analysis by Cook et al.[83] has indicated that endoscopic therapy can significantly reduce mortality (odds ratio 0.55; confidence interval 0.40–0.76).

Making a decision as to which type of endoscopic therapy to use is more difficult, however, and when appraising the different trials it is very important to take account of the type of lesion that has been treated. In trials in which the control patients were treated non-surgically until they fulfilled criteria that were independent of endoscopic appearances, it is found that approximately 60% of patients with active arterial bleeding came to surgery.[14] Approximately 25% and 40% of those with active oozing or a non-bleeding visible vessel, respectively, required surgery. When the results of adequately documented trials are put together, it becomes clear that whereas laser photocoagulation for active arterial bleeding is associated with an emergency surgery rate of about 40%, diathermy and injection techniques can reduce it to around 15%.[14]

In addition to this type of analysis, there have now been a very large number of trials comparing one method of endoscopic therapy with another, and these are summarised in **Table 7.2**. It can be seen that very few of the trials showed any difference between the techniques studied, with the exception that laser therapy seems to be the least favourable. Fibrin glue and endoclips look promising, but these are highly specialised techniques requiring considerable expertise, which is not currently widely available. It would therefore seem that the choice of therapeutic modality remains largely personal, based on training and experience. The current

author's preference and reasons for his choice are given in the Key points section at the end of the chapter.

SURGICAL TREATMENT

Despite the important advances in endoscopic intervention outlined above, there remains a small group of patients who will require surgical intervention as a life-saving procedure. This is becoming a major problem, as few surgeons in this country now have extensive experience of operating for peptic ulcer disease, and the emergency that does not respond to endoscopic treatment usually represents a significant surgical challenge. It is therefore vital that surgery for upper gastrointestinal bleeding is carried out by an experienced surgeon who is used to operating on the stomach and duodenum and is not delegated to a junior member of staff.

This section looks at the indications for surgery in peptic ulcer bleeding and then examines specific techniques for dealing with duodenal, gastric and oesophageal ulcers. Finally, the choice of procedure and the role of vagotomy is considered.

Indications for surgery

Before the introduction of endoscopic haemostasis, the decision whether or not to operate for bleeding peptic ulcer could be difficult. When active bleeding was seen at endoscopy this was usually taken as an absolute indication to proceed. However, it was more common to find that the patient had stopped bleeding at the time of endoscopy, and the surgeon had to decide between waiting for clinical evidence of rebleeding and performing 'prophylactic' surgery.

The most important factors in predicting rebleeding appeared to be the presence of significant endoscopic stigmata of recent haemorrhage, an ulcer on the posterior wall of the duodenum or high on the lesser curve of the stomach, age over 60 years and shock or anaemia on admission.[84,85] In 1984, Morris and others published the results of a randomised study comparing a policy of delayed surgery with early surgery.[86] The criteria for early surgery were one rebleed in hospital, four units of plasma expander or blood in 24 hours, endoscopic stigmata or a previous history of peptic ulcer with bleeding. In the delayed group, the criteria consisted of two rebleeds in hospital or eight units of blood or plasma expander in 24 hours. For patients over the age of 60 years, early surgery was associated with a lower mortality, and despite doubts as to the appropriateness of the endoscopic stigmata chosen and the very high operation rate, this study did emphasise the need for prompt surgical intervention in high-risk elderly patients.

Since the widespread adoption of endoscopic haemostasis, it can be argued that the decision about when to operate has become easier to make. If initial control of active bleeding is impossible endoscopically, then surgery is mandatory. If rebleeding occurs after successful delivery of endoscopic treatment, then immediate surgery should be undertaken unless the patient is deemed unfit.

Some endoscopists consider that retreatment after clinical rebleeding is safe,[87] and a recent randomised trial of endoscopic retreatment compared with immediate surgery has demonstrated a reduction in the need for surgery, with fewer complications and no increase in the risk of death.[88]

However, unless there is a high degree of cooperation between endoscopist and surgeon, a policy of endoscopic retreatment for recurrent bleeding can be very dangerous, not infrequently leading to patients being presented for surgery in less than optimal condition.

Some endoscopists follow a policy of routine re-endoscopy within 24 hours of endoscopic haemostasis, with retreatment if indicated.[53] This policy has been tested in several small randomised trials,[89–91] with conflicting results as to its effectiveness in preventing rebleeding. It is possible that this approach might improve the results of endoscopic treatment. This must not, however, be confused with the retreatment of overt clinical rebleeding. Another recent trial compared repeated fibrin glue injection versus early elective surgery following successful control of ulcer haemorrhage. While early surgery reduced the rate of rebleeding, mortality was the same in the two groups.[92]

If clinical rebleeding is to be used as an indication for surgery, it is very important to have clear definitive criteria, especially as melaena can continue for several days following a major bleed. If a patient remains haemodynamically stable without aggressive fluid replacement and does not have a fresh haematemesis or a substantial drop in haemoglobin after initial resuscitation, then rebleeding can be discounted. If there is any doubt as to whether a patient has rebled, then a check endoscopy should be carried out before committing the patient to surgery.

Techniques

THE BLEEDING DUODENAL ULCER

The majority of bleeding duodenal ulcers that require surgery are chronic posterior wall ulcers involving the gastroduodenal artery. The first step is to make a longitudinal duodenotomy immediately distal to the pyloric ring and, if there is active arterial bleeding, to obtain immediate haemostasis with finger pressure. It may then be necessary to extend the duodenotomy proximally through the pyloric ring in order to obtain adequate access. The pylorus should be preserved if possible to minimise the subsequent problems related to bile reflux.

The next stage is to clear the stomach and duodenum of blood and clot with suction to obtain an optimal view of the bleeding site. If access is still difficult, mobilisation of the duodenum laterally (Kocher's manoeuvre) may help, and taking a firm grasp of the posterior duodenal mucosa distal to the ulcer with Babcock's forceps can allow the ulcer to be drawn up into the operative field.

Regardless of whether there is active bleeding or a non-bleeding exposed artery, it is then important to obtain secure control of the vessel. This is best achieved using a small (1 cm diameter), heavy, round-bodied or taper-cut semicircular needle with 0 or No. 1 size suture material. This type of needle is ideal for the relatively restricted space and the tough fibrous tissue encountered at the base of a chronic ulcer. The material can be absorbable but of reasonable strength duration, e.g. Vicryl or PDS (polydioxanone, Ethicon UK Ltd) or Dexon (Davis and Geck, USA). The vessel must be under-run using two deeply placed sutures: one above the bleeding point and one below (Fig. 7.7). Use of the small needle suggested above will minimise the risk of damaging underlying structures such as the bile duct.

The duodenotomy may then be closed in the same direction as it was made. If the pyloric ring has been divided, the defect is closed vertically in the Heineke–Mickulicz fashion. If, however, a very long duodenotomy has been necessary in addition to division of the pyloric ring, this may be impossible to achieve safely. In this case, the duodenotomy can be closed longitudinally and a gastrojejunostomy performed if there is clinical concern that the diameter of the duodenum will be compromised. Alternatively, a Finney pyloroplasty can be fashioned by approximating the adjacent walls of the first and second parts of the duodenum as the posterior wall of the new lumen (Fig. 7.8).

Occasionally, the first part of the duodenum will be virtually destroyed by a giant ulcer and, once opened, it will be impossible to repair. In this case, it is necessary to proceed to a partial gastrectomy once the vessel has been secured. The right gastric and gastroepiploic vessels are ligated and divided, and the stomach is separated from the ulcer with a combination of sharp and blunt dissection. The stomach is then divided at a level that will represent an antrectomy, and continuity restored by a gastrojejunostomy. The difficulty then lies in closing the duodenal stump. Although this may be achieved by pinching the second part of the duodenum away

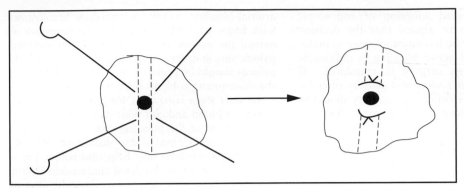

Figure 7.7 • Placement of sutures above and below a visible vessel in a posterior duodenal ulcer.

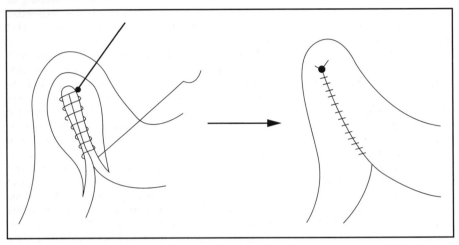

Figure 7.8 • A Finney pyloroplasty.

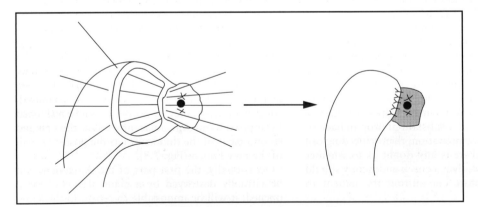

Figure 7.9 • The Nissen method for closing a difficult duodenal stump.

from the ulcer to allow conventional closure, this is generally hazardous and should not be attempted. Rather, it is preferable to employ Nissen's method, where the anterior wall of the duodenum is sutured onto the edge of the fibrotic ulcer base with interrupted sutures. A second layer of sutures is then inserted in the same way, rolling the anterior wall of the duodenum onto the ulcer base (**Fig. 7.9**). Drainage of the blind duodenal stump by means of one or two large tube drains is then advisable. Occasionally, it might be necessary to actually drain the duodenal stump and this is most conveniently achieved by means of a T-tube brought out through the healthy side wall of the second part of the

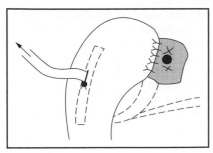

Figure 7.10 • Use of a T-tube for draining the duodenal stump.

duodenum (**Fig. 7.10**). Alternative methods include closure of the duodenal stump over a tube drain or large Foley catheter introduced through the anterior abdominal wall, creating a 'controlled fistula'.

THE BLEEDING GASTRIC ULCER

Conventionally, the bleeding gastric ulcer is treated by means of a partial gastrectomy, and for a sizeable antral ulcer this is often the best approach. However, with effective endoscopic haemostasis, by far the commonest situation requiring surgery is the chronic high lesser curve ulcer involving the left gastric artery. The important part of the procedure is then either excision of the lesser curve (Pauchet's manoeuvre) or simple under-running with large sutures and biopsy from the edge. If either of these techniques fails, formal gastrectomy may be necessary.

For the high lesser curve ulcer, therefore, simple ulcer excision is often the treatment of choice. However, this is not a minor procedure and has to be carried out with great care. The lesser curve has to be mobilised completely, often pinching the ulcer off the posterior abdominal wall and dividing the left gastric vessels. The stomach wall is then divided around the ulcer, making the incision in healthy tissue. If an anterior gastrotomy has to be made initially in order to find the ulcer or to obtain initial haemostasis, it should be made so that it can be incorporated in the excision. The defect in the lesser curve can then be closed with a continuous suture. This is best achieved with an initial mucosal suture to obtain secure haemostasis followed by a separate serosubmucosal suture. When excising the ulcer, the technique of stitch, excise a little of the ulcer, stitch a bit more, excise a bit more stops the stomach defect retracting away following excision of the ulcer.

In a patient with a large gastric ulcer with a visible vessel, simple ulcer excision may well not be possible as the ulcer base is often the anterior surface of the body of pancreas. In this situation, the choice is either gastrectomy or merely to under-run the bleeding vessel. An alternative approach is to open

the lesser sac through the gastrocolic omentum and then pinch the stomach off the anterior surface of the pancreas. This gives exposure to the bleeding vessel, usually a branch of the splenic artery which can be under-run. The ulcer in the stomach can then be excised. The final decision rests with the surgeon; however, a total gastrectomy performed on a sick elderly patient in the middle of the night is fraught with difficulty and simple under-running may be the best option. The tiny ulcer with an exposed vessel – the Dieulafoy lesion – can be treated very adequately in this way. In this latter condition, the ulcer can be very difficult to find at operation even if it has been well seen at endoscopy. Rather than trying to see the lesion, it is better to feel the suspicious area with the tips of the fingers and the vessel will usually declare itself as a distinct 'bristle'.

Occasionally, with multiple erosions throughout the stomach, it will be necessary to carry out a total gastrectomy. In this case, the site of bleeding is unclear and it is important to reduce gastric blood flow as quickly as possible. The first steps should therefore be to ligate and divide the right gastric and gastroepiploic vessels, divide the duodenum, lift up the stomach and ligate and divide the left gastric vessels. The rest of the operation can then be done at relative leisure. If the patient remains grossly coagulopathic following resection of part or all of the stomach, the principles of damage limitation surgery apply (see Chapter 13). Leave a large-bore nasogastric tube in the oesophagus or gastric remnant and return the patient to the intensive care unit. When the coagulopathy has been corrected (usually within a few days) the patient can return to theatre for restoration of intestinal continuity.

THE BLEEDING OESOPHAGEAL ULCER

Arterial bleeding from the oesophagus is usually caused by reflux oesophagitis or a Mallory–Weiss tear. It is very unusual for either of these to come to surgery as both tend to settle spontaneously and even if they do not, adrenaline injection almost always achieves permanent haemostasis.[93]

However, if a Mallory–Weiss tear does require surgery, it is nearly always possible to gain access through the abdomen, certainly in a thin patient. The oesophagus is mobilised, and the gastro-oesophageal junction is opened anteriorly by means of a longitudinal incision. It is then possible to see and under-run the tear in the mucosa. In the obese patient, access to the lower oesophagus may be easier through a left thoracotomy or thoraco-abdominal incision, and this approach should certainly be used for true lower oesophageal bleeding from oesophagitis. In this case, it may be possible to gain control via an oesophagotomy, but in some patients oesophagectomy may be necessary.

THE ROLE OF VAGOTOMY

For many years, the standard treatment for a bleeding duodenal ulcer was truncal vagotomy and drainage, and when a gastrectomy was necessary a vagotomy was often added. The rationale behind this approach was to provide definitive therapy and thereby minimise the risk of life-threatening recurrence. During the 1990s, however, changes in the management of peptic ulcer disease brought about a sea change in attitude to this problem.

First, the side effects of truncal vagotomy prompted the development of the highly selective vagotomy (HSV),[94] and it has been suggested that, after local control of bleeding, HSV should be the definitive procedure.[95] However, the results of HSV are highly operator dependent, and few surgeons now have extensive experience of the operation. This, along with the time-consuming nature of the operation, makes it impractical in most emergency situations.

More importantly, the medical treatment of peptic ulcer has improved immeasurably over the years. Although ineffective in stopping bleeding, antisecretory therapy in the form of the H_2 receptor antagonists or the proton pump inhibitors is highly effective in securing ulcer healing. In addition, the pathogenic role of *Helicobacter pylori* is now firmly established, and successful eradication therapy reduces the risk of recurrent ulcer to very acceptable levels.[96]

For these reasons, the use of truncal vagotomy in acute bleeding may now be seriously questioned. It is the author's view that secure haemostasis is sufficient in the majority of patients in the acute situation. Of course, it is then mandatory to ensure that the patient is properly treated and investigated postoperatively; this implies starting intravenous proton pump inhibitors after surgery followed by *H. pylori* eradication therapy and the cessation, where possible, of ulcerogenic drugs. Follow-up for gastric ulcer mandates a repeat endoscopy at 4–8 weeks to ensure healing of the ulcer. The follow-up of duodenal ulcers is less clear. Options include no follow-up or the selective follow-up of 'high-risk' cases, either by check endoscopy or urea breath test to ensure *H. pylori* eradication.

Occasionally, the surgeon will encounter the patient who has had multiple courses of treatment and attempts at *H. pylori* eradication who then bleeds from an ulcer. In this case definitive surgery with vagotomy and/or antrectomy is definitely indicated, but should only be carried out by a surgeon experienced in the technique.

Summary of control of ulcer bleeding

In the duodenum, control of bleeding inevitably involves under-running of the bleeding vessel and,

vagotomy aside, the only choice then is between closure of the duodenotomy and antrectomy. The ideal course of action is usually obvious and determined by the size of the ulcer, as outlined above. In gastric ulcer, the decision can be more difficult. Two groups have found that simple under-running for bleeding gastric ulcer produced satisfactory results.[97,98] However, in a randomised trial comparing minimal surgery with conventional ulcer surgery, Poxon and others found that patients treated by under-running alone were more likely to suffer fatal rebleeding.[99] The ideal operation for bleeding peptic ulcer is highly individual and must vary with the clinical situation and the experience of the surgeon. The main aim is to save life; this requires secure haemostasis by whatever means are appropriate; all other considerations are secondary.

FUTURE DIRECTIONS

Future developments in the management of non-variceal upper gastrointestinal bleeding will attempt to improve mortality rates and to reduce the need for emergency surgery. To this end, it is possible that improved medical treatment and new methods of endoscopic haemostasis may make contributions.

However, perhaps the most pressing immediate need is to improve the definition of stigmata of recent haemorrhage. Several studies have demonstrated that, apart from active arterial (spurting) bleeding, there is huge variation in the interpretation of the endoscopic appearances of the peptic ulcer that has bled, even among very experienced endoscopists.[11–13] This makes the results of many of the trials of endoscopic haemostasis difficult to assess, and the true value of treating a non-bleeding lesion is therefore still unclear. A simple, purely descriptive classification is given in **Box 7.1**.

Another difficult and related area is the problem of identifying those lesions that are at high risk of rebleeding after apparently successful endoscopic haemostasis. This can be fully resolved only when agreement is reached on endoscopic appearances, but there is now evidence that Doppler ultrasound may be useful in indicating the presence of a large vessel in an ulcer.[100] This might provide a more objective measure of risk and could be used to identify those patients who should go for early surgery. In one recent study,[101] all patients with a persistent flow through the vessel following the 'completion' of endoscopic therapy rebled. This compares with a rebleed rate of 11% when the Doppler signal was abolished at the 'completion' of endoscopic therapy.

Real improvements in the care of patients with upper gastrointestinal haemorrhage have been seen in recent years, particularly in centres that have developed bleeding units. There can be no substitute for enthusiasm and dedication in the management of this demanding problem, and the real challenge for the future is to ensure widespread cooperation between interested specialists in acute hospitals. Only in this way can a coordinated and effective response to gastrointestinal bleeding be achieved.

Box 7.1 • Descriptive definitions for the endoscopic appearances of the bleeding peptic ulcer

Definitions	Stigmata
Arterial bleeding: spurting blood	1. Arterial bleeding
Oozing: blood trickling from the ulcer base	2. Visible vessel with oozing
Visible vessel: a protruding discoloured lesion arising from the ulcer base, but not fleshy clot	3. Adherent clot with oozing
	4. Non-bleeding visible vessel
Adherent clot: fleshy clot on the ulcer base which cannot be washed away	5. Non-bleeding adherent clot

NB: other appearances *not* included as too vague and of doubtful prognostic significance.

Key points

The reasons for the following recommendations are elaborated in the main text of this chapter, but a brief outline is given with each one.

- A gastrointestinal bleeding unit should be formed in all acute hospitals. Interested surgeons, gastroenterologists and radiologists should be prepared to work closely together. Only in this way will patients receive optimal care. There is good evidence that this approach reduces mortality.
- The patient with upper gastrointestinal bleeding should have prompt endoscopy. This maximises the chance of making a diagnosis, provides prognostic information and allows endoscopic treatment. In the high-risk patient, it is very important to document the precise location of the ulcer; ideally, the endoscopy should be carried out by, or with the assistance of, the surgeon who will be operating if it becomes necessary. If video-endoscopy is available, a record of the exact ulcer location can be taken.
- In massive bleeding where endoscopy fails to provide a diagnosis, urgent mesenteric angiography should be arranged. It is very important to have a clear idea of the source of bleeding before embarking on a laparotomy.
- Medical therapy should not be relied on for control of bleeding. Good supportive care is obviously very important, but specific pharmacological treatment does not have a major effect on the outcome.
- For active ulcer bleeding and visible vessels, endoscopic haemostasis with injection of 1 in 10 000 adrenaline is recommended. Although heat probe, BICAP and injection sclerotherapy have all been shown to be effective, adrenaline is often used with these modalities, and the available trials indicate that adrenaline alone is equally effective. In addition, adrenaline appears to be associated with the lowest incidence of adverse effects and is easy to administer. Repeated injection of fibrin glue or the application of endoclips may be seen as optimal in specialist centres, but both require special expertise. Laser therapy cannot now be recommended.
- Surgical intervention is indicated when endoscopic therapy fails to control active bleeding, or at the first clinical rebleed after apparently successful endoscopic treatment. Although routine repeat endoscopy within 24 hours with reinjection if appropriate may be of value, reinjection for clinical rebleeding should be avoided unless special expertise is available.
- The aim of surgery is to obtain secure haemostasis. Unless the patient has a long history of failed medical management, including attempted *H. pylori* eradication, vagotomy should be avoided. For gastric ulcer, the ideal treatment is often formal ulcer excision.

REFERENCES

1. Rockall TA, Logan RFA, Devlin HB, Northfield TC. Incidence of and mortality from acute upper gastrointestinal haemorrhage in the United Kingdom. Br Med J 1995; 311:222–6.

   This audit provides the most accurate picture of acute upper gastrointestinal bleeding in the UK.

2. Schiller KFR, Truelove SC, Williams DG. Haematemesis and melaena, with special reference to factors influencing the outcome. Br Med J 1970; ii:7–14.

3. Johnston SJ, Jones PF, Kyle J, Needham CD. Epidemiology and course of gastrointestinal haemorrhage in North-East Scotland. Br Med J 1973; iii:655–60.

4. Dronfield MW. Special units for acute upper gastrointestinal bleeding. Br Med J 1987; 294:1308–9.

5. Swain CP, Salmon PR, Northfield TC. Does ulcer position influence presentation or prognosis of upper gastrointestinal bleeding? Gut 1986; 27:A632.

6. Cooper GS, Chak A, Way LE, Hammar PJ, Harper DL, Rosenthal GE. Early endoscopy in upper gastrointestinal haemorrhage: associations with recurrent bleeding, surgery, and length of hospital stay. Gastrointest Endosc 1999; 49:145–52.

7. Foster DN, Miloszewski KJ, Losowsky MS. Stigmata of recent haemorrhage in diagnosis and prognosis of upper gastrointestinal bleeding. Br Med J 1978; i:1173–7.

8. Griffiths WJ, Neumann DA, Welsh JD. The visible vessel as an indicator of a controlled or recurrent gastrointestinal haemorrhage. N Engl J Med 1979; 300:1411–13.

9. Storey DW, Bown SJ, Swain CP, Salmon PR, Kirkham JS, Northfield TC. Endoscopic prediction of recurrent bleeding in peptic ulcers. N Engl J Med 1981; 305:915–16.

10. Wara P. Endoscopic prediction of major rebleeding: a prospective study of stigmata of haemorrhage in bleeding ulcer. Gastroenterology 1985; 88:1209–14.

11. Lau YWJ, Sung JYJ, Chan CWJ et al. Stigmata of haemorrhage in bleeding peptic ulcers: an interobserver agreement study among international experts. Gastrointest Endosc 1997; 46:33–6.

12. Laine L, Freeman M, Cohen H. Lack of uniformity in evaluation of endoscopic prognostic features of bleeding ulcers. Gastrointest Endosc 1994; 40:411–17.

13. Moorman PW, Siersema PD, van Ginneken AM. Descriptive features of gastric ulcers: do endoscopists agree on what they see? Gastrointest Endosc 1995; 42:555–9.

   These three papers[11–13] demonstrate that expert endoscopists do not necessarily agree on the appearances that constitute the various stigmata of haemorrhage. This calls into question the results of many trials of

endoscopic haemostasis, demanding considerable caution in their interpretation.

14. Steele RJC. Endoscopic haemostasis for nonvariceal upper gastrointestinal haemorrhage. Br J Surg 1989; 76:219–25.

15. Yang CC, Shin JS, Lin XZ, Hsu PI, Chen KW, Lin CY. The natural history (fading time) of stigmata of recent haemorrhage in peptic ulcer disease. Gastrointest Endosc 1994; 40:562–6.

16. Thomson JN, Salem RR, Hemingway AP et al. Specialist investigation of obscure gastrointestinal bleeding. Gut 1987; 28:47–51.

17. Winzelberg GG, McKusick KA, Froelich JW et al. Detection of gastrointestinal bleeding with ^{99m}Tc-labelled red blood cells. Semin Nucl Med 1982; 12:126–38.

18. Desa LA, Ohri SK, Hutton KAR, Lee H, Spencer J. Role of intraoperative enteroscopy in obscure gastrointestinal bleeding of small bowel origin. Br J Surg 1991; 78:192–5.

19. Berry AR, Campbell WB, Kettlewell MGW. Management of major colonic haemorrhage. Br J Surg 1988; 7:637–40.

20. Collins R, Langman M. Treatment with histamine H_2 antagonists in acute upper gastrointestinal haemorrhage. Implications of randomised trials. N Engl J Med 1985; 313:660–6.

21. Walt RP, Cottrell J, Mann SG et al. Randomised, double blind, controlled trial of intravenous famotidine infusion in 1005 patients with peptic ulcer bleeding. Lancet 1992; 340:1058–62.

22. Khuroo MS, Yattoo GN, Javid G et al. A comparison of omeprazole and placebo for bleeding peptic ulcer. N Engl J Med 1997; 336:1054–8.

   This is the first trial to demonstrate a convincing effect of acid suppression on the outcome in acute gastrointestinal haemorrhage. It should be pointed out that, unlike the previous two trials,[21,22] this study was confined to peptic ulcer bleeding.

23. Lau JJW, Sung JJY, Lee KKC et al. Effect of intravenous omeprazole on recurrent bleeding after endoscopic treatment of bleeding ulcers. N Engl J Med 2000; 342:310–16.

24. Kaviani MJ, Hashemi MR, Kazemifar AR et al. Effect of oral omeprazole in reducing re-bleeding in bleeding peptic ulcers: a prospective, double-blind, randomised, clinical trial. Aliment Pharmacol Ther 2003; 17:211–16.

25. Hasselgren G, Lind T, Lundell L et al. Continuous intravenous infusion of omeprazole in elderly patients with peptic ulcer bleeding. Results of a placebo-controlled multicenter study. Scand J Gastroenterol 1997; 32:396–8.

26. Udd M, Miettinen P, Palmu A et al. Regular-dose versus high-dose omeprazole in peptic ulcer bleeding: a prospective randomised double-blind study. Scand J Gastroenterol 2001; 36:1332–8.

27. Barer D, Ogilvie A, Henry D et al. Cimetidine and tranexamic acid in the treatment of acute upper gastrointestinal tract bleeding. N Engl J Med 1983; 308:1571–5.

28. Henry DA, O'Connell DL. Effects of fibrinolytic inhibitors on mortality from upper gastrointestinal haemorrhage. Br Med J 1989; 298:1142–6.

29. Roudebush Veterans Affairs (Indianapolis, IA, USA). Somatostatin or octreotide compared with H$_2$ antagonists and placebo in the management of acute nonvariceal upper gastrointestinal haemorrhage: a meta-analysis. Ann Intern Med 1997; 127:1062–71.

> This meta-analysis indicates that somatostatin may have a role in peptic ulcer bleeding.

30. Birnie GC, Fenn GC, Shield MJ et al. Double blind comparative study of misoprostol with placebo in acute upper gastrointestinal bleeding. Gut 1991; 32:A1246.

31. Pinkas H, McAllister E, Norman J, Robinson B, Brady PG, Dawson PJ. Prolonged evaluation of epinephrine and normal saline solution injections in an acute ulcer model with a single bleeding artery. Gastrointest Endosc 1995; 41:51–5.

32. Levy J, Khakoo S, Barton R, Vicary R. Fatal injection sclerotherapy of a bleeding peptic ulcer. Lancet 1991; 37:504.

33. Fromm D. Endoscopic coagulation for gastrointestinal bleeding. N Engl J Med 1987; 316:1652–4.

34. Rockall TA. Management and outcome of patients undegoing surgery after acute upper gastrointestinal haemorrhage. Steering Group for the National Audit of Acute Upper Gastrointestinal Haemorrhage. J R Soc Med 1998; 91:518–23.

35. Laurence BH, Cotton PB. Bleeding gastroduodenal ulcers: non-operative treatment. World J Surg 1987; 11:295–303.

36. Matthewson K, Swain CP, Bland M, Kirkham JS, Bown SG, Northfield TC. Randomised comparison of NdYAG laser, heater probe and no endoscopic therapy for bleeding peptic ulcers. Gastroenterology 1990; 98:1239–44.

37. Rutgeerts P, van Trappen G, Broeckaert L et al. Controlled trial of YAG laser treatment of upper digestive haemorrhage. Gastroenterology 1982; 83:410–16.

38. MacLeod IA, Mills PR, MacKenzie JF et al. Neodymium yttrium aluminium garnet laser photocoagulation for major haemorrhage from peptic ulcers and single vessels: a single double blind controlled study. Br Med J 1983; 286:345–8.

39. Swain CP, Kirkham JS, Salmon PR et al. Controlled trial of Nd-YAG laser photocoagulation in bleeding peptic ulcers. Lancet 1986; i:1113–16.

40. Krejs GJ, Little KH, Westergaard H et al. Laser photocoagulation for the treatment of acute peptic-ulcer bleeding. N Engl J Med 1987; 316:1618–21.

41. Goudie BM, Mitchell KG, Birnie GC et al. Controlled trial of endoscopic bipolar electrocoagulation in the treatment of bleeding peptic ulcers. Gut 1984; 25:A1185.

42. Kernohan RM, Anderson JR, McKelvey STD et al. A controlled trial of bipolar electrocoagulation in patients with upper gastrointestinal bleeding. Br J Surg 1984; 71:889–91.

43. Brearly S, Hawker PC, Dykes PW et al. Perendoscopic bipolar diathermy coagulation of visible vessel using a 3.2 mm probe: a randomised clinical trial. Endoscopy 1987; 19:160–3.

44. O'Brien JD, Day SJ, Burnham WR. Controlled trial of small bipolar probe in bleeding peptic ulcers. Lancet 1986; i:464–7.

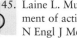

45. Laine L. Multipolar electrocoagulation in the treatment of active upper gastrointestinal haemorrhage. N Engl J Med 1987; 316:1613–17.

46. Laine L. Multipolar electrocoagulation for the treatment of ulcers with non-bleeding visible vessels: a prospective, controlled trial. Gastroenterology 1988; 94:A246.

> Laine's work is the most convincing evidence of the effectiveness of BICAP and emphasises the importance of individual expertise in this area.

47. Avgerinos A, Rekoumis G, Argirakis G et al. Randomised comparison of endoscopic heater probe electrocoagulation, injection of adrenaline and no endoscopic therapy for bleeding peptic ulcers. Gastroenterology 1989; 98:A18.

48. Fullarton GM, Birnie GC, MacDonald A et al. Controlled trial of heater probe treatment in bleeding peptic ulcers. Br J Surg 1989; 76:541–4.

49. Jensen DM. Heat probe for haemostasis of bleeding peptic ulcers: techniques and results of randomised controlled trials. Gastrointest Endosc 1990; 36:S42–S49

50. Rutgeerts P, van Trappen G, Brieckaert L et al. A new and effective technique of Yag laser photocoagulation for severe upper gastrointestinal bleeding. Endoscopy 1984; 16:115–17.

51. Soehendra N, Grimm H, Stenzel M. Injection of nonvariceal bleeding lesions of the upper gastrointestinal tract. Endoscopy 1985; 17:129–32.

52. Chung SCS, Sung JY, Lai CW, Ng EKW, Chan KL, Yung MY. Epinephrine injection alone or epinephrine injection plus heater probe treatment for bleeding ulcers. Gastrointest Endosc 1994; 40:A271.

53. Chung SCS, Leong HT, Chan AC et al. Epinephrine or epinephrine plus alcohol for injection of bleeding ulcers: a prospective randomised trial. Gastrointest Endosc 1996; 43:591–5.

54. Chung SCS, Leung JWC, Steele RJC et al. Endoscopic adrenaline injection for actively bleeding ulcers: a randomised trial. Br Med J 1988; 296:1631–3.

This trial provides good evidence for the effectiveness of adrenaline injection alone in the treatment of active bleeding from peptic ulcer.

55. Johnston JH, Sones JQ, Long BW, Posey LE. Comparison of heater probe and YAG laser in endoscopic treatment of major bleeding from peptic ulcers. Gastrointest Endosc 1985; 31:175–80.

56. Goff JS. Bipolar electrocoagulation versus Nd-YAG laser photocoagulation for upper gastrointestinal bleeding lesions. Dig Dis Sci 1986; 31:906–10.

57. Rutgeerts P, van Trappen G, van Hootegem P et al. Neodymium–YAG laser photocoagulation versus multipolar electrocoagulation for the treatment of severely bleeding peptic ulcers: a randomised comparison. Gastrointest Endosc 1987; 33:199–202.

58. Rutgeerts P, van Trappen G, Broechaert L, Coremans G, Janssens J, Hiele M. Comparison of endoscopic polidocanol injection and YAG laser therapy for bleeding peptic ulcers. Lancet 1989; i:1164–7.

59. Chiezzini G, Bortoluzzi F, Pallin D et al. Controlled trial of absolute ethanol vs epinephrine as injection agent in gastrointestinal bleeding. Gastroenterology 1989; 96:A86.

60. Loizou IA, Bown SG. Endoscopic treatment for bleeding peptic ulcers: randomised comparison of adrenaline injection and adrenaline injection + Nd:YAG laser. Gut 1991; 32:1100–3.

61. Hui WM, Ng MMT, Lok ASF, Lai CL, Lau YN, Lam SK. A randomised comparative study of laser photocoagulation, heater probe and bipolar electrocoagulation in the treatment of actively bleeding ulcers. Gastrointest Endosc 1991; 37:299–304.

62. Lin HI, Lee FY, Kang WM, Tsai YT, Lee SD, Lee CH. Heat probe thermocoagulation and pure alcohol injection in massive peptic ulcer haemorrhage: a prospective, randomised controlled trial. Gut 1990; 31:753–7.

63. Laine L. Multipolar electrocoagulation versus injection therapy in the treatment of bleeding peptic ulcers. Gastroenterology 1990; 99:1303–6.

64. Chung SCS, Leung JWC, Sung JY, Lo KK, Li AKC. Injection or heat probe for bleeding ulcer. Gastroenterology 1991; 100:30–7.

65. Waring JP, Sanowski RA, Sawyer RL, Woods CA, Foutch PG. A randomised comparison of multipolar electrocoagulation and injection sclerosis for the treatment of bleeding peptic ulcer. Gastrointest Endosc 1991; 37:295–8.

66. Choudari CD, Rajgopal C, Palmer KR. Comparison of endoscopic injection therapy versus the heater probe in major peptic ulcer haemorrhage. Gut 1992; 33:1159–61.

67. Chung SCS, Leung JWC, Leong HT, Lo KK, Li AKC. Adding a sclerosant to endoscopic epinephrine injection in actively bleeding ulcers: a randomised trial. Gastrointest Endosc 1993; 39:611–15.

68. Lin HI, Perng CL, Lee FY et al. Endoscopic injection for the arrest of peptic ulcer haemorrhage: final results of a prospective, randomised comparative trial. Gastrointest Endosc 1993; 39:15–19.

69. Choudari CP, Palmer KR. Endoscopic injection therapy for bleeding peptic ulcer: a comparison of adrenaline alone with adrenaline plus ethanolamine oleate. Gut 1994; 35:608–10.

70. Jensen DM, Kovacs T, Randall G, Smith J, Freenan M, Jutabha R. Prospective study of thermal coagulation (gold probe – GP) vs combination injection and thermal (Ing + GP) treatment of high risk patients with severe ulcer or Mallory Weiss (MW) bleeding. Gastrointest Endosc 1994; 40:A42.

71. Rutgeerts P, Rauws E, Wara P et al. Randomised trial of single and repeated fibrin glue compared with injection of polidocanol in treatment of bleeding peptic ulcer. Lancet 1997; 350:692–6.

72. Chung IK, Ham JS, Kim HS, Park SH, Lee MH, Kim SJ. Comparison of the haemostatic efficacy of the endoscopic haemoclip method with hypertonic saline–epinephrine injection and a combination of the two for the management of bleeding peptic ulcers. Gastrointest Endosc 1999; 49:13–18.

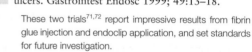

These two trials[71,72] report impressive results from fibrin glue injection and endoclip application, and set standards for future investigation.

73. Cipolletta L, Bianco MA, Marmo R et al. Endoclips versus heater probe in preventing early recurrent bleeding from peptic ulcer: a prospective and randomised trial. Gastrointest Endosc 2001; 53:147–51.

74. Pescatore P, Jornod P, Borovicka J et al. Epinephrine versus epinephrine plus fibrin glue in peptic ulcer bleeding: a prospective randomised trial. Gastrointest Endosc 2002; 55:348–53.

75. Lin HJ, Hsieh YH, Tseng GY, Perng CL, Chang FY, Lee SD. Endoscopic injection with fibrin sealant versus epinephrine in the arrest of peptic ulcer bleeding: a randomised, comparative trial. J Clin Gastroenterol 2002; 35:218–21.

76. Asaki S. Endoscopic haemostasis by local absolute alcohol injection for upper gastrointestinal tract bleeding: a multicentre study. In: Okabe H, Honda T, Ohshiba S (eds) Endoscopic surgery. New York: Elsevier, 1984; pp. 105–16.

77. Pascu O, Draghici A, Acalovachi I. The effect of endoscopic haemostasis with alcohol on the mortality rate of nonvariceal upper gastrointestinal haemorrhage: a randomised prospective study. Endoscopy 1989; 36:S53–S55.

78. Koyama T, Fukimoto K, Iwakiri R et al. Prevention of recurrent bleeding from gastric ulcer with a nonbleeding visible vessel by the endoscopic injection of absolute ethanol: a prospective, controlled trial. Gastrointest Endosc 1995; 42:128–31.

137

References

79. Panes J, Viver J, Forne M et al. Controlled trial of endoscopic sclerosis in bleeding peptic ulcers. Lancet 1987; ii:1292–4.

80. Balanzo J, Sainz S, Such J et al. Endoscopic haemostasis by local injection of epinephrine and polidocanol in bleeding ulcer. A prospective, randomised trial. Endoscopy 1988; 20:298–291.

81. Rajgopal C, Palmer KR. Endoscopic injection sclerosis: effective therapy for bleeding peptic ulcer. Gut 1991; 32:727–9.

82. Oxner RBG, Simmonds NJ, Gertner DJ, Nightingale JMD, Burnham WR. Controlled trial of endoscopic injection treatment for bleeding from peptic ulcers with visible vessels. Lancet 1992; 339:966–8.

83. Cook DJ, Guyatt GH, Salena BJ et al. Endoscopic therapy for acute non-variceal upper gastrointestinal haemorrhage: a meta-analysis. Gastroenterology 1992; 102:139–48.

    Although a few years old now, this meta-analysis provides very convincing evidence that the concept of endoscopic haemostasis is sound.

84. Clason AE, Macleod DAD, Elton RA. Clinical factors in the prediction of further haemorrhage or mortality in acute upper gastrointestinal haemorrhage. Br J Surg 1986; 73:985–7.

85. Hunt PS. Bleeding gastroduodenal ulcers: selection of patients for surgery. World J Surg 1987; 11:289–94.

86. Morris DL. Hawker PC, Brearley S et al. Optimal timing of operation for bleeding peptic ulcer: prospective randomised trial. Br Med J 1984; 288:1277–80.

87. Palmer KR, Choudari CP. Endoscopic intervention in bleeding peptic ulcer. Gut 1995; 37:161–4.

88. Lau JY, Sung JJ, Lam YH et al. Endoscopic retreatment compared with surgery in patients with recurrent bleeding after initial endoscopic control of bleeding ulcers. N Engl J Med 1999; 340:751–6.

    This important study challenges the concept that retreatment is more dangerous than immediate surgery when rebleeding occurs after endoscopic haemostasis.

89. Villanueva C, Balanzo J, Torras X, Soriano G, Sainz S, Vilardell F. Value of second-look endoscopy after injection therapy for bleeding peptic ulcer: a prospective and randomised trial. Gastrointest Endosc 1994; 40:34–9.

90. Saeed Z, Cole RA, Ramirez FC et al. Endoscopic retreatment after successful initial hemostasis prevents ulcer rebleeding: a prospective randomised trial. Endoscopy 1996; 28:288–94.

91. Messmann H, Schaller P, Andus T et al. Effect of programmed endoscopic follow-up examination on the rebleeding rate of gastric or duodenal peptic ulcers treated by injection therapy: a prospective, randomised controlled trial. Endoscopy 1998; 30:583–9.

92. Imhof M, Ohmann C, Roher HD, Glutig H; DUESUC study group. Endoscopic versus operative treatment in high-risk ulcer bleeding patients: results of a randomised study. Langenbecks Arch Surg 2003; 387:327–36.

93. Park KGM, Steele RJC, Masson J. Endoscopic adrenaline injection for benign oesophageal ulcer haemorrhage. Br J Surg 1994; 81:1317–18.

94. Johnston D. Operative mortality and postoperative morbidity of highly selective vagotomy. Br Med J 1975; 4:545–7.

95. Miedema BW, Torres PR, Farnell MB et al. Proximal gastric vagotomy in the emergency treatment of bleeding duodenal ulcer. Am J Surg 1991; 162:64–7.

96. Moss S, Calam J. Helicobacter pylori and peptic ulcers: the present position. Gut 1992; 33:289–92.

97. Teenan RP, Murray WR. Late outcome of undersewing alone for gastric ulcer haemorrhage. Br J Surg 1990; 77:811–12.

98. Schein M, Gecelter G. Apache II score in massive upper gastrointestinal haemorrhage from peptic ulcer: prognostic value and potential clinical applications. Br J Surg 1989; 76:733–6.

99. Poxon VA, Keighley MRB, Dykes PW et al. Comparison of minimal and conventional surgery in patients with bleeding peptic ulcer: a multicentre trial. Br J Surg 1991; 78:1344–5.

100. Fullerton GM, Murray WR. Prediction of rebleeding in peptic ulcers by visual stigmata and endoscopic doppler ultrasound criteria. Endoscopy 1990; 22:68–71.

101. Wong RC, Chak A, Kobayashi K et al. Role of Doppler US in acute peptic ulcer hemorrhage: can it predict failure of endoscopic therapy? Gastrointest Endosc 2000; 52:315–21.

Eight

Pancreaticobiliary emergencies

James J. Powell and
Rowan W. Parks

INTRODUCTION

Increasing specialisation in surgical practice has produced a trend towards concentration of elective pancreatic and complex biliary surgery in the hands of 'upper' gastrointestinal surgeons. However, the nature of surgical service provision often demands that pancreaticobiliary emergencies be treated by surgeons with principal specialist interests outwith the upper gastrointestinal tract. Thus the aim of this chapter is to provide an overview of current evidence guiding the treatment of the more commonly encountered pancreaticobiliary emergencies. To this end, the chapter addresses the management of acute cholecystitis, acute cholangitis and acute pancreatitis.

BILIARY COLIC AND ACUTE CHOLECYSTITIS

The majority of acute gallbladder problems are the consequence of gallstones and have a range of clinical presentations.

Pathogenesis

Symptomatic cholelithiasis presents with a range of clinical syndromes. In the emergency setting the patient is most likely to present with either biliary colic or acute cholecystitis. It is often difficult at the initial assessment to distinguish between the two conditions because it is likely that biliary colic and acute cholecystitis form part of a spectrum. Biliary colic is thought to occur following the impaction of a gallstone within the cystic duct or gallbladder infundibulum, leading to gallbladder obstruction.[1] In a functioning gallbladder, obstruction results in marked gallbladder contraction with the perception of pain. Following disimpaction of the stone, pain subsides. Disimpacted gallstones can either fall back into the gallbladder or pass into the common bile duct.

Conventional models of the pathophysiology of acute cholecystitis suggest that continued gallbladder obstruction gives rise to an acute inflammatory process, although it should be borne in mind that there is often a poor correlation between the clinical presentation and the histopathological features of acute and chronic inflammation in the gallbladder wall.[1] Initially in acute cholecystitis the inflammatory process within the gallbladder is sterile; however, bacterial colonisation of the obstructed bile and inflamed tissue occurs and may result in an empyema of the gallbladder. Further, if the inflammatory process is particularly severe, gallbladder ischaemia and necrosis can occur, with the consequent risk of gallbladder perforation and subsequent biliary peritonitis.

Clinical presentation

Biliary colic presents with severe upper abdominal pain in the epigastric and right upper quadrant regions often radiating to the back or shoulders. Although termed 'colic', the pain is often constant but remits after a period of minutes to hours. It may be provoked by eating, and the patient may describe an association with ingestion of fatty foods. A history of previous similar episodes may be obtained. On examination during the acute episode the patient may be distressed because of the pain.

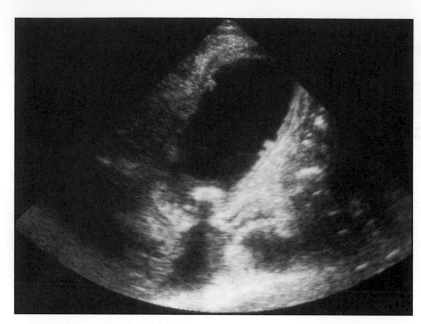

Figure 8.1 • Ultrasound of acute cholecystitis. Note the thickened gallbladder wall, the acoustic shadow produced by the gallstone in the neck and the surrounding pericystic fluid. This patient was also tender on pressing the transducer onto the gallbladder (sonographic Murphy's sign). With thanks to Dr Paul Allan, Consultant Radiologist, Royal Infirmary, Edinburgh.

Palpation of the abdomen may reveal epigastric/right upper quadrant tenderness but no evidence of peritoneal irritation. Blood investigations are usually normal.

In acute cholecystitis the pain is localised to the right upper quadrant, and may radiate through to the back or right shoulder tip. Because of peritoneal irritation the pain is exacerbated by movement and breathing. Typically, the patient is nauseated and may have vomited. On examination, patients demonstrate systemic signs of inflammation including tachycardia and pyrexia. Abdominal examination demonstrates right upper quadrant tenderness with signs of localised peritonitis. Classically, Murphy's sign (pain on deep inspiration during palpation at the tip of the right ninth rib) can be elicited in patients with acute cholecystitis. A tender mass may be palpable in the right upper quadrant. Haematological investigations typically demonstrate a leucocytosis. Liver function tests may be deranged. An obstructive picture to the liver function tests may be a consequence of common bile duct stones but may also be a consequence of impacted gallstones in Hartmann's pouch pressing on or eroding into the common hepatic duct (Mirizzi's syndrome)[2] or contiguous inflammation affecting the common bile duct or adjacent hepatic parenchyma.

Initial radiological imaging

Transabdominal ultrasonography is the initial investigation of choice in both biliary colic and acute cholecystitis. Standard grey-scale ultrasound has a sensitivity of greater than 95% for detecting gallstones.[3] In addition, ultrasound can demonstrate signs of acute inflammation such as gallbladder wall thickening, pericholecystic fluid and a sonographic Murphy's sign (**Fig. 8.1**). Ultrasound is also able to visualise gas in the gallbladder wall in those patients with emphysematous cholecystitis. Newer techniques of colour velocity imaging and power Doppler sonography have greater accuracy than grey-scale ultrasonography in detecting acute cholecystitis,[4] and may therefore be used to distinguish patients with true acute cholecystitis from those with upper abdominal pain and incidental chronic cholelithiasis. In addition, transabdominal ultrasound can detect the presence of biliary tree dilatation, suggesting choledocholithiasis.

Other imaging techniques exist. Radionuclide scans have been reported to have greater accuracy in diagnosing acute cholecystitis than standard ultrasound techniques.[5-7] However, these techniques are time-consuming and involve the use of a radiopharmaceutical. Therefore the use of radionuclide scanning is probably restricted to those individuals who are clinically suspected of having acute cholecystitis but who have inconclusive or normal ultrasound scans.

Management of patients with acute gallbladder disease and suspected bile duct stones

In patients with obstructive liver function tests, ultrasonographic evidence of biliary dilatation and/or evidence of ductal calculi, preoperative assessment of the bile duct is established practice. However, in the acute setting several additional factors complicate the decision-making process.

Most importantly, if there are signs of generalised peritonitis then operative intervention cannot be deferred and investigation for common bile duct calculi becomes a secondary issue. In this situation, ductal stones can be dealt with if they are encountered at surgery. It is also important to bear in mind the clinical overlap between acute cholangitis and acute cholecystitis. Patients with sepsis secondary to impacted common bile duct calculi may have upper abdominal tenderness and guarding. Clearly, an appropriate index of suspicion together with findings on ultrasonography should result in such individuals being appropriately treated for their ductal calculi.

In the majority of patients with acute cholecystitis and deranged liver function tests there will be an opportunity to assess the common bile duct. The usual management strategy includes preoperative endoscopic retrograde cholangiopancreatography (ERCP). Increasing use is being made of magnetic resonance cholangiopancreatography (MRCP), as this investigation has the advantage that it is a non-invasive modality that may be as accurate as ERCP in detecting bile duct stones (**Fig. 8.2**),[8,9] although small stones may be missed.[10] In current practice, ERCP is widely used as it combines the opportunity for therapeutic intervention with diagnosis (**Fig. 8.3**).

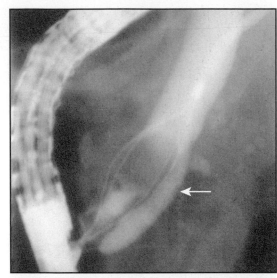

Figure 8.3 • Basket extraction of common bile duct calculi at endoscopic retrograde cholangiopancreatography. With thanks to Dr Kel Palmer, Consultant Gastroenterologist, Western General Hospital, Edinburgh, UK.

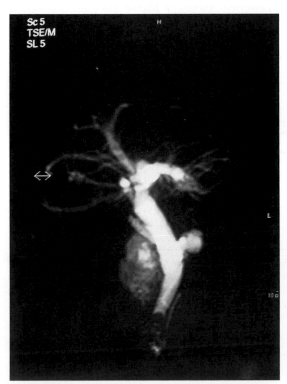

Figure 8.2 • Magnetic resonance cholangiogram demonstrating a single calculus in the distal common bile duct.

Other management strategies include intraoperative cholangiography during cholecystectomy (**Fig. 8.4**). If an impacted stone (with proximal duct dilatation and obstruction to flow of contrast into the duodenum) is demonstrated on intraoperative cholangiography, this constitutes an indication for common bile duct exploration. However, treatment of a non-obstructing calculus may be deferred at the time of initial surgery, with postoperative ERCP and stone extraction being undertaken. The main risk with adoption of a postoperative ERCP strategy is that failure to cannulate at endoscopy leaves the patient at risk of requiring a second surgical procedure.

Given that many surgeons would no longer regard acute cholecystitis as a contraindication to the laparoscopic approach, a logical extension to the procedure is to combine laparoscopic cholecystectomy with laparoscopic exploration of the common bile duct for the treatment of ductal stones. Studies from Australia[11] and Norwich[12] support such an approach. However, it should be noted that these studies are single-centre reports by enthusiastic advocates of laparoscopic bile duct exploration and application of their techniques outwith carefully evaluated programmes is likely to produce appreciably poorer outcomes.

Figure 8.5 illustrates our current algorithm for the investigation and management of patients with biliary colic or acute cholecystitis and suspected bile duct stones.

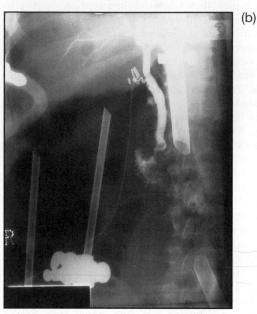

Figure 8.4 • Operative cholangiograms obtained during laparoscopic cholecystectomy demonstrating a non-obstructing calculus in **(a)** cystic duct and **(b)** distal common bile duct.

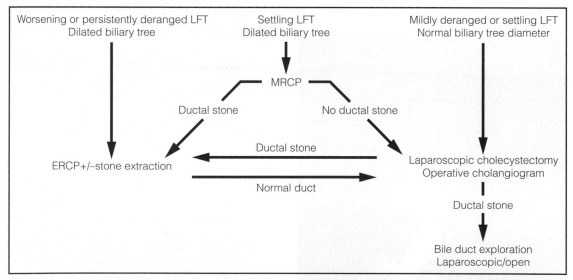

Figure 8.5 • Investigation and management of patients with biliary colic or acute cholecystitis and suspected bile duct stones. ERCP, endoscopic retrograde cholangiopancreatography; LFT, liver function tests; MRCP, magnetic resonance cholangiopancreatography.

Treatment

BILIARY COLIC

The initial treatment for biliary colic consists of adequate analgesia and antiemetics. Although opiate analgesia is widely prescribed, non-steroidal anti-inflammatory drugs (NSAIDs) are also effective in relieving pain.[13–15] Moreover, studies have suggested that NSAIDs can reduce the number of patients progressing from biliary colic to acute cholecystitis.[14,16] Following symptom resolution,

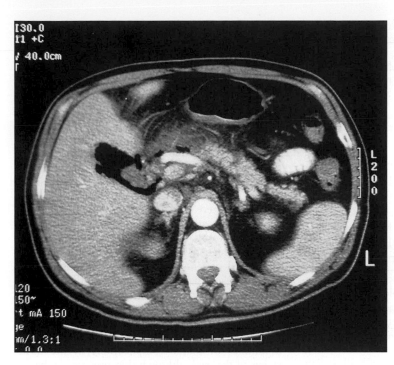

Figure 8.6 • Computed tomography of emphysematous cholecystitis demonstrating gas in the gallbladder wall with extension into the hepatoduodenal ligament.

optimal definitive therapy in the form of laparoscopic cholecystectomy should be undertaken. Although it is preferable to undertake surgery during the index admission, patients may be discharged with plans for an interval procedure, but at the risk of recurrent symptoms.

ACUTE CHOLECYSTITIS

Initial therapy in acute cholecystitis includes intravenous fluid resuscitation, analgesia, a nil-by-mouth regimen and administration of intravenous antibiotics. Although the initial inflammation is sterile, secondary infection with aerobic Gram-negative organisms (48%), enterococci (31%) and anaerobes (15%) occurs.[17] *Clostridium perfringens* infection of the necrotic gallbladder may be a particular complication in the diabetic patient. Few data exist to support the optimum antibiotic regimen, although a second- or third-generation cephalosporin combined with metronidazole is frequently prescribed.

Urgent surgical intervention is indicated in those patients with generalised peritonitis arising from a gallbladder perforation or in those with emphysematous cholecystitis (**Fig. 8.6**). Outwith these circumstances, the therapeutic options are to remove the gallbladder either during the index admission or electively at a later admission. Early operation has the advantage of prompt definitive therapy but surgical intervention may be technically more difficult. The rationale for deferred surgery is

to allow for resolution of inflammation, but the patient remains at risk of exacerbations during the 'waiting' period and subsequent 'delayed' surgery may still be very difficult.

Recent randomised controlled trials comparing early versus late laparoscopic cholecystectomy for acute cholecystitis have now confirmed that early laparoscopic cholecystectomy is both safe and has significant benefits for patients. Conversion rate, hospital stay and complications are all significantly lower in the early surgery group.[18–20]

The benefits of early laparoscopic cholecystectomy over early open cholecystectomy have also been assessed.[21] A total of 63 patients with acute cholecystitis were randomised to either early laparoscopic cholecystectomy ($n = 32$) or early open cholecystectomy ($n = 31$). Conversion to the open procedure was required in five patients randomised to laparoscopic cholecystectomy. Although there were no deaths or bile-duct injuries in either group, the postoperative complication rate was significantly higher in the open group ($P = 0.0048$): seven patients (23%) had major and six (19%) had minor complications after open cholecystectomy, whereas only one (3%) minor complication occurred after the laparoscopic procedure. Both the postoperative hospital stay (median 4 days vs. 6 days; $P = 0.0063$) and duration of sick leave (mean 13.9 days vs. 30.1 days; $P < 0.0001$) were significantly shorter in the laparoscopic group.

As a result, early laparoscopic cholecystectomy should be attempted in all patients with acute cholecystitis who are fit for surgery, recognising that there will be some in whom the acute inflammation prevents adequate visualisation of the anatomy and conversion will be required.

ANTIBIOTIC COVER FOR URGENT CHOLECYSTECTOMY

Antibiotic therapy following successful early cholecystectomy for acute non-gangrenous cholecystitis does not need to be continued beyond 12 hours.[22]

NON-SURGICAL OPTIONS FOR DECOMPRESSING THE GALLBLADDER IN ACUTE CHOLECYSTITIS

Although early laparoscopic cholecystectomy is optimal management in acute cholecystitis, surgery may not be feasible in some patients because of comorbid conditions. In these patients ultrasound-guided percutaneous cholecystostomy is a useful alternative (Fig. 8.7). If the diagnosis is in doubt, such as might be the case in the critically ill patient on the intensive care unit, percutaneous cholecystostomy can also be diagnostic,[23–26] with successful drainage of the gallbladder possible in up to 90% of patients.[23,25] Although cannulation of the gallbladder may be achieved through a transperitoneal approach, a transhepatic approach is to be preferred because of the lower risk of biliary peritonitis and the earlier maturation of the cholecystostomy tract.[27] Following insertion of the drainage tube into the gallbladder, free drainage is established, although antibiotic instillation may also be carried out.[28] It has also been suggested that simple aspiration of the gallbladder is as effective as formal cholecystostomy drainage.[29] Signs of effective

intervention usually occur within 24–48 hours;[23,24] therefore in those in whom rapid improvement does not occur, a complication of either the acute cholecystitis (gallbladder necrosis, perforation) or of the insertion of the cholecystostomy tube (bile leak, visceral perforation) should be presumed and surgical intervention should be reconsidered. The cholecystostomy tube should be maintained until a mature fistula tract is achieved. Contrast radiology in the form of a 'tubogram' may be undertaken in order to confirm drain position, cystic and common bile duct patency, as well as the presence and site of calculi.

To date there has only been one randomised clinical trial assessing the role of percutaneous cholecystostomy in patients with acute cholecystitis who are high-risk surgical candidates.[30] In this study, 123 patients with acute cholecystitis and an Acute Physiological and Chronic Health Evaluation (APACHE) II score of 12 or greater were randomised to either percutaneous cholecystostomy (PC, $n = 60$) or to conservative therapy (C, $n = 63$). Percutaneous cholecystostomy was associated with a number of major complications in the initial stages of the trial, although this appeared to be due to the use of non-locking drains inserted under computed tomography (CT) guidance. A change in technique to ultrasound-guided transhepatic placement of locking drains helped to lower procedure-related complications. Nevertheless, in this trial rates of clinical resolution (PC 86% vs. C 87%) and mortality (PC 17.5% vs. C 13%) were similar between the percutaneous cholecystostomy and conservative therapy groups. As a result, percutaneous cholecystostomy should be used in those patients not fit for surgery whose symptoms do not improve rapidly on standard conventional therapy.

Following disease resolution, definitive therapy directed towards the gallbladder needs to be

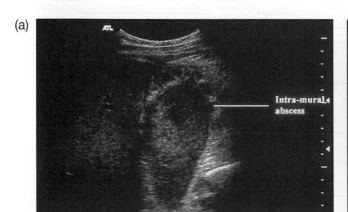
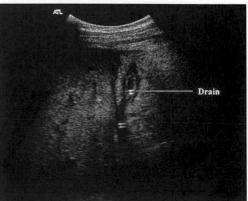

(a)   (b)

Intra-mural abscess

Drain

Figure 8.7 • Ultrasound of a patient with acute cholecystitis. **(a)** Before treatment; note the microabscesses within the thickened gallbladder wall. **(b)** After successful percutaneous transhepatic drainage. With thanks to Dr Paul Allan, Consultant Radiologist, Royal Infirmary, Edinburgh.

considered. Recurrent symptoms will occur in approximately one-third of patients who have previously had acute calculous cholecystitis and have not undergone definitive treatment.[31] Therefore interval cholecystectomy following optimisation of medical therapy treating comorbid disease should be considered. In those patients in whom surgical intervention is absolutely contraindicated, the cholecystostomy tube may be left in situ for a prolonged period.[32] Cholelithiasis may also be treated by percutaneous extraction of the gallstone or direct dissolution with a solvent such as methyl-*tert*-butyl ether. However, recurrence of gallstones following these therapies is common, with studies suggesting that 10–20% of all patients treated by these methods develop further symptoms.[33–35]

ACUTE ACALCULOUS CHOLECYSTITIS

Acute inflammation of the gallbladder can occur in the absence of gallstones and is termed acute acalculous cholecystitis (AAC). Although AAC may present as a complication of a number of clinical conditions, it occurs most frequently in the critically ill or postoperative patient. Despite the fact that AAC is an uncommon entity, it appears to be increasing in frequency.[36] Observational studies have suggested that AAC occurs in 0.004–0.05% of patients undergoing surgery.[37,38] However, although it is rarer than gallstone-induced acute cholecystitis, the mortality rate of AAC is significantly higher.[36]

The pathogenetic mechanisms in AAC are not clear. Most recent evidence suggests that AAC is a consequence of microvascular ischaemia resulting in gallbladder inflammation. Studies have demonstrated that the gallbladder arterial and capillary network is reduced and irregular in AAC compared with that in acute cholecystitis.[39,40] Further, in animal models the induction of a vasculitic process through the activation of factor XII causes AAC.[41] As indirect evidence, AAC can occur as a consequence of systemic lupus erythematosus, polyarteritis nodosa and antiphospholipid syndrome.[42–44] In critical illness states, gallbladder microvascular ischaemia probably occurs as a manifestation of the systemic inflammatory response syndrome.

The diagnosis of AAC is often difficult. Because it occurs principally in critically ill patients and in those who have recently had abdominal surgery, the symptoms and signs may be masked by coexisting problems. The critically ill patient may be sedated and/or ventilated, limiting history-taking, and abdominal signs may be masked by sedation or drug-induced paralysis. In the postoperative patient, abdominal signs may be limited by wound pain, and other more operation-specific complications

may be considered as a cause for changes in the clinical condition.

Unfortunately, diagnostic imaging may also be unhelpful. Although ultrasonographic signs of AAC have been described (dilated gallbladder, gallbladder wall thickening, pericholecystic fluid and gallbladder sludge), these are not diagnostic.[45] In a prospective series of 21 critically ill patients, all study subjects had gallbladder abnormalities on at least one occasion during serial ultrasound examinations; however, only four patients required intervention for AAC.[45] Similarly, although CT may demonstrate gallbladder abnormalities, these signs may again be non-diagnostic. Cholescintigraphy may be the most accurate method of identifying AAC. In a retrospective study of 27 patients with AAC, cholescintigraphy detected AAC in 9 of 10 patients (90%) whereas CT detected AAC in 8 of 12 (67%) and ultrasound detected AAC in 2 of 7 (29%).[46] However, these results must be viewed cautiously as all patients did not undergo all investigations. Moreover, other series have suggested a high incidence of false-positive cholescintigraphy scans in critically ill patients.[47] Because of the inaccuracy of imaging studies, the definitive diagnosis of AAC may only be made at laparotomy or diagnostic laparoscopy.[48] AAC must therefore be considered in all critically ill or postoperative patients with right upper quadrant pain, deranged liver function tests or unexplained sepsis. With the difficulty of diagnosis in mind, one prospective study assessed the benefit of percutaneous cholecystostomy in 82 critically ill patients with unexplained sepsis.[49] In 48 patients (59%) there was rapid improvement in the clinical condition within 48 hours but ultrasound did not predict which patients would respond to cholecystostomy. This study confirms the view that a low index of suspicion is required for the diagnosis of AAC in critically ill patients.

The optimal therapeutic strategy in AAC is not clear. In all patients, broad-spectrum antibiotic therapy should be instituted as 65% of bile cultures will be positive, with *Escherichia coli* the most common organism.[50] Therapeutic interventions include cholecystostomy with or without interval cholecystectomy, or early cholecystectomy. Several series have demonstrated that percutaneous cholecystostomy is not only an effective immediate intervention but may also constitute definitive treatment as the likelihood of recurrent episodes is small.[51,52] However, early cholecystectomy has been advocated because necrosis of the gallbladder may occur in up to 63% of cases,[46,53] with perforation occurring in approximately 15%. It would therefore appear reasonable to manage AAC in critically ill patients with initial percutaneous cholecystostomy, but in the absence of rapid clinical improvement a complication should be presumed and cholecystectomy carried out. In those patients managed successfully by percutaneous cholecystostomy there does not appear to be an absolute requirement for interval cholecystectomy.

ACUTE CHOLANGITIS

Acute cholangitis may be defined as an acute pyogenic infection within the biliary tree. Because of the possibility of rapid disease progression, acute cholangitis is a potentially life-threatening condition that requires urgent therapeutic intervention.

Pathogenesis

Acute cholangitis arises as a consequence of biliary stasis with subsequent bacterial infection. Although a number of pathological processes may lead to biliary stasis, the most common underlying causes of acute cholangitis are bile duct calculi, malignant bile duct obstruction and biliary stent occlusion. Biliary obstruction need not be complete as acute cholangitis can arise in a partially obstructed biliary system. Under normal conditions bile is sterile; however, in 58% of individuals with asymptomatic ductal calculi, bile cultures will be positive indicating bacterial colonisation.[54] In those progressing to acute cholangitis, cholangiovenous reflux of bacteria and bacterial products occurs because of increasing hydrostatic pressure within the biliary tree.[55,56] This cholangiovenous reflux results in bacteraemia and the induction of a systemic inflammatory response, and it is this response, leading to organ dysfunction, that is responsible for the morbidity and mortality in acute cholangitis. Decompression of the biliary tree removes the inflammatory insult.[57]

Aerobic Gram-negative bacilli (*E. coli*, *Klebsiella*, *Pseudomonas* species), enterococcus and anaerobes are the most common organisms cultured from the bile of patients with acute cholangitis.[54,58] In up to 50% of patients, anaerobic organisms may be associated with aerobic organisms.[59] In the elderly, polymicrobial infection is more common than monomicrobial infection, and again concomitant anaerobic infection occurs in the majority.[60] In approximately 35% of patients, blood cultures will be positive for the same organisms that are found in the bile.[58] The route of bacterial biliary colonisation is not clear; however, the types of bacteria involved suggest that they are derived from the intestinal tract.

Presentation

The presentation of acute cholangitis can be variable, ranging from mild symptoms and signs to overwhelming septic shock. Classically, patients with acute cholangitis present with the symptoms and signs that constitute Charcot's triad: upper abdominal pain, jaundice and pyrexia. However, the complete triad may be present in as few as 22% of patients.[61] Especially in the elderly patient, the presentation may be subtle, with signs of an acute confusional state being common,[62] with deranged liver function tests being the only pointer to the diagnosis. Similarly, acute cholangitis must be included in the differential diagnosis for any patient presenting with rigors. It is not uncommon for patients who have previously had endoscopic biliary stents to present with a rigor as the major feature of an obstructed infected stent. At the other end of the spectrum, acute cholangitis can present with signs of septic shock and evidence of multiple organ dysfunction. Because the progression to septic shock can be rapid in patients with biliary obstruction, the diagnosis of acute cholangitis must be considered in any patient presenting with jaundice and signs of sepsis.

Investigation

Cholestatic liver function tests are found in the majority of patients with acute cholangitis, demonstrating elevated bilirubin, alkaline phosphatase and gamma-glutamyl transferase. However, serum bilirubin may be normal in acute cholangitis arising in a partly obstructed biliary tree because the remaining unobstructed liver is able to compensate. A neutrophilia is typical and serum amylase may also be raised. Deranged coagulation tests can occur, either as a consequence of prolonged biliary obstruction resulting in vitamin K deficiency, or due to disseminated intravascular coagulation. Blood cultures must always be taken.

The initial radiological investigation of choice is transabdominal ultrasonography. This will demonstrate signs of bile duct obstruction, although false-negative scans can occur. Ultrasound may also determine the underlying pathology.

CT can identify biliary dilatation in 78% of patients with acute cholangitis as well as the level of obstruction in 65% and the cause of the obstruction in 61%;[63] however, the initial information obtained is no greater than with ultrasonography.

Although the determination of the exact site and nature of the bile duct obstruction may require direct visualisation with either ERCP or percutaneous transhepatic cholangiography (PTC), the true value of these procedures is their potential for therapeutic intervention. For this reason, although MRCP has recently been reported to be accurate in identifying biliary obstruction and the underlying obstructing lesion,[9] it does not have an early role in managing patients with acute cholangitis.

Management

Initial resuscitation aims to achieve adequate oxygen delivery, administration of an appropriate volume of intravenous fluid and appropriate analgesia. Efficacy of therapy is assessed by close monitoring of vital signs and, because of the potential for rapid decompensation, management of the patient in a high-dependency unit is usually required.

Aerobic Gram-negative bacilli are the most common organisms in acute cholangitis, and therefore empirical therapy with antibiotics covering these bacteria should be commenced. In addition, because anaerobic bacteria, although rarely cultured from blood, are frequently found in bile cultures in association with aerobic bacteria, antibiotic regimens should also have anaerobic activity. Piperacillin is an extended-spectrum penicillin with activity against aerobic Gram-negative bacilli, enterococcus and anaerobes. The addition of the β-lactamase inhibitor tazobactam increases the spectrum of activity.

In a randomised clinical trial involving 96 patients with acute cholangitis, piperacillin had similar efficacy to combination therapy with ampicillin and tobramycin, achieving clinical cure or significant improvement in 70% of patients.[64] In another randomised trial assessing single antibiotic therapy, Sung et al.[58] demonstrated that intravenous ciprofloxacin alone improved the clinical condition in 85% of cases and had similar efficacy to a combination of ceftazidime, ampicillin and metronidazole.

Although appropriate antibiotic therapy is important, relief of biliary obstruction is crucial to successful disease resolution. Emergency operative intervention is associated with significant risk, with a reported mortality of 20% and a 50% complication rate for patients with severe acute cholangitis.[65] As a result, the mainstay of treatment now is endoscopic bile duct drainage, with improved results compared with surgical intervention.[66]

The benefits of endoscopic therapy over surgery have been confirmed in a randomised controlled trial, with significantly fewer complications and lower mortality in those undergoing endoscopic drainage.[67]

The method used to achieve non-surgical biliary drainage would appear to be less important than simply achieving adequate drainage. Within the confines of a randomised trial, Lee et al.[68] demonstrated that biliary decompression in acute cholangitis with a biliary stent inserted without a sphincterotomy was as efficacious as insertion of a nasobiliary drain. In patients in whom ERCP is unsuccessful, drainage by PTC should be undertaken in the acute situation, even in patients who do not have a dilated intrahepatic biliary tree.[69] External drainage should be achieved in the first instance, with placement of a biliary stent as a staged procedure.

In the case of gallstone-related acute cholangitis, following resolution of the episode of acute cholangitis, adequate clearance of the bile duct should be confirmed by direct cholangiography, ERCP, high-quality MRCP or operative cholangiography. Cholecystectomy should be undertaken if there are no contraindications in order to reduce the risk of further gallstone-related problems.[70,71]

In summary, effective management in patients with acute cholangitis requires both antibiotic therapy and relief of biliary obstruction. Endoscopic and percutaneous drainage techniques are effective in the early stages but may also provide definitive therapy in certain patients.

ACUTE PANCREATITIS

Acute pancreatitis is defined as an acute inflammatory process of the pancreas, with variable involvement of other regional or remote organ systems.[72] It is a common acute illness, with epidemiological data from the Health Service Statistics Division in Scotland reporting an annual incidence of 318 cases per million (365 cases per million in men, 275 cases per million for women).[73] Analysis of patterns of incidence in this particular population (which has remained relatively constant over the past decade) suggests an increase in the incidence of acute pancreatitis, particularly in those over 40 years of age. Similar increases in the incidence of acute pancreatitis have also been observed in Germany,[74] Finland[75] and Denmark.[76] The factors giving rise to the observed increased incidences are not clear; however, at least in Finland, the increase in the incidence of acute pancreatitis is strongly correlated with an increase in alcohol consumption.

In practical terms the management of acute pancreatitis can be divided into two broad phases. The first phase includes the establishment of diagnosis, severity stratification, initial resuscitation and the choice of appropriate disease-specific initial therapy. The second phase relates to those with severe disease who will usually require further intervention for intra-abdominal complications or support for ongoing multiple organ failure. Recent guidelines[77–79] suggest that patients with complications arising from severe acute pancreatitis are most appropriately managed in a unit with specialist expertise and therefore this chapter only focuses on the initial phase of management. In this context, the

Box 8.1 • Terminology relating to acute pancreatitis as defined by the Atlanta consensus conference

Mild acute pancreatitis

Minimal organ dysfunction and an uneventful recovery

Severe acute pancreatitis

Associated with organ failure and/or local complications such as necrosis, abscess or pseudocyst

Acute fluid collections

Occur early in the course of acute pancreatitis, are situated in or near the pancreas, and always lack a wall of granulation or fibrous tissue

Pancreatic necrosis

Diffuse or focal areas of non-viable pancreatic parenchyma, typically associated with peripancreatic fat necrosis

Acute pseudocysts

Collection of pancreatic juice surrounded by a wall of fibrous or granulation tissue

Pancreatic abscess

Circumscribed intra-abdominal collection of pus arising in close proximity to the pancreas, but containing little or no pancreatic necrosis, which arises as a consequence of acute pancreatitis

Box 8.2 • Aetiological agents in acute pancreatitis

COMMON

Gallstones
Alcohol

UNCOMMON
Trauma

Endoscopic retrograde cholangiopancreatography
Sphincterotomy
Biliary manometry
Pancreatic duct obstruction
Ampulla of Vater neoplasia

Drugs

Azathioprine

Metabolic

Hypercalcaemia
Hyperlipidaemia

Infection

Mumps
Coxsackie B
HIV

Vascular

Vasculitis
Cardiopulmonary bypass

Hereditary pancreatitis

question of timing of transfer to a specialist unit should be addressed. Although there are data from a retrospective case series suggesting that delay in transfer may adversely affect outcome,[80] there are as yet no prospective comparative studies demonstrating a difference in mortality between patients admitted de novo to specialist units and those admitted to general surgical units.

Within this chapter the terminology used to describe patients with acute pancreatitis is in keeping with definitions agreed by the 1992 Atlanta consensus conference (**Box 8.1**).[78] Before this conference the terminology relating to acute pancreatitis was often confusing and imprecise, leading to difficulty in comparing data between centres. The Atlanta terminology is robust and relevant to biological disease patterns in acute pancreatitis and is now well established.

Aetiology

Acute pancreatitis may be caused by a wide variety of aetiological agents (**Box 8.2**), although the majority of cases are due to either gallstones or alcohol excess. Recent epidemiological studies have demonstrated that alcohol excess is an increasingly frequent cause of acute pancreatitis.[74,81] The prevalence of idiopathic acute pancreatitis varies between reported series and is probably a function of the degree of investigation undertaken to identify a cause. Recent UK guidelines state that no more than 20–25% of patients should be labelled as having idiopathic acute pancreatitis.[79]

Pathogenesis

The mechanisms through which each aetiological agent causes pancreatic acinar cell injury are not clear. However, after the initial pancreatic insult, it is believed that regardless of the aetiological agent the pathogenetic mechanisms of disease progression in acute pancreatitis are similar. Following pancreatic acinar cell injury, local pancreatic inflammation occurs. Although the inflammatory process may remain confined to the pancreas and peripancreatic tissues, a systemic inflammatory response may be triggered. This systemic inflammatory response is characterised by the systemic activation of leucocytes and endothelial cells and the secretion of proinflammatory cytokines, and is responsible for the development of the organ dysfunction that characterises severe acute pancreatitis.[82,83] It is not clear why some patients develop severe acute pancreatitis whilst others with similar aetiological agents develop mild acute pancreatitis; however, there is evidence to implicate both excessive pro-inflammatory mediators[84,85] and decreased anti-inflammatory mechanisms.[86]

Clinical presentation

Presenting symptoms may range from mild discomfort to overwhelming abdominal pain. Typically, patients present with increasing epigastric/central abdominal pain radiating through to the back. This pain may be eased by sitting forward. Nausea is a predominant early symptom, with associated vomiting or retching. Before presenting with gallstone-induced acute pancreatitis, patients may have had symptoms consistent with biliary colic. Likewise, in alcohol-induced acute pancreatitis, patients will have a long history of alcohol ingestion and/or recent binge drinking.

Signs of cardiovascular and respiratory dysfunction may be present. Examination may reveal abdominal signs ranging from localised epigastric tenderness to generalised peritonitis. More specific signs of severe acute pancreatitis include periumbilical bruising (Cullen's sign) and flank bruising (Grey Turner's sign) (**Fig. 8.8**; see also Plate 1, facing p. 116).

Diagnosis (see also Chapter 5)

Traditionally, the diagnosis of acute pancreatitis has depended on the detection of a serum amylase concentration more than three times the upper limit of normal. However, hyperamylasaemia may occur in several other conditions (**Box 8.3**), and a serum amylase concentration above the 'diagnostic' threshold does not definitely indicate acute pancreatitis. Conversely, acute pancreatitis may exist with serum amylase concentrations below this threshold. In those patients with a prolonged history prior to admission to hospital, serum amylase concentrations may have normalised. Amylase measurement therefore needs to be timely. Serum amylase levels do not provide prognostic information, nor can they be followed in order to monitor the early disease process.[87] However, very high levels of serum amylase on admission are suggestive of a gallstone aetiology.[88]

Because of the limitations of the serum amylase test, other markers have been used to diagnose acute pancreatitis. Serum lipase is perhaps the most common and is more sensitive and specific than

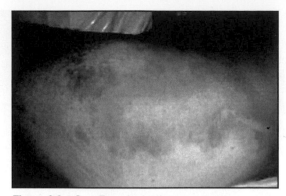

Figure 8.8 • Grey Turner's sign in severe acute pancreatitis. Reproduced from Hospital Medicine 2003; 64:150–5.

Box 8.3 • Main differential diagnoses of hyperamylasaemia

Acute pancreatitis
Pancreatic pseudocyst
Mesenteric infarction
Perforated viscus
Acute cholecystitis
Diabetic ketoacidosis

serum amylase. Moreover, because of its longer half-life, serum lipase is more accurate if there has been a delay in obtaining the initial sample.[77] However, as with serum amylase, serum lipase concentrations do not correlate with disease severity. In contrast, newer markers such as urinary trypsinogen activation peptide (TAP)[89] and serum carboxy-peptide B activation peptide (CAPAP-B)[90] provide both diagnostic and prognostic information.[91]

Although the vast majority of cases of acute pancreatitis can be diagnosed on the basis of clinical, biochemical and plain radiological findings, contrast-enhanced CT may be required in equivocal cases (**Fig. 8.9**).

Finally, in a few patients laparotomy may be required to confirm the diagnosis of acute pancreatitis while refuting other potential diagnoses such as acute mesenteric ischaemia or a perforated posterior duodenal ulcer. The decision to undertake diagnostic laparotomy is not made lightly as there is evidence that early operation has an adverse effect on outcome in acute pancreatitis.[92] In contrast, patients with acute intestinal ischaemia may present with abdominal pain and hyperamylasaemia and diagnostic delay may be critical. In the authors' unit, we have evolved the management strategy that if diagnostic uncertainty remains after assessment

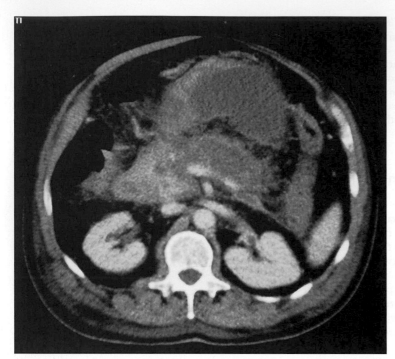

Figure 8.9 • Contrast-enhanced computed tomography of severe acute pancreatitis demonstrating a non-enhancing body of pancreas with an associated acute fluid collection.

of clinical, biochemical and plain radiological findings, contrast-enhanced CT is undertaken.[93] If the pancreas appears normal on CT, and in the absence of a firm diagnosis, we would proceed to laparoscopy or laparotomy if there are ongoing signs of peritonitis. Clearly, access to CT on a 24-hour basis is a prerequisite for this strategy.

Establishment of aetiology

Following diagnosis, usually confirmed biochemically, transabdominal ultrasound should be undertaken in all patients with acute pancreatitis to determine the presence or absence of gallstones.[79] For those patients in whom alcohol is thought to be the causative agent, an accurate history must be taken, with collaborative information being obtained from other sources if necessary.

Management

GENERAL GUIDELINES

Guidelines for the initial management of acute pancreatitis have been published by the British Society of Gastroenterology,[79] the American College of Gastroenterology,[78] the 1997 Santorini consensus conference,[77] the Japanese Society of Abdominal Emergency Medicine[94] and the International Association of Pancreatology.[95] Their recommendations are broadly similar.

INITIAL RESUSCITATION

As in other acute abdominal emergencies, initial therapy is aimed at adequate resuscitation. Provision of oxygen to maintain arterial oxygen saturation, intravenous fluid therapy and adequate analgesia constitute the mainstays of therapy. In addition, the correction of metabolic abnormalities such as hyperglycaemia or hypocalcaemia may require administration of intravenous insulin or calcium. Patients with acute pancreatitis should be started on some form of thromboprophylaxis (see also Chapter 14).[96] Antacid therapy with H_2 antagonists, proton pump inhibitors or other gastroprotective agents may be commenced as prophylaxis against upper gastrointestinal haemorrhage in those patients with severe disease.

SEVERITY STRATIFICATION

Following resuscitation, patients should be categorised into either prognostically mild or severe disease, allowing decisions to be taken regarding the degree of monitoring, supportive care and intervention appropriate for each patient. Subjective clinical assessment of prognosis is inaccurate and a validated prognostic scoring system should be used.[97] A number of systems currently exist and can be divided as follows.

- Multiple factor scoring systems: Glasgow,[98–100] Ranson[101] and APACHE II.[102]

- Biochemical scoring systems: C-reactive peptide (CRP)[103,104] and the Hong Kong system based on glucose and urea.[105]
- Immunological scoring: interleukin (IL)-6.[103,104]
- Radiological scoring: Balthazar[106] and Helsinki.[107]

It should be noted that the Ranson score is based on a North American population with alcohol as the predominant aetiological agent, whereas the Glasgow score is designed for use in a typical British population of gallstone-predominant disease. Further, practical confusion can result from the fact that there are at least three versions of the 'Glasgow' score: the original publication in 1978[98] and subsequent modifications in 1981[100] and 1984.[99] An APACHE II score of 9 or more has been validated for predicting prognostic severity in acute pancreatitis,[108] although a number of clinical trials have used lower cut-off points in order to predict severe disease, resulting in lower positive predictive values. Although an APACHE II score can be generated soon after admission, unlike the Ranson and Glasgow systems, it has the disadvantage of requiring collation of a sizeable number of variables. However, comparative studies have demonstrated that no single system is superior to the others.[109] It is also important to recognise that these scoring systems achieve approximately 80% accuracy in predicting prognosis. Finally, it should be noted that the currently used prognostic systems are a one-off or static assessment and that serial or dynamic assessment may provide a more accurate determination of outcome. Indeed, it would appear that it is not the presence of organ dysfunction at presentation that is important in determining outcome, rather it is the response to initial resuscitation. Buter et al.[110] have demonstrated that clinical outcome is worst in patients with persistent organ dysfunction, as manifested by worsening or static organ dysfunction scores following initial resuscitation, compared with patients whose organ dysfunction scores improve.

IMAGING IN ACUTE PANCREATITIS

As already mentioned, ultrasound should be performed in order to confirm or exclude the presence of gallstones. Following this, all patients with prognostically severe acute pancreatitis should undergo contrast-enhanced CT between the third and tenth day of admission to determine the presence of pancreatic necrosis.[79]

Specific therapies for acute pancreatitis

The majority of patients (74%) recover from an episode of acute pancreatitis without complication[111]

and require little intervention. However, despite intense biomedical research activity there remains a dearth of effective specific therapies for severe acute pancreatitis. The importance of vigorous volume resuscitation and careful monitoring and treatment for metabolic, respiratory, renal and cardiac complications cannot be overemphasised. However, in addition to this supportive care, the therapeutic options are limited. Randomised controlled trials have suggested evidence of benefit in severe acute pancreatitis in two areas of therapy: early ERCP and prophylactic antibiotics. However, controversy still persists regarding the relative values of both these therapeutic options. These treatments, together with other potential therapeutic options, are reviewed below.

EARLY ERCP

Early ERCP with endoscopic sphincterotomy (ES) in gallstone-induced acute pancreatitis aims to remove impacted ductal gallstones, thereby eliminating the initiating stimulus and hopefully reducing pancreatic inflammation. Three randomised trials assessing early ERCP have been published. They have produced some conflicting results so it is worth discussing the results in some detail.

Neoptolemos et al.[112] randomised 121 patients with gallstone-induced acute pancreatitis, 53 of whom had prognostically severe disease, to either early ERCP (n = 59) or conventional therapy (n = 62). Although there was no difference in mortality between the two groups (1 for ERCP vs. 5 for conservative therapy; P = 0.23), there was a significant reduction in total complications (17% ERCP vs. 34% conservative; P = 0.03) and duration of hospital stay (median 9.5, range 6–36, days ERCP vs. 17.0, range 4–74, days; P = 0.035) in those patients with prognostically severe disease. Similarly, Fan et al.[113] randomised 195 patients with acute pancreatitis, of whom only 127 had gallstone-induced disease and 81 prognostically severe disease, to either early ERCP (n = 97) or conventional therapy (n = 98). Again, there was no significant difference in mortality rates between the two groups (5 for ERCP vs. 9 for conservative therapy; P = 0.276). However, there was a significant reduction in the incidence of biliary sepsis following ERCP in those with prognostically severe acute pancreatitis (0% ERCP vs. 20% conservative; P = 0.008). Moreover, in those patients with gallstones a significant reduction in overall morbidity was obtained (16% ERCP vs. 33% conservative; P = 0.003).

In contrast, a multicentre trial undertaken by Fölsch et al.[114] randomised 238 patients with gallstone-induced acute pancreatitis but without evidence of biliary obstruction to undergo either early ERCP (n = 126) or conservative management (n = 112). In total 46 patients had prognostically severe disease. In contrast to the previous studies, the mortality rate was higher in the groups undergoing ERCP (10 for ERCP vs. 4 for conservative therapy; odds ratio 4.57, 95% CI 0.67–62.7, P = 0.16). Furthermore, ERCP was associated with an increased rate of respiratory failure (15 for ERCP vs. 5 for conservative; odds ratio 5.16, 95% CI 1.63–22.9, P = 0.03). Because of the trend towards increased mortality and the significantly increased rate of respiratory failure in those undergoing ERCP, the trial supervisory committee terminated the study early.

One further study exists that appears to support early ERCP/ES, although the results of this trial have to date only been published in abstract form. While the results suggest that early ERCP/ES is beneficial in patients with gallstone-induced acute pancreatitis, the conclusions that can be drawn must remain guarded as precise details regarding the study are limited.[115]

Rationalisation of the results of the three fully reported trials suggests that early ERCP/ES is of benefit in patients with prognostically severe gallstone-induced acute pancreatitis with evidence of cholangitis or biochemical evidence of obstructive liver function tests (serum bilirubin >90 μmol/L).

ANTIBIOTIC THERAPY

The administration of prophylactic antibiotics in acute pancreatitis is based on the hypothesis that the prevention of infected pancreatic necrosis would improve outcome; however, initial trials failed to demonstrate benefit.[116–118] The failure of these trials was probably not because the hypothesis was false but rather because ampicillin was used, which is now known not to penetrate pancreatic tissue. Furthermore, these studies did not restrict entry to patients with prognostically severe acute pancreatitis; thus the inclusion of patients with mild disease, who rarely develop pancreatic infection and improve regardless of intervention, reduced the ability of these studies to detect any potential benefit from treatment. More recent trials have now demonstrated improved outcome measures in patients with severe acute pancreatitis following the administration of prophylactic antibiotics.

In a multicentre trial, Pederzoli et al.[119] randomised 74 patients with CT-proven pancreatic necrosis to receive either imipenem or no initial antibiotic therapy. In the control group 30% developed pancreatic infection, whereas only 12% of patients treated with imipenem developed pancreatic infection (P < 0.001). Furthermore, rates of non-pancreatic infection were also significantly reduced in the antibiotic-treated group. However, antibiotic therapy had no effect on the development of multiple organ failure, the need for operative intervention or on the mortality rate. In another multicentre, randomised, controlled trial involving 60 patients with pancreatic necrosis, Bassi et al.[120] observed that intravenous perfloxacin was less effective than imipenem at reducing rates of both infected pancreatic necrosis (34% perfloxacin vs. 10% imipenem; P = 0.034) and extrapancreatic infection (44% perfloxacin vs. 20% imipenem; P = 0.059). There was no difference in mortality rates between the two groups.

The use of imipenem has been further studied by Nordback et al.[121] who undertook a randomised trial comparing the prophylactic use of imipenem with therapeutic use of imipenem in patients with severe acute pancreatitis and CT-proven pancreatic necrosis. Patients enrolled in the prophylactic arm received imipenem from the time of admission, whereas patients in the therapeutic arm only commenced imipenem following the development of signs suggesting the development of infected pancreatic necrosis (pyrexia, leucocytosis, raised CRP, in the absence of another source of infection). Although 90 patients were initially randomised, 32 patients were excluded from the final analysis (26 patients because when the initial CT was re-examined it was deemed not to demonstrate pancreatic necrosis, five because they were aged over 70 and were therefore felt not to be suitable for surgical intervention, and one because of inappropriate antibiotic administration). This resulted in 25 patients receiving prophylactic imipenem. In the opposite arm of the study, 14 of 33 patients received therapeutic imipenem following the development of signs of infected pancreatic necrosis. There was no significant difference in the number of patients requiring necrosectomy (2 prophylactic vs. 5 therapeutic; P = 0.41) or in the mortality rate (2 prophylactic vs. 5 therapeutic; P = 0.41) between the two groups. There are a number of significant concerns regarding this trial. Firstly, a large number (36%) of patients were excluded from the final data analysis. Secondly, the reported statistical analysis was not undertaken on an intention-to-treat basis. Thirdly, although the authors suggested that there was a significant reduction in major organ complications, the endpoints used to define organ complications were not entirely appropriate. The results of this trial must therefore be viewed with caution.

Sainio et al.[122] randomised 60 patients with CT-proven pancreatic necrosis to receive either intravenous cefuroxime or antibiotics only when there were clinical indications of infection. Although there was no difference in the rates of pancreatic infections between the two groups (30% cefuroxime vs. 40% control), prophylactic intravenous cefuroxime significantly reduced the mean number of infectious complications per patient (1.0 vs. 1.8; $P < 0.01$), mainly through a marked fall in the number of urinary tract infections. Most importantly, there was a significant reduction in the number of deaths in patients treated with cefuroxime (1 vs. 7; $P = 0.028$).

Delcenserie et al.[123] randomised 23 patients with alcohol-induced severe acute pancreatitis to either standard medical therapy or standard medical therapy plus intravenous ceftazidime, amikacin and metronidazole. Antibiotic therapy resulted in a significant reduction in the number of patients with proven infections (0 vs. 7; $P < 0.03$), but there was no significant reduction in mortality rates. Schwarz et al.[124] reported a randomised controlled trial of 26 patients with CT-proven pancreatic necrosis in which the combination of ofloxacin and metronidazole lessened the physiological disturbance found in severe acute pancreatitis, but did not prevent or delay the development of infected pancreatic necrosis. The small size of these last two studies precludes the drawing of any meaningful conclusions.

Using a different strategy aimed at eliminating the reservoir from which bacteria arise to colonise pancreatic necrosis, Luiten et al.[125] evaluated the role of selective gut decontamination. In a multi-centre trial, 102 patients with prognostically severe acute pancreatitis were randomised to either conventional therapy or conventional therapy supplemented with selective gut decontamination using oral and rectal colistin, amphotericin and norfloxacin. In addition, patients in the selective gut decontamination group received intravenous cefotaxime until aerobic Gram-negative bacteria were eliminated from the oral cavity and rectum. Encouragingly, selective gut decontamination reduced rates of pancreatic infection compared with the control group (38% vs. 18%; $P = 0.03$). Although there was a reduction in mortality from 35% in the control group to 22% in the selective decontamination group, it did not reach significance ($P = 0.19$). However, when allowing for differences in disease severity, multivariate analysis suggested a significant survival benefit following gut decontamination ($P = 0.048$).

These studies taken together suggest that prophylactic therapy in the form of intravenous antibiotics or selective gut decontamination may be beneficial in severe acute pancreatitis.[126] Indeed, intravenous antibiotic therapy is currently recommended for those with severe disease.[77–79,94,95] In line with this, a questionnaire survey found that 88% of surgeons in the UK prescribe prophylactic antibiotic therapy in acute pancreatitis.[97]

In order to present a balanced perspective it should be appreciated that although published guidelines call for the use of antibiotics in patients with severe acute pancreatitis, none of the published randomised trials is in itself of sufficient power to mandate antibiotic prophylaxis. In an attempt to strengthen the evidence regarding the use of antibiotic prophylaxis in acute pancreatitis, two meta-analyses have been performed. In 1998, Golub et al.[127] undertook a meta-analysis of all trials that had been published up to that point, including the original trials involving ampicillin,[116–118] and suggested that antibiotic prophylaxis was beneficial in reducing mortality. Furthermore, when separate analysis was performed on the trials which utilised broad-spectrum antibiotics in patients with severe disease,[119,122–124] the risk of death fell from 18.2% in patients not receiving antibiotic prophylaxis to 5.3% in those receiving prophylaxis (log odds ratio −0.32 to −2.44, $P = 0.008$). Similarly, Sharma and Howden[128] undertook a meta-analysis of three of the trials utilising broad-spectrum antibiotics in patients with severe disease.[119,122,124] They suggested that antibiotic prophylaxis resulted in a 12.3% (95% CI 2.7–22%) absolute risk reduction in mortality rate, with eight (95% CI 5–37) patients needing treatment to prevent one death.

However, in spite of the results of all these studies suggesting benefit from the use of antibiotic prophylaxis, concern still exists that the use of antibiotics will increase the rate of fungal-associated infected pancreatic necrosis and in turn adversely affect outcome. Although it has been reported that the use of antibiotic therapy alters the organisms involved in the development of infected pancreatic necrosis,[129,130] there is no definite evidence that rates of fungal infection have increased. Moreover, it is still not certain that fungal-associated infected pancreatic necrosis is associated with increased mortality when compared with bacterial-associated infected pancreatic necrosis.[131–134]

Further trials are therefore needed to clarify the role of antibiotic prophylaxis in acute pancreatitis. Such trials should have sufficient power to definitively determine whether prophylactic antibiotics reduce mortality, with subsequent work being performed to identify the optimal antibiotic regimen.

EARLY ENTERAL NUTRITION

In those patients with severe acute pancreatitis the systemic inflammatory response may be maintained by intestinal dysfunction, leading to bacterial translocation from the intestinal lumen. Intestinal dysfunction may in part be a consequence of the nil-by-mouth regimen, leading to a loss of luminal nutrition in the intestine. The provision of enteral nutrition aims to ameliorate intestinal dysfunction, thereby reducing the systemic inflammatory response and improving outcome.

McClave et al.[135] randomised 32 patients with acute pancreatitis to receive either early enteral nutrition through an endoscopically placed feeding tube or parenteral nutrition following central or peripheral venous cannulation. Enteral nutrition appeared to be well tolerated, with no patients developing a significant complication from the study intervention. Importantly, enteral nutrition was able to supply a similar caloric intake to parenteral nutrition. However, the patients in the study had relatively mild disease and thus no significant differences in clinical outcome were observed, although enteral nutrition was associated with a significant reduction in the cost of patient care.

A similar study that randomised 34 patients with acute pancreatitis to receive, in addition to standard therapy, either early enteral nutrition or parenteral nutrition demonstrated that the introduction of early enteral nutrition was associated with a significant reduction in CRP and APACHE II scores.[136] Furthermore, in those receiving parenteral nutrition, serum anti-endotoxin IgM antibody levels increased whereas they remained unchanged in those receiving enteral nutrition.

In contrast to the previous two studies, all patients in the randomised controlled trial reported by Kalfarentzos et al.[137] had prognostically severe disease. In total, 38 patients were randomised to receive either enteral nutrition or parenteral nutrition. Enteral nutrition was delivered distal to the ligament of Treitz through a radiologically screened feeding tube. Even in this population of patients with severe disease, enteral nutrition was well tolerated, with the protein and caloric intake equalling that administered to the patients receiving parenteral nutrition. This ability to provide adequate nutrition via the enteral route appeared to translate into a clinical benefit. In those patients receiving enteral nutrition there were significantly fewer complications and a significant reduction in the number of infectious episodes. Further, the cost of nutritional support in the enteral feeding group was one-third of that in the parenteral nutrition group.

A slightly different study randomised 27 patients with prognostically severe acute pancreatitis to either enteral nutrition or standard care, where parenteral nutrition was not instituted from the outset.[138] Although no major complications arose from the provision of enteral nutrition, it was not possible to meet full nutritional requirements. In contrast to previous studies, enteral nutrition did not appear to affect markers of the inflammatory response (IL-6, tumour necrosis factor receptors, CRP). Moreover, the institution of enteral nutrition was associated with a significant deterioration in gut barrier function.

In an attempt to determine the efficacy of both enteral nutrition and antibiotic prophylaxis, Olah et al.[139] undertook a two-phase study. In the first phase, patients within 72 hours of the onset of prognostically severe acute pancreatitis were 'randomised' to either parenteral nutrition or enteral nutrition delivered by a nasojejunal feeding tube. In this phase of the study there was no significant difference in the rates of septic complications between the two treatment groups. The second phase of the study was a prospective cohort study, with all patients being given enteral nutrition and imipenem with prophylactic intent, with subsequent comparison of outcome measures obtained in phase 2 with those obtained in phase 1. Following their analysis, the authors of this study stated that the combination of enteral nutrition and antibiotic prophylaxis significantly reduced the rate of septic complications and the requirement for surgical intervention when compared with parenteral nutrition. However, the results of the study have to be interpreted with caution. The initial phase of the study was not truly 'randomised', with patients being allocated to treatment groups according to date of birth, whereas the second phase involved comparison of historical cohorts. Both of these flaws may result in bias.

Another small study randomised 17 patients with prognostically severe acute pancreatitis (APACHE II score ≥ 6) to either enteral nutrition through a nasojejunal tube ($n = 8$) or parenteral nutrition ($n = 9$).[140] Not surprisingly, given the small numbers enrolled in the trial, there was no significant difference in morbidity between the two treatment groups, although the use of enteral nutrition was associated with an earlier institution of normal diet and resumption of normal bowel opening.

The interpretation of the results of all the published trials assessing the role of enteral nutrition and the subsequent translation of these into evidence-based clinical practice is difficult. Firstly, all the trials have insufficient power to determine the effects of enteral nutrition on the most relevant outcome measures of morbidity and mortality. Although a meta-analysis has been undertaken,[141] only the trials by McClave et al.[135] and Kalfarentzos et al.[137] met the study inclusion criteria and were used in the analysis. This meta-analysis observed that there was a trend to improved outcome following the use of enteral nutrition instead of parenteral nutrition, although the numbers included were small. Therefore, at present, there appears to be insufficient data upon which to make firm judgements. Secondly, all the randomised trials to date have delivered enteral nutrition through a nasojejunal feeding tube requiring either radiological or endoscopic placement. However, a prospective observational study has reported that successful nasogastric feeding can be achieved in patients with severe acute pancreatitis.[142] Thirdly, other than the trial conducted by Powell et al.,[138] enteral nutrition was compared with early parenteral nutrition. In general, it is not standard practice to commence parenteral nutrition immediately after admission with acute pancreatitis. Furthermore, it is possible that the observed 'benefits' from the institution of enteral nutrition, as compared with parenteral nutrition, are in fact due to the induction of deleterious effects by parenteral nutrition. Fong et al.[143] have demonstrated that a nil-by-mouth regimen and the institution of parenteral nutrition in normal volunteers is associated with an increased inflammatory response following a stimulus and malnourished patients have an impairment of intestinal function and increased markers of the acute-phase response.[144] Furthermore, the use of parenteral nutrition in acute pancreatitis is associated with a significant increase in line sepsis when compared with standard management.[145]

Although there is no definitive evidence demonstrating that early enteral nutrition improves outcome in severe acute pancreatitis, all published studies demonstrate that enteral nutrition is feasible, safe and does not exacerbate the disease process. Further trials are required to determine the impact of early enteral nutrition in predicted severe acute pancreatitis on infectious complications and disease outcome.

OTHER POTENTIAL TREATMENT STRATEGIES

Probiotic therapy

The use of probiotic therapy in acute pancreatitis is based on the hypothesis that colonisation of the proximal gastrointestinal tract by pathogenic bacteria is a precursor to the development of infected pancreatic necrosis. Probiotic therapy therefore aims to establish colonisation of the gastrointestinal tract by non-pathogenic bacteria, thereby reducing the risk of infective complications. This hypothesis was tested by randomising 45 patients with acute pancreatitis, 32 of whom had severe disease, to receive either live *Lactobacillus plantarum* ($n = 22$) or killed *Lactobacillus plantarum* ($n = 23$) delivered via a nasojejunal feeding tube, along with oat fibre as a bacterial substrate.[146] All patients received a standard enteral nutrition formula in addition to the live or killed *Lactobacillus plantarum*. Within this trial, probiotic therapy appeared to reduce the risk of developing either infected pancreatic necrosis or abscess. One patient who received live *Lactobacillus plantarum* developed pancreatic infection compared with seven patients in the control group ($P = 0.023$). Although these are encouraging results suggesting benefit from probiotic therapy, further trials are required.

Anticytokine therapy

With increased understanding of the pathogenetic mechanisms in acute pancreatitis, it is hoped that novel therapies will be developed that can perturb these mechanisms and improve outcome. Indeed a large number of agents that either antagonise the proinflammatory response or augment the anti-inflammatory response have been demonstrated to ameliorate disease severity in animal models of acute pancreatitis. However, it should be noted that in these studies the agent is usually administered before or immediately after the induction of acute pancreatitis, a scenario that does not translate to the clinical situation. One such agent to undergo clinical trials is lexipafant, a high-affinity platelet-activating factor receptor antagonist which acts as a general down-regulator of the proinflammatory cytokine response. On the basis of encouraging results from initial trials,[147–150] a large multicentre trial recruiting 1500 patients was undertaken. Although the trial results have not been formally reported, it is widely known that there was no improvement in mortality following the use of lexipafant, and that the manufacturers are now no longer pursuing this drug as a treatment for severe acute pancreatitis.

It is expected that further drugs perturbing the pathogenetic mechanisms of acute pancreatitis will be developed and will undergo clinical trials.

Prognosis

Current UK guidelines provide targets for mortality rates in acute pancreatitis.[79] These guidelines state that overall mortality should be less than 10% of patients admitted with acute pancreatitis, with a mortality rate less than 30% in those with prognostically severe acute pancreatitis. Encouragingly, recent epidemiological data have suggested that there has been a reduction in mortality rates over recent years.[73]

Treatment of gallstones in acute gallstone pancreatitis

In 1988, before laparoscopic surgery, Kelly and Wagner[151] randomised 165 patients with gallstone-induced acute pancreatitis to either early ($n = 83$) or late ($n = 82$) biliary surgery, with early surgery being undertaken within 48 hours of admission. In those with mild acute pancreatitis ($n = 125$) there was no significant difference in outcome between the two groups (morbidity: early 6.7% vs. late 3.3%, $P > 0.10$; mortality: early 3.1% vs. late 0%, $P > 0.10$). However, in those with severe acute pancreatitis ($n = 40$) early biliary surgery resulted in a significant increase in morbidity and mortality (morbidity: early 82.6% vs. late 17.6%, $P < 0.001$; mortality: early 47.8% vs. late 11%, $P < 0.025$).

It would therefore seem appropriate for patients with gallstone-induced mild acute pancreatitis to undergo cholecystectomy during the index admission; indeed the British Society of Gastroenterology guidelines recommend that this group of patients should undergo cholecystectomy (now using the laparoscopic technique) within 2–4 weeks of disease onset.[79] In

patients with severe comorbid disease contraindicating cholecystectomy, definitive treatment may be provided by ES.[152] In those with gallstone-induced severe disease, cholecystectomy should be delayed until disease resolution or undertaken as an additional procedure during surgery for a complication of acute pancreatitis.

Key points

- Laparoscopic cholecystectomy is the gold standard intervention for the management of biliary colic and acute cholecystitis.
- Laparoscopic cholecystectomy during the index admission is both feasible and safe in patients with acute cholecystitis.
- Percutaneous cholecystostomy may be undertaken in those patients with acute cholecystitis who do not respond to conservative management and have significant comorbidity contraindicating emergency surgical intervention.
- Percutaneous cholecystostomy may be definitive therapy in patients with acute acalculous cholecystitis.
- Intravenous antibiotics and endoscopic drainage of the biliary tree form the basis of management for patients with acute cholangitis.
- Definitive management of acute cholangitis secondary to choledocholithiasis includes cholecystectomy in order to reduce the risk of further gallstone-related complications.
- Acute pancreatitis is an increasingly common life-threatening illness.
- Initial management of severe acute pancreatitis involves appropriate resuscitation and organ support.
- Prophylactic broad-spectrum antibiotics may reduce mortality and morbidity in severe acute pancreatitis.
- Early ERCP and ES should be undertaken in patients with gallstone-induced severe acute pancreatitis and evidence of either acute cholangitis or significant biliary obstruction (serum bilirubin > 90 μmol/L).
- Surgery has little role in the initial management of severe acute pancreatitis.
- Cholecystectomy should be undertaken in patients with gallstone-induced acute pancreatitis.
- Complicated severe acute pancreatitis should be managed in a specialist unit.

REFERENCES

1. Nathanson LK. Gallstones. In: Garden OJ (ed.) Hepatobiliary and pancreatic surgery, 2nd edn. Edinburgh: WB Saunders, 2001; pp. 213–40.

2. Mirizzi PL. Sindrome del conducto hepatico. J Int Chir 1948; 8:731–2.

3. Cooperberg PL, Gibney RG. Imaging of the gallbladder, 1987. Radiology 1987; 163:605–13.

4. Soyer P, Brouland JP, Boudiaf M et al. Color velocity imaging and power Doppler sonography of the gallbladder wall: a new look at sonographic diagnosis of acute cholecystitis. Am J Roentgenol 1998; 171:183–8.

5. Samuels BI, Freitas JE, Bree RL, Schwab RE, Heller ST. A comparison of radionuclide hepatobiliary imaging and real-time ultrasound for the detection of acute cholecystitis. Radiology 1983; 147:207–10.

6. Fink-Bennett D, Freitas JE, Ripley SD, Bree RL. The sensitivity of hepatobiliary imaging and real-time ultrasonography in the detection of acute cholecystitis. Arch Surg 1985; 120:904–6.

7. Flancbaum L, Choban PS, Sinha R, Jonasson O. Morphine cholescintigraphy in the evaluation of hospitalized patients with suspected acute cholecystitis. Ann Surg 1994; 220:25–31.

8. Magnuson TH, Bender JS, Duncan MD, Ahrendt SA, Harmon JW, Regan F. Utility of magnetic resonance cholangiography in the evaluation of biliary obstruction. J Am Coll Surg 1999; 189:63–71; discussion 71–2.

9. Varghese JC, Farrell MA, Courtney G, Osborne H, Murray FE, Lee MJ. A prospective comparison of magnetic resonance cholangiopancreatography with endoscopic retrograde cholangiopancreatography in the evaluation of patients with suspected biliary tract disease. Clin Radiol 1999; 54:513–20.

10. Zidi SH, Prat F, Le Guen O et al. Use of magnetic resonance cholangiography in the diagnosis of choledocholithiasis: prospective comparison with a reference imaging method. Gut 1999; 44:118–22.

11. Martin IJ, Bailey IS, Rhodes M, O'Rourke N, Nathanson L, Fielding G. Towards T-tube free laparoscopic bile duct exploration: a methodologic evolution during 300 consecutive procedures. Ann Surg 1998; 228:29–34.

12. Rhodes M, Sussman L, Cohen L, Lewis MP. Randomised trial of laparoscopic exploration of common bile duct versus postoperative endoscopic retrograde cholangiography for common bile duct stones. Lancet 1998; 351:159–61.

Evidence relating to the safety and efficacy of laparoscopic bile duct exploration in the management of choledocholithiasis.

13. Broggini M, Corbetta E, Grossi E, Borghi C. Diclofenac sodium in biliary colic: a double blind trial. Br Med J (Clin Res Ed) 1984; 288:1042.

14. Goldman G, Kahn PJ, Alon R, Wiznitzer T. Biliary colic treatment and acute cholecystitis prevention by prostaglandin inhibitor. Dig Dis Sci 1989; 34:809–11.

15. Magrini M, Rivolta G, Movilia PG, Moretti MP, Liverta C, Bruni G. Successful treatment of biliary colic with intravenous ketoprofen or lysine acetylsalicylate. Curr Med Res Opin 1985; 9:454–60.

16. Akriviadis EA, Hatzigavriel M, Kapnias D, Kirimlidis J, Markantas A, Garyfallos A. Treatment of biliary colic with diclofenac: a randomized, double-blind, placebo-controlled study. Gastroenterology 1997; 113:225–31.

17. Claesson BE, Holmlund DE, Matzsch TW. Microflora of the gallbladder related to duration of acute cholecystitis. Surg Gynecol Obstet 1986; 162:531–5.

18. Lo CM, Liu CL, Fan ST, Lai EC, Wong J. Prospective randomized study of early versus delayed laparoscopic cholecystectomy for acute cholecystitis. Ann Surg 1998; 227:461–7.

Randomised study of 99 patients to either early (within 72 hours) or delayed laparoscopic cholecystectomy. Early surgery was associated with a lower conversion rate (early 11% vs. delayed 23%; $P = 0.174$), lower complication rate (early 13% vs. delayed 29%; $P = 0.07$), shorter total hospital stay (early 6 days vs. delayed 11 days; $P < 0.001$) and shorter recuperation period (early 12 days vs. delayed 19 days; $P < 0.001$).

19. Lai PB, Kwong KH, Leung KL et al. Randomized trial of early versus delayed laparoscopic cholecystectomy for acute cholecystitis. Br J Surg 1998; 85:764–7.

Randomised study of 104 patients to either early ($n = 53$) or delayed ($n = 51$) laparoscopic cholecystectomy. Surgery would appear to have been more difficult in the early group as manifested by significantly longer operating times (123 vs. 107 min; $P = 0.04$); however, this did not translate into a higher conversion rate (early 21% vs. delayed 24%; $P = 0.74$). Morbidity rates were similar between the two groups, with no bile duct injuries reported. Early surgery was associated with a significant reduction in overall hospital stay (7.6 vs. 11.6 days; $P < 0.001$).

20. Johansson M, Thune A, Blomqvist A, Nelvin L, Lundell L. Management of acute cholecystitis in the laparoscopic era: results of a prospective, randomized clinical trial. J Gastrointest Surg 2003; 7:642–5.

Study of 145 patients randomised to early laparoscopic cholecystectomy within the first 7 days (early, *n* = 71) or to interval cholecystectomy at 6–8 weeks (late, *n* = 74). In the late group, 26% failed conservative therapy and required urgent laparoscopic cholecystectomy. On an intention-to-treat basis, analysis demonstrated no significant difference in conversion rates (early 31% vs. delayed 29%; *P* = 0.78) or complications, although one major bile duct injury occurred in the delayed group. There was a reduction in overall hospital stay [early 5 (range 3–63) days vs. delayed 8 (range 4–50) days; *P* < 0.05].

21. Kiviluoto T, Siren J, Luukkonen P, Kivilaakso E. Randomised trial of laparoscopic versus open cholecystectomy for acute and gangrenous cholecystitis. Lancet 1998; 351:321–5.

    Significantly lower complication rate in laparoscopic group, with shorter hospital stay and quicker return to work.

22. Lau WY, Yuen WK, Chu KW, Chong KK, Li AK. Systemic antibiotic regimens for acute cholecystitis treated by early cholecystectomy. Aust NZ J Surg 1990; 60:539–43.

    In a randomised trial of 203 patients, the continuation of cefamandole for 12 hours after surgery had equal efficacy with a prolonged dosage schedule of 7 days but was associated with less adverse drug reactions.

23. Werbel GB, Nahrwold DL, Joehl RJ, Vogelzang RL, Rege RV. Percutaneous cholecystostomy in the diagnosis and treatment of acute cholecystitis in the high-risk patient. Arch Surg 1989; 124:782–5; discussion 785–6.

24. Vauthey JN, Lerut J, Martini M, Becker C, Gertsch P, Blumgart LH. Indications and limitations of percutaneous cholecystostomy for acute cholecystitis. Surg Gynecol Obstet 1993; 176:49–54.

25. McGahan JP, Lindfors KK. Percutaneous cholecystostomy: an alternative to surgical cholecystostomy for acute cholecystitis? Radiology 1989; 173:481–5.

26. Lo LD, Vogelzang RL, Braun MA, Nemcek AA Jr. Percutaneous cholecystostomy for the diagnosis and treatment of acute calculous and acalculous cholecystitis. J Vasc Intervent Radiol 1995; 6:629–34.

27. Hatjidakis AA, Karampekios S, Prassopoulos P et al. Maturation of the tract after percutaneous cholecystostomy with regard to the access route. Cardiovasc Intervent Radiol 1998; 21:36–40.

28. Salim AS. Percutaneous aspiration, lavage and antibiotic instillation. New approach in the management of acute calculous cholecystitis. HPB Surg 1991; 3:167–75; discussion 175–6.

29. Chopra S, Dodd GD III, Mumbower AL et al. Treatment of acute cholecystitis in non-critically ill patients at high surgical risk: comparison of clinical outcomes after gallbladder aspiration and after percutaneous cholecystostomy. Am J Roentgenol 2001; 176:1025–31.

30. Hatzidakis AA, Prassopoulos P, Petinarakis I et al. Acute cholecystitis in high-risk patients: percutaneous cholecystostomy vs conservative treatment. Eur Radiol 2002; 12:1778–84.

31. Vetrhus M, Soreide O, Nesvik I, Sondenaa K. Acute cholecystitis: delayed surgery or observation. A randomized clinical trial. Scand J Gastroenterol 2003; 38:985–90.

32. Boland GW, Lee MJ, Mueller PR et al. Gallstones in critically ill patients with acute calculous cholecystitis treated by percutaneous cholecystostomy: nonsurgical therapeutic options. Am J Roentgenol 1994; 162:1101–3.

33. McDermott VG, Arger P, Cope C. Gallstone recurrence and gallbladder function following percutaneous cholecystolithotomy. J Vasc Intervent Radiol 1994; 5:473–8.

34. Courtois CS, Picus DD, Hicks ME et al. Percutaneous gallstone removal: long-term follow-up. J Vasc Intervent Radiol 1996; 7:229–34.

35. Hellstern A, Leuschner U, Benjaminov A et al. Dissolution of gallbladder stones with methyl *tert*-butyl ether and stone recurrence: a European survey. Dig Dis Sci 1998; 43:911–20.

36. Glenn F, Becker CG. Acute acalculous cholecystitis. An increasing entity. Ann Surg 1982; 195:131–6.

37. Inoue T, Mishima Y. Postoperative acute cholecystitis: a collective review of 494 cases in Japan. Jpn J Surg 1988; 18:35–42.

38. Devine RM, Farnell MB, Mucha P Jr. Acute cholecystitis as a complication in surgical patients. Arch Surg 1984; 119:1389–93.

39. Hakala T, Nuutinen PJ, Ruokonen ET, Alhava E. Microangiopathy in acute acalculous cholecystitis. Br J Surg 1997; 84:1249–52.

40. Warren BL. Small vessel occlusion in acute acalculous cholecystitis. Surgery 1992; 111:163–8.

41. Becker CG, Dubin T, Glenn F. Induction of acute cholecystitis by activation of factor XII. J Exp Med 1980; 151:81–90.

42. Kamimura T, Mimori A, Takeda A et al. Acute acalculous cholecystitis in systemic lupus erythematosus: a case report and review of the literature. Lupus 1998; 7:361–3.

43. Dessailloud R, Papo T, Vaneecloo S, Gamblin C, Vanhille P, Piette JC. Acalculous ischemic gallbladder necrosis in the catastrophic antiphospholipid syndrome. Arthritis Rheum 1998; 41:1318–20.

44. Parangi S, Oz MC, Blume RS et al. Hepatobiliary complications of polyarteritis nodosa. Arch Surg 1991; 126:909–12.

45. Helbich TH, Mallek R, Madl C et al. Sono-morphology of the gallbladder in critically ill patients. Value of a scoring system and follow-up examinations. Acta Radiol 1997; 38:129–34.

46. Kalliafas S, Ziegler DW, Flancbaum L, Choban PS. Acute acalculous cholecystitis: incidence, risk factors, diagnosis, and outcome. Am Surg 1998; 64:471–5.

47. Kalff V, Froelich JW, Lloyd R, Thrall JH. Predictive value of an abnormal hepatobiliary scan in patients with severe intercurrent illness. Radiology 1983; 146:191–4.

48. Almeida J, Sleeman D, Sosa JL, Puente I, McKenney M, Martin L. Acalculous chole-cystitis: the use of diagnostic laparoscopy. J Laparoendosc Surg 1995; 5:227–31.

49. Boland GW, Lee MJ, Leung J, Mueller PR. Percutaneous cholecystostomy in critically ill patients: early response and final outcome in 82 patients. Am J Roentgenol 1994; 163:339–42.

50. Howard RJ. Acute acalculous cholecystitis. Am J Surg 1981; 141:194–8.

51. Shirai Y, Tsukada K, Kawaguchi H, Ohtani T, Muto T, Hatakeyama K. Percutaneous trans-hepatic cholecystostomy for acute acalculous cholecystitis. Br J Surg 1993; 80:1440–2.

52. Sugiyama M, Tokuhara M, Atomi Y. Is percu-taneous cholecystostomy the optimal treatment for acute cholecystitis in the very elderly? World J Surg 1998; 22:459–63.

53. Shapiro MJ, Luchtefeld WB, Kurzweil S, Kaminski DL, Durham RM, Mazuski JE. Acute acalculous cholecystitis in the critically ill. Am Surg 1994; 60:335–9.

54. Csendes A, Burdiles P, Maluenda F, Diaz JC, Csendes P, Mitru N. Simultaneous bacteriologic assessment of bile from gallbladder and common bile duct in control subjects and patients with gallstones and common duct stones. Arch Surg 1996; 131:389–94.

55. Huang T, Bass JA, Williams RD. The signifi-cance of biliary pressure in cholangitis. Arch Surg 1969; 98:629–32.

56. Lygidakis NJ, Brummelkamp WH. The signifi-cance of intrabiliary pressure in acute cholangitis. Surg Gynecol Obstet 1985; 161:465–9.

57. Lau JY, Chung SC, Leung JW, Ling TK, Yung MY, Li AK. Endoscopic drainage aborts endotoxaemia in acute cholangitis. Br J Surg 1996; 83:181–4.

58. Sung JJ, Lyon DJ, Suen R et al. Intravenous ciprofloxacin as treatment for patients with acute suppurative cholangitis: a randomized, controlled clinical trial. J Antimicrob Chemother 1995; 35:855–64.

59. Marne C, Pallares R, Martin R, Sitges-Serra A. Gangrenous cholecystitis and acute cholangitis associated with anaerobic bacteria in bile. Eur J Clin Microbiol 1986; 5:35–9.

60. Shimada K, Noro T, Inamatsu T, Urayama K, Adachi K. Bacteriology of acute obstructive suppurative cholangitis of the aged. J Clin Microbiol 1981; 14:522–6.

61. Csendes A, Diaz JC, Burdiles P, Maluenda F, Morales E. Risk factors and classification of acute suppurative cholangitis. Br J Surg 1992; 79:655–8.

62. Sugiyama M, Atomi Y. Treatment of acute cholangitis due to choledocholithiasis in elderly and younger patients. Arch Surg 1997; 132: 1129–33.

63. Balthazar EJ, Birnbaum BA, Naidich M. Acute cholangitis: CT evaluation. J Comput Assist Tomogr 1993; 17:283–9.

64. Thompson JE Jr, Pitt HA, Doty JE, Coleman J, Irving C. Broad spectrum penicillin as an adequate therapy for acute cholangitis. Surg Gynecol Obstet 1990; 171:275–82.

65. Lai EC, Tam PC, Paterson IA et al. Emergency surgery for severe acute cholangitis. The high-risk patients. Ann Surg 1990; 211:55–9.

66. Leese T, Neoptolemos JP, Baker AR, Carr-Locke DL. Management of acute cholangitis and the impact of endoscopic sphincterotomy. Br J Surg 1986; 73:988–92.

67. Lai EC, Mok FP, Tan ES et al. Endoscopic biliary drainage for severe acute cholangitis. N Engl J Med 1992; 326:1582–6.

A randomised controlled trial comparing endoscopic biliary drainage with surgical decompression in 82 patients with severe acute cholangitis as manifested by signs of shock or progression of the disease despite appropriate antibiotics. In those undergoing endoscopic therapy there were fewer complications (34% vs. 66%; $P > 0.05$) but more importantly a significant reduction in mortality (10% vs. 32%; $P < 0.03$).

68. Lee DW, Chan AC, Lam YH et al. Biliary decompression by nasobiliary catheter or biliary stent in acute suppurative cholangitis: a prospective randomized trial. Gastrointest Endosc 2002; 56:361–5.

69. Pessa ME, Hawkins IF, Vogel SB. The treatment of acute cholangitis. Percutaneous transhepatic biliary drainage before definitive therapy. Ann Surg 1987; 205:389–92.

70. Boerma D, Rauws EA, Keulemans YC et al. Wait-and-see policy or laparoscopic chole-cystectomy after endoscopic sphincterotomy for bile-duct stones: a randomised trial. Lancet 2002; 360:761–5.

Evidence regarding the management of cholelithiasis following successful treatment of choledocholithiasis.

71. Targarona EM, Ayuso RM, Bordas JM et al. Randomised trial of endoscopic sphincterotomy with gallbladder left in situ versus open surgery for common bileduct calculi in high-risk patients. Lancet 1996; 347:926–9.

72. Bradley ELD. A clinically based classification system for acute pancreatitis. Summary of the International Symposium on Acute Pancreatitis, Atlanta, Ga, September 11 through 13, 1992. Arch Surg 1993; 128:586–90.

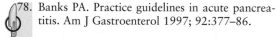

Consensus conference which defines the current terminology in acute pancreatitis.

73. McKay CJ, Evans S, Sinclair M, Carter CR, Imrie CW. High early mortality rate from acute pancreatitis in Scotland, 1984–1995. Br J Surg 1999; 86:1302–5.

74. Lankisch PG, Schirren CA, Schmidt H, Schonfelder G, Creutzfeldt W. Etiology and incidence of acute pancreatitis: a 20-year study in a single institution. Digestion 1989; 44:20–5.

75. Jaakkola M, Nordback I. Pancreatitis in Finland between 1970 and 1989. Gut 1993; 34:1255–60.

76. Floyd A, Pedersen L, Nielsen GL, Thorladcius-Ussing O, Sorensen HT. Secular trends in incidence and 30-day case fatality of acute pancreatitis in North Jutland County, Denmark: a register-based study from 1981–2000. Scand J Gastroenterol 2002; 37:1461–5.

77. Dervenis C, Johnson CD, Bassi C et al. Diagnosis, objective assessment of severity, and management of acute pancreatitis. Santorini consensus conference. Int J Pancreatol 1999; 25:195–210.

78. Banks PA. Practice guidelines in acute pancreatitis. Am J Gastroenterol 1997; 92:377–86.

79. Glazer G, Mann DV. United Kingdom guidelines for the management of acute pancreatitis. Gut 1998; 42(Suppl. 2):S1–S13.

80. de Beaux AC, Palmer KR, Carter DC. Factors influencing morbidity and mortality in acute pancreatitis: an analysis of 279 cases. Gut 1995; 37:121–6.

81. Mero M. Changing aetiology of acute pancreatitis. Ann Chir Gynaecol 1982; 71:126–9.

82. Kingsnorth A. Role of cytokines and their inhibitors in acute pancreatitis. Gut 1997; 40:1–4.

83. Norman J. The role of cytokines in the pathogenesis of acute pancreatitis. Am J Surg 1998; 175:76–83.

84. McKay CJ, Gallagher G, Brooks B, Imrie CW, Baxter JN. Increased monocyte cytokine production in association with systemic complications in acute pancreatitis. Br J Surg 1996; 83:919–23.

85. de Beaux AC, Goldie AS, Ross JA, Carter DC, Fearon KC. Serum concentrations of inflammatory mediators related to organ failure in patients with acute pancreatitis. Br J Surg 1996; 83:349–53.

86. Pezzilli R, Billi P, Miniero R, Barakat B. Serum interleukin-10 in human acute pancreatitis. Dig Dis Sci 1997; 42:1469–72.

87. Imrie CW, Wilson C. Evaluation of severity in acute pancreatitis and the need for early surgery. In: Carter DC, Warshaw AL (eds) Pancreatitis. Edinburgh: Churchill Livingstone, 1989; pp. 31–43.

88. Davidson BR, Neoptolemos JP, Leese T, Carr-Locke DL. Biochemical prediction of gallstones in acute pancreatitis: a prospective study of three systems. Br J Surg 1988; 75:213–15.

89. Gudgeon AM, Heath DI, Hurley P et al. Trypsinogen activation peptides assay in the early prediction of severity of acute pancreatitis. Lancet 1990; 335:4–8.

90. Appelros S, Thim L, Borgstrom A. Activation peptide of carboxypeptidase B in serum and urine in acute pancreatitis. Gut 1998; 42:97–102.

91. Buchler MW, Uhl W, Andren-Sandberg A. CAPAP in acute pancreatitis: just another marker or real progress? Gut 1998; 42:8–9.

92. Mier J, Leon EL, Castillo A, Robledo F, Blanco R. Early versus late necrosectomy in severe necrotizing pancreatitis. Am J Surg 1997; 173:71–5.

93. Powell JJ, Siriwardena AK. Management strategy for differentiating between acute intestinal ischaemia and acute pancreatitis. Eur J Surg 2000; 166:823–5.

94. Mayumi T, Ura H, Arata S et al. Evidence-based clinical practice guidelines for acute pancreatitis: proposals. J Hepatobiliary Pancreat Surg 2002; 9:413–22.

95. Uhl W, Warshaw A, Imrie C et al. IAP guidelines for the surgical management of acute pancreatitis. Pancreatology 2002; 2:565–73.

96. Prophylaxis of venous thromboembolism. Scottish Intercollegiate Guidelines Network, 2002.

97. Powell JJ, Campbell E, Johnson CD, Siriwardena AK. Survey of antibiotic prophylaxis in acute pancreatitis in the UK and Ireland. Br J Surg 1999; 86:320–2.

98. Imrie CW, Benjamin IS, Ferguson JC et al. A single-centre double-blind trial of Trasylol therapy in primary acute pancreatitis. Br J Surg 1978; 65:337–41.

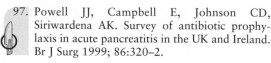
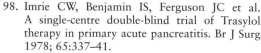

99. Blamey SL, Imrie CW, O'Neill J, Gilmour WH, Carter DC. Prognostic factors in acute pancreatitis. Gut 1984; 25:1340–6.

100. Osborne DH, Imrie CW, Carter DC. Biliary surgery in the same admission for gallstone-associated acute pancreatitis. Br J Surg 1981; 68:758–61.

101. Ranson JH, Rifkind KM, Roses DF, Fink SD, Eng K, Spencer FC. Prognostic signs and the role of operative management in acute pancreatitis. Surg Gynecol Obstet 1974; 139:69–81.

102. Knaus WA, Draper EA, Wagner DP, Zimmerman JE. APACHE II: a severity of disease classification system. Crit Care Med 1985; 13:818–29.

103. Leser HG, Gross V, Scheibenbogen C et al. Elevation of serum interleukin-6 concentration precedes acute-phase response and reflects severity in acute pancreatitis. Gastroenterology 1991; 101:782–5.

104. Pezzilli R, Billi P, Miniero R et al. Serum interleukin-6, interleukin-8, and beta 2-microglobulin in early assessment of severity of acute pancreatitis. Comparison with serum C-reactive protein. Dig Dis Sci 1995; 40:2341–8.

105. Fan ST, Lai EC, Mok FP, Lo CM, Zheng SS, Wong J. Prediction of the severity of acute pancreatitis. Am J Surg 1993; 166:262–8; discussion 269.

106. Balthazar EJ, Robinson DL, Megibow AJ, Ranson JH. Acute pancreatitis: value of CT in establishing prognosis. Radiology 1990; 174:331–6.

107. Schroder T, Kivisaari L, Somer K, Standertskjold-Nordenstam CG, Kivilaakso E, Lempinen M. Significance of extrapancreatic findings in computed tomography (CT) of acute pancreatitis. Eur J Radiol 1985; 5:273–5.

108. Larvin M, McMahon MJ. APACHE-II score for assessment and monitoring of acute pancreatitis. Lancet 1989; ii:201–5.

109. Wilson C, Heath DI, Imrie CW. Prediction of outcome in acute pancreatitis: a comparative study of APACHE II, clinical assessment and multiple factor scoring systems. Br J Surg 1990; 77:1260–4.

110. Buter A, Imrie CW, Carter CR, Evans S, McKay CJ. Dynamic nature of early organ dysfunction determines outcome in acute pancreatitis. Br J Surg 2002; 89:298–302.

111. Heath D, Alexander D, Wilson C, Larvin M, Imrie CW, McMahon MJ. Which complications of acute pancreatitis are the most lethal? A prospective multi-centre clinical study of 719 episodes. Gut 1995; 36:478.

112. Neoptolemos JP, Carr-Locke DL, London NJ, Bailey IA, James D, Fossard DP. Controlled trial of urgent endoscopic retrograde cholangio-pancreatography and endoscopic sphincterotomy versus conservative treatment for acute pancreatitis due to gallstones. Lancet 1988; ii:979–83.

113. Fan ST, Lai EC, Mok FP, Lo CM, Zheng SS, Wong J. Early treatment of acute biliary pancreatitis by endoscopic papillotomy. N Engl J Med 1993; 328:228–32.

114. Fölsch UR, Nitsche R, Ludtke R, Hilgers RA, Creutzfeldt W. Early ERCP and papillotomy compared with conservative treatment for acute biliary pancreatitis. The German Study Group on Acute Biliary Pancreatitis. N Engl J Med 1997; 336:237–42.

115. Nowak A, Nowakowska-Dulawa E, Marek T, Rybicka J. Final results of the prospective, randomized, controlled study on endoscopic sphincterotomy versus conventional management in acute biliary pancreatitis. [Abstract] Gastroenterology 1995; 108:A380.

116. Howes R, Zuidema GD, Cameron JL. Evaluation of prophylactic antibiotics in acute pancreatitis. J Surg Res 1975; 18:197–200.

117. Finch WT, Sawyers JL, Schenker S. A prospective study to determine the efficacy of antibiotics in acute pancreatitis. Ann Surg 1976; 183:667–71.

118. Craig RM, Dordal E, Myles L. The use of ampicillin in acute pancreatitis. [Letter] Ann Intern Med 1975; 83:831–2.

119. Pederzoli P, Bassi C, Vesentini S, Campedelli A. A randomized multicenter clinical trial of antibiotic prophylaxis of septic complications in acute necrotizing pancreatitis with imipenem. Surg Gynecol Obstet 1993; 176:480–3.

120. Bassi C, Falconi M, Talamini G et al. Controlled clinical trial of perfloxacin versus imipenem in severe acute pancreatitis. Gastroenterology 1998; 115:1513–17.

121. Nordback I, Sand J, Saaristo R, Paajanen H. Early treatment with antibiotics reduces the need for surgery in acute necrotizing pancreatitis: a single-center randomized study. J Gastrointest Surg 2001; 5:113–18; discussion 118–20.

122. Sainio V, Kemppainen E, Puolakkainen P et al. Early antibiotic treatment in acute necrotising pancreatitis. Lancet 1995; 346:663–7.

123. Delcenserie R, Yzet T, Ducroix JP. Prophylactic antibiotics in treatment of severe acute alcoholic pancreatitis. Pancreas 1996; 13:198–201.

124. Schwarz M, Isenmann R, Meyer H, Beger HG. Antibiotic use in necrotizing pancreatitis. Results of a controlled study. [In German] Dtsch Med Wochenschr 1997; 122:356–61.

125. Luiten EJ, Hop WC, Lange JF, Bruining HA. Controlled clinical trial of selective decontamination for the treatment of severe acute pancreatitis. Ann Surg 1995; 222:57–65.

126. Powell JJ, Miles R, Siriwardena AK. Antibiotic prophylaxis in the initial management of severe acute pancreatitis. Br J Surg 1998; 85:582–7.

127. Golub R, Siddiqi F, Pohl D. Role of antibiotics in acute pancreatitis: a meta-analysis. J Gastrointest Surg 1998; 2:496–503.

128. Sharma VK, Howden CW. Prophylactic antibiotic administration reduces sepsis and mortality in acute necrotizing pancreatitis: a meta-analysis. Pancreas 2001; 22:28–31.

129. Howard TJ, Temple MB. Prophylactic antibiotics alter the bacteriology of infected necrosis in severe acute pancreatitis. J Am Coll Surg 2002; 195:759–67.

130. Buchler MW, Gloor B, Muller CA, Friess H, Seiler CA, Uhl W. Acute necrotizing pancreatitis: treatment strategy according to the status of infection. Ann Surg 2000; 232:619–26.

131. De Waele JJ, Vogelaers D, Blot S, Colardyn F. Fungal infections in patients with severe acute pancreatitis and the use of prophylactic therapy. Clin Infect Dis 2003; 37:208–13.

132. Gotzinger P, Wamser P, Barlan M, Sautner T, Jakesz R, Fugger R. Candida infection of local necrosis in severe acute pancreatitis is associated with increased mortality. Shock 2000; 14:320–3; discussion 323–4.

133. Gloor B, Muller CA, Worni M et al. Pancreatic infection in severe pancreatitis: the role of fungus and multiresistant organisms. Arch Surg 2001; 136:592–6.

134. Isenmann R, Schwarz M, Rau B, Trautmann M, Schober W, Beger HG. Characteristics of infection with Candida species in patients with necrotizing pancreatitis. World J Surg 2002; 26:372–6.

135. McClave SA, Greene LM, Snider HL et al. Comparison of the safety of early enteral vs parenteral nutrition in mild acute pancreatitis. J Parenter Enteral Nutr 1997; 21:14–20.

136. Windsor AC, Kanwar S, Li AG et al. Compared with parenteral nutrition, enteral feeding attenuates the acute phase response and improves disease severity in acute pancreatitis. Gut 1998; 42:431–5.

137. Kalfarentzos F, Kehagias J, Mead N, Kokkinis K, Gogos CA. Enteral nutrition is superior to parenteral nutrition in severe acute pancreatitis: results of a randomized prospective trial. Br J Surg 1997; 84:1665–9.

138. Powell JJ, Murchison JT, Fearon KC, Ross JA, Siriwardena AK. Randomized controlled trial of the effect of early enteral nutrition on markers of the inflammatory response in predicted severe acute pancreatitis. Br J Surg 2000; 87:1375–81.

139. Olah A, Pardavi G, Belagyi T, Nagy A, Issekutz A, Mohamed GE. Early nasojejunal feeding in acute pancreatitis is associated with a lower complication rate. Nutrition 2002; 18:259–62.

140. Gupta R, Patel K, Calder PC, Yaqoob P, Primrose JN, Johnson CD. A randomised clinical trial to assess the effect of total enteral and total parenteral nutritional support on metabolic, inflammatory and oxidative markers in patients with predicted severe acute pancreatitis (APACHE II ≥6). Pancreatology 2003; 3:406–13.

141. Al-Omran M, Groof A, Wilke D. Enteral versus parenteral nutrition for acute pancreatitis. Cochrane Database Syst Rev 2003:CD002837.

142. Eatock FC, Brombacher GD, Steven A, Imrie CW, McKay CJ, Carter R. Nasogastric feeding in severe acute pancreatitis may be practical and safe. Int J Pancreatol 2000; 28:25–31.

143. Fong YM, Marano MA, Barber A et al. Total parenteral nutrition and bowel rest modify the metabolic response to endotoxin in humans. Ann Surg 1989; 210:449–56; discussion 456–7.

144. Welsh FK, Farmery SM, MacLennan K et al. Gut barrier function in malnourished patients. Gut 1998; 42:396–401.

145. Sax HC, Warner BW, Talamini MA et al. Early total parenteral nutrition in acute pancreatitis: lack of beneficial effects. Am J Surg 1987; 153:117–24.

146. Olah A, Belagyi T, Issekutz A, Gamal ME, Bengmark S. Randomized clinical trial of specific Lactobacillus and fibre supplement to early enteral nutrition in patients with acute pancreatitis. Br J Surg 2002; 89:1103–7.

147. Kald B, Kald A, Ihse I, Tagesson C. Release of platelet-activating factor in acute experimental pancreatitis. Pancreas 1993; 8:440–2.

148. Kingsnorth AN. Early treatment with lexipafant, a platelet activating factor antagonist, reduces mortality in acute pancreatitis: a double blind, randomized, placebo controlled study. Gastroenterology 1997; 112:A452.

149. Kingsnorth AN, Galloway SW, Formela LJ. Randomized, double-blind phase II trial of

Lexipafant, a platelet-activating factor antagonist, in human acute pancreatitis. Br J Surg 1995; 82:1414–20.

150. McKay CJ, Curran F, Sharples C, Baxter JN, Imrie CW. Prospective placebo-controlled randomized trial of lexipafant in predicted severe acute pancreatitis. Br J Surg 1997; 84:1239–43.

151. Kelly TR, Wagner DS. Gallstone pancreatitis: a prospective randomized trial of the timing of surgery. Surgery 1988; 104:600–5.

152. Uomo G, Manes G, Laccetti M, Cavallera A, Rabitti PG. Endoscopic sphincterotomy and recurrence of acute pancreatitis in gallstone patients considered unfit for surgery. Pancreas 1997; 14:28–31.

Nine

Acute conditions of the small bowel and appendix

Simon Paterson-Brown

INTRODUCTION

Acute disease of the small bowel, from which appendicitis is considered separately, contributes substantially to the workload of the general surgeon and many patients will present as emergencies. There are many causes of acute small bowel disease and, because of the mobility and position of the bowel within the abdominal cavity, disease in any intra-abdominal organ or any part of the investing layers of the abdominal cavity may involve the small bowel secondarily. The pattern of acute small bowel disease varies with the age of the patient: some conditions are more common in young people, others in an older population. The incidence of acute surgical small bowel pathology is difficult to estimate overall but is probably second to appendicitis as the site of disease requiring urgent surgical intervention. Acute small bowel disease manifests itself in one of three main ways: (i) obstruction, (ii) peritonitis and (iii) haemorrhage. These categories are not mutually exclusive and more than one type of pathological process may exist in each clinical episode. Usually one category predominates but the clinical picture may change if the presentation or treatment is delayed.

Treatment of small bowel disease may be operative or conservative and the timing of any surgical intervention requires as much consideration as the causes and specific treatment of small bowel disease.

SMALL BOWEL OBSTRUCTION

Although there are many causes of small bowel obstruction (**Box 9.1**), the commonest cause in the USA and Europe is adhesions secondary to previous surgery, followed by malignancy. By comparison, in the developing world the most common cause is hernia. A large retrospective study using the Scottish National Health Service medical linkage system estimated that 5.7% of all hospital readmissions following abdominal and pelvic surgery over a 10-year period were directly related to adhesions.[1] In order to avoid unnecessary surgery and to ensure the correct surgical approach is employed, an attempt should be made to diagnose the cause of the obstruction preoperatively where possible or at least to eliminate conditions that might require special treatment. In practice, however, the cause of the obstruction is often diagnosed at operation.

Mechanism

The small bowel will respond to obstruction by the onset of vigorous peristalsis. This produces colicky abdominal pain usually in the central abdomen as the small bowel is of midgut embryological origin. As the obstruction develops, the proximal intestine dilates and fills with fluid, producing systemic hypovolaemia. Further fluid is lost through vomiting,

Box 9.1 • Causes of small bowel obstruction

Within the lumen
Gallstone
Food bolus
Bezoars
Parasites (e.g. *Ascaris*)
Enterolith
Foreign body

Within the wall
Tumour
Primary
Small bowel tumour
Carcinoma
Lymphoma
Sarcoma
Carcinoma of caecum
Secondary
Inflammation
Crohn's disease
Radiation enteritis
Postoperative stricture
Potassium chloride stricture
Vascultides (e.g. scleroderma)

Outside the wall
Adhesions
Congenital
Bands
Acquired
Postoperative
Inflammatory
Neoplastic
Chemical (e.g. starch, talc)
Pharmacological (e.g. practolol)
Hernia
Primary
Congenital (e.g. diaphragmatic)
Acquired (e.g. inguinal, femoral, etc.)
Secondary
Incisional hernia
Internal postoperative hernia (e.g. lateral space, mesenteric defect)

which occurs early if the obstruction is proximal. As the process continues, the risk of complications increases. If the blood supply is compromised, infarction and perforation will occur. If the blood supply remains intact and the bowel is readily decompressed by vomiting and subsequent naso-gastric suction, the peristalsis will eventually stop leaving grossly dilated, non-functioning bowel;

auscultation will reveal a silent abdomen. In the former scenario the pain, initially colicky, will become continuous, whereas in the latter even the colicky pain may cease as peristalsis ceases. The aim of management must be to identify possible strangulation before gangrene and perforation occurs, so that early surgery can be arranged. There is less urgency in the recognition of non-strangulating obstruction, and a period of decompression and intravenous fluid resuscitation may allow resolution to occur without surgery. However, failure of the obstruction to resolve after 24–48 hours is usually an indication for surgical intervention.

Presentation

The typical clinical presentation of small bowel obstruction is central abdominal colicky pain, vomiting (which is often bile-stained), abdominal distension and a reduction or absence of flatus. Vomiting may be less of a feature and a greater degree of abdominal distension observed if the blockage is in the distal ileum. Bowel sounds increase and may be audible to the patient. Localised peritonitic pain and tenderness may develop and suggests incipient strangulation. In some patients there may be an obvious causative feature such as an irreducible hernia. The presence of surgical scars is important, as is any history of previous intra-abdominal pathology.

Although small bowel obstruction can occur without development of abdominal pain, the absence of this symptom should be viewed with caution. This is particularly the case in postoperative patients where small bowel obstruction and intestinal ileus can be difficult to differentiate. The history and examination of the patient should be sufficiently detailed to allow a diagnosis of small bowel obstruction and to determine possible causes. Complicated small bowel obstruction, with ischaemia or perforation, should be readily detectable by marked abdominal tenderness. It is essential to assess the patient's general state, particularly the degree of dehydration and its effect on the patient so that adequate resuscitation is undertaken prior to any planned surgical treatment.

Investigation

The investigations undertaken in patients with small bowel obstruction are aimed at:

1. assessing the general state of the patient;
2. confirming the diagnosis of small bowel obstruction;
3. identifying, if possible, which patients should undergo early surgery (those with a high risk of strangulation) and those in whom a non-operative approach is appropriate.

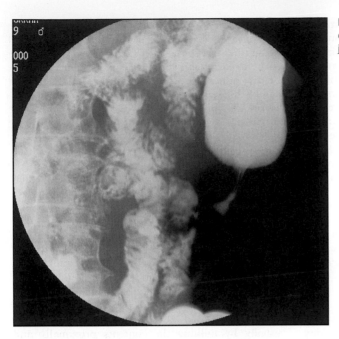

Figure 9.1 • Small bowel follow-through demonstrating a benign stricture in the proximal jejunum with gross proximal dilatation.

These investigations have been discussed in detail in Chapter 5 and, apart from emphasising the value of contrast studies (**Fig. 9.1**), they will not be repeated here, except to reinforce the current view that to date identifying those patients with possible strangulation remains difficult, irrespective of which tests are used, and the surgeon must base most of his or her decision-making on clinical assessment.

Management

GENERAL MANAGEMENT

As in all patients admitted to hospital with an abdominal emergency, the first step in management is fluid resuscitation. Patients usually need several litres of normal saline with potassium supplementation in the first few hours after admission. There remains controversy as to whether colloid or crystalloid fluid is most suitable and each unit will have its own protocols. As a rule of thumb, patients without significant clinical signs of hypovolaemia can usually be adequately resuscitated with normal saline. However, those who present with hypotension and tachycardia on admission will benefit from the addition of colloids as well as oxygen. Patients with a long history are likely to be severely dehydrated, with an alkalosis and associated hypokalaemia, the former due to loss of hydrogen ions in the vomit and the latter from renal compensation. Urinary catheterisation is essential to monitor response to resuscitation and measurement of central venous pressure can be very helpful in the elderly, particularly in those patients with coexist-

ing morbidity. Adequate fluid replacement must be given before any surgical intervention is planned and can be given rapidly if required, even in the elderly, provided appropriate monitoring is used (see also Chapter 16).

Decompression of the stomach with a nasogastric tube will reduce vomiting in most patients, decompress the bowel and reduce the risk of airway contamination from aspiration. Fluid lost from the nasogastric tube should be replaced with additional intravenous crystalloids (normal saline) and potassium supplements. Analgesia should be given early and in adequate doses, with opiates the most commonly used. This will not mask signs of localised or generalised peritonitis and there is no justification for withholding adequate analgesia while waiting for further clinical assessment. However, the analgesia requirement needs to be reviewed regularly, especially in the early stages of management, as a persistent and recurrent requirement for increasing amounts of opiate analgesia is a strong sign that underlying strangulation is a possibility and surgery indicated. Again, as in all emergency patients, anti-thromboembolic prophylaxis should be commenced early and continued until resolution (see Chapter 14), particularly in elderly patients and those with malignancy.

NON-OPERATIVE MANAGEMENT

Intravenous fluids and nasogastric aspiration are the two components of the 'drip and suck' regimen, which is the first-line treatment for most patients with obstruction, particularly when the underlying cause is thought to be adhesions, as spontaneous resolution will occur in the majority. As mentioned earlier, this treatment plan should be abandoned at the first suggestion of underlying strangulation. Although non-operative management can be continued for several days in the absence of any suggestion of strangulation, surgical exploration is generally indicated if the obstruction fails to resolve after 24–48 hours. In some patients with known extensive adhesions from multiple previous explorations, it might be worth waiting longer and if so attention should be paid to nutritional support, sometimes necessitating insertion of a central line for parenteral feeding (see Chapter 17).

SURGICAL MANAGEMENT

The particular circumstances of any given case determine the relative need for surgical intervention but some of the commonest features in decision-making are listed in **Box 9.2**.

Operative principles

Once a decision to operate has been made, patients should be fully resuscitated, treatment of comorbidity optimised and the stomach emptied with a nasogastric tube. The wide range of possible surgical procedures should be explained to the patient. Prophylactic antibiotics and anti-thromboembolic prophylaxis should be administered.

Generally, a midline incision is the most flexible when the diagnosis is unknown. If the patient has a previous midline incision, this should be excised

---

Box 9.2 • Small bowel obstruction: indications for surgery

Absolute indication (surgery as soon as patient resuscitated)
Generalised peritonitis
Visceral perforation
Irreducible hernia
Localised peritonitis

Relative indication (surgery within 24 hours)
Palpable mass lesion
'Virgin' abdomen
Failure to improve (continuing pain, high nasogastric aspirates)

Trial of conservatism (wait and see and/or investigate)
Incomplete obstruction
Previous surgery
Advanced malignancy
Diagnostic doubt (possible ileus)

---

and extended cranially or caudally so that the peritoneal cavity can be entered through a virgin area rather than directly through the back of the old scar. In particular, loops of small bowel may be densely adherent to the back of the old scar and it can be difficult to recognize a change in tissue plane before the lumen of the bowel is entered. Although this is not a major problem if the small bowel is normal, it is clearly best avoided if the bowel wall is grossly distended, friable and diseased (such as from previous irradiation).

Having entered the abdominal cavity, the first step is to identify the point at which the dilated bowel proximal to the obstruction changes to collapsed distal bowel. It is important to demonstrate that such a change is present as this confirms the diagnosis of mechanical obstruction and identifies the obstructing point. The presence of uniformly dilated small bowel, or no definite point of change in diameter of the bowel, suggests that the clinical diagnosis of mechanical obstruction may be incorrect. Dilated bowel can be decompressed, usually by milking the contents proximally and aspirating via the nasogastric tube, which should be of a large size. If the small bowel contents are thick and will not easily pass retrogradely to the stomach or if the bowel is so friable that retrograde decompression might produce a tear, then a suction catheter may be inserted through a small enterotomy. Decompression is particularly useful in a distal obstruction as a large number of dilated loops can be difficult to handle. The large amount of fluid within the bowel makes it heavy and if it is removed from the abdominal cavity, it should be supported so that the mesentery is not stretched or damaged. The large surface area of dilated loops results in considerable insensible fluid loss. If it is anticipated that the viscera will lie outside the abdominal cavity for a significant length of time, it should be placed in a waterproof 'bowel' bag or wrapped in moist swabs. The dilated bowel may be friable and should be handled with care.

Having identified the point of obstruction, the cause is dealt with. If it is due to adhesions, they should be divided as completely as possible, although it is not necessary or helpful to divide every last adhesion within the abdomen as these will inevitably re-form. It is essential to recognise the patient in whom the clinical diagnosis of mechanical small bowel obstruction is incorrect, and the presence of adhesions does not, in itself, confirm the diagnosis.

The small bowel should be resected if it is clearly ischaemic or there is disease in the bowel at the point of obstruction. Anastomosis may be carried out if both ends of the bowel are healthy. However, exteriorisation of the bowel is indicated if there is generalised disease of the bowel with obstruction at one point, as anastomotic dehiscence is more likely. An ileostomy may be indicated in patients with Crohn's disease as part of their long-term management, and the possibility of such a step should be recognised, considered and discussed with the patient before undertaking the exploratory laparotomy.

Closure should always be carried out using a mass closure technique. Although continuous sutures are most popular, in those patients in whom closure is difficult or in whom healing might be reduced, interrupted closure should be considered. There are some patients with gross obstruction in whom, even after relief, closure is clearly going to be very difficult and dehiscence a significant risk, irrespective of the method of closure. In these patients the use of a prosthetic mesh to allow temporary closure, with subsequent removal and formal closure a few days later, should be seriously considered. If at subsequent surgery it is still not possible to approximate the fascial edges, then the mesh can be left in situ and the wound edges mobilised and closed over the top.

Special conditions

RADIATION ENTERITIS

Patients can present with an acute abdomen during radiotherapy due to radiation enteritis or with acute-on-chronic attacks many years later. Patients in the former scenario can present considerable diagnostic difficulties as they are often neutropenic or suffering other side effects of their treatment. The possibility of a primary pathology, such as acute appendicitis, arising during the course of radiotherapy must also be borne in mind but, where possible, surgical exploration is best avoided.

A more common acute presentation is with adhesions due to previous radiotherapy and these patients normally have obstructive symptoms. Again, a conservative management policy is the best course as the laparotomy is fraught with difficulty. The adhesions are often dense and, if the small bowel is inadvertently injured during mobilisation, it is very likely that it will not heal whether it is repaired or anastomosed.

MALIGNANT OBSTRUCTION

Primary tumours of the small bowel are rare but can be the cause of acute small bowel obstruction. A diagnosis in such situations is rarely made preoperatively and surgical management at laparotomy will depend on the exact nature of the disease.

A more common problem is the patient with advanced intra-abdominal malignancy, with or without a past history of surgical treatment for intra-abdominal malignancy, who presents with bowel obstruction. These patients usually respond to initial conservative management and thus emergency laparotomy is less likely to be carried out. If the obstruction fails to settle or rapidly recurs, there is usually time to carry out appropriate investigations to determine the extent of the disease. Ascites can be a confusing clinical factor in such a patient. When surgery is necessary, the exact procedure will depend on the operative findings. The choice usually lies between resection or bypass.

However, it is important to recognise that not all patients have obstruction due to their malignant process. One study of patients who presented with obstruction following previous treatment of intra-abdominal malignancy, either by surgery or radiotherapy, reported that in around one-third of such patients the obstruction was due to a cause other than secondary malignancy.[2] In a study from Japan of 85 patients who had previously undergone surgery for gastric cancer and who were subsequently readmitted to hospital with intestinal obstruction, the cause was benign adhesions in 20%.[3]

The results of bypass entero-enterostomy for malignant adhesions are generally poor, with short periods of patient survival. For this reason there is growing expertise among palliative care physicians in the medical management of intestinal obstruction.[4] The principles involve the use of fluid diet, steroids and octreotide. The results of such management are variable but it does offer the opportunity to spare a patient the morbidity of laparotomy in the terminal phase of their disease.

A third option of surgical management, which is appropriate in a small minority of patients, is placement of percutaneous gastrostomy and feeding jejunostomy to decompress the bowel proximal to an obstructing point and maintain nutrition. The jejunostomy must obviously be placed distal to the obstruction and will usually require a small laparotomy incision. Gastrostomy tube drainage is certainly highly effective at decompressing an obstructed stomach and is more acceptable than the use of a long-term nasogastric tube. Total parenteral nutrition may be required in place of a jejunostomy depending on the extent of obstruction. Advanced malignancy is a common indication for total parenteral nutrition in the USA but is less popular in the UK unless facilities exist to manage the patient at home.

GROIN HERNIA

Any hernia can present with intestinal obstruction. If presentation is delayed, gangrene may have occurred and a bowel resection may be necessary. A Richter's hernia involves part of the circumference of the bowel wall and the lumen is not obstructed. Infarction of the trapped bowel wall segment can still occur and there will be exquisite localised tenderness over a potential hernia site; the indication for surgical intervention is usually clinically apparent.

Any patient with acute symptoms of a hernia that is irreducible should have urgent surgery, with repair carried out in the usual way. In the presence of obstruction necessitating bowel resection, it is probably best to avoid use of a prosthetic mesh. When there has been gross contamination of the surrounding area, the risk of complications is obviously increased and a full treatment course of antibiotics should be given. In most cases, direct approach to the hernia is appropriate. The incarcerated tissue may reduce under anaesthesia and it is unlikely, should this occur, that there will have been strangulation. However, all possible attempts should be made to inspect the bowel loops from within the hernia sac to ensure that a gangrenous loop of bowel has not dropped back into the abdominal cavity. If this is not confirmed, then it will usually become readily apparent in the early postoperative period.

A final consideration is the patient who has an asymptomatic hernia who develops acute intestinal obstruction and who then may demonstrate signs of an apparently irreducible swelling. The intestinal obstruction raises intra-abdominal pressure and this will, in turn, produce the irreducible hernia. The unwary may find the hernia difficult to reduce and, in their efforts to do so, elicit tenderness. This is likely to occur in patients with ascites and large bowel obstruction due to colorectal cancer. Thus, it is worth obtaining a plain abdominal radiograph in all patients with an irreducible hernia and apparent bowel obstruction. The absence of dilated small bowel loops, or the presence of a dilated colon, should suggest the possibility that the apparently 'incarcerated' hernia is a secondary effect of some other intra-abdominal pathology. If in doubt the groin hernia should be explored and, in the absence of conclusive evidence that this is the cause of obstruction, a full laparotomy carried out.

ENTEROLITH OBSTRUCTION

Enterolith obstruction is rare: the commonest types are gallstone ileus and bezoars. Gallstone ileus typically occurs in the elderly female and is due to the development of a cholecystoduodenal fistula after an episode of acute cholecystitis. The gallstone may be visible on a plain abdominal radiograph and gas can often be seen within the biliary tree. At surgery the stone should be removed by proximal enterotomy and the intestine proximal to the obstruction carefully palpated to exclude the presence of a second large gallstone. In these circumstances the gallbladder should be left alone, as cholecystectomy can be not only difficult and hazardous but usually unnecessary.

Bezoars may arise in psychiatric patients, the normal population who have over-indulged in particular types of food (e.g. peanuts) and those who have ingested a foreign body. Rarely, they can occur with material that is collected within a jejunal diverticulum.

INTUSSUSCEPTION

This form of obstruction is rarely diagnosed preoperatively in adults. In children, acute presentation is usually to the paediatric department and the main differential diagnosis is gastrointestinal infection. This is discussed in more detail in Chapter 12. Intussusception in adults is usually caused by benign or malignant tumours of the bowel, which should be treated on their merits once detected at laparotomy.

CONNECTIVE TISSUE DISORDERS

There are several systemic connective tissue disorders that can affect the gastrointestinal tract and result in a loss of peristaltic power. These patients generally present with chronic symptoms and the presence of the underlying disorder is established. Occasionally, symptoms suggesting acute gastrointestinal obstruction are present and the differentiation between full mechanical obstruction and ileus can be difficult. Expectant management of these patients should be pursued whenever possible. The obstructed episode may progress to perforation of the bowel and the patient can present with free gas visible on erect chest radiographs.

Surgical intervention should be based on the clinical condition of the patient and a laparotomy is not always necessary. If peritonitis is present, the perforated bowel should be resected and consideration given to bringing the proximal bowel out as an ileostomy depending on the site and state of disease. In addition, postoperative ileus is common and the differentiation of a further episode of mechanical obstruction or continuing ileus presents a major diagnostic challenge.

INTESTINAL OBSTRUCTION IN THE EARLY POSTOPERATIVE PERIOD

Gastrointestinal ileus can occur after any intra-abdominal operation. The surgeon may also be asked to see patients who have undergone orthopaedic or gynaecological procedures who have apparent bowel obstruction. Each case must be judged on its merits but the differentiation between true mechanical obstruction and paralytic ileus can be difficult. In patients who genuinely have a mechanical obstruction, appropriate surgical intervention is frequently delayed as a result of this diagnostic dilemma. In these patients, the use of dilute barium or water-soluble contrast small bowel studies is often helpful and should be considered early.[5,6] Ultrasound is also useful as it may demonstrate lack of peristalsis, which would support the diagnosis of an ileus.[7]

LAPAROSCOPY

Following the introduction and development of laparoscopic surgery, there have been a few reports regarding the use of laparoscopy and laparoscopic surgery in the treatment of small bowel obstruction and the division of band adhesions.[8] It must be pointed out, however, that this is a risky procedure because of the distended loops of small bowel, and laparoscopy must be performed with great care and using an 'open' technique. It is probably most appropriate when the cause of the adhesive obstruction is likely to be a single band, such as might occur in a patient who has previously had an appendicectomy but no other major abdominal surgery. Unless the surgeon has extensive experience in laparoscopic surgery, conventional open surgery should be the choice for the treatment of intestinal obstruction that requires operation.

PERITONITIS

Small bowel pathology may present as an acute abdomen, with either localised or generalised peritonitis. This may represent the end stage of any condition causing obstruction, but this section considers those conditions that present with primarily inflammatory signs.

Crohn's disease

Crohn's disease is a chronic relapsing inflammatory disease that can affect any part of the gastrointestinal tract. A common presentation is inflammation of the terminal ileum and this occasionally presents as an acute abdomen. The small bowel alone is affected in approximately 30% of patients and the small bowel and colon together in 50%. The incidence of Crohn's disease is highest in the USA, the UK and Scandinavia and is rare in Asia and Africa, suggesting that dietary factors may be important. Similar to appendicitis, the disease can appear at any age but is most frequent in young adults and there may be a familial tendency. It is thought that the disease is most likely an immunological disorder, although the exact mechanism remains unclear. The final pathway is probably a microvasculitis in the bowel wall. Where possible, the management of patients with Crohn's disease should be undertaken by a surgeon with a special interest in this condition and the reader is referred to the much more detailed account of this disease in the *Colorectal Surgery* volume of the *Companion*

to Specialist Surgical Practice series.[9] Only first principles for managing an acute episode are discussed in this chapter.

PRESENTATION

A typical acute clinical episode presents with abdominal pain, diarrhoea and possible fever. These symptoms can be acute in onset in a patient who has previously been entirely well. An acute presentation is more likely in young adults, hence the differential diagnosis of Crohn's disease in patients with suspected appendicitis.

Two other clinical presentations occur, although they are less likely to be acute. First, resolving Crohn's disease will produce fibrosis in the ileum that can cause obstructive symptoms. These tend to be subacute or chronic and an acute presentation with small bowel obstruction is rare. Second, enteroenteric or entero-cutaneous fistula occurs in Crohn's disease because of the transmural inflammation that is a characteristic histological finding.

INVESTIGATION

A patient who presents with right iliac fossa pain, but in whom the symptoms are more insidious than typical appendicitis, should give rise to clinical suspicion. Non-specific inflammatory markers may be markedly elevated (white cell count, platelet count, alkaline phosphatase, erythrocyte sedimentation rate). However, these markers can be raised in acute appendicitis and will not differentiate Crohn's disease. An ultrasound scan may show thickening of the bowel wall or a mass, and if these signs are present further investigation should be undertaken. A radiolabelled white cell scan or small bowel enema can suggest the diagnosis.

SURGERY FOR ACUTE CROHN'S DISEASE PRESENTING DE NOVO

If a patient with known Crohn's disease presents with an acute flare-up or during first presentation, and the diagnosis of Crohn's disease is established before surgery, the patient should be referred to a surgeon with a special interest in this condition. However, during the first presentation of this condition, the diagnosis is often only suspected at the time of laparotomy and the surgeon must proceed according to first principles. In the presence of a localised inflammatory mass or stricture, resection and primary anastomosis are appropriate. If surgery has been carried out for suspected appendicitis and a normal appendix with ileocaecal Crohn's disease is discovered, the appendix should be removed with careful repair of the caecum. No further action needs to be taken at this time for the Crohn's disease and appropriate treatment can be started in the postoperative period. Fortunately, extensive

Crohn's disease affecting the entire small bowel is an uncommon finding at laparotomy, but in this situation the bare minimum should be carried out once the diagnosis has been established and any acute pathology (such as stricture) dealt with. If a stricture is found it should be resected, both to treat the problem and to confirm the diagnosis. If multiple strictures are found, and this will be rare in the acute first presentation, resection of one and multiple stricturoplasties of the others should be carried out. The differential diagnosis of lymphoma should of course be considered and frozen section may help confirm the cause.

Mesenteric ischaemia

Mesenteric ischaemia can be due to embolism or thrombosis, arterial or venous, and may be acute or chronic. Chronic mesenteric ischaemia is also termed 'mesenteric claudication' and is usually caused by a stenosis in the proximal part of the superior mesenteric artery. Patients develop cramp-like abdominal pains after eating, caused by the increased oxygen requirements to the small intestine, which cannot be met by increased blood flow because of the stenosis. The disease is usually associated with atherosclerosis and the investigation of choice is mesenteric angiography. Further management should be transferred to a specialist vascular surgeon and is not discussed further here.

Acute mesenteric ischaemia can affect any part of the gastrointestinal tract, but is most common in the small bowel and colon. Acute ischaemia to the small bowel will usually produce infarction, whereas ischaemia to the large bowel may present less dramatically with bloody diarrhoea and abdominal pain, which often settles over the course of a few days and is often termed 'ischaemic colitis'. Delayed strictures may occur.

Acute small bowel ischaemia is caused by either thrombosis or embolus. Thrombosis may occur in the superior mesenteric artery or its branches, usually associated with underlying atherosclerosis. Embolus is often associated with atrial fibrillation, when the patient may have mural thrombosis in the atrium that dislodges and impacts itself somewhere in the superior mesenteric artery distribution. Venous thrombosis in the distribution of the superior mesenteric vein is a less common cause of acute small bowel ischaemia but may be related to increased blood coagulability, portal vein thrombosis, dehydration, infection, compression and vaso-constricting drugs.

Early detection of acute mesenteric ischaemia is difficult (see Chapter 5) and failure to detect this condition early continues to be one of the major causes of morbidity and mortality. The diagnosis is usually more common in the elderly patient who gives a history of vague abdominal pain getting worse, often colicky in nature. There may be a background history of atherosclerosis, but not invariably so. Examination findings are often unremarkable, lulling the clinician into a false sense of security. Detection of atrial fibrillation or decreased peripheral pulses should alert the clinician to an underlying vascular problem, but even then early diagnosis remains the exception rather than the rule.

The investigations for possible mesenteric ischaemia have been discussed in detail in Chapter 5 and are not repeated here. Angiography may be useful if the diagnosis is suspected, but by this stage a more appropriate investigation is likely to be laparoscopy or laparotomy. Patients in whom a diagnosis is suspected should be resuscitated and prepared for abdominal surgery. Once the diagnosis has been confirmed, a decision needs to be made as to whether the ischaemic bowel is salvageable by vascular reconstruction. If the underlying cause is thrombosis, then resection should be performed; however, if an embolus is present, then exploration of the superior mesenteric artery with removal of the embolus may save an extended small bowel resection. This procedure is difficult and may require associated vascular reconstruction. Advice should be sought from a specialist vascular surgeon.

If surgical resection is carried out, primary anastomosis may be performed providing the blood supply to both proximal and distal margins is adequate. If embolectomy and reconstruction have been performed, then both distal and proximal ends should be brought out as stomas with repeat laparotomy performed in 48 hours. There is a tendency among some surgeons to staple off the proximal and distal ends of bowel, forcing the surgeon to re-explore the patient in 48 hours, rather than performing an anastomosis and basing further management on clinical condition. Following straightforward thrombosis, it is safe to perform primary anastomosis providing good pulses are evident in both proximal and distal resection margins. Attention must still be given in the post-operative period to the general condition of the patient in order that any possible secondary ischaemic event can be detected early.

Unfortunately, the majority of patients with mesenteric ischaemia only have the diagnosis made at laparotomy and the small intestine is invariably beyond salvage and requires resection. If the whole of the superior mesenteric artery has been affected, the majority of small bowel and part of the proximal colon will often be involved and no resection should be performed. These patients should receive intravenous opiates and be kept well sedated, as death will occur shortly afterwards.

Meckel's diverticulum

Meckel's diverticulum is a remnant of the omphalo-mesenteric or vitelline duct. It arises from the antimesenteric border of the distal ileum approximately 60 cm from the iliocaecal valve. It may contain ectopic tissue, usually gastric, and is estimated to be found in approximately 2% of patients. Meckel's diverticulum may remain completely asymptomatic throughout life, particularly if it has a broad base and does not contain ectopic gastric mucosa. Occasionally, a band may exist between the Meckel's diverticulum and the umbilicus, which can cause small bowel obstruction. This should be treated as for a congenital band adhesion, although resection of the diverticulum should accompany division of the band. Occasionally, the diverticulum may intussuscept, also causing obstruction. Again this will require reduction and excision. The other two common complications of Meckel's diverticulum are inflammation, when the patient presents with signs and symptoms similar to acute appendicitis, and haemorrhage. Acute inflammation is rarely suspected before surgery and the patient is usually diagnosed on the operating table once a normal appendix has been found through a right iliac fossa incision or at laparoscopy. In the presence of inflammation the Meckel's diverticulum should be excised and the small bowel repaired. Occult gastrointestinal bleeding may occur from a Meckel's diverticulum that contains ectopic gastric mucosa and the diagnosis is usually established by isotope scan. The treatment is surgical resection.

HAEMORRHAGE

Disease of the small intestine is an occasional cause of acute gastrointestinal haemorrhage. There are no specific clinical features that distinguish the small bowel as the source rather than the colon, except that the blood loss may be less 'fresh' and more like melaena. As discussed in Chapter 7, it is important to exclude bleeding from a gastroduodenal source at an early stage by upper gastrointestinal endoscopy. The most commonly encountered causes are vascular malformation, peptic ulceration in a Meckel's diverticulum and small bowel tumour. These are all treated by resection.

One of the major problems at operation is that a vascular abnormality may produce no external signs. The mobility and variable anatomical layout of the small bowel means that it can be difficult to identify a bleeding point that has been demonstrated by red cell scan or angiography. In the latter case, a catheter should be passed by the radiologist into the mesenteric branches as close as possible to the bleeding point to aid surgical localisation. If this

has not been possible, intraoperative enteroscopy may be helpful. Occasionally, the only option is to place segmental soft bowel clamps throughout the small intestine, resecting the segment that fills up with blood after a period of waiting. However, blind resection is often unrewarding and the risks of rebleeding are high. If no bleeding point can be identified, the surgeon can either close and await events, hoping that further bleeding does not occur (and this can often be the case), or divide the small bowel around its midpoint, bringing out two stomas. Subsequent bleeding can then be identified to one or other side and enteroscopy used to localise it further.

ACUTE APPENDICITIS

Acute appendicitis is the most common intra-abdominal surgical emergency that requires operation and has an incidence of 7–12% in the population of USA and Europe. Although frequently described as a childhood illness, the peak incidence is towards 30 years of age. It is slightly more common in males (1.3–1.6:1) but the operation of appendicectomy is more common in women because of other mimicking conditions (see below and also Chapter 5). The reader is referred to Chapter 5 for description of some of the general features and investigation of patients with acute abdominal pain, many of which relate directly to acute appendicitis.

Pathology

The aetiology of acute appendicitis is bacterial infection secondary to blockage of the lumen by faecoliths, parasitic worms, tumours of caecum or the appendix itself and enlargement of lymphoid aggregates within the appendix wall. In many cases, however, the cause of the obstruction is unknown. Barium contrast studies typically fail to demonstrate an appendiceal lumen in patients with acute appendicitis, and they are no longer used in the acute setting to make the diagnosis. There is little seasonal variation but there may be a familial tendency. The incidence has been falling since the 1930s, presumably because of improved living standards and general hygiene. Changes in dietary habits, such as an increase in dietary fibre, may also be a factor as appendicitis is less common in those countries with a high roughage diet (e.g. Central Africa).

The pathology of acute appendicitis is classically described as suppurative, gangrenous or perforated. Typically, there is full-thickness inflammation of the appendix wall; as the disease progresses, adjacent tissues, particularly the omentum, may also become inflamed. Haemorrhagic ulceration and necrosis in the wall indicate gangrenous appendicitis, and subsequent perforation may be associated with a localised peri-appendiceal mass/abscess or generalised peritonitis.

Clinical features

The presentation of acute appendicitis varies widely but the classical history is of central abdominal pain over 12–24 hours shifting to the right iliac fossa. Nausea and vomiting are common but diarrhoea less so. On examination, the patient usually exhibits a low-grade pyrexia and localised peritonism in the right lower quadrant. Rebound tenderness may be effectively demonstrated by percussion of the abdominal wall rather than the crude method of deep palpation and sudden release.

Appendicitis can occur at any age; although the main peak is in young adults, there is a second peak around the seventh decade. The condition is most difficult to diagnose at the extremes of age: in the very young because of the lack of history and frequent late presentation and in the elderly because of a wider list of differential diagnoses and often less impressive physical signs. Acute appendicitis should be considered in the differential diagnosis of virtually any patient with an acute abdomen.

A further factor that may produce atypical signs is the variation in the position of the appendix. A retrocaecal appendix can give rise to tenderness in the right loin and/or right upper quadrant, whereas a pelvic appendix may be associated with very little abdominal discomfort but marked tenderness on rectal examination and a history of diarrhoea. Rectal examination tends to be of little value in the diagnosis of acute appendicitis unless the organ lies in the pelvis. If the diagnosis has been established from abdominal examination, rectal examination contributes very little additional information in the male patient[10] but obviously can be useful in the female to identify other possible pelvic conditions. Clearly, if a pelvic abscess is suspected a rectal examination is mandatory.

Acute appendicitis is one of a relatively dwindling number of conditions in which a decision to operate may be based solely on clinical findings. In this context, the description of classic history and/or the presence of localised peritonism are highly predictive of acute appendicitis. Features such as high fever, non-localising abdominal tenderness or prolonged history tend to make the diagnosis less likely. The risk of morbidity and mortality is significantly increased if the appendix perforates; thus, to err on the side of overdiagnosing acute appendicitis remains accepted best surgical practice. As discussed in Chapter 5, if in doubt, laparoscopy offers an alternative to what may turn out to be an unnecessary laparotomy.

Investigations

The majority of these investigations have been discussed at length in Chapter 5.

Urinalysis is helpful. Although pus cells and microscopic haematuria can occur in appendicitis, their absence may be useful in excluding significant urinary tract disease from a list of differential diagnoses. However, in the presence of signs of peritoneal irritation and pus cells without significant bacteria in the urine, urgent investigation of the renal tract is indicated to exclude pyelonephritis or pyonephrosis. If these diagnoses are excluded, an acutely inflamed retrocaecal appendix remains the most likely cause and appendicectomy is indicated.

Plain abdominal radiographs are virtually of no help in the diagnosis of acute appendicitis and are not routinely indicated. Barium enema can be carried out on an urgent basis without bowel preparation. Its value lies in the ability to exclude appendicitis rather than to confirm the diagnosis, as complete filling of the appendiceal lumen rarely occurs in acute appendicitis whereas failure to fill the lumen is less predictive. This, together with the practicalities of arranging an urgent barium enema, the lack of bowel preparation and its relatively invasive nature, particularly for young patients, limits its practical application. More recently, computed tomography (CT) has been used to identify acute appendicitis[11] but is probably best left for those patients in whom diagnostic doubt remains and laparoscopy is likely to be difficult (such as patients with multiple abdominal scars and those on the intensive care unit). As already mesntioned, the reader is referred to Chapter 5 for a more detailed list of possible investigations and their usefulness.

Differential diagnosis

Just as appendicitis should be considered in any patient with abdominal pain, virtually every other abdominal emergency can be considered in the differential diagnosis of acute appendicitis. Some of the more common conditions that present in a similar fashion include gastroenteritis and mesenteric lymphadenitis, gynaecological diseases, right-sided urinary tract disease and disease of the distal small bowel. Gynaecological disorders are probably the most important group because the removal of a normal appendix is highest in young women. Acute salpingitis, Mittelschmerz pain and complications of ovarian cyst may all be difficult to differentiate. Torsion of an ovarian cyst usually presents with a notable acute onset of pain and may sometimes be distinguished on clinical grounds. It is important to recognise ruptured ectopic pregnancy, and females of childbearing age should routinely have a pregnancy test (although it must be remembered that appendicitis is not uncommon in the first trimester of pregnancy).

The continuing development of ultrasound techniques and laparoscopic surgery has prompted the view that the proportion of normal appendices removed (typically up to 20% of patients operated on) is unacceptably high. Although it is clearly advantageous to spare patients unnecessary surgery, the morbidity and mortality of failing to diagnose appendicitis until perforation has occurred is greater than that associated with the removal of a normal appendix. If the diagnostic tools discussed in Chapter 5 are not readily available, the best policy remains early surgery when there is clinical suspicion of acute appendicitis.

Management

A positive diagnosis of acute appendicitis requires urgent surgery as any further delay will result in a higher proportion of perforation.[12,13] Where the diagnosis is in doubt, in patients who are systemically well and/or have mild signs, early exploration in the middle of the night is not indicated and these patients can be safely observed with regular review or investigations as described in Chapter 5. The incidence of perforation in this subgroup of patients is no higher than if they are taken to theatre for early exploration.[14,15] All patients should be resuscitated with intravenous fluids and adequate analgesia.

Published data support the view that treatment with narcotic analgesia does not adversely affect the ability to diagnose appendicitis on clinical grounds and, indeed, may assist diagnosis by relieving the patient's anxiety.[16,17] Analgesia should therefore not be withheld pending clinical review.

Intravenous antibiotics may be given once a decision has been made to operate or to actively treat acute appendicitis non-operatively (see below).

SURGICAL TREATMENT

Conventional appendicectomy

A classical appendicectomy incision is made over the point of maximum tenderness and this usually lies on a line between the anterior superior iliac spine and umbilicus in the right iliac fossa. The skin incision should be horizontal and placed in a skin crease if possible to achieve a satisfactory cosmetic result. The abdominal wall muscles may be separated in the traditional 'muscle splitting' fashion or the abdominal cavity may be entered at the lateral margin of the rectus muscle, with retraction of the muscle fibres medially. This lateral rectal approach may be associated with less postoperative discomfort. A right-sided Pfannenstiel incision is used by some surgeons in female patients because it allows ready access to the pelvis for the diagnosis and treatment of gynaecological conditions should these be present. This incision is inconvenient, however, if the caecum lies outside the pelvis or the appendix is retrocaecal. The need for such an approach has been replaced by the wider availability of diagnostic laparoscopy and this incision is no longer recommended.

Once the abdominal cavity has been entered, the appendix should be located by gentle palpation and it may be most easily mobilised from the inflammatory adhesions by finger dissection. If it is obviously inflamed, it should be removed, lavage performed and no further laparotomy carried out. If the appendix is macroscopically normal, examination should be undertaken of the terminal ileum (for at least 60 cm to exclude an inflamed Meckel's diverticulum) and small bowel mesentery and pelvis, both by palpation and direct visualisation with retraction of the abdominal wall. Any free peritoneal fluid should be examined and cultured. The presence of bile staining indicates bowel perforation at some point, such as perforated peptic ulcer, and faecal fluid indicates a colonic perforation. In both cases a full laparotomy is indicated. In the former situation, it is best to close the right iliac fossa incision in preference to an upper midline, but in the latter condition some surgeons advocate extending the right iliac fossa incision across to the left as a muscle-cutting lower abdominal transverse incision. If in doubt, a midline incision is best.

It used to be traditional to bury the appendix stump but there is now general recognition that simple ligation of the stump is adequate.[18] However, if the appendix is perforated at the base, formal repair of the caecal pole is advised. Leaving an excessively long stump should be avoided as this will inevitably become ischaemic and can produce symptoms postoperatively. Peritoneal lavage should always be carried out but surgical drains are unnecessary unless there is an established abscess cavity.

All patients should receive prophylactic antibiotics against the risk of wound infection, which is the commonest complication of appendicectomy. Regimens vary but the two most common are metronidazole alone or in combination with a broad-spectrum cephalosporin or penicillin. A single dose is as effective as three doses for wound prophylaxis. In perforated appendicitis, however, a policy of instituting a full treatment course over

5 days is adopted by many surgeons, although there are no good data to support this view. Although the risk of deep vein thrombosis is relatively low in young patients, prophylaxis is best administered as a routine as not all patients will make a swift recovery and early postoperative mobilisation may be delayed. It goes without saying that it should be routinely employed in older patients.

Laparoscopic appendicectomy

The advantages of laparoscopic appendicectomy over the open approach have been extensively studied over the last 15 years, although many individual studies have produced conflicting results.[19–28]

Two recent meta-analyses have confirmed the benefit of the laparoscopic approach in relation to less pain, faster recovery and a lower incidence of wound infections.[29,30] However, the recently published Cochrane database systematic review of over 4000 patients suggested that there was a threefold increase in intra-abdominal abscesses and a longer operating time (16 minutes) in those patients undergoing the laparoscopic procedure.[31]

This may of course reflect either problems with surgical technique or poor patient selection. There is no rational reason why the laparoscopic approach should have a higher complication rate, if performed correctly, and indeed it brings with it the possibility of performing a better lavage than at open surgery.

As skill in laparoscopic techniques becomes increasingly more widespread, it is inevitable that laparoscopic appendicectomy will become more common. It would therefore be reasonable to proceed with laparoscopic appendicectomy in any patient in whom an acutely inflamed appendix is discovered during diagnostic laparoscopy, providing the surgeon has the relevant skills. Likewise, in the other patients, and these will usually be men, offering the laparoscopic approach will depend on the surgical expertise available. Large and obese patients probably benefit more from the laparoscopic approach due to the larger wound required at open surgery.

Technique The basic principles of laparoscopic appendicectomy mirror those of conventional open surgery. The appendix mesentery is usually divided first and may be cauterised with electrocoagulation at the level of the appendix, tied in continuity with ligatures or controlled by application of haemostatic clips. The appendix itself is usually ligated with a preformed loop ligature. An alternative, highly effective and rapid technique is to apply an endoscopic stapling device[32] using vascular staples

to the mesoappendix, which is divided as the first step. The appendix can then be removed after further application of the stapler or by using a pretied ligature. Unfortunately, the stapling device is expensive.

The inflamed appendix should be removed through an endoscopic port or, if it is excessively swollen, placed in a bag for retrieval as it is essential to remove the appendix through the abdominal wall without contaminating the soft tissues. This minimises the risk of wound infection, which appears to be significantly lower than after conventional surgery.[30] A very friable and perforated appendix should be handled very gently and care taken to remove all debris, including any loose faecolith. If manipulation of the swollen appendix is likely to result in perforation, conversion to an open operation should be considered. In this situation the laparoscope can be used to transilluminate the abdominal wall, allowing accurate placement of a conventional surgical incision, which it may be possible to keep to a smaller size than would otherwise have been used. A thorough lavage is essential in contaminated cases to prevent postoperative abscess formation. In patients with generalised peritonitis from a perforated appendix, it must be remembered that the advantages of the laparoscopic approach over the open approach are small, as even if the operation can be completed laparoscopically these patients rarely recover quickly due to the systemic nature of their disease.

There have been various descriptions of operative technique for laparoscopic appendicectomy and different positions for port placement are used. If ports are placed low in the abdominal wall, the cosmetic result may be improved, although some surgeons prefer to place one port in the right upper quadrant and one in the lower abdomen to allow the classical positioning of the long axis of laparoscopic instruments at right angles to each other. However, there is no evidence to suggest that one approach is better than another.

A technique of laparoscopic-assisted appendicectomy has been described whereby the appendix is approached through a small incision in the right iliac fossa.[33] Under laparoscopic view the appendix and caecal pole are delivered onto the abdominal wall after release of the pneumoperitoneum and appendicectomy carried out. Once the stump has been closed, the caecum is returned to the peritoneal cavity, the abdominal incision closed and laparoscopic inspection then carried out after reproducing the pneumoperitoneum.

One of the reported complications of laparoscopic appendicectomy is leaving too long a stump and risking recurrent symptoms.[34] Care must be taken to ensure that the entire appendix has been fully mobilised to avoid this complication.

The normal appendix

If a standard incision is made, conventional teaching dictates that a normal appendix should be removed to prevent confusion in the future should right iliac fossa pain recur. On the one hand, this hypothesis has never been fully tested and one would imagine that most patients are capable of understanding whether their appendix had been removed, provided they are given this information. On the other hand, removal of a normal appendix is associated with minimal morbidity, although the wound infection rate is the same for removal of a normal appendix as for a non-perforated inflamed appendix. In practice, a normal appendix should probably be removed in every patient, including those with Crohn's disease that affects the caecum at the base of the appendix, in order to prevent future diagnostic dilemma. The main longer-term complication of removing a normal appendix is small bowel obstruction. This has been examined in a historical cohort study of 245 400 patients in Sweden with population-based matched controls.[35] This study calculated the cumulative risk of surgically treated small bowel obstruction following open appendicectomy to be 1.3% after 30 years compared with 0.21% for non-operated controls. Higher risk was associated with those patients undergoing appendicectomy for other conditions, a perforated appendix and a normal appendix.

Removal of a normal appendix at diagnostic laparoscopy is not mandatory and should not be undertaken if a definitive diagnosis for the patient's symptoms, such as pelvic inflammatory disease, can be established. If no cause for symptoms is discovered, there are two arguments in favour of removing the appendix: (i) there is a small incidence of appendicitis on histological examination of a macroscopically normal appendix;[36] and (ii) the removal of the appendix prevents the development of a diagnostic dilemma in a patient who continues to suffer from abdominal symptoms and signs following laparoscopy. It could also be argued that a major advantage of laparoscopy in suspected appendicitis is the ability to remove a normal appendix easily and with very low morbidity.

However, the counter-argument suggests that all operative interventions or procedures are associated with some form of risk and if the appendix is normal at laparoscopy there needs to be a good reason to remove it. Surgeons will no doubt have their own thoughts on this matter and decisions may vary between patients and the clinical presentation.

NON-SURGICAL TREATMENT

It has been suspected for many years that not only can acute appendicitis settle spontaneously, returning with recurrent symptoms at a later date, but that it can also be successfully treated with antibiotics, providing there are no signs of overt peritonitis. The former is supported by a study which reported that 71 of 1084 patients (6.5%) who underwent appendicectomy for acute appendicitis admitted to similar symptoms 3 weeks to 12 years previously.[37] The latter is supported by a randomised controlled study comparing antibiotic treatment versus appendicectomy in 40 patients with suspected appendicitis.[38] The problem with this method of treatment is the high recurrence rate in the antibiotic-treated group (7 of 20 patients within 12 months). However, only 1 of the 20 patients treated non-operatively failed to resolve and required appendicectomy after 12 hours. It therefore follows that when a diagnosis of acute appendicitis is suspected, and in the absence of overt peritonitis, it is reasonable to treat the patient with antibiotics if there are other factors that favour a non-operative approach. This decision is obviously made in the full knowledge that regular review is essential, that immediate operation is indicated if resolution does not take place within 12–24 hours or the patient's symptoms deteriorate and that there is a significant risk of recurrent symptoms during the course of the next 12 months.

Treatment of atypical presentation of acute appendicitis

APPENDIX MASS

The natural history of acute appendicitis left untreated is that it will resolve, become gangrenous and perforate, or will become surrounded by a mass of omentum and small bowel that walls off the inflammatory process and prevents inflammation spreading to the abdominal cavity yet resolution of the condtion is delayed. Such a patient usually presents with a longer history (1 week or more) of right lower quadrant abdominal pain, appears systemically well and has a tender palpable mass in the right iliac fossa. This condition is best managed conservatively as the risk of perforation has passed and removal of the appendix at this late stage can be difficult and is associated with a significant complication rate.[39] The differential diagnosis includes Crohn's disease in younger patients and carcinoma of the caecum in older patients. Confirmation is obtained from ultrasound or CT, and it is not uncommon for these investigations to reveal an underlying abscess.[40] However, if the patient remains systemically well, non-operative treatment can still be pursued. Following resolution of the symptoms and mass, further investigations, which might include ultrasound, CT, barium enema and colonoscopy, must be used to exclude these other conditions.

In the past, routine interval appendicectomy (6 weeks to 3 months) was considered essential to prevent recurrent symptoms in the young and to exclude carcinoma in the elderly. However, providing carcinoma can be excluded by other means, routine interval appendicectomy is no longer considered essential. In the majority of cases the appendix has been destroyed and in one study only 9% of patients treated non-operatively for an appendix mass subsequently developed recurrent symptoms and all did so within 5 months.[40] In another study of 30 patients with an appendix mass, of whom three underwent early appendicectomy, only two delayed appendicectomies were carried out (at 2 and 3 months) for recurrent symptoms, with follow-up ranging from 6 months to 3 years.[41]

APPENDIX ABSCESS

In some patients the appendix becomes walled off by omentum but has perforated and an abscess will develop localised to the peri-appendiceal region. This may be in the right paracolic gutter, the subcaecal area or the pelvis. There may be a mass but, unlike a simple 'appendix mass', the patient is systemically unwell with significant abdominal tenderness. As is the case in all abscesses, drainage is the best treatment, either under radiological control or surgically. The advantage of the latter is that through a standard right iliac fossa incision the residual necrotic appendix can be found and resected along with the

inevitable faecolith, which if left contributes to a long and protracted recovery. There is no doubt, however, that surgical drainage can be associated with significant complications, not least because tissues and organs adjacent to the abscess will be friable and must be handled with great care. The alternative of non-operative management using radiologically guided drainage has been reported to produce significantly lower complications and equivalent early operation/reoperation rates.[42,43] It would therefore seem reasonable to use the non-operative approach in any patient who remains systemically well and in whom overt signs of peritonitis are absent.

CHRONIC APPENDICITIS

As mentioned above, there is certainly a group of patients who suffer from recurrent appendicitis[37] and who benefit from appendicectomy. Similarly, there are some patients who, having recovered from an acute attack of appendicitis, go on to suffer from recurrent less-acute episodes of abdominal pain. These also benefit from appendicectomy, usually as an elective procedure and increasingly carried out laparoscopically. In these patients, the macroscopic appearance of the appendix is abnormal; thus, when in doubt, laparoscopy is the best investigation, following which the appendix can be removed. Assessment in difficult cases can be helped by a barium enema, which reveals a non-filling appendix lumen (**Fig. 9.2**), or even by CT (**Fig. 9.3**).

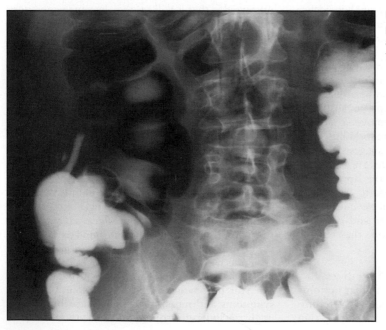

Figure 9.2 • Barium enema in a patient with recurrent right-sided abdominal pain showing non-filling of the distal appendix lumen.

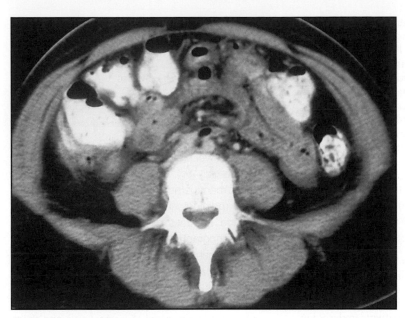

Figure 9.3 • Computed tomography scan of the same patient as in Fig. 9.2 showing an abnormal and thickened tip of appendix without contrast. These findings were confirmed at appendicectomy when a grossly abnormal distal half of appendix was found.

Postoperative complications and outcome

HOSPITAL STAY

The duration of hospital stay depends on local resources, policies, the patient's general condition and any coexisting disease. It is now fairly clear that laparoscopic appendicectomy is associated with a more rapid return to normal activities[29,30] than conventional surgery, but this does not necessarily relate to a shorter hospital stay. Much may depend on local factors and reports of routine early discharge (24–48 hours) after conventional appendicectomy[44] suggest that a full diet and early mobilisation are well tolerated by the majority of patients.

WOUND INFECTION

This is the commonest postoperative complication, occurring in around 15% of patients following a conventional right iliac fossa incision. In most patients there is superficial inflammation, which responds to antibiotics. In a smaller number there will be dehiscence of the wound and purulent discharge. Occasionally, surgical intervention may be required to drain a collection in the abdominal wall. The current practice of early discharge results in many wound infections developing once the patient is at home and the possibility of this complication should always be discussed with the patient. As already discussed, wound infection appears to be significantly less following laparoscopic appendicectomy.[29,30]

There is no clear evidence that injection of local anaesthetic into the wound is associated with any alteration in the incidence of wound infection but there is also minimal benefit in reducing postoperative wound pain.[45,46] The skin may be closed with interrupted stitches or a continuous suture and this does not appear to affect wound infection rates or subsequent management. Some surgeons prefer to leave the skin incision open if there has been gross contamination of the wound in perforated appendicitis. The subsequent cosmetic result of such a scar is usually entirely satisfactory but healing takes several weeks.

OTHER SEPTIC COMPLICATIONS

Pericaecal fluid collections are relatively common and are usually indicated by the presence of abdominal discomfort and a low-grade pyrexia. They can be diagnosed by ultrasound and treated by antibiotics, especially in children,[47] or occasionally aspiration; formal drainage is rarely necessary. Pelvic abscess is an uncommon complication that presents with lower abdominal discomfort and swinging pyrexia. The symptoms may be delayed by 10 days or more and a soft tender mass may be palpable on rectal examination, but this is not always the case. Again, ultrasound or even CT diagnosis is required and, if pus is aspirated, a percutaneous drain should be placed if possible. Occasionally, a pelvic abscess may be difficult to drain percutaneously and in this situation the options are between antibiotics, drainage of the abscess into the rectum or to proceed to surgical drainage through the abdomen. The decision is influenced by the local circumstances and general condition of the patient. Prolonged use of antibiotics should be avoided and further attempts made for drainage if the collection is not resolving on repeated ultrasound examinations.

In patients who have undergone laparoscopic appendicectomy for a perforated appendicitis, signs of generalised peritonitis can develop in the first 48 hours. This may be due to dissemination of infected fluid through the abdominal cavity, possibly by circulation of the carbon dioxide used to create the pneumoperitoneum. The main differential diagnosis in this situation is iatrogenic injury to the intestine and, if in doubt, re-laparoscopy is indicated.

PROGNOSIS

The mortality of appendicitis is associated with the age of the patient and delayed diagnosis (perforated appendix). The report from the Royal College of Surgeons of England showed a mortality of 0.24% and morbidity of 7.7% in 6596 patients undergoing open appendicectomy between 1990 and 1992.[48] A further prognostic consideration is the incidence of subsequent tubal infertility after appendicectomy. Although one report suggested that the increased risk of tubal infertility following perforated appendicitis was 4.8 in nulliparous women and 3.2 in multiparous women,[49] a more recent historical cohort study revealed no long-term consequence on fertility.[50] This latest study is another factor which opposes the view that it is better to carry out an unnecessary appendicectomy than risk delaying surgery, with the possible increased risk of perforation in particular, for acute appendicitis. As already discussed, a period of close observation with regular review in hospital is not associated with an increased risk of perforation, while the early and late complications of removing a normal appendix (using conventional surgery) range from 13 to 17%.[51,52]

Key points

- The main emergency conditions affecting the small bowel are obstruction, haemorrhage and ischaemia.
- Early management requires adequate clinical and radiological assessment, which might include contrast radiology and, increasingly, ultrasonography (see also Chapter 5).
- Early appendicectomy for acute appendicitis is better than non-operative treatment with antibiotics because of high recurrence rate.
- Laparoscopic appendicectomy results in less pain and faster return to normal activities than open appendicectomy but hospital stay remains similar and there is a higher risk of postoperative abscess formation.
- Non-operative approach is indicated in the majority of patients with appendix mass or abscess, with radiological drainage as required. Subsequent interval appendicectomy is only indicated in those patients with recurrent symptoms. However, care must be taken to ensure that underlying disease other than appendicitis has been excluded (e.g. caecal carcinoma and Crohn's disease).

REFERENCES

1. Ellis H, Thompson JN, Parker MC et al. Adhesion-related hospital re-admissions after abdominal and pelvic surgery: a retrospective study. Lancet 1999; 353:1476–9.

2. Walsh HPJ, Schofield PE. Is laparotomy for small bowel obstruction justified in patients with previously treated malignancy? Br J Surg 1984; 71:933–5.

3. Nakane Y, Okumura S, Akehira K et al. Management of intestinal obstruction after gastrectomy for carcinoma. Br J Surg 1996; 83:133.

4. Parker MC, Baines MJ. Intestinal obstruction in patients with advanced malignant disease. Br J Surg 1996; 83:12.

5. Chen S-C, Lin F-Y, Lee P-H, YU S-C, Wang S-M, Chang J-J. Water soluble contrast study predicts the need for early surgery in adhesive small bowel obstruction. Br J Surg 1999; 86:1692–8.

6. Brochwocz MJ, Paterson-Brown S, Murchison JT. Small bowel obstruction: the water-soluble follow-through revisited. Clin Radiol 2003; 58:393–7.

7. Ogata M, Mateer JR, Condon RE. Prospective evaluation of abdominal sonography for the diagnosis of bowel obstruction. Ann Surg 1996; 223:237–41.

8. Paterson-Brown S. Emergency laparoscopic surgery. Br J Surg 1993; 80:279–83.

9. Thompson-Fawcett MW, Mortensen NJMcC. Crohn's disease. In: Phillips RKS (ed.) Colorectal surgery, 3rd edn. Edinburgh: Elsevier, 2005; pp. 163–92.

10. Dixon JM, Elton RA, Rainey IB, Macleod DAD. Rectal examination in patients with pain in the right lower quadrant of the abdomen. Br Med J 1991; 302:386–8.

11. Rao PM, Rhea JT, Novelline RA, Mostafavi AA, McCabe CJ. Effect of computed tomography of the appendix on treatment of patients and use of hospital resources. N Engl J Med 1998; 338:141–6.

12. Moss JG, Barrie JL, Gunn AA. Delay in surgery for acute appendicitis. J R Coll Surg Edinb 1985: 30:290–3.

13. Temple CL, Huchcroft SA, Temple WJ. The natural history of appendicitis in adults. A prospective study. Ann Surg 1995; 221:278–81.

14. McLean AD, Stonebridge PA, Bradbury AW, Rainey JB, McLeod DAD. Time of presentation, time of operation, and unnecessary appendicectomy. Br Med J 1993; 306:307.

15. Surana R, Quinn F, Puri P. Is it necessary to perform appendicectomy in the middle of the night in children? Br Med J 1993; 306:1168.

16. Attard AR, Corlett MJ, Kidner NJ, Leslie AL, Fraser IA. Safety of early pain relief for acute abdominal pain. Br Med J 1992; 30:554–6.

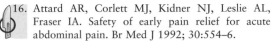

Assessment of patients with acute abdominal pain is not affected adversely by early analgesia.

17. Thomas SH, Cheema F, Reisner A et al. Effects of morphine analgesia on diagnostic accuracy in emergency department patients with abdominal pain: a prospective randomized trial. J Am Coll Surg 2003; 196:18–31.

A randomised study of 74 patients who received either morphine or placebo. The diagnostic accuracy was not affected by morphine.

18. Engstrom L, Fenvo G. Appendicectomy: assessment of stump invagination: a prospective, randomised trial. Br J Surg 1985; 72:971–2.

19. Kum CK, Ngoi SS, Goh PMY, Tekant Y, Isaac JR. Randomized controlled trial comparing laparoscopic and open appendicectomy. Br J Surg 1993; 80:1599–600.

20. McAnena OJ, Austin O, O'Connell PR, Hederman WP, Gorey TF, Fitzpatrick J. Laparoscopic versus open appendicectomy: a prospective evaluation. Br J Surg 1992; 79:818–20.

21. Cox MR, McCall JL, Toouli J et al. Prospective randomized comparison of open versus laparoscopic appendectomy in men. World J Surg 1996; 20:263–6.

22. Tate JJT, Dawson IW, Chung SCS, Lau WY, Li AKC. Laparoscopic versus open appendicectomy: prospective randomised trial. Lancet 1993; 342:633–7.

23. Martin LC, Puente I, Sosa JL et al. Open versus laparoscopic appendectomy. Ann Surg 1995; 222:256–62.

24. Hansen JB, Smithers BM, Schache D, Wall DR, Miller BJ. Laparoscopic versus open appendectomy: prospective randomised trial. World J Surg 1996; 20:17–21.

25. Minne L, Burnell A, Ratzer E, Clark J, Haun W. Laparoscopic vs open appendectomy. Arch Surg 1997; 132:708–12.

26. Reiertsen O, Larsen S, Trondsen E, Edwin B, Faerden AE, Rosseland AR. Randomised controlled trial with sequential design of laparoscopic versus conventional appendicectomy. Br J Surg 1997; 84:842–7.

27. Hellberg A, Rudberg C, Kullman E et al. Prospective randomised multicentre study of laparoscopic versus open appendicectomy. Br J Surg 1999; 86:48–53.

28. Lintula H, Kokki H, Vanamo K. Single-blind randomised clinical trial of laparoscopic versus open appendicectomy in children. Br J Surg 2001; 88:510–14.

29. Sauerland S, Lefering R, Holthausen U, Neugebauer E. A meta-analysis of studies comparing laparoscopic with conventional appendectomy. In: Krahenbuhl L, Frei E, Klaiber Ch, Buchler MW (eds) Acute appendicitis: standard treatment or laparoscopic surgery? Basel: Karger, 1998; pp. 109–114.

Less pain and earlier return to normal activity after the laparoscopic approach.

30. Golub R, Siddiqui F, Pohl D. Laparoscopic versus open appendectomy: a metaanalysis. J Am Coll Surg 1998; 186:545–53.

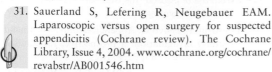
Analysis of 1682 patients. Less postoperative pain, shorter hospital stay, faster return to normal activities and less wound infections following laparoscopic appendicectomy.

31. Sauerland S, Lefering R, Neugebauer EAM. Laparoscopic versus open surgery for suspected appendicitis (Cochrane review). The Cochrane Library, Issue 4, 2004. www.cochrane.org/cochrane/revabstr/AB001546.htm

32. Olsen DO. Laparoscopic appendectomy using a linear stapling device. Surg Rounds 1991; 37:873–83.

33. Byrne DS, Bell G, Morrice JJ, Orr G. Technique for laparoscopic appendicectomy. Br J Surg 1992; 79:574–5.

34. Milne AA, Bradbury AW. 'Residual' appendicitis following incomplete laparoscopic appendicectomy. Br J Surg 1996; 83:217.

35. Andersson REB. Small bowel obstruction after appendicectomy. Br J Surg 2001; 88:1387–91.

36. Lau WY, Fan S-T, Yiu T-F, Chu K-W, Suen H-C, Wong K-K. The clinical significance of routine histopathologic study of the resected appendix and safety of appendiceal inversion. Surg Gynecol Obstet 1986; 162:256–8.

37. Barber MD, McLaren J, Rainey JB. Recurrent appendicitis. Br J Surg 1997; 84:110–12.

38. Eriksson S, Granstrom L. Randomised controlled trial of appendicectomy versus antibiotic therapy for acute appendicitis. Br J Surg 1995; 82:166–9.

39. De U, Ghosh S. Acute appendicectomy for appendicular mass: a study of 87 patients. Ceylon Med J 2002; 47:117–18.

40. Bagi P, Dueholm S. Nonoperative management of the ultrasonically evaluated appendiceal mass. Surgery 1987; 101:602–5.

41. Adalla SA. Appendiceal mass: interval appendicectomy should not be the rule. Br J Clin Pract 1996; 50:168–9.

42. Hurme T, Nyalamo E. Conservative versus operative treatment of appendicular abscess. Ann Chir Gynaecol 1995; 84:33–6.

43. Oliak D, Yamini D, Udani VM et al. Initial nonoperative management for periappendiceal abscess. Dis Colon Rectum 2001; 44:936–41.

44. Salam IMA, Fallouji MA, El Ashaal YI et al. Early patient discharge following appendicectomy: safety and feasibility. J R Coll Surg Edinb 1995; 40:300–2.

45. Dahl IB, Moiniche S, Kehle H. Wound infiltration with local anaesthetics for post-operative pain relief. Acta Anaesthesiol Scand 1994; 38:7–14.

46. Turner GA, Chalkiadis G. Comparison of pre-operative with postoperative lignocaine infiltration on postoperative analgesic requirements. Br J Anaesth 1994; 72:541–3.

47. Okoye BO, Rampersad B, Marantos A, Abernethy LJ, Losty PD, Lloyd DA. Abscess after appendicectomy in children: the role of conservative management. Br J Surg 1998; 85:1111–13.

48. Baigrie RJ, Dehn TCB, Fowler SM, Dunn DC. Analysis of 8651 appendicectomies in England and Wales during 1992. Br J Surg 1995; 82:933.

49. Mueller BA, Daling JR, Moore DE et al. Appendectomy and the risk of tubal infertility. N Engl J Med 1986; 315:1506–7.

50. Andersson R, Lambe M, Bergstrom R. Fertility patterns after appendicectomy: historical cohort study. Br Med J 1999; 318:963–7.

51. Chang FC, Hogie HH, Welling DR. The fate of the negative appendix. Am J Surg 1973; 126:752–4.

52. Deutsch AA, Shani N, Reiss R. Are some appendicectomies unnecessary? J R Coll Surg Edinb 1983; 28:35–40.

Ten

Colonic emergencies

Faisal Abbasakoor and
Carolynne Vaizey

INTRODUCTION

Emergency conditions of the large bowel are a common reason for admission to general surgical units and there have been a number of interesting changes in the philosophy of their surgical management in recent years. Instead of rushing the patient to the operating theatre after a token resuscitation, the current trend is towards a much more detailed assessment using ultrasound, computerised tomography (CT), contrast enemas and angiography.

Many patients can be treated conservatively using antibiotic therapy and intravenous fluids, with nasogastric suction and blood transfusion when necessary. Time is taken to ensure that medical problems such as cardiac arrhythmias, cardiac failure, respiratory problems and diabetes mellitus are treated adequately. Patients are closely monitored using central venous pressure or pulmonary artery pressure measurement; oxygen saturation is measured with a pulse oximeter and hourly urine volumes are observed in addition to other standard parameters. The decision about whether the patient is looked after in a high-dependency unit or intensive care unit should be made on the basis of clinical need. If facilities are not available, transfer to a larger centre may be necessary. Most large district general hospitals and teaching hospitals now have dedicated emergency theatres available around the clock, so that lack of theatre availability is no longer a reason for operating during the night.

The operative mortality for emergency colon resection is two to three times as high as for elective resection. As a result, surgeons have been investigating ways of reducing the need for emergency resection by introducing alternative interventions that allow the condition to settle completely or that lead to sufficient improvement to permit later elective resection. The former approach is typified by increased use of conservative methods to treat some cases of perforated diverticulitis, and the latter by the use of expandable metal stents for the initial treatment of patients with left-sided malignant large bowel obstruction.

The decision about whether to operate may be difficult but can become clearer after several visits to observe and re-examine the patient (active observation). Asking a consultant colleague for a second opinion is no longer regarded as demeaning, and indeed in many hospitals is a regular feature of clinical care. There is general agreement that consultant surgeons should be involved in both the assessment and the operative procedure in this very challenging group of patients.

When emergency operation is necessary, there has been a very clear trend towards single rather than staged procedures for large bowel disorders. This approach reduces the length of hospital stay and avoids the risks of multiple operations, but is not suitable for all patients. In some unfit or acutely septic patients, a staged approach may still be preferable.

Preparation for operation

The patient must be informed of the likely diagnosis and the possible methods of surgical management and risks of surgery, including the possibility of anastomotic dehiscence. If the patient is well enough to understand the implications of stoma formation, this should be explained carefully. If there is a reasonable prospect that a stoma will be necessary, the stoma therapist should visit the patient before operation if possible. Optimum stoma sites on either the right or left iliac fossa are selected and marked clearly preoperatively.

The risk of postoperative deep vein thrombosis and pulmonary embolus is substantial in this group of patients, and prophylactic measures are therefore essential. Subcutaneous low-molecular-weight heparin is commenced soon after admission and continued during the patient's stay. It is also common practice in many units to use intermittent pneumatic calf compression during all major operative procedures.

The case for prophylactic antibiotic therapy is well recognised in both elective and emergency large bowel surgery. Single-dose therapy is as effective as multiple-dose regimens, but if there is peritoneal contamination at the time of operation, antibiotics should be continued for several days at the surgeon's discretion.

VOLVULUS OF THE COLON

Colonic volvulus can be defined as an axial rotation around its mesentery. In a recent review article, it was noted that the sigmoid colon was involved in 76% of cases, the caecum in 22% and the transverse colon in 2%.[1] Another report suggests that 40–60% of patients have had previous episodes of obstruction.[2]

Sigmoid volvulus

There is marked variation in the incidence of sigmoid volvulus throughout the world. In industrialised countries, typical incidence figures are 1.7 per 100 000 in the east of Scotland[3] and 1.47 per 100 000 in Olmsted County, Minnesota, USA.[4] In contrast, in the Brong Ahafo region of Ghana the incidence rises to 12 per 100 000.[5] Patients who develop sigmoid volvulus in the industrialised world tend to be older, and one-third either have mental illness or are institutionalised.[6] This is not a feature of patients with sigmoid volvulus in Africa.[7]

The sigmoid colon rotates through 180–720° in either a clockwise or anticlockwise direction to produce the volvulus.[8] A narrowed sigmoid mesocolon provides a pedicle for rotation. The condition is occasionally associated with Chagas' disease and Hirschsprung's disease, in which redundancy of the colon is a feature. Non-specific motility disorders of the colon may be a significant predisposing factor.[6] It has also been reported following laparoscopic cholecystectomy and may be caused by a combi-

nation of the pneumoperitoneum, lateral tilt of the table together with a long redundant sigmoid colon.[9]

PRESENTATION

A typical patient with a sigmoid volvulus presents with abdominal pain, constipation and feeling bloated. On examination there is marked distension, which is often asymmetrical. Severe pain and tenderness, associated with tachycardia and hypotension, may suggest colonic ischaemia. About 50% of patients have a history of previous attacks.

INVESTIGATION

Findings on the plain abdominal radiograph are often characteristic. Massive distension of the sigmoid colon is visible; the bowel loses its haustration and extends in an inverted U from the pelvis to the right upper quadrant of the abdomen (**Fig. 10.1**). Wide fluid levels are seen in both limbs of the loop on the erect film, commonly at different levels ('pair of scales').[10] In one-third of patients, the appearances are not typical and an emergency contrast enema should be carried out. This may demonstrate narrowing of the contrast column at the point of twisting, which has been described as resembling the beak of a bird of prey.[11]

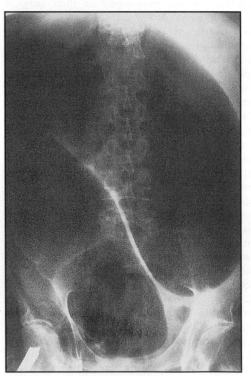

Figure 10.1 • Plain abdominal radiograph of sigmoid volvulus. Radiograph kindly provided by Dr D. Nicholls, Consultant Radiologist, Raigmore Hospital, Inverness.

MANAGEMENT

It is important to stress that despite the fact that many of these patients can be managed conservatively, there may still be considerable fluid and electrolyte deficit, which requires careful correction.

Non-operative decompression

Since Bruusgaard reported sigmoidoscopic decompression in 124 patients in 1947, the endoscopic route has become firmly established as the treatment of choice.[12] If this method is to be used, it is important that the patient does not have clinical features suggestive of colonic strangulation. A simple technique involves pushing a soft catheter, such as a wide-bore chest drain, through the twisted segment into the sigmoid loop using a rigid sigmoidoscope. When the sigmoid loop decompresses it usually derotates and success has been reported in more than 80% of patients.[12,13] Most surgeons suggest that the catheter should be left in situ for at least 24 hours, secured in place by a suture to the perineal skin.

However, there are limitations and disadvantages to this technique. First, there is the risk of reduction of gangrenous sigmoid colon.[14] This risk may be minimised by performing laparotomy when (i) the bowel content draining through the rectal catheter is blood-stained or (ii) gangrenous patches are seen on the mucosa of the sigmoid colon. Second, there is a small risk of perforation of the colon.[15] The endoscopic method of decompression has been refined by the use of the flexible colonoscope instead of the rigid sigmoidoscope.[16] The potential advantages are that decompression can be done under vision, increasing the accuracy of insertion through the twisted segment in the sigmoid colon. In addition, the mucosa of the whole sigmoid loop can be visualised directly. The experience of colonoscopic reduction of sigmoid volvulus has been encouraging. A report from Nigeria on 92 patients with sigmoid volvulus has shown that decompression was achieved in 83 patients using colonoscopy. The remaining nine patients were noted to have ischaemic changes and therefore underwent operation. All patients in this series survived.[17]

Operative management

If symptoms and signs at the time of presentation suggest ischaemia of the colon, laparotomy should be undertaken when the patient has been adequately resuscitated. Likewise, the patient who has unsuccessful non-operative treatment and those who have clinical features suggestive of colonic ischaemia at colonoscopy should also undergo emergency laparotomy. Since it is likely that resection will be required, the patient should be placed in the lithotomy/Trendelenburg position on the operating table. If colonic distension makes it difficult to handle the colon, a needle inserted obliquely through a taenia attached to a suction apparatus aids decompression. If the colon is gangrenous, it should be resected with as little manipulation as possible; the most widely recommended procedure is Hartmann's operation with an end colostomy and closure of the rectal stump.[3,5] In a prospective randomised trial from West Africa, Bagarani et al. compared the operative treatment in 31 patients with or without gangrene.[18] When gangrene was present, the mortality for Hartmann's procedure was 12.5% compared with 33.3% when resection and anastomosis was performed.

A small number of surgeons have described resection and primary anastomosis with good results. A recent study from India reported 197 patients with acute sigmoid volvulus treated by single-stage resection and anastomosis, 23 of whom had gangrene of the bowel.[19] Only two patients had anastomotic leaks, both of which responded to conservative management. The two mortalities occurred in elderly patients who presented with perforations. A study from Ghana reported 21 patients with acute sigmoid volvulus treated by single-stage resection and anastomosis, 15 of whom had gangrene of the bowel.[20] Only one patient had a minor anastomotic leak, which responded to conservative management. However, it is important to stress that the majority of the patients in these studies were young and these results may not be applicable to the typical Western patient. In contrast, a series from the USA with 228 patients reported a mortality rate of 24% for emergency operations and 6% for elective operations. This study found mortality to correlate with emergency surgery and necrotic colon.[21]

Intraoperative colonic irrigation may facilitate primary anastomosis in patients with sigmoid volvulus who require emergency operation, since faecal loading proximal to the volvulus may increase the risk of anastomotic dehiscence. However, it is still important that only patients who are generally fit and without systemic sepsis and peritoneal contamination are selected for this procedure.

Elective resection

Because the risk of recurrent volvulus after decompression and derotation has been reported to be between 40 and 60%,[2] elective surgery to prevent further volvulus should always be considered. The most widely accepted procedure is resection, which is now associated with an operative mortality of 2–3%. The operation may be performed as a laparoscopic-assisted procedure[22] but can also be performed through a small incision under local anaesthesia, especially in the elderly patient.[23]

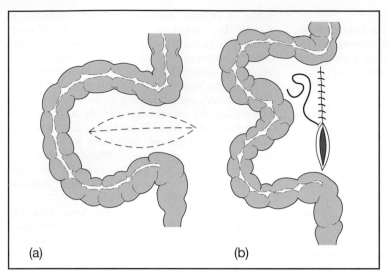

Figure 10.2 • The technique of mesosigmoidoplasty.

(a)   (b)

A variety of fixation procedures have been described but have been associated with high recurrence rates. An exception to this poor outcome has recently been reported with mesosigmoplasty.[24] The technique consists of shortening and broadening the sigmoid mesocolon by making an incision in the peritoneum from root to apex; the peritoneum is then mobilised and closed in a transverse direction (**Fig. 10.2**). The same procedure is then performed on the opposite side of the mesocolon. Recurrence was seen in only 2 of 125 patients followed for a mean of 8.2 years.

There are anecdotal reports of both laparoscopic and endoscopic sigmoidopexy and these techniques may be appropriate in the unfit patient.[25–27]

Ileosigmoid knotting

Ileosigmoid knotting is a variant of sigmoid volvulus in which the ileum twists around the base of the mesocolon (**Fig. 10.3**). It is also known as double volvulus. Three factors are responsible for ileosigmoid knotting: (i) a long small bowel mesentery and freely mobile small bowel, (ii) a long sigmoid colon on a narrow pedicle and (iii) ingestion of high-bulk diet in the presence of empty small bowel.[28,29] It has been suggested that when a large semiliquid bulky meal empties into the proximal jejunum it increases the motility of the intestine and the heavy segment of the bowel falls into the left lower quadrant. The empty loops of ileum and jejunum are thereby forced into a clockwise rotation towards the right upper quadrant around the base of a narrow sigmoid mesocolon. Further peristalsis forms an ileosigmoid knot with two closed loops, one affecting the small bowel and the other in the sigmoid colon.[28,29]

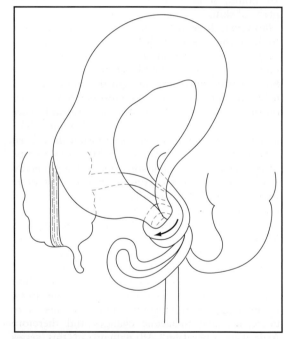

Figure 10.3 • Ileosigmoid knotting.

The condition is characterised by very acute onset of agonising generalised abdominal pain and repeated vomiting. Gangrene of the ileum and sigmoid colon is common. Generalised peritonitis, sepsis and dehydration are recognised complications, with hypovolaemic shock occurring early. The erect plain abdominal radiograph shows a dilated sigmoid colon and fluid levels in the small bowel.

Initial management consists of resuscitation and administration of antibiotics followed by surgical intervention. Resection and anastomosis of the terminal ileum and a Hartmann's procedure is the most commonly performed operation. Recent reports suggest that primary colonic anastomosis can be undertaken safely when there is a short history and the colon is clean and well vascularised. The condition unfortunately carries a very high mortality rate, ranging from 15 to 73%.[28,30]

Volvulus of the transverse colon

Volvulus affecting the transverse colon is much less common than sigmoid volvulus, accounting for only 2.6% of all cases of colonic volvulus in one series.[31] Predisposing conditions include pregnancy, chronic constipation, distal colonic obstruction and previous gastric surgery. There are two reports of familial tranverse colon volvulus, one of twins and the other of two brothers.[32,33] The plain abdominal radiograph usually shows gas-filled loops of large intestine with wide fluid levels. The condition is often mistaken for sigmoid volvulus and the diagnosis is rarely made preoperatively. After the operative diagnosis is made and the transverse colon untwisted, evidence of distal obstruction should be sought. The choice of treatment is either an emergency excision of the transverse colon or an extended right hemicolectomy.

The rarity of the condition makes definitive statements difficult to support from the published literature but, in general, a primary anastomosis after resection is probably safe. An alternative method of treatment advocated by Mortensen and Hoffman[34] consists of suturing the right side of the transverse colon to the ascending colon with a similar procedure on the left side, thus shortening the unattached transverse colon. In the presence of gangrenous bowel and significant peritoneal contamination, the safest approach may be to resect the affected colon and exteriorise both ends.

Caecal volvulus

Volvulus of the caecum is much less common than volvulus of the sigmoid colon, representing 28% of all cases of colonic volvulus reported over a 10-year period in Edinburgh.[35] It is likely that incomplete rotation of the midgut leaves the caecum and ascending colon inadequately fixed to the posterior abdominal wall with a substantial length of mesentery. Conditions that alter the normal anatomy may predispose to caecal volvulus. There is an increased risk of caecal volvulus in pregnancy, and some patients are found to have adhesions from previous surgery. There is also an association with distal colonic obstruction. Volvulus usually takes place in a clockwise direction around the ileocolic vessels. Although the term 'caecal volvulus' is used, the condition also involves the ascending colon and ileum. As it twists, the caecum comes to occupy a position above and to the left of its original position. A similar condition, which is seen very occasionally, is 'caecal bascule'. In this condition, the caecum folds upwards on itself, producing a sharp kink in the ascending colon.[36]

PRESENTATION

It is not usually possible to differentiate between caecal volvulus and other forms of proximal large bowel obstruction on clinical grounds. Some patients will have a previous history of episodes of obstruction that subsequently settled with conservative treatment. The main presenting symptoms are colicky abdominal pain and vomiting. A tympanitic abdominal swelling will usually be present in the mid-abdomen.

INVESTIGATION

The radiographic features of caecal volvulus have been reviewed by Anderson and Mills.[37] On the supine film, a comma-shaped caecal shadow in the mid-abdomen or left upper quadrant with a concavity to the right iliac fossa is diagnostic (**Fig. 10.4**) and there may be small bowel loops lying to the right side of the caecum. A single, long fluid level on the erect film is characteristic. If doubt persists, a contrast enema will show a beaked appearance in the ascending colon at the site of the volvulus.

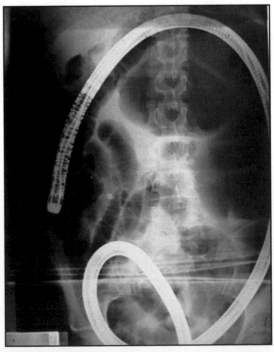

Figure 10.4 • Plain abdominal radiograph demonstrating a caecal volvulus with colonoscope in situ.

MANAGEMENT

Management of caecal volvulus will depend to some extent on the clinical picture. The patient who is unfit for surgical treatment can be considered for colonoscopy since occasional successes have been reported using this method.[38] However, laparotomy is necessary in most patients. If the right colon is gangrenous at operation, the treatment of choice is a right hemicolectomy. A primary anastomosis should be possible in most cases even in the presence of contamination of the peritoneal cavity. It should be remembered that there is a markedly increased mortality in patients who have caecal gangrene. A report from the Mayo Clinic had a mortality rate of 12% in patients with caecal volvulus with a viable caecum, rising to 33% if there was colonic gangrene.[4]

There is much more controversy about the procedure of choice in patients who have a viable caecum after reduction of the volvulus. Derotation alone is associated with a high recurrence rate. Resection avoids all risk of recurrence but carries a small risk of anastomotic leak. In a study of 22 patients there was no mortality and no anastomotic leaks. A 14% morbidity included one abdominal wall abscess, one intra-abdominal abscess and one medical complication.[39] The other two procedures commonly performed for caecal volvulus are caecostomy and caecopexy. Reports on the use of caecostomy demonstrate a wide variation in terms of both recurrence (0–25%) and mortality (0–33%). Some authors express concern over the morbidity of caecostomy and the very occasional serious complication of abdominal wall sepsis and fasciitis, in addition to the potential for a persistent fistula.

The treatment of caecal volvulus has been reviewed in a large study comprising 561 published cases.[40] This review showed that caecopexy was associated with a mortality rate of 10% and a recurrence rate of 13%. Anderson and Welch described a combined technique using caecopexy and caecostomy.[41] Using this technique, they reported no recurrence after a mean follow-up of 9.8 years. If all circumstances are favourable, resection appears to be a justifiable procedure with minimal risk of recurrence, accepting that there may be a small number of patients who will have increased bowel frequency. In other circumstances, the minimum procedure compatible with survival becomes the goal.

ACUTE COLONIC PSEUDO-OBSTRUCTION

Acute colonic pseudo-obstruction (ACPO) is the term used to describe the syndrome in which patients present with symptoms and signs of large bowel obstruction but in whom no mechanical

Box 10.1 • Predisposing conditions in acute colonic pseudo-obstruction

Chest infection
Myocardial infarction
Cerebrovascular accident
Renal failure
Puerperium
Retroperitoneal malignancy (Ogilvie's syndrome)
Orthopaedic trauma
Myxoedema
Electrolyte disturbance

cause can be demonstrated at contrast radiology. In more than 80% of patients with ACPO, an underlying precipitating condition exists, of which at least 50 have been described.[42] The most common of these associated conditions are metabolic disorders, trauma and cardiorespiratory disorders (**Box 10.1**). The term 'Ogilvie's syndrome' is loosely used in the literature as a synonym for ACPO. Ogilvie's original description was of two patients, a doctor and a solicitor, who had extensive malignant disease infiltrating the retroperitoneum and affecting the function of the sympathetic nerve supply to the gut.[43] Ogilvie's syndrome is therefore one of the causes of ACPO. The mortality rate of ACPO is high, partly as a result of the underlying disorders but also related to failure to recognise the condition, leading to inappropriate operation. The true incidence is hard to ascertain since a number of unrecognised cases are likely to resolve spontaneously, but it has been estimated that some 200 deaths per annum in the UK may result from ACPO.[44]

Aetiology

The state of colonic motility at any point in time is determined by a balance of the inhibitory influence of the sympathetic nervous supply and the stimulatory effect of the parasympathetic system. It has been suggested that 'neuropraxia' of the sacral parasympathetic nerves may be a factor in the aetiology of ACPO, leading to a failure of propulsion in the left colon. This would also explain the 'cut-off' between dilated and collapsed bowel, which is located on the left side of the large bowel in 82% of patients.[45] It is well recognised that sepsis is a potent stimulus of sympathetic activity and was noted by Jetmore et al. in 42% of their patients.[46] Many of the conditions commonly associated with ACPO are likely to result in sympathetic overactivity.

Presentation

The clinical features of ACPO are almost identical to those of mechanical large bowel obstruction,[47] making differentiation on clinical grounds alone almost impossible. Vanek and Al-Salti reviewed 400 cases and noted that the clinical features of ACPO are abdominal pain (83%), constipation (51%), diarrhoea (41%), fever (37%) and abdominal distension (100%).[45] On examination, the abdomen is generally very distended and tympanitic, but tenderness is often less than expected. The majority of patients will already have had operative procedures or have been hospitalised for some time because of some other disorder. Serum electrolytes are often abnormal.

Investigation

Plain radiographs of the abdomen in ACPO typically show gross distension of the large bowel with cut-off at the splenic flexure, rectosigmoid junction or, less commonly, the hepatic flexure (**Fig. 10.5**). Gas–fluid levels are less commonly seen on the plain radiograph in patients with ACPO compared with those presenting with mechanical obstruction.[48,49] It has been suggested that a prone lateral view of the rectum may be useful in making the diagnosis since gaseous filling of the rectum will tend to exclude mechanical obstruction.[50] The caecal diameter should be measured on sequential abdominal radiographs since it is believed that the risk of caecal rupture increases greatly with increasing caecal diameter.[48,49]

There is now overwhelming support for the use of a contrast enema in all patients with suspected ACPO in order to establish the diagnosis, since the differentiation from mechanical obstruction can be extremely difficult. This is well illustrated in a study reported by Koruth et al., who performed a contrast enema on 91 patients with suspected large bowel obstruction.[51] Of the 79 patients who were thought clinically to have mechanical obstruction, the diagnosis was confirmed in 50. There was free flow of contrast to the caecum in the remaining 29 patients. Of these 29, 11 had non-obstructing colonic pathology such as diverticular disease and ulcerative colitis and 18 patients had pseudo-obstruction. Of the 12 patients who were thought to have pseudo-obstruction before the water-soluble contrast enema, two were shown to have carcinoma of the colon.

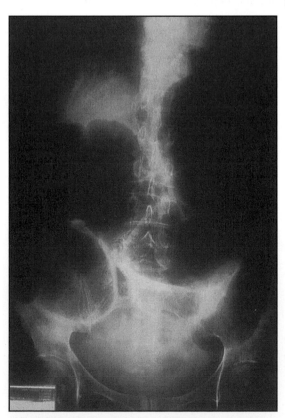

Figure 10.5 • Plain abdominal radiograph of a patient with acute colonic pseudo-obstruction.

Management

NON-OPERATIVE MANAGEMENT

The initial management of ACPO is non-operative and the underlying cause is treated if possible. Any medications that cause gut stasis should be discontinued, particularly analgesics. A nasogastric tube is routinely inserted to prevent swallowed air from entering the intestine. The use of enemas and flatus tubes is said to be of value in the treatment of early colonic pseudo-obstruction; in a number of patients the water-soluble contrast enema itself may have a useful therapeutic effect. In most patients, the condition will resolve without intervention. Bachulis and Smith found that it took an average of 6.5 days for complete resolution to take place in a group of 26 patients treated medically.[48] Progress should be checked by serial examination of the abdomen and by abdominal radiographs.

It is only when the risk of perforation increases substantially that more active intervention becomes necessary. The risk of perforation is approximately 3%[52] and Johnson et al.[53] showed a correlation between perforation and the duration of distension, with a mean duration of distension of 6 days in the group of patients who went on to perforate compared with a mean duration of 2 days in the group that did not progress to perforation.

Neely and Catchpole were the first to describe the restoration of alimentary tract motility by pharmacological means.[54] Hutchinson and Griffiths used 20 mg guanethidine (an adrenergic blocker) in 100 mL normal saline infused intravenously over 40 minutes.[55] During this time, recordings of blood pressure and pulse were made every 10 minutes and then 2.5 mg neostigmine was given over 1 minute after the guanethidine infusion. They found that improvement occurred only after neostigmine was given. Two patients had a problem that may have been attributed to the treatment: one patient experienced postural hypotension and another excessive salivation.

In a more recent randomised, double-blind, controlled trial of neostigmine only, 10 of 11 patients who were treated with intravenous neostigmine had prompt passage of flatus or stool, with reduced abdominal distension, compared with none of 10 patients who received placebo injection.[56]

These results were mirrored in a trial of 28 patients, with rapid resolution in 26. Time to pass flatus varied from 30 seconds to 10 minutes. In the two patients who failed to resolve, one was found to have a sigmoid cancer and the other died of multi-organ failure.[57] There is a risk of bradycardia with cholinergic agonists, and it has been suggested that patients with cardiac instability should not be treated with neostigmine. Interestingly, there is anecdotal evidence that the concomitant administration of glycopyrrolate with neostigmine seems to offset the risk of bradycardia and may be considered in patients with cardiac instability.[58]

Epidural anaesthesia blocks sympathetic outflow, and improvement has been observed in a number of patients with ACPO who have had this form of treatment.[59]

COLONOSCOPY

The use of colonoscopy to decompress the colon in ACPO has become well established since it was first suggested by Kukora and Dent,[60] and it is successful in 73–90% of patients.[61–63] The procedure can be difficult and tedious, requiring a skilled colonoscopist, and air insufflation must be kept to a minimum. Frequent small-volume irrigation is required to ensure good visibility in the colon and maintain the patency of the colonoscope suction channel.

A further advantage of colonoscopy is that necrotic patches can be identified on the colonic mucosa, allowing pre-emptive surgical treatment before perforation supervenes.[64] The risk of perforation of the colon during colonoscopy for this condition has been estimated at around 3%,[63] and other complications are very unusual. It should be emphasised, however, that radiographs taken after successful clinical response often fail to show complete resolution of caecal distension, and one disadvantage of colonoscopic treatment is the tendency for the condition to recur. The overall rate of recurrence following initial colonoscopic decompression varies from 15 to 29%.[46,60,62] There is some difference of opinion about the best method of management of recurrent ACPO, but the safety and efficacy of repeat colonic decompression has now been reported.[42,46,62] A potential means of avoiding recurrence is intubation of the caecum with a long intestinal tube passed alongside the colonoscope.[65]

OPERATIVE MANAGEMENT

The indications for surgery include the following.

1. Caecal distension: the extent of distension varies between authors, from 9 cm[66] to 10 cm[67] and more recently 12 cm,[68] the threshold rising with increasing availability of medical therapy.
2. Continuing caecal distension beyond 48–72 hours despite maximum medical therapy.
3. Pain over the right iliac fossa, i.e. the caecum.
4. Pneumoperitoneum.

There are doctors who recommend percutaneous caecostomies,[69] where a tube is inserted into the caecum using radiological guidance for the purpose of decompression. A trephine caecostomy performed surgically is a relatively minor procedure that may be performed under local anaesthesia.[70] To avoid contamination, the caecum can be sutured to the incised external or internal oblique muscles and only opened when the peritoneal cavity is sealed off. Only when perforation of the caecum is suspected should a full laparotomy be performed. If a perforation or necrosis of the caecum has already occurred, a full laparotomy is necessary and a right hemicolectomy is the treatment of choice. When resection of the right colon is required, it is probably safest to bring out an ileostomy and mucous fistula and re-anastomose the two ends of bowel at a later date. Primary anastomosis may be feasible if contamination of the peritoneal cavity is not a feature and the remaining colon looks healthy.

MALIGNANT LARGE BOWEL OBSTRUCTION

Malignant large bowel obstruction generally occurs in the elderly patient; of 168 patients with this condition reported by Gerber et al., 63% were more than 70 years of age.[71] Although carcinoma of the colon is the most common cause of large bowel obstruction in Europe and North America, only 8–29% of patients with colorectal carcinoma present with intestinal obstruction,[72–75] accounting for 85% of colonic emergencies due to colon cancer.[76] Presentation is with obstruction in approximately half of splenic flexure malignant tumours, 25% of those on the left colon, 6% of rectosigmoid lesions[72,77] and 8–30% of right-sided carcinomas.[78] Both obstruction and perforation occur together in approximately 1% of all colon cancers, but in patients who have an obstruction caused by cancer, 12–19% will have a perforation.[79,80] The perforation may either be at the site of the tumour or in the caecum, caused by back pressure from the distal obstructing lesion.

The influence of obstruction on prognosis is controversial. Some studies suggest that the apparent adverse effect of obstruction on prognosis is a consequence of the stage of the disease rather than obstruction itself, as 27% have liver metastasis at the time of operation.[72] Other reports suggest that obstruction is an independent predictor of poor prognosis.[74,81]

Presentation

The symptoms experienced by patients with large bowel obstruction to some extent reflect the site of the tumour. In right-sided obstruction, particularly at the level of the ileocaecal valve, the onset of colicky central abdominal pain may be quite sudden and vomiting is a relatively early feature. If the obstruction is at the rectosigmoid junction, there may be a history of a change in bowel habit and of per rectal bleeding. In these distal tumours, vomiting is rare.

On examination, abdominal distension is the most notable feature and the distribution of distension can be an indicator of the level of obstruction. A tympanitic swelling, particularly noted in the right lower quadrant, may signify caecal distension. Signs of peritoneal irritation suggest that perforation is either imminent or may have already occurred. Palpation of an irregular liver edge suggests that liver metastasis may be present and a palpable mass on rectal examination is likely to be a carcinoma of the rectum or, on occasion, involvement of the anterior rectal wall by a sigmoid carcinoma prolapsing into the pelvis.

Investigation

Plain abdominal radiography will usually provide the diagnosis of large bowel obstruction. The pattern of gas distribution in both the small and large bowel will depend on the site of obstruction and also on whether the ileocaecal valve is competent.

All patients with suspected large bowel obstruction without evidence of perforation should undergo a water-soluble contrast enema (**Fig. 10.6**) because plain film radiography can be misleading.[51]

This investigation will exclude other conditions such as volvulus or pseudo-obstruction and, in addition, may go some way to cleansing the colon distal to the obstructing lesion. Sigmoidoscopy or colonoscopy can be useful, particularly if the suspected obstructing lesion is in the distal colon. In addition, either technique can be used to exclude synchronous carcinoma or adenoma below the level of obstruction. CT with intravenous and water-soluble rectal contrast is increasingly used in the emergency setting and this has the added advantage of providing information on the spread of disease preoperatively (**Fig. 10.7**).

Management

NON-OPERATIVE MANAGEMENT

There is good evidence that the morbidity and mortality rate associated with emergency procedures for obstruction of the colon is at least twice that for elective surgery. In recent years, a number of techniques have been used to allow patients presenting with obstruction to be operated on electively. The decompression techniques that deserve serious

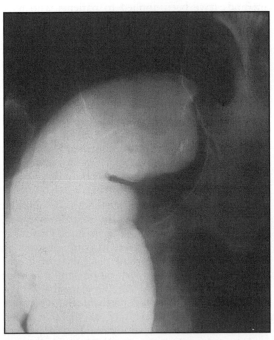

Figure 10.6 • Water-soluble contrast enema demonstrating complete obstruction in the proximal sigmoid colon.

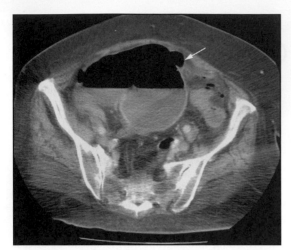

Figure 10.7 • Computed tomography scan of a patient with a perforated caecum (perforation indicated by arrow). The scan also revealed an obstructing splenic flexure tumour and extensive liver metastases.

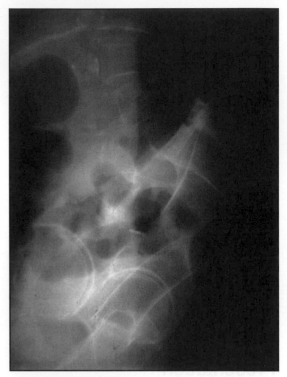

Figure 10.8 • Plain abdominal radiograph showing colonic stent in situ in a patient with a sigmoid tumour who was unfit for surgery.

consideration are: (i) laser therapy, particularly the neodymium–yttrium aluminium garnet (Nd-YAG) laser; (ii) use of an expandable metal stent (**Fig. 10.8**); and (iii) use of a transanal endoscopic decompression tube.

Experience with the first two techniques was initially confined to patients who had inoperable distal colonic carcinoma, but more recently these methods have been applied to patients who have operable distal large bowel obstruction. Using the Nd-YAG laser, Kiefhaber et al. reported successful recanalisation in 57 of 75 patients with obstructing carcinoma.[82] No patient died but there were two cases of laser-related perforation. Postoperative mortality was 3.7% of those patients who subsequently had resection and primary anastomosis. Eckhauser and Mansour reported a series of 46 patients with obstructing colorectal carcinoma of whom 29 had laser therapy before curative resection.[83] There was one case of laser-related perforation and postoperative mortality was 3.4% in those who had a subsequent resection.

A self-expanding metal stent can be inserted radiologically, endoscopically or, alternatively, using a combination of both techniques. One study reports a series of 15 patients with obstructing colonic carcinoma who had placement of a self-expanding stent;[84] two perforations and one stent displacement occurred. All 12 patients with a successful stent tolerated mechanical preparation before surgery. Preoperative expandable metal stenting was used successfully in 35 of 38 patients with large bowel obstruction.[85] The mortality rate after stent insertion and subsequent resection was 2.6%. A comparative study of preoperative stenting versus emergency operation concluded that stent placement prevented unnecessary operations in 17 of 18 patients found to have metastatic disease and 'a large number of colostomies';[86] the rate of primary anastomosis in the emergency setting will of course vary from study to study. A further study successfully used stenting to palliate 13 of 15 patients,[87] but late complications included stent migration in two patients and tumour ingrowth in three.

Two recent papers have evaluated transanal decompression.[88,89] The tube is placed transanally over a guidewire inserted through a colonoscope. After proximal colon decompression, colonic lavage can be performed by oral administration of polyethylene glycol solution or via the tube itself. In the first study of five patients the mean time from insertion of the tube to operation was 4.2 days (range 3–5 days) and there were no anastomotic leaks after primary anastomosis. The second study reported success in 34 of 36 patients.

OPERATIVE MANAGEMENT

Patients with right-sided obstruction should be positioned flat on the operating table. Those with left-sided large bowel obstruction are placed in the lithotomy/Trendelenburg position to allow access to the anus during the procedure for purposes of irrigation of the rectal stump or anal insertion of a surgical stapling instrument. It also allows the surgical assistant the option of standing between the patient's legs.

The abdomen is opened through a midline incision. If the bowel is tense, it should be decompressed: first, to improve visualisation of the rest of the abdomen and, second, to prevent spillage of faecal content. The large bowel can be decompressed by inserting a 16G intravenous catheter obliquely through the colonic wall, following which suction is applied. This is often enough to make it possible to handle the large bowel without fear of rupture as the distension is mainly gas. After localisation of the primary tumour, synchronous tumours should be excluded. The presence of direct spread to adjacent structures should also be assessed, in addition to any peritoneal seedlings and the presence of liver secondaries. Based on these observations, a decision can be made as to whether the operation is potentially curative or palliative.

When there is a prospect of curative resection, standard techniques of radical cancer therapy should be employed, including wide excision of the lesion en bloc with the appropriate blood vessels and mesentery. If the lesion is adherent to other structures, an attempt should be made to resect the affected part of these structures with the resected specimen where this is feasible. High cure rates are possible with locally advanced tumours if the lymph nodes are not involved and there are no distant metastases, but this is only achieved if a radical approach to resection is adopted and clear resection margins obtained. The presence of liver or peritoneal metastases does not preclude resection of the primary carcinoma. When it is deemed that the operation is palliative, gastrointestinal continuity should be restored if at all possible and staged procedures avoided.

Right-sided obstruction

If there is a closed loop obstruction because of competence of the ileocaecal valve, the caecum and right colon may be very tense. Complete decompression can be achieved as a preliminary to resection by making a small enterotomy in the terminal ileum and passing a Foley catheter through the ileocaecal valve into the caecum. This technique is particularly useful in situations where there is splitting of the taenia on the caecum, indicating impending rupture. The range of operations available for treatment of right-sided tumours causing obstruction includes right hemicolectomy with primary anastomosis, right hemicolectomy with exteriorisation of both ends of the large bowel, and ileo-transverse colon bypass. There is general agreement that a right hemicolectomy with primary anastomosis is the treatment of choice in most patients; however, this procedure is by no means free of complications. One report noted an operative mortality rate of 17% in 195 patients who had

emergency right hemicolectomy with primary anastomosis for obstructing colonic carcinoma.[90] In addition, a leak rate of 10% was noted in 179 patients who had a right hemicolectomy and primary anastomosis for obstruction. This compares with a leak rate of 6% in 579 patients with right colon cancer who did not have an obstruction.[90] Other studies have shown similar mortality rates, and many of the deaths resulted from anastomotic failure. This suggests that instead of subjecting all patients with obstruction to right hemicolectomy with primary anastomosis, it may be wiser to use a policy of selection, subjecting patients with good risk status to primary anastomosis and managing patients with risk factors for anastomotic failure by resection and exteriorisation of the bowel ends.

The anastomotic technique used will depend on the surgeon's preference. If the obstructed bowel is very thickened and oedematous, care should be taken with the use of stapling instruments since there is a tendency for the instruments to cut through oedematous bowel. Only on the relatively rare occasion when locally advanced disease is unresectable should the patient be subjected to an ileo-transverse colon bypass procedure. There is almost no place for caecostomy in the current management of right-sided large bowel obstruction; trephine ileostomy, which can usually be achieved under local anaesthesia, affords better palliation in very sick patients not fit for operation under general anaesthesia.

Transverse colon obstruction

Most surgeons would advocate an extended right hemicolectomy for patients with transverse colon carcinoma, and decompression of the colon may be necessary to facilitate mobilisation. For the patient who has a large carcinoma obstructing the transverse colon, achieving clearance may be difficult because of involvement of the transverse mesocolon and adjacent organs. The splenic flexure will require to be mobilised and a primary anastomosis between ileum and upper descending colon will usually be possible. In the sick patient who already has a perforated caecum, exteriorisation may be appropriate.

Left-sided obstruction

There is an increasing trend towards resection and primary anastomosis for obstructing left-sided tumours of the colon. Previously the debate centred around whether primary resection of the obstructing carcinoma (Hartmann's procedure) or simple decompression using a loop stoma should be performed at the time of presentation. Subsequently, interest has focused on whether primary anastomosis after resection performed as an emergency operation is as safe as a two-stage procedure. The current focus of interest centres on which single-stage operation is best.

Three-stage procedure For many years, this was the standard approach to the treatment of left-sided large bowel obstruction. It consists of a defunctioning colostomy, usually in the transverse colon, resection of the tumour at a second stage, with the third stage consisting of colostomy closure. The theoretical advantages of this approach are that a colostomy is a relatively minor procedure in patients who are often frail and that the anastomosis fashioned at the second operation is protected by the transverse colostomy. However, in practice there are a number of disadvantages. First, a transverse colostomy is not an easy stoma for the patient to manage, particularly if it is situated in the right upper quadrant.[91,92] Second, there is a higher incidence of herniation in the transverse stoma group, both parastomal and incisional.[93] This is a particular problem for the 25% of patients with left-sided obstruction who are not fit enough to have further surgery for their neoplasm and therefore have a permanent transverse colostomy. Third, these patients have a combined hospital stay of 30–55 days.[94] Although mortality rates of 20% were common in the 1970s with this three-stage approach, the combined mortality in reports from the surgical literature from the late 1980s and early 1990s showed an operative mortality of 11%,[95–98] which is similar to the operative mortality of two-stage and single-stage operations. Most reports show decreased long-term survival in patients who have three-stage procedures compared with primary resection and delayed anastomosis.[99,100]

Two-stage procedure The suggested advantages of a two-stage procedure over the three-stage technique are that (i) the tumour itself is removed at the first operation, thereby possibly conferring a better prognosis; (ii) two operations instead of three are necessary, thus reducing the time in hospital; and (iii) an anastomosis with its attendant risks of failure are avoided. The operation became popular during the 1970s and remains the procedure of choice for many surgeons. The overall mortality of the two-stage procedure is around 10%.[80,97] The mean hospital stay is shorter than for the three-stage procedure, ranging from 17 days[101] to 30 days.[95] However, one of the main disadvantages of this approach is that only around 60% of patients will have continuity restored at a later date, leaving 40% of patients with a permanent stoma and the attendant problems.

The second stage of the two-stage operation may be difficult because of adhesions. If the rectal stump has been divided intraperitoneally, restoration of bowel continuity is not as much of a problem as it

is when the rectum has had to be divided below the peritoneal reflection. The timing of the second stage is also important. In a study of 80 patients undergoing re-anastomosis after Hartmann's procedure,[102] the most important variable was the length of time between the primary operation and the second stage. There was no anastomotic leakage or mortality in the patients who had the second stage performed more than 6 months after the Hartmann's resection.

The second stage of the two-stage procedure is increasingly being performed using laparoscopic techniques. Early results suggest that hospital stay may be reduced by performing the procedure laparoscopically, but it should be remembered that, as with conventional surgery, the second stage may be very difficult indeed and conversion to open surgery may be necessary.

Single-stage procedure Although isolated reports of primary resection with anastomosis in the treatment of left-sided malignant large bowel obstruction have appeared in the surgical literature since the 1950s, this approach only started to become popular in the 1980s. Increasingly, there have been reports demonstrating the advantage of primary resection and anastomosis, based on a possible shorter hospital stay, reduced mortality and morbidity and the avoidance of a stoma. The choice of procedure depends on surgeon preference. Subtotal colectomy followed by ileosigmoid or ileorectal anastomosis has been reported to have a low operative mortality of 3–11%[94] and a hospital stay of around 15–20 days.[103–105] Segmental colectomy (left hemicolectomy, sigmoid colectomy or anterior resection of the rectosigmoid) with on-table irrigation followed by primary anastomosis has a reported operative mortality rate around 10%,[106,107] anastomotic leakage around 4%[108] and hospital stay of approximately 20 days.

A recent retrospective study of 243 patients who underwent emergency operation for obstructing colorectal cancers showed that primary resection and anastomosis for left-sided malignant obstruction either by segmental resection with on-table lavage or by subtotal colectomy was not more hazardous than primary anastomosis for right-sided obstruction.[109]

More recent papers have described segmental resection and primary anastomosis without any attempt to clean the bowel. One study reported only one leak and one postoperative death in 58 consecutive patients with left-sided malignant colonic obstruction who underwent bowel decompression without irrigation, followed by resection and primary colocolic anastomosis.[110] The patients had a mean age of 63 (range 54–89) years, the leak occurring in a 61 year old with a sigmoid carcinoma and the death in an 80 year old due to myocardial infarction. None of the carcinomas described were rectosigmoid or rectal. A further study of left-sided obstruction in which 40 of 60 patients had carcinoma compared one-stage resection with Hartmann's procedure.[111] There was no significant difference in outcome or time taken to complete the operation, with the only death being in the Hartmann's group. Again none of the tumours described was more distal than the sigmoid colon.

In certain circumstances one of these procedures may be preferable to the other. For example, segmental resection is preferable in the elderly. Subtotal colectomy is the procedure of choice if there are synchronous tumours in the colon.

If subtotal colectomy with ileorectal anastomosis is selected as the operation of choice, the whole colon will require to be mobilised in the usual way and the rectum washed out as for elective surgery. After resection of the colon, an ileorectal or ileosigmoid anastomosis is performed using either a sutured or stapled end-to-end technique. The first randomised trial comparing subtotal versus segmental resection was reported in 1995.[112] This study involved 91 eligible patients recruited by 18 consultant surgeons in 12 centres; 47 were randomised to subtotal colectomy and 44 to on-table irrigation and segmental colectomy. There was no significant difference in operative mortality, hospital stay, anastomotic leakage or wound sepsis between the two groups. There was a significantly higher permanent stoma rate in the subtotal colectomy group compared with the segmental colectomy group (7 vs. 1). The high permanent stoma rate in the subtotal colectomy group was partly accounted for by four patients who were randomised to subtotal colectomy but who underwent Hartmann's procedure because this was thought clinically more appropriate by the operating surgeon. Two additional patients had the anastomosis taken down at a later date and a stoma formed. At follow-up 4 months after the operation, there was a significantly greater number of patients who had three or more bowel movements a day after subtotal colectomy than after segmental resection (14 of 35 vs. 4 of 35). One patient had 12 bowel movements per day after subtotal colectomy. Nearly one-third of patients randomised to subtotal colectomy had night-time bowel movements during the first few months after operation. In contrast, less than 10% of those who had segmental resection had this problem.

The authors concluded that although the results of both techniques were acceptable, segmental resection following intraoperative irrigation was the preferred treatment for left-sided malignant colonic obstruction.[112]

Although the study addressed the immediate and early results after these two procedures, it did not investigate the long-term implications of either procedure. It has been argued that there are advantages in performing a subtotal colectomy rather than segmental resection because synchronous tumours will be removed along with the obstructing lesion and, since the length of colon left is small, there should be less risk of developing a metachronous tumour.

ACUTE COLONIC BLEEDING

Bleeding from the colon and rectum accounts for about 20% of all cases of acute gastrointestinal haemorrhage. The majority of patients are elderly, with a mean age of 66 years reported in one series of 153 patients.[113] The site and source of haemorrhage in the lower gastrointestinal tract is considerably less easy to determine than in the upper gastrointestinal tract, and because bleeding settles without intervention in the majority of patients, the cause is often never satisfactorily resolved. Even after examination of a surgically resected specimen, the final diagnosis may remain uncertain.

Severity of acute lower gastrointestinal haemorrhage has been classified as mild, moderate and massive. Mild haemorrhage involves loss of less than 20% of blood volume, moderate haemorrhage loss of 20–40% of blood volume, and massive haemorrhage loss of greater than 40% of blood volume.

Causes

DIVERTICULOSIS

The introduction of selective angiography and colonoscopy has made an important contribution to defining the source of acute colonic bleeding. Before these investigations were commonplace, reliance on sigmoidoscopy and barium enema led to the perception that diverticular disease was the cause of severe colonic haemorrhage in 70% of patients.[114] More recent reports attribute only about 50% to diverticular problems.[115] Although most diverticula occur in the sigmoid colon, approximately 60% of patients who have bleeding of diverticular origin are bleeding from the right colon.[116] Diverticula develop at the site of penetration of nutrient vessels in the colon, and bleeding occurs as a result of arterial rupture into the diverticulum. It has been suggested that the tendency for right-sided diverticula to bleed results from the wider necks and domes of these diverticula compared with those on the left side of the colon, leading to thinning of the mucosa overlying the vasa recta.[117] The bleeding tends to be large and continuous rather than the intermittent bleeding of vascular ectasia.

ANGIODYSPLASIA

Since the 1970s, malformation of intestinal blood vessels, which is known as vascular ectasia or angiodysplasia, has been diagnosed with increasing frequency as a cause of intermittent bleeding from the large bowel. It has been suggested that angiodysplasia may be acquired through repeated partial low-grade obstruction of submucosal veins, which in turn leads to the formation of arteriovenous shunts. Although in 80% of patients angiodysplasia affects the terminal ileum, caecum, ascending colon or hepatic flexure,[118] in 20% it occurs in the descending colon and sigmoid.[119] Association with coagulopathy and cardiac valvular disease is frequently quoted; in one study these conditions were noted in 28% and 25% of patients respectively.[120] It has been suggested that the relationship between aortic valve stenosis and angiodysplasia could be explained by a deficiency of von Willebrand factor,[121] and aortic valve replacement has been shown to stop gastrointestinal haemorrhage in most patients.[122] Angiodysplasia causes a spectrum of presentation ranging from unexplained iron-deficiency anaemia to acute colonic haemorrhage. Dilated tortuous vessels and distinct 'cherry-red' areas are typical features on colonoscopy. In the acute setting and without optimal bowel preparation, the relatively subtle appearances are easily missed and the diagnosis is often dependent on arteriography. The angiographic features consist of early filling, tortuous arteries; in the capillary phase, dilated lakes of contrast are noted in the wall of the bowel and these drain into large veins, which fill earlier than usual (**Fig. 10.9**). There is a clinical dilemma when angiodysplasia is found in a patient with a significant bleed but no active bleeding from the site, as it is notoriously difficult to demonstrate actual bleeding from angiodyplasia either at angiography or colonoscopy. Additionally, angiodysplasia is a common finding at routine colonoscopy, quoted at 3–6% but in up to 25% of the elderly group of patients.[116]

OTHER CAUSES OF BLEEDING

Although diverticulosis and vascular ectasia are important causes of colonic bleeding in the elderly patient, other causes are occasionally seen. Carcinoma of the left colon sometimes causes acute haemorrhage. Patients with inflammatory bowel disease rarely have a severe lower gastrointestinal bleed that necessitates surgery. Ischaemic colitis is also a well-recognised cause of rectal bleeding. In

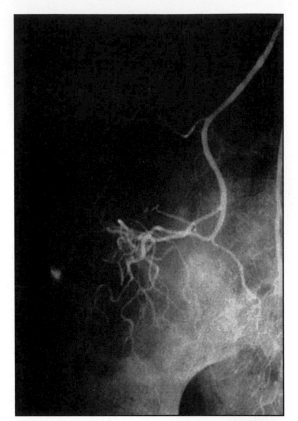

Figure 10.9 • Mesenteric angiography demonstrating angiodysplasia in the area of the caecum. Radiograph kindly provided by Dr D. Nicholls, Consultant Radiologist, Raigmore Hospital, Inverness.

patients suspected of having, or diagnosed with, AIDS there may be a different spectrum of underlying causes.[123] In a study of 18 patients with AIDS, lower gastrointestinal bleeding was due to human immunodeficiency virus (HIV) type 1-associated disorders in 72%, including cytomegalovirus in seven, idiopathic colonic ulcers in five, intestinal Kaposi's sarcoma in one and HIV-associated thrombocytopenia in two. Cytomegalovirus infections should also be excluded in other patients with immunosuppression, such as those on chemotherapy.

Presentation

The nature of bleeding ascertained on detailed history and examination may provide clues about the site. Melaena usually signifies bleeding from the upper gastrointestinal tract but can occasionally occur from small bowel and the proximal colon. Large-volume fresh bleeding often indicates a colonic cause, but can result from a brisk upper gastrointestinal source. A history of previous aortic surgery with the insertion of a graft increases the possibility of an aorto-enteric fistula. Abdominal pain may be associated with ischaemic colitis or inflammatory bowel disease. Bloody diarrhoea suggests inflammatory bowel disease or an infective colitis, whereas a history of anal symptoms might suggest haemorrhoids. Digital examination of the rectum and inspection of the blood are mandatory.

Initial management

Two main patterns are seen in massive colonic haemorrhage. One group of patients, after a significant initial bleed, settle down, allowing investigation to proceed in a more leisurely fashion. A second group shows evidence of continued haemorrhage or rebleeding after initial cessation and requires urgent investigation. However, in the majority of patients the bleeding will ultimately stop spontaneously.

Patients require thorough assessment of their haemodynamic status on admission. The overtly shocked clearly require prompt resuscitation. Elderly patients and those with underlying systemic disorders will tolerate considerably lesser degrees of blood loss than the younger and fitter patient. After establishing good venous access, a full blood count and coagulation study should be done. Any coagulation defects should be vigorously corrected. In acute colonic haemorrhage, monitoring of urine output will generally be required and insertion of a central venous catheter will aid in monitoring intravascular volume replacement. Nasogastric intubation and stomach lavage may be helpful in highlighting the possibility of upper gastrointestinal haemorrhage, but a negative lavage occurs in up to 16% of patients with significant upper gastrointestinal bleeding. Upper gastrointestinal endoscopy is therefore the most direct way of excluding bleeding from the upper gastrointestinal tract (see also Chapter 7).

Investigation

The aim of investigation is to localise the site of haemorrhage. The methods in common use are colonoscopy, arteriography and radionuclide scanning. A few centres have built up a large experience of this problem and claim that the use of investigative techniques has increased the accuracy of localisation of the bleeding site to around 90%. The majority of patients are looked after by clinicians who have much less experience of the condition and have less easy access to investigative expertise. Localisation of the bleeding site is often elusive, making the management of these patients quite demanding.

COLONOSCOPY

This was initially thought by most clinicians to have little place in the management of patients with acute colorectal bleeding because of difficulty in visualisation in the presence of faeces and blood clot. Provided there is an endoscopist of sufficient skill and experience, colonoscopy now forms a part of the protocol for the management of acute bleeding from the large bowel. It can be used immediately after resuscitation in patients who have severe haemorrhage, since the blood acts as a cathartic; if examination is performed when bleeding is active, the diagnostic yield may be as high as 76%.[124] A bowel lavage may be given to help clear the lower bowel of stool and blood clot. However, the views can still be poor, with faecal material and blood often absorbing most of the available light. Even when pathology is identified, establishing the presence of stigmata of recent haemorrhage is more difficult than in the upper gastrointestinal tract. In addition, colonoscopy is associated with a risk of complications such as perforation. Inconclusive findings owing to technically unsatisfactory results are frequent and failure to achieve a firm diagnosis may reflect stricter diagnostic criteria rather than inferior diagnostic skill.

As in elective colonoscopy, the patient should be closely monitored and receive oxygen therapy. Sedation should be carefully titrated to maintain a cooperative patient. A colonoscope with wide-bore suction channel is required and excessive insufflation should be avoided since colonic wall distension can exacerbate haemorrhage. It may be useful to perform rigid sigmoidoscopy beforehand to remove blood clots from the rectal ampulla. Therapeutic manoeuvres include injection of vasoconstrictor substances and coagulation by laser, diathermy or heater probe to areas of angiodysplasia and polyp sites.

In those patients who have stopped bleeding a gentle bowel preparation may be given orally and colonoscopy performed during the same hospital admission.

ANGIOGRAPHY

This is extremely helpful when it demonstrates extravasation of contrast into the bowel lumen, allowing therapeutic embolisation or guiding surgery. This requires that the patient is actively bleeding at a rate of 1–1.5 mL/min. Elective angiography of the superior mesenteric artery is performed first, since the source of bleeding lies most commonly in the distribution of this vessel. If no bleeding point is seen, an inferior mesenteric angiogram should then be performed. Superselective catheterisation of branch arteries and multiple injections of contrast may be required to examine the entire territory. It is important to take late films in the venous phase as they may demonstrate abnormalities that may not be seen in the arterial phase. If a bleeding point is not visualised and angiodysplasia is noted on an arteriogram, it should not necessarily be assumed that this is the site of bleeding. In one study, angiography correctly identified the site of bleeding in 58–86% of patients.[115] Major complications of diagnostic arteriography include arterial thrombosis, embolisation and renal failure caused by the contrast material.

Superselective angiography can be useful in certain circumstances when standard angiographic techniques have failed to demonstrate the bleeding lesion. Occasionally, intraoperative angiography is helpful, and this may be supplemented by injecting methylene blue after superselective catheterisation to demonstrate a bleeding point.

One of the arguments used to support routine use of angiography is its therapeutic potential. Intraarterial vasopressin therapy can arrest haemorrhage and in a proportion prevent the need for surgery. In one series of 22 patients, control of haemorrhage was obtained in 20 using vasopressin; although 50% rebled at varying times afterwards, it was felt that this allowed surgery to be performed electively in 57% of the patients.[115]

The high rebleeding rate with vasopressin has led to other more definitive therapeutic manoeuvres during angiography such as superselective embolisation, which is effective in controlling colonic haemorrhage and is associated with a low rate of postembolisation colonic ischaemia. In a study of 27 patients, all were initially controlled with arterial embolisation but six rebled, five of these needing surgical intervention.[125]

A recent study looked at the morphological and histopathological changes in the bowel after superselective embolisation with gelatin sponge particles and/or microcoils. Fourteen patients were reviewed, 11 of whom had a colonic source of bleeding. Embolisation was successful in arresting haemorrhage in all of them, with no recurrence of bleeding. There was no significant bowel damage in 13 patients (93%). One patient treated with numerous gelatin particles delivered from the proximal arcade of the superior mesenteric artery developed significant muscular fibrosis.[126]

RADIONUCLIDE SCANNING

The introduction of technetium-99m (^{99m}Tc) sulphur colloid and ^{99m}Tc-labelled red cell scintigraphy to the investigation of gastrointestinal haemorrhage was particularly important because these are relatively non-invasive investigations and can detect the source of bleeding where blood loss is as low as 0.05–0.1 mL/min. The ^{99m}Tc-sulphur colloid undergoes rapid clearance from the blood and has high background activity in the liver and spleen; consequently, it has largely been replaced by ^{99m}Tc-labelled red cells. This allows the patient to be monitored for up to 24 hours after a single injection and may be of value in patients who have intermittent bleeding. Although the technique can be sensitive, rapid movement of extravasated blood along the bowel lumen contributes to inaccuracy in localisation in intermittent imaging, and intestinal irritation from blood in the lumen probably contributes to retrograde as well as antegrade movement. Because some scans show bleeding but cannot localise it, and no confirmatory evidence is found in other patients whose bleeding settles, the results of scintigraphy overall are difficult to quantify. Data from six reports that included 641 patients showed that confirmation of scintigraphic diagnosis ranged from 42 to 97%, the correct localisation from 40 to 97% and incorrect localisation from 3 to 59%.[127]

Some clinicians feel that scintigraphic imaging is useful as a screening test for patients who have acute lower gastrointestinal bleeding; however, a major disadvantage of scintigraphy with ^{99m}Tc-labelled red cells is that it only localises the bleeding to an area of the abdomen. Other disadvantages include poor resolution and it is of little or no value in patients who have stopped bleeding.

OVERALL DIAGNOSTIC APPROACH

The methods chosen for investigation of patients with acute colonic bleeding will be determined first by the severity of bleeding and second by the expertise available locally. The approach of the authors is to exclude upper gastrointestinal bleeding as the initial step. If this is even a remote possibility, then upper gastrointestinal endoscopy is carried out. Rigid sigmoidoscopy can exclude a local anorectal bleed and can also be used to remove blood clot prior to colonoscopy. In around 80% of patients who present with acute colonic bleeding, the haemorrhage will cease spontaneously and in these patients investigation can proceed electively. This usually takes the form of colonoscopy after a gentle bowel preparation. If the bleeding is ongoing, angiography is requested. Colonoscopy is also attempted if the bleeding source is not obvious on angiography. We would reserve the use of radionuclide scanning for patients who are haemodynamically stable, when there is a lack of vascular radiology expertise and failure to localise bleeding using endoscopy. Patients require surgical intervention if they continue to bleed profusely and medical, endoscopic and angiographic interventions have failed.

Control of bleeding

As colonoscopy is a first-line investigation, it can also be used as a first-line treatment. Monopolar or bipolar diathermy, argon plasma coagulation, Nd-YAG laser and the heater probe have all been described in the successful management of angiodysplasia. Not surprisingly, there is a small risk of perforation with these techniques, particularly with monopolar diathermy.[128] The heater probe has been used to treat bleeding diverticula.[129]

Although vasopressin can be infused at angiography and is effective in stopping bleeding in up to 90% of patients with either angiodysplasia or diverticula, it should be regarded as a temporising procedure because rebleeding commonly occurs once the vasospasm wears off and most of these patients will require surgical management. For patients who are not fit for surgery, selective arterial embolisation should still be considered.[130]

The rate of blood loss from the colon will determine the urgency of the need for operation. If the bleeding source has been identified, either by angiography or colonoscopy, and haemorrhage continues, laparotomy and segmental excision can be performed with a low operative mortality and risk of recurrent haemorrhage.[93] The use of on-table irrigation and intraoperative colonoscopy allows a further opportunity to localise the bleeding site as well as prepare the colon for primary anastomosis in the patient who has vigorous colonic bleeding. Indeed, laparotomy, high-flow antegrade irrigation and intraoperative colonoscopy have been advocated as the management of choice in patients who continue to bleed after resuscitation. In one report, this approach identified the bleeding site in seven of nine patients.[131] There is controversy about what to do if, for example, a vascular malformation is demonstrated in the right colon, diverticula are noted in the remaining colon but no active bleeding site is demonstrated. Although subtotal colectomy would appear to be a sensible option, the patient can continue to bleed postoperatively, with the bleeding source being sited in the small bowel or rectum. Careful proctography of a thoroughly cleaned rectum and on-table enteroscopy will minimise this risk. In the emergency setting the colonoscope can be passed into the small bowel either retrogradely from the terminal ileum at the time of laparotomy or antegradely through the mouth, manipulated onwards through the stomach, duodenum and small bowel by the operating surgeon.

Intraoperative angiography merits mention as another potential technique in difficult cases. Methylene blue injected into an appropriate artery while the surgeon has the bowel exposed has been described. Another procedure that can be performed during operation to identify the site of bleeding is transillumination of the bowel with an endoscope and the theatre lights turned down.

ACUTE COLONIC DIVERTICULITIS

Diverticula are found in the colon more commonly with increasing age. It has been estimated that one-third of the population will have colonic diverticula by the age of 50 years and two-thirds after 80 years.[132,133] Although the vast majority of individuals with colonic diverticula are asymptomatic, most patients who require surgical care do so because of an inflammatory complication. Acute diverticulitis can affect any part of the colon; in western Europe and North America, the left side is more commonly affected, whereas in Japan and China right-sided diverticulitis is more commonly seen.[133,134]

Symptomatic complications of diverticulitis occur in 10–30% of patients.[135,136] Although 15–30% of patients who were admitted with acute diverticulitis required operation in the 1960s,[137] operation for acute diverticulitis is now less common.

Presentation

Diverticulitis is thought to result from inspissation of stool in the neck of a diverticulum, with consequent inflammation and possible microperforation. This results in local bacterial proliferation, leading to inflammation in the surrounding colonic wall and mesentery (acute phlegmonous diverticulitis). A collection of pus may form either in the mesentery of the colon or adjacent to the colonic wall. As the collection of pus enlarges, it becomes walled-off by loops of small bowel or the peritoneum of the pelvis. Occasionally, free perforation into the peritoneal cavity occurs with consequent purulent or faecal peritonitis. The Hinchey grading system for acute diverticulitis has become fairly widely accepted, allowing more meaningful comparison between outcome studies (Box 10.2).[138]

From time to time other complications also arise. A fistula sometimes develops between bowel and another adjacent organ, for example the bladder.

Box 10.2 • Hinchey classification of peritoneal contamination in diverticulitis

Stage 1	Pericolic or mesenteric abscess
Stage 2	Walled-off pelvic abscess
Stage 3	Generalised purulent peritonitis
Stage 4	Generalised faecal peritonitis

Diverticular disease is responsible for around 10% of all cases of left-sided large bowel obstruction[139] and is frequently difficult to differentiate from malignant left-sided large bowel obstruction on clinical grounds. Bleeding is a rare complication.

There has been controversy regarding the virulence of diverticular disease in younger patients and the possible increase in need for surgical intervention in this group. Recently, Biondo et al. looked at 327 patients treated for acute left colonic diverticulitis and compared those aged 50 or less with those older than 50.[140] No difference was noted regarding severity or recurrence. Another study found that diverticulitis in the young does not follow a particularly aggressive course.[141] In general, there is a trend towards conservative management of acute diverticulitis, with early investigation and confirmation of the diagnosis being a fundamental part of this approach. The mortality and morbidity rates can be high if emergency surgery is necessary.[142]

Investigation

Acute right-sided diverticulitis, a rare condition in the Western world, can be confused with appendicitis as it occurs in a somewhat younger age group than left-sided disease.[143] Ultrasound has been reported to have a sensitivity of 91.3%, specificity of 99.8% and overall accuracy of 99.5% in the diagnosis of acute right-sided diverticulitis.[144]

In the more common left-sided disease, the plain abdominal radiograph may show non-specific abnormalities such as pneumoperitoneum in approximately 3–12% and intestinal obstruction or a soft tissue mass in 30–50% of patients with acute diverticulitis.[145,146] Pneumoperitoneum is indicated by Rigler's sign, where both sides of the bowel are outlined by gas, and by the characteristic appearances of the falciform ligament, which sometimes manifests as a linear density in the right upper quadrant, and the lateral umbilical ligaments, which are outlined as an inverted V shape over the sacrum.[147] There is debate regarding the nature of additional investigations. Some clinicians believe that initial evaluation will allow patients to be staged and the need for surgical intervention to be predicted. Others suggest that evaluation can usefully be deferred until conservative management has failed and complications require to be delineated and treated.

 CT is now the favoured modality for acute investigation.[148]

Features of acute diverticulitis include thickening of the bowel wall, increased soft tissue density within the pericolic fat secondary to inflammation and a soft tissue mass, which represents either a phlegmon or an abscess. Advantages of CT include the accurate assessment of the extent of pericolonic involvement and the diagnosis of abscess formation[149] or perforation (**Fig. 10.10**). It is also useful for tracking the therapeutic percutaneous drainage of any abscess. CT is the investigation of choice for those patients in whom delineation of the problem has not been clear on contrast enema and the decision about surgery is difficult. One study has suggested that CT might influence the management of patients with diverticulitis since patients with large soft tissue masses were more likely to require surgery.[149]

When CT is compared with barium enema, CT is no more accurate in terms of diagnosis but undoubtedly provides better definition of the extent and severity of the inflammatory process, which is of prognostic value in the short and long term.[150] Although ultrasonography has not been as widely used as CT for localised diverticulitis, recent studies support the use of ultrasonography as an initial investigation.[151] One recent study showed ultrasound to have a sensitivity of 85% and specificity of 80% compared with the final clinical diagnosis assessed by contrast study or surgical exploration.[152] Diagnostic criteria of ultrasound include thickening of the bowel wall more than 4 mm involving a segment of 5 cm or more in the left side of the abdomen and demonstration of diverticula or abscess adjacent to the bowel. A potential advantage of ultrasound is that it also has a therapeutic role in the management of abscesses.[153] The main disadvantages of ultrasonography are that assessment of bowel thickening is a non-specific finding and assessment is very operator dependent. In those cases with involvement of the lower sigmoid,

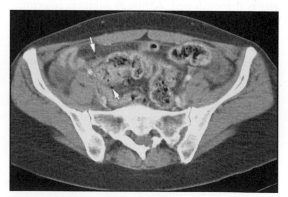

Figure 10.10 • Appearance of perforated sigmoid diverticular disease on computed tomography. The upper arrow shows a small pocket of free air and the lower arrow one of the diverticula.

transrectal ultrasound may provide additional information, increasing the accuracy of this investigation when combined with the transabdominal approach.[154]

An alternative investigation is contrast enema. Despite the extensive literature on the use of contrast enema in acute diverticulitis, there is no consensus on either the best contrast agent or the optimal timing of the examination. Although many advocate water-soluble contrast, others prefer barium, provided pneumoperitoneum is excluded.[155] Others advise against any enema examination during the acute phase or for up to 2 weeks after an acute episode.[156]

In many hospitals in the UK, water-soluble contrast enema is the favoured investigation in patients with acute symptoms, but no air contrast is used during the examination. The appearances of acute diverticulitis on water-soluble enema are (i) diverticulosis with or without spasm, (ii) peridiverticulitis and sigmoid irregularity with long strictures or obstruction and (iii) extravasation of contrast, which is the most reliable radiological sign of perforation. If there are no diverticula present, the diagnosis must be reviewed. The examination has been shown to be of importance in predicting the need for surgery. Only 3 of 30 patients who had diverticulosis with or without spasm detected by water-soluble contrast enema required surgery, whereas operation was necessary in 13 of 16 patients with extravasation or peridiverticulitis.[157]

Recently, there has been some interest with magnetic resonance imaging in the diagnosis of acute diverticulitis in the form of prospective observational studies. The results are encouraging but more formal evaluation is required.[158]

Management

RIGHT-SIDED DISEASE

Right-sided disease may be encountered unexpectedly at surgery or be operated on for a complication diagnosed preoperatively. The treatment options are controversial, ranging from appendicectomy to hemicolectomy. A conservative approach with appendicectomy and antibiotics has resulted in a similar mortatility, morbidity and recurrence as for resection of the diverticulum.[159] A Western surgeon unused to this condition would tend to be more aggressive, performing a limited ileocaecal resection for an isolated caecal diverticulum or right hemicolectomy in the presence of more extensive right-sided disease.[160] A right hemicolectomy is the correct operation when it is not possible to rule out the presence of a carcinoma.[161] On-table caecoscopy using a bronchoscope passed through the appendix stump has been used to confirm the diagnosis of

diverticulitis,[159] but this is probably only really practical in centres that deal with this condition on a regular basis.

LEFT-SIDED DISEASE

A typical patient with localised diverticulitis will complain of pain in the left iliac fossa and will be febrile. Examination reveals tenderness and sometimes a mass is palpable per abdomen or on rectal examination. In women, a vaginal examination should also be performed to help exclude gynaecological pathology. If sigmoidoscopy is performed, it should be done very gently with minimal insufflation of air.

In the absence of generalised peritonitis, a non-operative policy is adopted, with antibiotic therapy directed against Gram-negative and anaerobic bacteria. Most clinicians advocate bowel rest initially, with fluids and antibiotics given by the intravenous route. If the pain and fever settle within a few days, the patient can go home and barium enema and sigmoidoscopy or colonoscopy can be performed as an outpatient a few weeks later. This will exclude any possibility of malignancy.

If the patient continues to be pyrexial and the pain does not settle, or the lower abdominal mass is enlarging, CT should be requested. If this investigation is not available, ultrasound or even a water-soluble contrast enema may provide useful information at this stage. If there is an abscess, it can be drained percutaneously under radiological guidance. In the event of localised abdominal signs becoming more generalised or if there is a failure of the infective process to settle despite adequate conservative therapy, operation is indicated. In the small number of patients who require operation for localised diverticulitis, a policy of primary resection, on-table irrigation and primary anastomosis is becoming more popular.[162]

GENERALISED PERITONITIS

Pain from perforated sigmoid diverticulitis usually commences in the lower abdomen, mostly on the left side and gradually spreads throughout the abdomen. In 25% of patients, however, signs and symptoms are predominantly right-sided.[163] On examination, there are signs of generalised peritonitis including guarding and rebound tenderness. About one-quarter of all patients will have free gas under the diaphragm on abdominal radiography, and at operation purulent peritonitis is more common than faecal peritonitis. In a report of 93 consecutive patients with perforated diverticulitis and diffuse peritonitis, 18 had faecal peritonitis and 75 had purulent peritonitis.[163] The majority of patients presenting in this way will clearly require operation, and there is no merit in pursuing further specific investigations. The main priority at this stage is adequate resuscitation, as many of the patients are elderly with poor myocardial reserve. In this group, it is important to avoid miscalculation of fluid requirement by using central venous pressure measurement for estimation. A short time spent on resuscitation in a high-dependency unit will pay dividends in terms of patient survival and it is a great mistake to rush such patients to theatre immediately. The goals are to restore depleted intravascular and extracellular fluid volume, to re-establish urine output and maximise myocardial and respiratory function. Antibiotic therapy should be commenced early to cover both anaerobic organisms and Gram-negative bacteria.

Some patients will improve so much with conservative treatment that the surgeon can review the need for laparotomy. If the abdominal pain and signs improve significantly, it is appropriate to continue for a longer period with conservative therapy.

OPERATIVE MANAGEMENT

The patient is placed in the lithotomy/Trendelenburg position and good access is best obtained by using a long midline incision. Pus and faecal material should be removed from the peritoneal cavity and specimens sent for microscopy and both aerobic and anaerobic culture. The place of intraoperative irrigation of the peritoneal cavity remains controversial. Killingback suggested that the use of 6–10 L of warm saline solution is of value,[164] while the addition of topical antibiotics to the solution, although logical, remains to be generally accepted. Using tetracycline lavage (1 g tetracycline in 1 L 0.9% saline) as the method of treating intraperitoneal infection, Koruth et al. reported 82 consecutive emergency colon resections with a 2% residual intraperitoneal sepsis rate.[165] As tetracycline is no longer available, cephradine (cefradine) 1 g in 1 L of 0.9% saline can be used as an alternative.

In addition to treating the peritonitis, the main aim of surgical treatment is to minimise the risk of continued contamination of the peritoneal cavity. In the past, it was thought that resection of the colon was too major an undertaking to impose on the acutely ill patient. In fact, the converse appears to apply, in that mortality associated with failure to remove a diseased colon is very high. Krukowski and Matheson[142] analysed 57 reports on the treatment of acute diverticular disease and showed that the operative mortality rates from procedures that involve primary resection were less than half those from operations that did not include excision of the diseased segment of colon. The mortality rate for 295 patients with generalised purulent faecal peritonitis resulting from diverticular disease who

were subjected to primary excision was 10%, whereas mortality rose to 25% for 813 patients treated using a three-stage procedure.

A further reason for advocating primary resection is the difficulty experienced at the time of operation in deciding whether the lesion is a perforated carcinoma or an area of diverticulitis. At laparotomy, the appearance of both lesions may be similar when the colon is inflamed and oedematous. It has been estimated that as many as 25% of patients with a preoperative diagnosis of perforated diverticulitis may be found to have a perforated carcinoma. If there is reasonable suspicion of carcinoma, a radical resection of the lesion, together with the colonic mesentery, needs to be performed. Examination of the resected specimen at the earliest opportunity is recommended to aid further decision-making.

Failure to take the resection far enough distally beyond the sigmoid colon risks recurrence of diverticular disease. Therefore, Hartmann's resection with complete excision of the sigmoid and closure of the rectum, with formation of a left iliac fossa colostomy, has been the standard procedure advocated by most surgeons. If the operation is exceptionally difficult owing to the colon being very adherent to surrounding structures, making safe mobilisation impossible, it may be reasonable to create a proximal stoma, drain the area and transfer the patient to a tertiary referral centre.

Primary anastomosis

There has been an increase in the use of primary anastomosis in selected patients who have operations for acute diverticulitis. The main reasons are (i) that patients require one operation rather than two; (ii) after a Hartmann's operation many patients are left with a permanent stoma, either because of unwillingness or unfitness to have further surgery; and (iii) reversal operation after Hartmann's resection can be very difficult.

Gregg, in 1955, was the first to report resection and primary anastomosis in several patients with perforated diverticulitis without mortality or anastomotic leakage.[166] In their review of the surgical literature, Krukowski and Matheson collected 100 cases of resection with primary anastomosis.[142] The operative mortality rate was 9% compared with 12.2% for resection without anastomosis. However, they pointed out that the reported cases are likely to be highly selected and the good results may reflect the enthusiasm and skill of the surgeon performing these procedures rather than the intrinsic merit of the procedure itself. Biondo et al. used resection, intraoperative colonic lavage and primary anastomosis in 55 of 124 patients with complicated diverticular disease; 49 of the 55 had diverticulitis, 33 having localised and 16 generalised peritonitis.[167] Faecal peritonitis was considered a contraindication to a one-stage procedure. There were two anastomotic leakages and three abdominal wound dehiscences. Four patients died, one from an anastomotic leak.

 This study concluded that in selected patients a one-stage resection is feasible.[167]

A further study of primary anastomosis in emergency colorectal surgery showed no significant difference in the incidence of complications, even in patients with free peritonitis (21.9% perforation, 17.7% localised sepsis).[168] The necessity for intra-operative colonic lavage has also been challenged recently in a retrospective study of 33 patients undergoing resection, primary anastomosis without bowel preparation or on-table colonic lavage. There were 12 patients each in Hinchey grades 1 and 2, and seven patients and two patients respectively in Hinchey grades 3 and 4. There was one documented anastomotic leak and three deaths, one of whom was suspected to have had an anastomotic leak.[169] Despite an increasing trend to perform primary anastomosis in patients who have perforated diverticulitis, the number of patients who are suitable for such a procedure will be small.

NEUTROPENIC ENTEROCOLITIS

Neutropenic enterocolitis, also known as typhlitis, is a potentially life-threatening condition characterised by an inflammatory process that usually involves the caecum and ascending colon. It occurs most often as a complication of chemotherapy and can progress to necrosis and perforation. Although it can affect any part of the small and large intestine, the cause of its predisposition for the right colon is unclear.

Clinical features include nausea, vomiting, abdominal pain, distension and diarrhoea, which can be bloody. Right iliac fossa tenderness and pyrexia are quite common and in later stages peritonitis may be present. CT is the diagnostic modality of choice and may reveal right-sided colon wall thickening, mesenteric stranding, pneumatosis and ascites (**Fig. 10.11**).[170]

Management demands careful evaluation of the patient, with each case treated individually.[171] An initial conservative approach includes fluid and electrolyte replacement, broad-spectrum antibiotics, correction of any attendant coagulopathy and complete bowel rest with parenteral nutrition. The use of recombinant granulocyte colony-stimulating factor to correct chemotherapy-induced neutro-

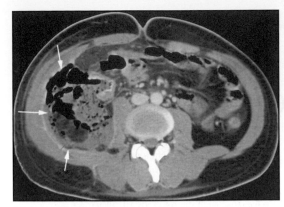

Figure 10.11 • Computed tomography scan showing large retroperitoneal collection (indicated by arrows) secondary to acute necrotising enterocolitis with a delayed perforation of the posterior wall of the caecum and ascending colon.

penia should be considered. Colonic perforation and generalised peritonitis are clear indications for surgery. The operative procedure of choice is a right hemicolectomy, with either exteriorisation of the bowel ends or a primary anastomosis depending on the extent of sepsis and peritoneal soiling.[172] In general, most cases can be managed conservatively.[173]

STERCORAL PERFORATION

The word *stercus* means dung or faeces. Perforation of the bowel caused by pressure necrosis from a faecal mass is a rare entity, first reported by Berry at the Pathological Society of London in 1894. Fewer than 100 cases have been reported in the literature, although this may reflect the poor outcome (with mortality rates approaching 50%), an increasing reluctance to publish case reports and ill-defined diagnostic criteria. There appears to be an equal incidence in men and women and the median age for these patients is said to be 60 years.[174]

Reported predisposing factors have included chronic constipation, megacolon, scleroderma, hypercalcaemia, renal failure and renal transplantation. Medications associated with stercoral perforation include narcotics, postoperative analgesia, antacids, calcium channel blockers and antidepressants.

Only 11% of cases are accurately diagnosed prior to operation,[175] with investigations frequently non-contributory. Perforations usually occur on the anti-mesenteric border, with the majority occurring in the sigmoid colon and rectosigmoid region. Multiple perforations are found in about one-fifth of patients, with the remaining patients usually having ulceration extending away from the perforation.

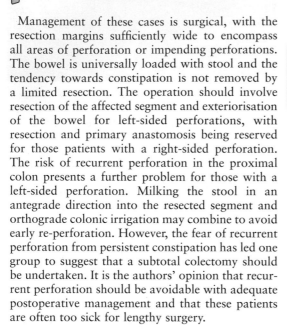

The suggested clinicopathological diagnostic criteria are:
- a round or ovoid colonic perforation exceeding 1 cm in diameter;
- faecolomas present within the colon;
- microscopic evidence of pressure necrosis or ulcer and chronic inflammatory reaction around the perforation site.[176]

Management of these cases is surgical, with the resection margins sufficiently wide to encompass all areas of perforation or impending perforations. The bowel is universally loaded with stool and the tendency towards constipation is not removed by a limited resection. The operation should involve resection of the affected segment and exteriorisation of the bowel for left-sided perforations, with resection and primary anastomosis being reserved for those patients with a right-sided perforation. The risk of recurrent perforation in the proximal colon presents a further problem for those with a left-sided perforation. Milking the stool in an antegrade direction into the resected segment and orthograde colonic irrigation may combine to avoid early re-perforation. However, the fear of recurrent perforation from persistent constipation has led one group to suggest that a subtotal colectomy should be undertaken. It is the authors' opinion that recurrent perforation should be avoidable with adequate postoperative management and that these patients are often too sick for lengthy surgery.

ANASTOMOTIC DEHISCENCE

Breakdown of an anastomosis is one of the most significant complications after large bowel surgery. The presentation can be insidious but more commonly the patient becomes dramatically unwell, particularly if there is generalised peritonitis. If the diagnosis is not made and appropriate treatment undertaken, death is likely to follow. There is no doubt that the presence of anastomotic leakage significantly increases mortality. Fielding et al. noted a mortality rate of 22% in 191 patients who had leakage after large bowel anastomosis compared with only 7.2% in 1275 patients without a leak.[177] In the patients who survive this serious complication, morbidity is greatly increased and prolonged hospital inpatient stay inevitable.

Causes

A variety of general and local causative factors of anastomotic dehiscence are described in most textbooks.[178] The general factors listed usually include poor nutritional state, anaemia, uraemia, diabetes, steroid administration and old age. It is also generally taught that local factors affecting the anastomosis contribute. Inadequate mobilisation of bowel ends producing tension on the anastomosis may well be a factor in dehiscence of low colorectal anastomoses. Experimental evidence favours the view that local infection around the anastomosis leads to breakdown rather than synthesis of collagen, collagen synthesis being an important factor in anastomotic healing.[179]

The risk of anastomotic leakage in low colorectal anastomosis is several times higher than in either ileocolic or colocolic anastomosis. In a recent study reported from Inverness and Aberdeen, the clinical leak rate for ileocolic and colocolic anastomosis was 0.4%, whereas the leak rate after low colorectal anastomosis was 4.7%.[180]

Another important factor in dehiscence is the oxygen tension at the bowel ends used for the anastomosis. In an elegant study reported in 1987, it was shown that if tissue oxygen tension in the ends of bowel to be anastomosed fell to less than 20 mmHg (2.66 kPa), there was a high likelihood of anastomotic breakdown.[181] However, perhaps the most common cause of anastomotic failure is poor surgical technique, whether it is a sutured or stapled anastomosis.

Presentation

In general, the clinical features of anastomotic dehiscence will depend on whether the leak is localised or more extensive, causing generalised peritonitis. At one end of the spectrum, when sepsis associated with the leak is localised, the patient may have minimal symptoms and only a few physical signs. There may be 'flu-like' symptoms of feeling vaguely unwell with shivering and nausea. If the anastomosis lies low in the pelvis, there may be some lower abdominal pain and tenderness and on rectal examination a defect can often be felt in the anastomosis. Tachycardia is a common general feature and is often associated with pyrexia. If a drain is still in situ, faecal material or pus may be seen.

At the other end of the spectrum is the scenario associated with a major leak, when faecal material or pus has leaked into the general peritoneal cavity. The effect on the patient is usually profound. Abdominal pain is difficult to control and tachycardia and tachypnoea are common. The temperature is raised and hypotension is often a feature. The patient is distressed and sweaty and on abdominal examination the abdomen is tender with abdominal guarding. Sometimes the features of even an extensive leak can be more insidious, with the patient not making progress as rapidly as expected and suffering abdominal pain that is vague rather than dramatic.

It is clear from the Annual Report of the Scottish Audit of Surgical Mortality that delay in diagnosis of large bowel anastomotic leakage is still a major problem and leads to increased morbidity and mortality.[182] It is crucial that surgeons are vigilant about deterioration in the condition of any patient who has a large bowel anastomosis and maintain a low threshold for ordering investigations to identify a leak. It should be remembered that the anastomosis may leak any time during the first 2–3 weeks after operation.

Investigations

Usually the white blood count is elevated, except in patients who have overwhelming sepsis, when it may be either normal or even low. Erect chest radiograph or abdominal films will sometimes show gas under the diaphragm, but this sign is of debatable significance in the first few days after the original operation because of the presence of intra-abdominal air introduced at the time of operation. The absence of this feature, however, should in no way discourage the clinician from pursuing investigations to check the integrity of the anastomosis.

Ultrasound examination can be helpful in the patient with a suspected collection of pus related to anastomotic leakage, but the value of this investigation is often impaired by the presence of dilated gas-filled loops of bowel, with dressings and drains on the abdomen further increasing technical difficulties. CT is the investigation of choice.

Water-soluble contrast enema is a simple investigation for assessing anastomotic leakage, particularly on the left side of the large bowel. In addition to demonstrating whether a leak has occurred, assessment of the extent of leakage is of value in deciding the overall management. It is important to be aware of two caveats, however; occasionally, when the contrast enema shows no leak, a later investigation will show one. The corollary of this is also rarely true. The enema may show a leak that is of no clinical consequence (radiological leak). It is therefore important to look at the overall clinical picture and attempt to assess all the clinical and radiological evidence before coming to a final conclusion about the presence of a clinically significant leak.

Management

Although the literature on colonic anastomotic leak rates is extensive, there is a paucity of information on how to treat the leakage. It is best to consider the management of localised leakage separate from those who present with generalised peritonitis.

LOCALISED LEAKAGE

Most patients with localised leakage can be treated conservatively with gut rest and antibiotic therapy. If there is a large collection of pus around the anastomosis, it is usual to drain this percutaneously under ultrasound control.

GENERALISED LEAKAGE

Patients with generalised peritonitis from a large bowel anastomotic leak are usually dramatically ill and require resuscitation. Assuming that investigations have been performed and the diagnosis confirmed, the next step is to improve the patient's condition for surgical intervention.

Haemodynamic status needs to be assessed and treatment given to improve cardiac and respiratory function. Monitoring the patient's condition by measurement of central venous pressure and hourly urine volumes is essential, as well as observing other routine clinical parameters. Parenteral antibiotic administration is a priority and inotropic support may be necessary. Adequate pain control for the patient is often neglected by medical staff in these circumstances, and if a place is available these patients are best managed in a high-dependency unit or intensive therapy unit. The anaesthetist on call is alerted at an early stage and only when the patient's condition is stabilised is operation undertaken.

The patient with a leaking colorectal anastomosis is usually best placed on the operating table in the lithotomy/Trendelenburg position. The previous midline incision is reopened and great care is taken not to damage adherent loops of small intestine. Bowel loops are dissected free and the area of anastomosis exposed. Faecal material and pus are removed from the peritoneal cavity and pelvis. Occlusion clamps are gently placed on bowel above and below the leaking anastomosis to limit further contamination. Extensive lavage of the peritoneal cavity is performed using copious antiseptic or antibiotic solution.

The next step will depend on the size of the defect in the anastomosis. In the majority of cases the best method of management is to take the anastomosis down and bring out the proximal end of bowel as an end stoma and the distal end as a mucous fistula. If the distal stump is not long enough to be brought out on the abdominal wall, it should be closed carefully using a series of interrupted seromuscular sutures. If the defect occurs in a low colorectal anastomosis, a defunctioning ileostomy should be created.

Very occasionally, the surgeon will see a very small defect in the anastomosis that has given rise to the deterioration in the patient's clinical condition. If the defect is 1 cm or less and the bowel ends are well vascularised, it may be possible either to close the defect or insert a Foley catheter into it to decompress the bowel and then bring the catheter out through the abdominal wall. In a review from Aberdeen and Inverness of 477 patients who had colonic or rectal resection with anastomosis, there were nine clinically significant leaks that required reoperation.[180] Four patients had the anastomosis taken down and a stoma fashioned. In five other patients in whom the defect was small with good vascularity of bowel ends, the anastomosis was salvaged. Endoanal closure of the defect was achieved in three of these patients, one had a Foley catheter inserted through the defect and the fifth patient had a drain placed at the site of the leak. Four of the five patients had a covering stoma fashioned. There were no deaths related to the anastomotic leakage and the small defects in the anastomosis all healed; the stomas were closed at a later date.

The main advantage of anastomotic salvage in patients with anastomotic leakage is in those with a small defect in a low colorectal anastomosis, in whom the alternative is to take the anastomosis down, close the rectal stump and create an end colostomy in the left iliac fossa. It is widely recognised that patients who are treated by dismantling the anastomosis will rarely have bowel continuity restored at a later date. However, in a patient who has already had an anastomotic leak it is poor practice to risk a further leak and the patient's safety should be the prime objective.

BOWEL DAMAGE AT COLONOSCOPY

The perforation rate at colonoscopy is now generally agreed to be about 1 in 500, varying with the level of intervention employed. There is no such agreement over the perforation rate at flexible sigmoidoscopy; in recent studies this has been variably quoted at between 1 in 1136 and 1 in 40 674.[183–185]

There are three possible mechanisms responsible for colonoscopic perforation:[186]

1. mechanical perforation directly from the colonoscope or biopsy forceps;
2. barotrauma from overzealous air insufflation;
3. perforations occurring as a result of therapeutic procedures.

Measurement of forces exerted during colonoscopy has only been reported in one paper from the Royal London Hospital,[183] where an electronic device was used in a research setting. The caecum and right colon are most susceptible to barotrauma, although diverticula can also be directly inflated. The use of carbon dioxide for insufflation may decrease perforation rates and increase levels of patient comfort. Therapeutic interventions, such as polyp removal with a hot biopsy or snare and balloon dilatation of strictures, are associated with a higher risk of perforation.

The most common site of perforation is the sigmoid colon.[182] Signs and symptoms of a perforation are not always obvious at the time of colonsocopy. In retrospective studies, the diagnosis of a perforation is delayed in about 50% of cases.[187,188] If the endoscopist is worried after an examination has been completed, an erect chest radiograph should be ordered as a screening test and the patient observed until symptoms have settled. In cases where there is a high index of suspicion, a water-soluble enema can be used to confirm the diagnosis.

Conservative treatment with close observation, intravenous fluids and antibiotics may be possible following colonoscopy where the bowel is clean after a full bowel preparation. This approach is usually confined to those cases where the perforation has been made at a therapeutic rather than a diagnostic colonoscopy.[189,190] This is because a perforation caused by the passage of a scope through the bowel wall is usually large and needs repair. A large defect with peritoneal contamination is usually treated operatively, with direct suture of the defect possible when the diagnosis has been made in the early stages. It may be possible to effect the repair laparoscopically. Delayed diagnosis usually results in a temporary defunctioning stoma because of the associated faecal soiling.

• **Key points**

- There has been a recent swing towards greater emphasis on preoperative investigations, especially CT, and daytime operating by specialist consultant surgeons for most emergency surgery. In cases of colonic emergencies where there is faecal contamination of the peritoneal cavity, out-of-hours surgery may still be life-saving.
- **Volvulus.** Emergency decompression using a long soft tube such as a chest drain or a colonoscope should, in most cases, be followed by elective definitive surgery.
- **Acute colonic pseudo-obstruction.** Some patients can be managed entirely conservatively, employing regular review and frequent plain abdominal radiographs to check caecal diameter. As caecal diameter increases, decompression is required. Many patients will respond to a trial of neostigmine. If this treatment is not successful, the colon can be decompressed with the colonoscope in the majority of patients, but failure will necessitate caecostomy. If perforation or necrosis is suspected, a full laparotomy is necessary.
- **Malignant disease.** Right hemicolectomy with primary anastomosis is the treatment of choice for most patients with right-sided or transverse colonic obstruction. A subtotal colectomy may be the preferred option for patients who have a lesion at the splenic flexure. Most other patients who have an obstructing carcinoma in the left colon will be best treated by segmental colectomy with primary anastomosis where possible. Patients who are thought to be particularly at risk from lengthy emergency operations are best served by either segmental resection or colostomy.
- **Bleeding.** After exclusion of upper gastrointestinal bleeding, the surgeon can allow most colonic bleeds to stop spontaneously. Thereafter full colonic investigation including colonoscopy can be performed. Continued or torrential bleeding is ideally investigated, and sometimes treated, angiographically where such expertise exists. If surgery is required, localisation of the bleeding can be a major problem.
- **Diverticulits.** CT is now the investigation of choice for those patients presenting as emergencies. Abscesses can then be drained percutaneously and perforations requiring surgery diagnosed early. One-stage surgery is ideal; however, in left-sided disease this is not appropriate for the unstable patient or in those with gross faecal contamination.
- **Typhlitis.** There should be a high index of suspicion for this condition in the neutropenic patient. The majority respond to conservative measures including antibiotics and complete bowel rest but perforation should be actively excluded along the course of the disease, preferably with CT.
- **Stercoral perforation.** This rare condition may be difficult to diagnose preoperatively. Awareness of the possibility of postoperative re-perforation, especially where limited resections have been performed, may be the key to a successful outcome.
- **Anastomotic leak.** Postoperative assessment of the abdomen is complex, with many signs being attributable to the surgery itself. In equivocal cases further investigations should be instigated where there is uncertainty. Active observation should be employed by senior surgical staff. In some instances, transfer to a specialist colorectal unit needs to be considered after initial resuscitation and assessment.
- **Colonoscopic damage.** Signs and symptoms of perforation are not always obvious at the time of colonoscopy. A high index of suspicion, especially following interventional procedures, may allow conservative management or primary repair if surgery is performed early.

REFERENCES

1. Ballantyne GH. Review of sigmoid volvulus: clinical pattern and pathogenesis. Dis Colon Rectum 1982; 36:508.
2. Gibney EJ. Volvulus of the sigmoid colon. Surg Gynecol Obstet 1991; 173:243–55.
3. Anderson JR, Lee D. The management of acute sigmoid volvulus. Br J Surg 1981; 68:117–20.
4. Ballantyne GH, Brandner MD, Beart RW, Ilstrup DM. Volvulus of the colon. Ann Surg 1985; 202:83–92.
5. Schagen van Leeuwen JH. Sigmoid volvulus in a West African population. Dis Colon Rectum 1985; 28:712–16.

6. Sonnenberg A, Tsou VT, Muller AD. The 'institutional colon': a frequent colonic dysmotility in psychiatric and neurologic disease. Am J Gastroenterol 1994; 89:62–6.

7. Shepherd JJ. The treatment of volvulus of sigmoid colon: a review of 425 cases. Br J Med 1968; 1:280–3.

8. Sutcliffe MML. Volvulus of the sigmoid colon. Br J Surg 1968; 55:903–10.

9. Walsh S, Lee J, Stokes M. Sigmoid volvulus after laparoscopic cholecystectomy. An unusual complication. Surg Endosc 2001; 15:218.

10. Andersen DA. Volvulus in Western India. Br J Surg 1956; 44:132–43.

11. Rigler LG, Lipschultz O. Roentgenologic findings in acute obstruction of the colon. Radiology 1940; 35:534–43.

12. Bruusgaard C. Volvulus of the sigmoid colon and its treatment. Surgery 1947; 22:466–78.

13. Mangiarte EC, Croce MA, Fabian TC et al. Sigmoid volvulus, a four decade experience. Am Surg 1989; 55:41–4.

14. Hinshaw DB, Carter R. Surgical management of acute volvulus of the sigmoid colon. Ann Surg 1957; 146:52–60.

15. Knight J, Bokey EL, Chapuis PH, Pheils MT. Sigmoidoscopic reduction of sigmoid volvulus. Med J Aust 1980; 2:627–8.

16. Starling JR. Initial treatment of sigmoid volvulus by colonoscopy. Ann Surg 1979; 190:36–9.

17. Arigbabu AO, Badejo OA, Akinola DO. Colonoscopy in the emergency treatment of colonic volvulus in Nigeria. Dis Colon Rectum 1985; 28:795–8.

18. Bagarani M, Conde AS, Longo R et al. Sigmoid volvulus in West Africa: a prospective study on surgical treatments. Dis Colon Rectum 1993; 36:186.

19. De U, Ghosh S. Single stage primary anastomosis without colonic lavage for left sided colonic obstruction due to acute sigmoid volvulus: a prospective study of one hundred and ninety seven cases. Aust NZ J Surg 2003; 73:390–2.

   A prospective study of 197 patients with acute sigmoid volvulus treated by single-stage resection and primary anastomosis, 23 of whom had gangrene of the bowel. Two patients had anastomotic leaks and were successfully managed conservatively. There were two deaths, both in elderly patients who presented with perforations.

20. Naeeder SB, Archampong EQ. One-stage resection of acute sigmoid volvulus. Br J Surg 1995; 82:1635–6.

21. Grossmann EM, Longo WE, Stratton MD, Virgo KS, Johnson FE. Sigmoid volvulus in Department of Veterans Affairs Medical Centers. Dis Colon Rectum 2000; 43:414–18.

22. Leach SD, Ballantyne GH. Laparoscopic management of sigmoid volvulus: modern management of an ancient disease. Semin Colon Rectal Surg 1993; 4:249–56.

23. Sharon N, Efrat Y, Charuzi I. A new operative approach to volvulus of sigmoid colon. Surg Gynecol Obstet 1985; 161:483–4.

24. Subrahmanyam M. Mesosigmoplasty as a definitive operation for sigmoid volvulus. Br J Surg 1992; 79:683–4.

25. Mehendale VG, Chaudhari NC, Mulchandani MH. Laparoscopic sigmoidopexy by extraperitonealization of sigmoid colon for sigmoid volvulus: two cases. Surg Laparosc Endosc Percutan Tech 2003; 13:283–5.

26. Pinedo G, Kirberg A. Percutaneous endoscopic sigmoidopexy in sigmoid volvulus with T-fasteners: report of two cases. Dis Colon Rectum 2001; 44:1867–9.

27. Choi D, Carter R. Endoscopic sigmoidopexy: a safer way to treat sigmoid volvulus. J R Coll Surg Edinb 1998; 43:64.

28. VerSteeg KR, Whitehead WA. Ileosigmoid knot. Arch Surg 1980; 115:761–3.

29. Akgun Y. Management of ileosigmoid knot. Br J Surg 1997; 84:672–3.

30. Miller BJ, Borrowdale RC. Ileosigmoid knotting: a case report and review. Aust NZ J Surg 1992; 62:402–4.

31. Anderson JR, Lee D, Taylor TV, Ross AH. Volvulus of the transverse colon. Br J Surg 1981; 7:12–18.

32. Pustorino S, Polimeni F, Migliorato D et al. Chronic idiopathic intestinal pseudo-obstruction associated with volvulus of the transverse colon. The identical mode of clinical presentation and of the intestinal manometric pattern in monozygotic twins. Minerva Gastroenterol Dietol 1994; 40:37–46.

33. Rangiah D, Schwartz P. Familial transverse colon volvulus. Aust NZ J Surg 2001; 71:329–30.

34. Mortensen NJMcC, Hoffman G. Volvulus of the transverse colon. Postgrad Med J 1979; 55:54–7.

35. Anderson JR, Lee D. Acute caecal volvulus. Br J Surg 1980; 67:39–41.

36. Weinstein M. Volvulus of the cecum and ascending colon. Ann Surg 1938; 107:248–59.

37. Anderson JR, Mills JOM. Caecal volvulus: a frequently missed diagnosis. Clin Radiol 1984; 35:65.

38. Anderson MJ, Okike N, Spencer RJ. The colonoscope in cecal volvulus: report of 3 cases. Dis Colon Rectum 1978; 21:71–4.

39. Tuech JJ, Pessaux P, Regenet N, Derouet N, Bergamaschi R, Arnaud JP. Results of resection for volvulus of the right colon. Tech Coloproctol 2002; 6:97–9.

40. Rabanovici R, Simansky DA, Kaplan O, Mavor E, Manny J. Cecal volvulus. Dis Colon Rectum 1990; 33:765–9.

41. Anderson JR, Welch GH. Acute volvulus of the right colon: an analysis of 69 patients. World J Surg 1986; 10:336–42.

42. Dorudi S, Berry AR, Kettewell MGW. Acute colonic pseudo-obstruction. Br J Surg 1992; 79:99–103.

43. Ogilvie H. Large intestine colic due to sympathetic deprivation: a new clinical syndrome. Br Med J 1948; 2:671–3.

44. Datta SN, Stephenson BM, Havard TJ, Salaman JR. Acute colonic pseudo-obstruction. Lancet 1993; 341:690.

45. Vanek VW, Al-Salti M. Acute pseudo-obstruction of the colon (Ogilvie's syndrome): an analysis of 400 cases. Dis Colon Rectum 1986; 29:203–10.

46. Jetmore AB, Timmcke AE, Gathright JB, Hicks TC, Ray JE, Baker JW. Ogilvie's syndrome: colonoscopic decompression and analysis of predisposing factors. Dis Colon Rectum 1992; 35:1135–42.

47. Dudley HAF, Paterson-Brown S. Pseudo-obstruction. Br J Surg 1986; 292:1157–8.

48. Bachulis BL, Smith PE. Pseudo-obstruction of the colon. Am J Surg 1978; 136:66–72.

49. Wanebo H, Mathewson C, Conolly B. Pseudo-obstruction in the colon. Surg Gynecol Obstet 1971; 133:44–8.

50. Low VH. Colonic pseudo-obstruction: value of prone lateral view of the rectum. Abdom Imaging 1995; 20:531–3.

51. Koruth NM, Koruth A, Matheson NA. The place of contrast enema in the management of large bowel obstruction. J R Coll Surg Edinb 1985; 30:258–60.

52. Laine L. Management of acute colonic pseudo-obstruction. N Engl J Med 1999; 341:192–3.

53. Johnson CD, Rice RP, Kelvin FM, Foster WL, Williford ME. The radiological evaluation of gross cecal distension. Emphasis on cecal ileus. Am J Radiol 1985; 145:1211–17.

54. Neely J, Catchpole B. Ileus: the restoration of alimentary-tract motility by pharmacological means. Br J Surg 1971; 58:21–8.

55. Hutchinson R, Griffiths C. Acute colonic pseudo-obstruction: a pharmacological approach. Ann R Coll Surg Engl 1992; 74:364–7.

56. Ponec RJ, Saunders MD, Kimmey MB. Neostigmine for the treatment of acute colonic pseudo-obstruction. N Engl J Med 1999; 341:137–41.

> Randomised study of 21 patients with acute ACPO in which 11 patients were randomised to receive neostigmine and 10 patients received intravenous saline. The study showed that where the conservative treatment of ACPO fails, intravenous injection of 2.0 mg neostigmine results in rapid decompression of the colon.

57. Trevisani GT, Hyman NH, Church JM. Neostigmine. Safe and effective treatment for acute colonic pseudo-obstruction. Dis Colon Rectum 2000; 43:599–603.

58. Abbasakoor F, Evans A, Stephenson BM. Neostigmine for acute colonic pseudo-obstruction. N Engl J Med 1999; 341:1622–3.

59. Lee JT, Taylor BM, Singleton BC. Epidural anaesthesia for acute pseudo-obstruction of the colon. Dis Colon Rectum 1988; 31:686–91.

60. Kukora JS, Dent TL. Colonoscopic decompression of massive non-obstructive cecal dilation. Arch Surg 1977; 112:512–17.

61. Nivatvongs SN, Vermeulen FD, Fang DT. Colonoscopic decompression of acute pseudo-obstruction of the colon. Ann Surg 1982; 196:98–100.

62. Strodel WE, Brothers T. Colonoscopic decompression of pseudo-obstruction and volvulus. Surg Clin North Am 1989; 69:1327–35.

63. Strodel WE, Norstrant TT, Eskhauser FE, Dent TL. Therapeutic and diagnostic colonoscopy in non obstructive colonic dilatation. Ann Surg 1983; 197:416–21.

64. Bernton E, Myers R, Reyna T. Pseudo-obstruction of the colon: case report including a new endoscopic treatment. Gastrointest Endosc 1982; 28:90–2.

65. Stephenson KR, Rodriguez-Bigas MA. Decompression of the large intestine in Ogilvie's syndrome by a colonoscopically placed long intestinal tube. Surg Endosc 1994; 8:116–17.

66. Hamed A, Dare F. Oglivie's syndrome. Int J Gynaecol Obstet 1992; 37:47–50.

67. Diethelm AG, Stanley RJ, Robbin ML. The acute abdomen. In: Sabiston's textbook of surgery. Philadelphia: WB Saunders, 1997; p. 842.

68. Laine L. Management of acute colonic pseudo-obstruction. N Engl J Med 1999; 341:192–3.

69. Chevallier P, Marcy P, Francois E et al. Controlled transperitoneal percutaneous cecostomy as a therapy alternative to the endoscopic decompression for Oglivie's syndrome. Am J Gastroenterol 2002; 97:471–4.

70. Gierson ED, Storm FK, Shaw W, Coyne SK. Caecal rupture due to colonic ileus. Br J Surg 1975; 62:383–6.

71. Gerber A, Thompson RJ, Reiswig OK, Vannix RS. Experiences with primary resection for acute obstruction of the large intestine. Surg Gynecol Obstet 1962; 115:593–8.

72. Phillips RK, Hittinger R, Fry JS, Fielding LP. Malignant large bowel obstruction. Br J Surg 1985; 72:296–302.

73. Fielding LP, Phillips RK, Fry JS, Hittinger R. Prediction of outcome after curative resection for large bowel cancer. Lancet 1986; ii:904–7.

74. Serpell JW, McDermott FT, Katrivessis H, Hughes ESR. Obstructing carcinomas of the colon. Br J Surg 1989; 76:965–9.

75. McKenzie S, Thomson SR, Baker LW. Management options in malignant obstruction of the left colon. Surg Gynecol Obstet 1992; 174:337–45.

76. Valerio D, Jones PF. Immediate resection in the treatment of large bowel emergencies. Br J Surg 1978; 65:712–16.

77. Rovito PF, Verazin T, Prorok JJ. Obstructing carcinoma of the caecum. J Surg Oncol 1990; 45:177–9.

78. Sjodahl R, Franzen T, Nystrom PO. Primary versus staged resection for acute obstructing colorectal carcinoma. Br J Surg 1992; 79:685–8.

79. Runkel NS, Schlag P, Schwarz V et al. Outcome after emergency surgery of the large intestine. Br J Surg 1991; 78:183–8.

80. Umpleby HC, Williamson RC. Survival in acute obstructing colorectal carcinoma. Dis Colon Rectum 1984; 27:299–304.

81. Crucitti F, Sofo L, Doglietto GB et al. Prognostic factors in colorectal cancer: current status and new trends. J Surg Oncol 1991; 2(Suppl.):76–82.

82. Kiefhaber P, Kiefhaber K, Huber F. Pre-operative neodymium YAG laser treatment of obstructive colon cancer. Endoscopy 1986; 18:44.

83. Eckhauser ML, Mansour EG. Endoscopic laser therapy for obstruction and/or bleeding colorectal carcinoma. Am Surg 1992; 58:358–63.

84. Saida PM, Sumiyama Y, Nagao J et al. Stent endoprosthesis for obstructing colorectal cancer. Dis Colon Rectum 1996; 39:552.

85. Tejero E, Mainar A, Fernandez L, Tobio R, de Gregorio MA. New procedure for the treatment of colorectal neoplastic obstruction. Dis Colon Rectum 1994; 37:1158–9.

86. Martinez-Santos C, Lobato RF, Fradejas JM, Pinto I, Ortega-Deballon P, Moreno-Azocoita M. Self-expandable stent before elective surgery vs. emergency surgery for the treatment of malignant colorectal obstructions: comparison of primary anastomosis and morbidity rates. Dis Colon Rectum 2002; 45:401–6.

87. Aviv RI, Shyamalani G, Watkinson A, Tibballs J, Ogunbaye G. Radiological palliation of malignant colonic obstruction. Clin Radiol 2002; 57:347–51.

88. Nozoe T, Matsumata T. Usefulness of preoperative colonic lavage using transanal ileus tube for obstructing carcinoma of left colon. J Clin Gastroenterol 2000; 31:156–8.

89. Tanaka T, Furukawa A, Murata K, Sakamoto T. Endoscopic transanal decompression with a drainage tube for acute colonic obstruction. Dis Colon Rectum 2001; 44:418–22.

90. Dudley H, Phillips R. Intraoperative techniques in large bowel obstruction: methods of management with bowel resection. In: Fielding LP, Welch J (eds) Intestinal obstruction. Edinburgh: Churchill Livingstone, 1987; pp. 139–52.

91. Gutman M, Kaplan O, Skornick Y, Greif F, Kahn P, Rozin RR. Proximal colostomy: still an effective emergency measure in obstructing carcinoma of the large bowel. J Surg Oncol 1989; 41:210–12.

92. Malafosse M, Goujard F, Gallot D, Sezeur A. Traitment des occlusions aigues par cancer du colon gauche. Chirurgie 1989; 115(Suppl. 2):123–5.

93. Edwards DP, Leppington-Clarke A, Sexton R, Heald RJ, Moran BJ. Stoma-related complications are more frequent after transverse colostomy than loop ileostomy: a prospective randomized clinical trial. Br J Surg 2001; 88:360–3.

94. Deans GT, Krukowski ZH, Irvin ST. Malignant obstruction of the left colon. Br J Surg 1994; 81:1270–6.

95. Ambrosetti P, Borst F, Robert J, Meyer P, Rohner A. L'excrese anastomose en un temps dans les occlusions coliques gauche operees en urgence. Chirurgie 1989; 115:(Suppl. 2):I–VI.

96. de Almeida AM, Gracias CW, dos Santos NM, Aldeia FJ. Surgical management of acute malignant obstruction of the left colon with colostomy. Acta Med Port 1991; 4:275–62.

97. Gandrup P, Lund L, Balslev I. Surgical treatment of acute malignant large bowel obstruction. Eur J Surg 1992; 158:427–30.

98. Sjodahl R, Franzen T, Nystrom PO. Primary versus staged resection for acute obstructing colorectal carcinoma. Br J Surg 1992; 79:685–8.

99. Irvin TT, Greaney MG. The treatment of colonic cancer presenting with intestinal obstruction. Br J Surg 1977; 64:741–4.

100. Carson SN, Poticha SM, Shields TW. Carcinoma obstructing the left side of the colon. Arch Surg 1977; 112:523–6.

101. Dixon AR, Holmes JT. Hartman's procedure for carcinoma of rectum and distal sigmoid colon. J R Coll Surg Edinb 1990; 35:166–8.

102. Pearce NW, Scott SD, Karran SJ. Timing and method of reversal of Hartmann's procedure. Br J Surg 1992; 79:839–41.

103. Dorudi S, Wilson NM, Heddle RM. Primary restorative colectomy in malignant left sided large bowel obstruction. Ann R Coll Surg Engl 1990; 72:393–5.

104. Stephenson BM, Shandall AA, Farouk R, Griffiths G. Malignant left-sided large bowel obstruction managed by subtotal/total colectomy. Br J Surg 1990; 77:1098–102.

105. Alle JL, Azagra JS, Elcheroth J, Cavenaile JC, Buchin R. La colectomie subtotale en un temps dans le traitement en urgence des neoplasies coliques gauches occlusives. Acta Chir Belg 1990; 90:86–8.

106. Murray JJ, Schoetz DJ, Coller JA, Roberts PL, Veidenheimer MC. Intra-operative colonic lavage and primary anastomosis in non-elective colon resection. Dis Colon Rectum 1991; 34:527–31.

107. Koruth NM, Krukowski ZH, Youngson GG et al. Intra-operative colonic irrigation in the management

of left sided large bowel emergencies. Br J Surg 1985; 72:708–11.

108. Konishi F, Muto T, Kanazawa K, Morioka Y. Intra-operative irrigation and primary resection for obstructing lesions of the left colon. Int J Colorectal Dis 1988; 3:204–6.

109. Lee YM, Law WL, Chu KW, Poon RT. Emergency surgery for obstructing colorectal cancers: a comparison between right-sided and left-sided lesions. J Am Coll Surg 2001; 192:719–25.

A retrospective study of 243 patients who underwent emergency operations for obstructing colorectal cancers. Single-stage resection with primary anastomosis was possible in 197 patients. Of the 101 patients with left-sided obstruction, segmental resection with on-table colonic lavage was performed in 75 patients and subtotal colectomy in 26. There were no differences in the mortality or leakage rates between patients with right-sided and left-sided lesions (mortality 7.3% vs. 8.9%; leakage 5.2% vs. 6.9% respectively).

110. Naraynsingh V, Rampaul R, Maharaj D, Kuruvilla T, Ramcharan K, Pouchet B. Prospective study of primary anastomosis without colonic lavage for patients with an obstructed left colon. Br J Surg 1999; 86:1341–3.

111. Turan M, Ok Engin, Sen M et al. A simplified operative technique for single-staged resection of left-sided colon obstructions: report of a 9-year experience. Surg Today 2002; 32:959–64.

112. The SCOTIA Study Group. Single stage treatment for malignant left sided colonic obstruction: a prospective randomised clinical trial comparing subtotal colectomy with segmental resection following intra-operative irrigation. Br J Surg 1995; 82:1622–7.

Multicentre, prospective, randomised trial comparing subtotal colectomy with segmental resection, intra-operative irrigation and primary anastomosis for left-sided malignant large bowel obstruction. Although post-operative mortality and length of stay in hospital were similar for both procedures, segmental resection with intraoperative colonic irrigation was superior to subtotal colectomy in terms of stoma rate and bowel function.

113. Dusold R, Burke K, Carpentier W, Dyck WP. The accuracy of technetium-99m-labelled red cell scintigraphy in localising gastrointestinal bleeding. Am J Gastroenterol 1994; 89:345–8.

114. Noer PF, Hamilton JE, Williams DJ, Broughton DS. Rectal hemorrhage: moderate and severe. Ann Surg 1962; 155:794–805.

115. Browder W, Cerise EJ, Litwin MS. Impact of emergency angiography in massive lower gastrointestinal bleeding. Ann Surg 1986; 204:530–6.

116. Demarkles MP, Murphy JR. Acute lower gastrointestinal bleeding. Med Clin North Am 1993; 77:1085–100.

117. Cavett CM, Selby H, Hamilton L, Williamson W. Arteriovenous malformation in chronic gastrointestinal bleeding. Ann Surg 1977; 185:116–21.

118. Lichtiger S, Kornbluth A, Salomon P et al. Lower gastrointestinal bleeding. In: Taylor MB, Gollan JL, Peppercorn MA (eds) Gastrointestinal emergencies. Baltimore: Williams & Wilkins, 1992; p. 358.

119. Santos JCM, Aprilli F, Guimaraes AS, Rocha JJR. Angiodysplasia of the colon: endoscopic diagnosis and treatment. Br J Surg 1988; 75:256–8.

120. Gupta N, Longo WE, Vernava AM. Angiodysplasia of the lower gastrointestinal tract: an entity readily diagnosed by colonoscopy and primarily managed non operatively. Dis Colon Rectum 1995; 38:979–82.

121. Warkentin TE, Moore JC, Morgan DG. Aortic stenosis and bleeding gastrointestinal angiodysplasia: is acquired von Willebrand disease the link? Lancet 1992; 340:35–7.

122. Cappell MS, Lebwohl O. Cessation of recurrent bleeding from gastrointestinal angiodysplasia after aortic valve replacement. Ann Intern Med 1986; 105:54–7.

123. Chalasani N, Wilcox CM. Etiology and outcome of lower gastrointestinal bleeding in patients with AIDS. Am J Gastroenterol 1998; 93:175–8.

124. Rossini FP, Ferrari A, Spandre M et al. Emergency colonoscopy. World J Surg 1989; 13:190.

125. DeBarros J, Rosas L, Cohen J, Vignati P, Sardella W, Hallisey M. The changing paradigm for the treatment of colonic hemorrhage: superselective angiographic embolisation. Dis Colon Rectum 2002; 45:802–8.

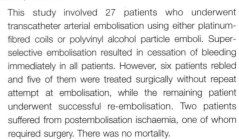

This study involved 27 patients who underwent transcatheter arterial embolisation using either platinum-fibred coils or polyvinyl alcohol particle emboli. Super-selective embolisation resulted in cessation of bleeding immediately in all patients. However, six patients rebled and five of them were treated surgically without repeat attempt at embolisation, while the remaining patient underwent successful re-embolisation. Two patients suffered from postembolisation ischaemia, one of whom required surgery. There was no mortality.

126. Horiguchi J, Naito A, Fukuda H et al. Morphologic and histopathologic changes in the bowel after super-selective transcatheter embolization for lower gastrointestinal hemorrhage. Acta Radiol 2003; 44:334–9.

127. Zuckerman DA, Bocchini TP, Birnbaum EH. Massive hemorrhage in the lower gastrointestinal tract in adults: diagnostic imaging and intervention. Am J Roentgenol 1993; 161:703–11.

128. Wadas DD, Sanowski RA. Complications of the hot biopsy forceps technique. Gastrointest Endosc 1988; 34:32.

129. Johnston J, Sones J. Endoscopic heater probe coagulation of the bleeding colonic diverticulum. Gastrointest Endosc 1986; 32:160.

130. Gomes AS, Lois JF, McCoy RD. Angiographic treatment of the gastrointestinal hemorrhage:

comparison of vasopressin infusion and embolization. Am J Roentgenol 1986; 146:1031–7.

131. Cussons PD, Berry AR. Comparison of the value of emergency mesenteric angiography and intra-operative colonoscopy with antegrade colonic irrigation in massive rectal haemorrhage. J R Coll Surg Edinb 1989; 34:91–3.

132. Mendeloff AL. Thoughts on the epidemiology of diverticular disease. Clin Gastroenterol 1986; 15:855–77.

133. Kirson SM. Diverticulitis: management patterns in a community hospital. South Med J 1988; 81:972–7.

134. Sugihara K, Muto T, Morioka Y et al. Diverticular disease of the colon in Japan. Dis Colon Rectum 1984; 27:531–7.

135. Almy TP, Howell DA. Diverticular disease of the colon. N Engl J Med 1980; 302:324–31.

136. Parks TG. Natural history of diverticular disease of the colon. Clin Gastroenterol 1975; 4:53–69.

137. Parks TG, Connel AM. The outcome in 455 patients admitted for the treatment of diverticular disease of the colon. Br J Surg 1970; 57:775–8.

138. Hinchey EJ, Schaal PG, Richards GK. Treatment of perforated diverticular disease of the colon. Adv Surg 1978; 12:85–109.

139. Greenlee HB, Pienkos FJ, Vanderbilt PC et al. Proceedings: acute large bowel obstruction. Comparison of county, veterans administration and community hospital publications. Arch Surg 1974; 108:470–6.

140. Biondo S, Pares D, Marti Rague J, Kreisler E, Fraccalvieri D, Jaurrieta E. Acute colonic diverticulitis in patients under 50 years of age. Br J Surg 2002; 89:1137–41.

141. Reisman Y, Ziv Y, Kravrovitic D, Negri M, Wolloch Y, Halevy A. Diverticulitis: the effect of age and location on the course of disease. Int J Colorectal Dis 1999; 14:250–4.

142. Krukowski ZH, Matheson NA. Emergency surgery for diverticular disease complicated by generalised and faecal peritonitis: a review. Br J Surg 1984; 71:921–7.

143. Shyung Li-Rung, Lin S-C, Kao C-R, Chou S-Y. Decision making in right-sided diverticulitis. World J Gastroenterol 2003; 9:606–8.

144. Chou Y, Chiou H, Tiu C et al. Sonography of acute right side colonic diverticulitis. Am J Surg 2001; 181:122–7.

145. Morris J, Stellato TA, Haaga JR, Lieberman J. The utility of computed tomography in colonic diverticulitis. Ann Surg 1986; 204:128–32.

146. Kourtesis GJ, Williams RA, Wilson SE. Acute diverticulitis: safety and value of contrast studies in predicting need for operation. Aust NZ J Surg 1988; 58:801–4.

147. Rice RP, Thomson WM, Gedgaudes RK. The diagnosis and significance of extraluminal gas in the abdomen. Radiol Clin North Am 1982; 20:819–37.

 148. Ambrosetti P, Becker C, Terrier F. Colonic diverticulitis: impact of imaging on surgical management. A prospective study of 542 patients. Eur Radiol 2002; 12:1145–9.

This study prospectively evaluated 420 patients who underwent both CT and water-soluble contrast enema in the evaluation of acute diverticulitis. The performance of CT was significantly higher than contrast enema both in terms of sensitivity (98% vs. 92%) and in the evaluation of the severity of the inflammation (26% vs. 9%). Furthermore, contrast enema picked up an abscess in 20 patients compared with 69 patients using CT.

149. Lieberman JM, Haaga JR. Computed tomography of diverticulitis. J Comput Assist Tomogr 1983; 7:431–3.

150. Hulnick DM, Megibow AJ, Balthazar EJ, Naidich DP, Bosniak MA. Computed tomography in the evaluation of diverticulitis. Radiology 1984; 152:491–5.

151. Wilson SR. The value of sonography in the diagnosis of acute diverticulitis of the colon. Am J Radiol 1990; 154:1199–202.

152. Verbanck J, Lambrecht S, Rutgeerts L et al. Can sonography diagnose acute colonic diverticulitis in patients with acute colonic inflammation? A prospective study. J Clin Ultrasound 1989; 17:661–6.

153. Neff CC, van Sonnenberg E, Casola G et al. Diverticular abscesses. Percutaneous drainage. Radiology 1987; 163:15–18.

154. Hollerweger A, Rettenbacher T, Macheiner P, Brunner W, Gritzmann N. Sigmoid diverticulitis: value of transrectal sonography in addition to transabdominal sonography. Am J Roentgenol 2000; 175:1155–60.

155. Stein GN. Radiology of colonic diverticular disease. Postgrad Med 1976; 60:95–102.

156. Grief J, Fried G, McSherry CK. Surgical treatment of perforated diverticulitis of sigmoid colon. Dis Colon Rectum 1980; 23:483–7.

157. Kourtesis GJ, Williams RA, Wilson SE. Surgical options in acute diverticulitis. Value of sigmoid resection in dealing with the septic focus. Aust NZ J Surg 1988; 58:955–9.

158. Heverhagen JT, Zielke A, Ishaque N, Bohrer T, El-Sheik M, Klose KJ. Acute colonic diverticulitis: visualization in magnetic resonance imaging. Magn Reson Imaging 2001; 19:1275–7.

159. Chiu P, Lam C, Lam S, Wu A, Kwok S. On-table cecoscopy. A novel diagnostic method in acute diverticulitis of the right colon. Dis Colon Rectum 2002; 45:611–14.

160. Junge K, Marx A, Peiper Ch, Klosterhalfen B, Schumpelick V. Caecal diverticulitis: a rare differential diagnosis for right-sided lower abdominal pain. Colorectal Dis 2003; 5:241–5.

161. Fang J, Chen R, Lin B, Hsu Y, Kao J, Chen M. Aggressive resection is indicated for cecal diverticulitis. Am J Surg 2003; 185:135–40.

162. Rothenberger DA, Wiltz O. Surgery for complicated diverticulitis. Surg Clin North Am 1993; 73:975–92.

163. Dawson JL, Hanon I, Roxburgh RA. Diverticulitis coli complicated by diffuse peritonitis. Br J Surg 1965; 52:354.

164. Killingback M. Management of perforative diverticulitis. Surg Clin North Am 1983; 63:97–115.

165. Koruth NM, Hunter DC, Krukowski ZH, Matheson NA. Immediate resection in emergency large bowel surgery: a 7 year audit. Br J Surg 1985; 72:703–7.

166. Gregg RO. The place of emergency resection in the management of obstructing and perforating lesions of the colon. Surgery 1955; 27:754–61.

167. Biondo S, Perea M, Ragué J, Pares D, Jaurrieta E. 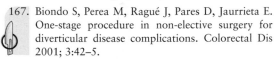 One-stage procedure in non-elective surgery for diverticular disease complications. Colorectal Dis 2001; 3:42–5.

This study investigated the efficacy and safety of one-stage resection, intraoperative colonic lavage and primary anastomosis in emergency surgery for complicated acute diverticulitis. Of 124 patients who underwent emergency operation for complicated diverticulitis, one-stage procedure was carried out on 55 patients, which included 33 patients with localized peritonitis and 16 patients with generalized purulent peritonitis. No patients with faecal peritonitis underwent a one-stage procedure. Major complications included two anastomotic leaks (one of which was successfully treated with parenteral nutrition), four reoperations (three for abdominal wound dehiscence and one for anastomotic leak) and four deaths (three of those who died were older than 70 years old). The study concluded that one-stage resection is feasible in selected patients.

168. Zorcolo L, Covotta L, Carlomagno N, Bartolo DCC. Safety of primary anastomosis in emergency colorectal surgery. Colorectal Dis 2003; 5:262–9.

169. Blair NP, Germann E. Surgical management of acute sigmoid diverticulitis. Am J Surg 2002; 183:525–8.

170. Kirkpatrick IDC, Greenberg HM. Gastrointestinal complications in the neutropenic patient: characterization and differentiation with abdominal CT. Radiology 2003; 226:668–74.

171. Avigan D, Richardson P, Elias A et al. Neutropenic enterocolitis as a complication of high dose chemotherapy with stem cell rescue in patients with solid tumors. Cancer 1998; 83:409–14.

172. Williams N, Scott ADN. Neutropenic colitis: a continuing surgical challenge. Br J Surg 1997; 84:1200–5.

173. Gomez L, Martino R, Rolston KV. Neutropenic enterocolitis: spectrum of the disease and comparison of definite and possible cases. Clin Infect Dis 1998; 27:695–9.

174. Dubinsky I. Stercoral perforation of the colon: case report and review of the literature. J Emerg Med 1996; 14:323–5.

175. Serpell JW, Nicholls RJ. Stercoral perforation of the colon. Br J Surg 1990; 77:1325–9.

176. Maurer CA, Renzulli P, Mazzucchelli L, Egger B, Seiler CA, Buchler MW. Use of accurate diagnostic criteria may increase incidence of stercoral perforation of the colon. Dis Colon Rectum 2000; 43:991–8.

This study, which constitutes one of the largest single-institution reports on stercoral perforation of the colon, defined strict clinical and pathological criteria for its diagnosis. Using these criteria stercoral perforation of the colon would appear to occur more frequently than previously reported in the literature.

177. Fielding LP, Stewart Brown S, Blesovsky L, Kearney G. Anastomotic integrity after operation for large bowel cancer: a multicentre study. Br Med J 1980; 282:411–14.

178. Keighley MRB, Williams NS. Surgical management of carcinoma of the colon and rectum. In: Keighley MRS, Williams NS (eds) Surgery of the anus, rectum and colon, 2nd edn. London: WB Saunders, 1999; p. 1100.

179. Irvin TT, Hunt TK. The effect of trauma on colonic healing. Br J Surg 1974; 61:430.

180. Watson AJ, Krukoswski ZH, Munro A. Salvage of large bowel anastomotic leaks. Br J Surg 1999; 86:499–500.

In a review of 477 large bowel anastomoses, which included 215 colorectal anastomoses, there were eight colorectal and one ileocolic leaks. All nine patients required laparotomy, and five (four colorectal and one ileocolic) of these nine were salvaged with no mortality. Three colorectal leaks (small posterior defects in stapled anastomoses) were closed with interrupted endoanal sutures and a proximal loop stoma fashioned in two patients who did not already have one. The other two leaks (defect in suture line attributable to a single suture cutting through) were managed by creating a controlled external fistula. None of these patients had further complications and all the stomas were subsequently closed. It is possible to salvage anastomotic leaks with a good outcome in selected patients with appropriate operative treatment.

181. Sheridan WG, Lowndes RH, Young HL. Tissue oxygen measurement as a predictor of colonic anastomotic healing. Dis Colon Rectum 1987; 30:867–71.

182. Scottish Audit of Surgical Mortality. Annual Report 1998. Glasgow: Royal College of Physicians and Surgeons of Glasgow; p. 25.

183. Anderson ML, Pasha TM, Leighton JA. Endoscopic perforation of the colon: lessons from a 10-year study. Am J Gastroenterol 2000; 95:3418–22.

184. Gatto NM, Frucht H, Sundararajan V, Jacobson J, Grann V, Neu A. Risk of perforation after

colonoscopy and sigmoidoscopy: a population based study. J Natl Cancer Inst 2003; 95:230–6.

185. UK Flexible Sigmoidoscopy Screening Trial Investigators. Single flexible sigmoidoscopy screening to prevent colorectal cancer: baseline findings of a UK multicentre randomised trial. Lancet 2002; 359:1291–300.

186. Appleyard MN, Mosse CA, Mills TN, Bell GD, Castillo FD, Swain CP. The measurement of forces exerted during colonoscopy. Gastrointest Endosc 2000; 52:237–40.

187. Damore LJ, Rantis PC, Vernava AM, Longo WE. Colonoscopic perforations. Dis Colon Rectum 1996; 39:1308–14.

188. Garbay JR, Suc B, Rotman N, Fourtanier G, Escat J. Multicentre study of surgical complications of colonoscopy. Br J Surg 1996; 83:42–4.

189. Orsoni P, Berdah S, Verrier C et al. Colonic perforation due to colonoscopy: a retrospective study of 48 cases. Endoscopy 1997; 29:160–4.

190. Soliman A, Grundman M. Conservative management of colonoscopic perforation can be misleading. Endoscopy 1998; 30:790–2.

Eleven

Anorectal emergencies

James B. Mander

INTRODUCTION

Anorectal emergencies form a significant proportion of any general surgical emergency workload. Patients may present with anal pain, overt sepsis, rectal bleeding, anorectal trauma or retained foreign bodies. Acute anal pain may be caused by anorectal sepsis, anal fissures or thrombosed haemorrhoids.

ANORECTAL ABSCESSES

Anorectal abscesses are among the commonest surgical emergencies. They predominantly occur in adults, may herald underlying disease and require prompt surgical drainage. They have a high propensity to recur and are frequently associated with fistula formation. Data from the 1960s suggest that the incidence in England and Wales may be as high as 1 per 1000 per year. The peak incidence is within the third and fourth decades and abscesses are three times more common in men than women.

An understanding of the anatomy of the anal canal is essential in order to understand the pathophysiology of abscess formation.

Anatomy

The anal canal is a 3–4 cm tube lined with epithelium that runs from the anorectal angle superiorly to the anal verge inferiorly (**Fig. 11.1**). It is surrounded by two rings of sphincter muscle vital to the continence mechanism. The innermost ring is the internal anal sphincter, formed as an extension of the circular muscle of the rectum. Beyond that is the external sphincter, formed from striated muscle, which becomes continuous superiorly with the levator plate. Between the two muscle layers is the intersphincteric space, which is the site of the anal glands. Ducts from these glands pass into the anal canal at the level of the dentate line. This marks the junction of the hindgut above, lined by columnar epithelium, and the proctodeum lined with squamous epithelium.

Aetiology

Primary anorectal abscesses arise as a result of anal gland infection (cryptoglandular), suppurating skin infections or pelvic pathology tracking through the levator plate. Cryptoglandular abscesses are believed to arise in anal glands found in the intersphincteric space.[1,2] These glands are connected to the anal epithelium at the dentate line. Support for the cryptoglandular theory comes from the observation that up to 60% of patients will have an associated internal opening at the dentate line.[3] The suppuration can spread in a number of directions, resulting in abscesses in a variety of anatomical spaces (**Fig. 11.1**). The frequency with which abscesses are found in different locations is shown in **Table 11.1**.[4]

Suppurative skin conditions include furuncles, carbuncles and infected apocrine glands. They account for approximately 10–25% of all anorectal sepsis and are invariably staphylococcal in origin.[5] Because there is no communication with the anal mucosa, they are rarely associated with subsequent fistula formation.

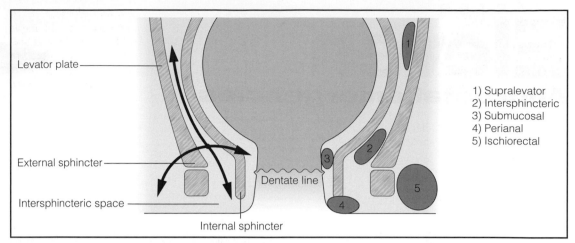

Figure 11.1 • The spread of anal gland infection and common sites of anorectal sepsis. Infection of the anal gland within the intersphincteric space can spread in a variety of directions (see left side of diagram), resulting in abscess in a number of classical sites: 1, supralevator; 2, intersphincteric; 3, submucosal; 4, perianal; 5, ischiorectal.

Table 11.1 • Location of anorectal sepsis by anatomical site

Anatomical site	Number	Percentage
Perianal abscess	437	42.7
Ischiorectal	233	22.8
Intersphincteric	219	21.4
Supralevator	75	7.3
Submucosal	59	5.8

From Ramunjam PS, Prasad MI, Abcarian H, Tan AB. Perianal abscesses and fistulae: a study of 1023 patients. Dis Colon Rectum 1984; 27:593–7, with permission.

Secondary anorectal abscesses arise as a manifestation of other conditions and account for approximately 10% of patients.[6] Diseases such as inflammatory bowel disease (especially Crohn's disease), colorectal neoplasia, diabetes mellitus, AIDS and tuberculosis are commonly implicated. Other potential causes of sepsis include local trauma arising from foreign bodies inserted into the rectum or passing through the gut (such as bones) and as a complication of the local treatment of haemorrhoids.

Natural history

It is likely that some patients with anorectal abscesses resolve spontaneously with or without antibiotics and it is probable that this group do not have a cryptoglandular abscess. In a few patients, particularly the immunocompromised and those with diabetes, the abscess may be associated with marked cellulitis that may progress to a life-threatening condition if not treated promptly.[7] A significant proportion of patients undergoing simple incision and drainage of abscesses represent with recurrent sepsis and an associated fistula. There is no good prospective study of the incidence of recurrence following a primary abscess and retrospective studies are limited by the short length of the follow-up period. Series of primary abscesses quote 30–40% of patients having had previous sepsis.[3,5] In over 80% the recurrence was found at the same site as the primary abscess. In a prospective study of 68 patients with recurrent abscesses, Chrabot et al. found an associated fistula in 53 (78%).[8]

Clinical features

Patients with anorectal abscesses present with signs and symptoms of acute inflammation. While perianal and ischiorectal abscesses are usually associated with a visible painful swelling, the same is not true of intersphincteric abscesses. These are usually not visible, but characteristically patients have severe anal pain and fever. Not surprisingly, digital examination is frequently impossible without anaesthesia. Supralevator abscesses may be felt bimanually or diagnosed on further imaging modalities. Patients with anorectal sepsis may occasionally present with necrotising infection. Such patients invariably have predisposing conditions, including diabetes, immunocompromise, obesity or chronic ill heath.

Investigation

Patients presenting with acute anorectal sepsis require appropriate work-up, with a full blood count and blood glucose assessment. All patients presenting with anorectal sepsis or severe anal pain warrant careful examination of the entire anorectum, including proctosigmoidoscopy. It is the author's opinion that a full examination can only be conducted under general anaesthesia (EUA). Although it is acknowledged that in the USA anorectal abscesses are often treated under local anaesthesia in the 'office' (a situation driven by financial pressures from insurance companies), formal EUA at the time of initial presentation is likely to be more cost-effective.[9]

ENDOANAL ULTRASOUND

In the majority of acute cases of anorectal sepsis there is little difficulty in identifying the abscess clinically and therefore the routine role of endoluminal sonography is debatable. Endoanal ultrasound is undoubtedly an extremely sensitive method of identifying collections of pus close to the anal canal. In one study of 22 patients with chronic sepsis, endosonography had a high sensitivity in demonstrating the presence of an intersphincteric abscess and the internal opening of an associated fistula.[10] Although standard endoanal probes lack the depth of resolution to image collections beyond the external sphincter, in cases of complex anorectal suppurative disease (e.g. Crohn's disease) or in the management of severe anal pain the technique can be very useful for identifying pockets of pus (**Fig. 11.2**). As endoanal ultrasound may often not be available or familiar to the operating surgeon, its use in the emergency setting is unlikely to become routine in the immediate future.

MAGNETIC RESONANCE IMAGING

Magnetic resonance imaging is very sensitive at delineating perianal sepsis and concomitant fistulas,[11] but at present has no role in the management of acute anorectal sepsis.

Treatment

The principles of treatment of anorectal sepsis are to drain the abscess, minimise hospital stay and time off work, and preserve continence.

ABSCESS DRAINAGE

In the vast majority of patients, simple drainage of the abscess is achieved with an incision over the swelling, gentle finger breakdown of the loculi and subsequent dressing (for details of the management of specific abscesses, see section Technical tips).

Deroofing of the abscess cavity results in a larger than necessary wound, which increases the postoperative stay and the need for time off work for regular dressings. The vogue for packing abscess cavities should be discontinued, as the only role of

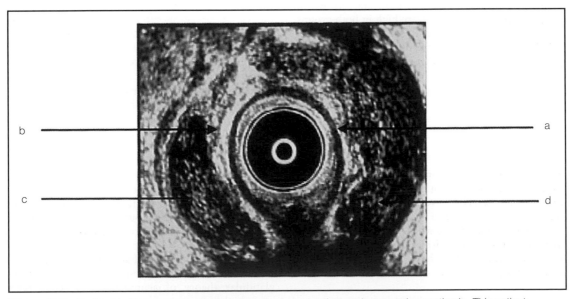

Figure 11.2 • Endoanal ultrasound examination carried out on a patient under general anaesthesia. This patient presented with severe anal pain and perianal induration but without any specific area of fluctuation. The ultrasound demonstrates an extensive ischiorectal abscess cavity (c) extending around the anal canal (a, internal sphincter; b, external sphincter). With thanks to Mr Mike Hulme-Moir, Clinical Fellow in Colorectal Surgery, Royal Infirmary, Edinburgh.

packing is to staunch haemorrhage. An alternative is to make a small stab incision and insert a small drainage catheter. Kyle and Ibister[12] compared a group of 91 patients who underwent this treatment with 54 who underwent more traditional incision and drainage.

The use of a small incision and catheter drainage resulted in a shorter hospital stay (mean 1.4 vs. 4.5 days) and less community nursing than traditional incision and drainage. There was no increase in the rate of subsequent fistula formation or failure to adequately drain the abscess.[12]

Primary closure

The rationale for primary closure after release of sepsis is that primary healing is common and further dressings are unnecessary. Simms et al. in Birmingham conducted a study in which soft tissue abscesses were drained under local anaesthetic in the accident and emergency department.[13] Patients were randomised to either incision and drainage alone or to incision and drainage and primary suture after drainage. Separating the anogenital abscesses as a subgroup, 17 patients were treated with primary suture as opposed to 22 with drainage. The time to healing was no different between the groups. There was a reported primary wound disruption rate of 35%. In contrast, Leaper et al. compared primary suture with drainage alone where there was confidence that no internal opening was present.[14] Healing times were marginally shorter in the primary suture group, with less time off work, although recurrence rates were high in both groups suggesting unidentified fistulas in many of the patients. Whatever benefit primary suture may hold in reducing time off work from repeated dressings is offset by the problems of failure to reduce the incidence of recurrent sepsis. This technique, and local anaesthetic management of abscesses in the accident and emergency setting, are therefore not recommended.

Role of antibiotics

There is no evidence supporting the use of antibiotics in the management of primary uncomplicated anorectal sepsis. However, they should be used during surgical drainage in patients at risk from bacteraemia (e.g. those with valve replacements) and in patients with florid cellulitis or necrotising infections. They also have a role in treating neutropenic patients.

DETERMINING THE LIKELIHOOD OF A CONCOMITANT FISTULA

As stated above, previous anorectal sepsis is frequently associated with an underlying fistula in

ano and gentle examination of the anal canal using a speculum while applying pressure to the abscess will frequently reveal pus at an internal opening. The chances of finding an internal opening are greater if there is an intersphincteric or supralevator abscess rather than a perianal or ischiorectal one.[4]

Microbiology

A sample of pus drained at the time of surgery should always be sent for culture. There is good evidence that when the principal organism in the pus is skin derived (usually *Staphylococcus aureus*), development of a subsequent fistula is extremely uncommon.[15,16] In the study by Grace et al., 156 patients with anorectal sepsis were examined by a single colorectal specialist.[15] Pus was sent for microbiological analysis and a fistula laid open if found. If no fistula was found, a second EUA was performed at 7–10 days.

In the 114 patients whose pus grew bowel-derived organisms, 62 (54%) had a fistula. In the 34 with skin-derived organisms, none had a fistula ($P < 0.0005$).[15]

An elegant study undertaken by Ekyn and Grace on 80 patients used the same surgical protocol but a considerably more elaborate bacteriological technique that differentiated gut-specific *Bacteroides* from other *Bacteroides*.[5] Of the 53 patients with a fistula, 45 (85%) grew *Escherichia coli* and 47 (89%) grew gut-specific *Bacteroides* in the cultured pus. In the 27 patients with no fistula, five (18%) grew gut-specific *Bacteroides* and five (18%) grew *E. coli*.

The presence of gut-specific anaerobes is 90% sensitive and 80% specific at predicting the presence of a fistula in ano.[5]

However, two problems exist with the use of pus culture to predict the likelihood of recurrent sepsis. First, without the sophisticated tests used in Ekyn and Grace's study to differentiate gut-derived from non-gut-derived anaerobes, the sensitivity of culture at predicting the presence of a fistula drops to 50–60%. Second, microbiological results are not immediately available and the patient may therefore require a second anaesthetic if no fistula is found initially and subsequent pus culture then suggests one is likely.

Assessment at the time of surgery

Lunnis and Phillips suggested that if the cryptoglandular theory of acute anorectal sepsis were correct, the presence of intersphincteric sepsis at the time of presentation might be a more sensitive indicator of an underlying fistula than microbiological analysis of the pus.[17] Their study included 22 patients in whom a radial incision was made over the apex of the abscess. This was extended medially to allow dissection of the intersphincteric space to determine the presence of intersphincteric sepsis. A careful examination was made to determine if a fistula was present. Patients were followed for a mean of 38 weeks.

Demonstration of intersphincteric sepsis in association with an anorectal abscess was 100% sensitive and 100% specific for the presence of an underlying fistula in ano.[17]

It should be acknowledged that two experienced colorectal surgeons performed this study. Although highly sensitive and specific, there is no evidence that this technique can be safely utilised by surgeons without specific training.

ROLE OF SYNCHRONOUS FISTULOTOMY

It is apparent that a significant proportion of patients with anorectal sepsis will have an associated fistula. If this can be dealt with simultaneously, then recurrence rates and patient inconvenience should be reduced. This potential benefit to the patient must be balanced against any risk of damage to the continence mechanism during definitive surgery. Furthermore, it may be difficult to delineate the anatomy of any fistulous track in the presence of gross oedema and inflammation.

There have been a number of randomised trials looking at the issue of the efficacy and safety of synchronous fistulotomy. Schouten and van Vroonhoven[18] studied 36 patients who underwent incision and drainage for anorectal abscesses accompanied by fistulotomy and 34 who underwent drainage alone.

After a median follow-up of 42.5 months there was an impressive reduction in recurrence rates in the synchronous fistulotomy group compared with those treated simply by incision and drainage (2.9% vs. 40.6%).[18]

There was a trend towards increased disturbance of continence in the fistulotomy group at 1 year (39.4% vs. 21.4 %) which did not reach statistical significance ($P < 0.106$). The observation that 20% of the incision and drainage group were classified as exhibiting disturbed continence suggests that their assessment of incontinence lacked specificity.

Two randomised trails from Singapore have also looked into the issue of concomitant treatment of an underlying fistula.[19,20] In the first study, consecutive patients with a perianal or ischiorectal abscess and a demonstrable internal opening were randomised to either incision and drainage alone (21 patients) or incision and drainage with concurrent fistulotomy (24 patients). There were proportionally more low transphincteric fistulas in the fistulotomy group than in the patients treated with incision and drainage (58% vs. 33%). At 1-year follow-up there were three recurrences in the incision and drainage group and none in the synchronous fistulotomy group ($P = 0.09$). There was no impaired continence in the fistulotomy group. The second study[20] included only perianal abscesses and randomised 52 consecutive patients to incision and drainage alone ($n = 28$) or incision and drainage with concomitant fistulotomy ($n = 24$).

At a mean follow-up of 16 months there were seven (25%) recurrent fistulas in the group treated with incision and drainage alone compared with none in the fistulotomy patients ($P < 0.009$). All patients were fully continent after surgery.[20]

TECHNICAL TIPS

The management of specific abscesses is shown diagrammatically in **Fig. 11.3**. Simple perianal abscesses should be drained and the cavity gently curetted (**Fig. 11.3a**). With ischiorectal abscesses, the cavity is often huge (**Fig. 11.3b**). The cavity should be incised as near to the anal verge as possible. This is to bring the external opening of any subsequent fistula close to the anal verge to minimise the trauma of subsequent fistulotomy should it be required. As mentioned earlier, the size of the drainage wound can be minimised if a drainage catheter is used. Intersphincteric abscesses require drainage into the anorectum, with excision of some of the internal sphincter (**Fig. 11.3c**). Submucosal abscesses, though rare, are drained into the anal canal. Supralevator or pelvic abscesses must be drained with care and ideally not through the perineum or a high fistula in ano will be created. In true pelvic abscesses unrelated to spread from the anal glands, drainage can be achieved into the rectum or vagina. If the abscess is related to pelvic pathology, the primary disease process will need to be excised along with the pus.

Management of secondary anal suppuration

MALIGNANT DISEASE

The abscess should be drained as per normal. It should be borne in mind that the presence of anorectal suppuration in these patients may well be caused by tumour extension beyond the bowel. This will have implications for the planning of definitive oncological treatment. If there is a significant malignant fistula, then the patient will require a defunctioning stoma.

INFLAMMATORY BOWEL DISEASE

Endoanal ultrasound is useful in identifying small collections in these patients. All collections of pus

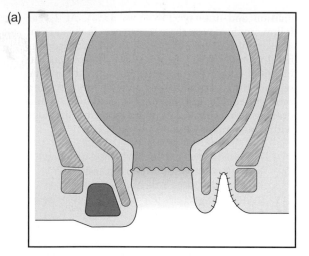

(a)

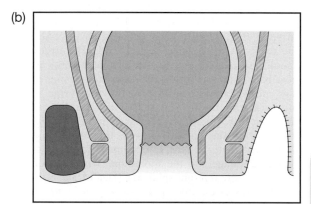

(b)

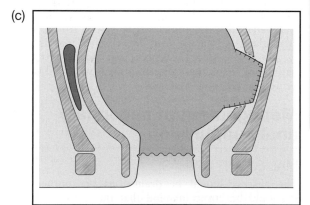

(c)

Figure 11.3 • Management of specific abscesses.
(a) Perianal abscess is treated by excision of a small disc of skin and curettage of the cavity. **(b)** Ischiorectal abscess is treated by excision of a substantial amount of tissue to facilitate drainage. The alternative is to introduce a drainage catheter through a small stab incision.
(c) Intersphincteric abscess is treated by excision of the mucosa and internal sphincter overlying the abscess. Such an abscess should not be drained through the perineal skin.

should be drained. In the majority of patients in the acute situation, setons should be placed across any fistulous openings.

NECROTISING FASCIITIS

Treatment involves drainage of the pus and debridement of all non-viable tissue as well as high-dose antibiotics (best chosen with local microbiological advice). A second-look EUA may be required and a proximal stoma is often needed to facilitate wound healing.

Anorectal sepsis in children

Anorectal sepsis in children is rare. The largest series in the literature is from Edinburgh, which reported 69 patients in a catchment population of 1 million over a 10-year period.[21] The median age for development of an abscess was 3 years (range 1 month to 12 years). The male to female ratio was 9:1. In total, 24 patients (38%) presented with recurrent sepsis after simple incision and drainage but in only half of these was a fistula found. The study was unable to relate pus culture to the presence of a fistula.

Recommendations

It is strongly recommended that acute anal suppuration be managed by early surgical intervention in the form of incision and drainage. Synchronous fistulotomy reduces the risk of recurrent sepsis. In experienced hands this can be achieved without damage to the continence mechanism. However, there is no conclusive evidence that this is a safe technique when undertaken by non-specialised surgeons and therefore cannot be recommended as primary treatment for all anorectal abscesses complicated by a fistula. It is strongly recommended that a pus swab be sent for culture to determine the likelihood of a subsequent fistula. If skin organisms are cultured, no further follow-up is necessary. If bowel organisms are grown, it is recommended that a further EUA should be undertaken.

PILONIDAL SEPSIS

A pilonidal sinus is a chronic inflammatory condition associated with hair and most commonly found in the natal cleft. Pilonidal abscesses are a common complication of the disease. Pilonidal abscesses usually present acutely with a tender, red, indurated swelling in or adjacent to the midline close to the natal cleft; midline pits are diagnostic of pilonidal disease. Not uncommonly, the abscess discharges spontaneously leaving a secondary track. The predominant organisms involved in pilonidal suppuration are staphylococcal but mixed anaerobes are also frequently cultured.[22]

As for all abscesses, the principles of treatment are drainage of the abscess and, if possible, eradication of the underlying disease while minimising the inconvenience to the patient. The surgical options include:

1. drainage of abscess and excision of disease at time of acute presentation;
2. drainage of abscess and staged definitive surgery;
3. drainage of abscess and staged definitive surgery only if required.

There are no good-quality randomised data on which approach is best. Attempts to excise the area surgically at the time of presentation are associated with high recurrence rates of up to 60%.[23] In addition, drainage alone may be a definitive treatment in itself. In a series of 73 patients treated with incision and drainage under local anaesthesia and followed for a median of 5 years, 42 patients (58%) healed primarily although nine (12%) subsequently developed a recurrence.[24] The likelihood of requiring a second procedure was increased if lateral tracts were present.

 Incision and drainage alone are sufficient to heal approximately half of all patients with pilonidal abscess without recurrence at 5 years.[24]

A comparative study from Israel assessed 58 patients with acute pilonidal abscess; 29 patients were treated with incision and drainage, the other 29 with wide excision (without closure). The results are displayed in **Table 11.2**.

 The risk of recurrent pilonidal suppuration is similar between patients undergoing incision and drainage with excision and those having incision and drainage alone, although those who underwent excision had a longer time off work.[25]

Recommendations

 As there is good evidence that simple incision and drainage will cure approximately 50% of all abscesses, it is strongly recommended that no excisional surgery is undertaken synchronously. Definitive surgery should be reserved for those who fail to heal or develop recurrence.

ACUTE ANAL FISSURE

Anal fissures usually present as a chronic entity in the outpatient setting, although occasionally a

Table 11.2 • Results of treatment for acute pilonidal abscess

	Excision	Incision and drainage	P value
Number	29	29	
Recurrence	12 (41)	16 (55)	NS
Hospital stay (days)	4	3	NS
Time off work (days)	14	7	0.06
Time to healing (days)	30	30	NS

Values expressed as medians; numbers in parentheses are percentages.
From Matter I, Kunin J, Schein M, Eldar S. Total excision versus non-resectional methods in the treatment of acute and chronic pilonidal disease. Br J Surg 1995; 82:752–3, with permission.

patient will present as an emergency with acute intractable anal pain. A primary fissure is a benign superficial ulcer within the anal canal. The patient characteristically presents with severe pain after defecation and there may be associated rectal bleeding. In the vast majority of patients it should be possible to diagnose the fissure simply by inspection. Gently parting the buttocks should reveal the lower edge of the fissure, usually in the midline posteriorly. It is often impossible to perform a digital rectal examination in these patients, although Larpent et al. used glyceryl trinitrate sublingually and were then able to exclude other pathology in 13 of 16 patients presenting acutely.[26] If it is impossible to adequately assess for the presence of a fissure, or the patient has returned with worsening or intractable pain, then an EUA should be undertaken to exclude the presence of other pathology.

In a study by Frezza et al.[27] of 308 patients with anal fissure, conservative therapy was compared with surgical treatment at the time of acute presentation.

 Nearly all (90%) acute fissures will heal without surgery and the time to healing is not altered by early surgical intervention.[27]

Lateral sphincterotomy was traditionally the mainstay of treatment for patients with anal fissures, with recurrence rates of the order of 0–2%.[28] However, the technique is associated with significant disturbances of continence in up to 6% of patients.[29] The pain from an acute fissure arises from internal sphincter spasm. This can be alleviated by topical preparations such as glyceryl trinitrate or diltiazem, both of which relax the anal sphincter.[30,31] Both have been shown to be efficacious in reducing sphincter pressure and healing chronic anal fissures,[32,33] although diltiazem has a lower side-effect profile.[34] Should a fissure be found acutely at EUA there is no place for acute sphincterotomy, but local anaesthetic infiltration will provide good symptomatic relief.

Recommendations

It is strongly recommended on the basis of a number of randomised trials that pharmacological agents should be used as first-line treatment for anal fissures, with surgery being reserved for those who fail to heal or recur.

THROMBOSED HAEMORRHOIDS

Uncomplicated haemorrhoidal disease is usually painless. The presence of severe pain usually points to another diagnosis or complication. Thrombosed prolapsed internal haemorrhoids are exquisitely tender and clinically obvious. Usually there is a history of a reducible prolapse prior to the onset of pain. Pain is so severe that the patient is often unable to sit, walk or defecate. The pain is caused by a combination of oedema of the perianal skin and thrombosis of the haemorrhoid. The condition, which is usually obvious on examination simply by parting the buttocks, may be further complicated by necrosis of the mucosa over the haemorrhoid.

The options for treatment are (i) conservative measures and (ii) emergency haemorrhoidectomy. Conservative therapy consists of adequate analgesia using topical and systemic preparations. There is little to be gained from the traditional regimen of ice packs and topical elevation. The rationale behind conservative measures is that although intensely painful the condition is usually self-limiting after 4–5 days and that haemorrhoidectomy itself is intensely painful for a similar period of time. The limitations of conservative treatment are apparent from a study of 117 patients at St Mark's Hospital, London, performed by Grace and Creed,[35] in which 92 patients were followed up after discharge.

Of 92 patients with thrombosed internal haemorrhoids treated conservatively, 87% continued to have symptoms of prolapse and bleeding after discharge and 10% had a further admission to hospital with thrombosis.[35]

The concerns regarding emergency surgery are that the operative field may be infected and that the

Table 11.3 • Results from comparative study on emergency and elective haemorrhoidectomy

	Elective surgery (n = 500)	Emergency surgery (n = 204)	P value
Haemorrhage	27 (5.4)	10 (4.9)	NS
Blood transfusion	10 (2)	4 (2)	NS
Anal stenosis	15 (3)	12 (5.9)	NS
Disturbance of continence	26 (5.2)	9 (4.4)	NS
Sepsis	0	0	NS
Recurrence	38 (7.6)	14 (6.8)	NS

Numbers in parentheses are percentages.
From Eu KW, Seow Choen F, Goh HS. Comparison of emergency and elective haemorrhoidectomy. Br J Surg 1994; 81:308–10, with permission.

massive swelling and oedema distorts the anatomy so much that haemorrhoidectomy is extremely difficult. The sequela of this is that too much tissue may be excised, with the subsequent risk of anal stenosis. In experienced hands, however, the results of early haemorrhoidectomy are good. Mazier reported a series of 400 patients who underwent haemorrhoidectomy for thrombosis.[36] Complications were stated to be no more frequent or serious than in the elective situation.

A case–control study from Singapore has compared 204 patients who underwent acute haemorrhoidectomy with 500 treated electively over the same time period. The clinical end points assessed were haemorrhage, anal stricture, recurrence of haemorrhoids, portal pyaemia and episodes of incontinence (**Table 11.3**). There was no difference in the profile or frequency of these complications between the two groups.[37]

Recommendations

There is good evidence that patients who present with acutely thrombosed haemorrhoids have a high risk of recurrent symptoms and will subsequently undergo haemorrhoidectomy. Emergency haemorrhoidectomy can be performed and has a complications profile similar to that seen with elective haemorrhoidectomy when undertaken by an appropriately skilled coloproctologist. Currently, the case is unproven as to whether all patients with thrombosed haemorrhoids should undergo definitive surgery in the acute setting.

ANORECTAL HAEMORRHAGE

Massive per rectal bleeding from an anorectal source is extremely rare. Nonetheless, proctosigmoidoscopy should always be undertaken to exclude bleeding from this area. In a series of 98 patients over the age of 65 presenting with major colonic haemorrhage, an anorectal source was responsible in only four.[38] The pathologies implicated were rectal carcinoma, rectal prolapse, haemorrhoids and solitary rectal ulcer. Other anorectal pathologies occasionally reported as causes of major haemorrhage include cavernous haemangiomas of the rectum, anal fissures, rectal varices and proctitis.

ANORECTAL TRAUMA

The rectum may be injured in its peritoneal or extra-peritoneal parts by penetrating trauma, iatrogenic injuries or from inserted foreign bodies. Injuries to the intraperitoneal rectum can be primarily repaired.[39] However, where there are large injuries, significant contamination, devascularisation of the tissues or open fractures, resection and diversion should be considered. Injuries to the extraperitoneal rectum are treated by primary repair if possible or by proximal diversion, rectal washout and a pre-sacral drain.[40] Sigmoidoscopy should be performed in cases of trauma where blood is found in the rectal lumen or if an extraperitoneal haematoma is found adjacent to the rectum at laparotomy.

Anal injuries may complicate childbirth, with 0.4% of all vaginal deliveries associated with a third-degree (into the external sphincter) or fourth-degree (into the anal canal) tear.[41] However, prospective studies using endoanal ultrasound suggest that up to 35% of women may have ultrasound evidence of internal or external anal sphincter damage following vaginal delivery.[42] Traditionally, obstetricians in the labour suite manage such tears by approximating the sphincter with interrupted sutures. However, results following repair of such injuries are disappointing. Of 34 women with a third-degree tear who underwent primary repair, 16 had significant problems with incontinence and urgency and 85% still had a sphincter defect on endosonography.[43] It is possible that the overlapping repair technique favoured by colorectal surgeons may improve these results.

FOREIGN BODIES

The literature contains a large number of case reports of a vast array of foreign bodies inserted into the rectum for sexual gratification and there are a similarly large array of innovative techniques described to extract them safely.

The largest single series is from San Diego (but also including some patients from the Hammersmith Hospital in London) reported by Cohen and Sackier.[44] Of 64 patients presenting with rectal foreign bodies, it was possible to remove the object in the emergency department under sedation in 31 (61%). Three patients with impacted bars of soap were successfully treated with admission and enemas, while 18 patients required EUA. Of these, five underwent laparotomy for rectal perforation, one required repair of a sphincter laceration and the other 12 underwent successful extraction.

The authors of this study recommended that patients should undergo visualisation of the rectum after extraction to ensure there is no associated full-thickness injury. The likelihood of requiring an EUA was increased if the lesion was high up within the rectum on clinical examination or plain abdominal radiograph.

Key points

- Anorectal sepsis should be managed by prompt drainage of pus using sound anatomical principles.
- The management of a synchronous fistula in ano should only be undertaken by an experienced coloproctologist.
- In the acute setting, pilonidal disease should be managed simply by incision and drainage.
- The first-line treatment of an acute anal fissure is pharmacological, with surgery being reserved for those that fail to heal.
- Thrombosed haemorrhoids should be managed conservatively unless experienced colorectal help is available.
- The management of patients with anorectal trauma and retained foreign bodies is determined principally by the site of injury or impaction.

REFERENCES

1. Eisenhammer S. The internal anal sphincter and the ano-rectal abscess. Surg Gynecol Obstet 1956; 103:501–6.

2. Parks AG. Pathogenesis and treatment of fistula in ano. Br Med J 1961; 1:63–9.

3. Buchan R, Grace RH. Anorectal suppuration: the results of treatment and the factors affecting the recurrence rate. Br J Surg 1973; 60:537–40.

4. Ramunjam PS, Prasad Ml, Abcarian H, Tan AB. Perianal abscesses and fistulae: a study of 1023 patients. Dis Colon Rectum 1984; 27:593–7.

5. Ekyn SJ, Grace RH. The relevance of microbiology in the management of anorectal sepsis. Ann R Coll Surg Engl 1986; 62:364–72.

> Seminal paper using detailed microbiological techniques to correlate the presence of a fistula in ano with gut-derived organisms. The technique is highly sensitive but not readily transferable to non-academic microbiological departments.

6. Winslett MC, Allan A, Ambrose NS. Anorectal sepsis as a presentation of occult rectal and systemic disease. Dis Colon Rectum 1988; 31:597–600.

7. Badrinath K, Jairam N, Ravi HR. Spreading extra-peritoneal cellulitis following perirectal sepsis. Br J Surg 1994; 81:297-8.

8. Chrabot CM, Prasad ML, Abcarian H. Recurrent anorectal abscesses. Dis Colon Rectum 1983; 26:105–8.

9. Abcarian H. Editorial comment to Winslett et al. Dis Colon Rectum 1988; 31:601.

10. Law PJ, Talbot RW, Bartram CI. Anal endo-sonography in the evaluation of perianal sepsis and fistula in ano. Br J Surg 1989; 7:752–5.

11. Lunnis PJ, Barker PG, Sultan AH et al. Magnetic resonance imaging of fistula in ano. Dis Colon Rectum 1994; 81:368–9.

12. Kyle S, Ibister WH. Management of anorectal abscesses: comparison between traditional incision and packing and dePezza catheter drainage. Aust NZ J Surg 1990; 60:129–31.

> A case–control study comparing 91 patients treated with stab incision and catheter drainage with 54 patients treated with radical incision and drainage. The study suggests considerable advantages from a minimally invasive approach and indwelling catheter.

13. Simms MH, Curran F, Johnson RA et al. Treatment of acute abscesses in the casualty department. Br Med J 1982; 284:1827–9.

14. Leaper DJ, Page RE, Bartram CI, Rosenburg IL, Wilson DH, Goligher JC. A controlled study comparing conventional treatment of idiopathic anorectal abscess with that of incision, curettage and primary suture under systemic antibiotic cover. Dis Colon Rectum 1976; 19:46–50.

15. Grace RH, Harper IA, Thompson RG. Anorectal sepsis: microbiology related to fistula-in-ano. Br J Surg 1982; 69:401–3.

> The first study to analyse microbiological data in acute anorectal sepsis. The presence of skin organisms in the cultured pus effectively excludes the presence of a fistula.

16. Whitehead SM, Leach RD, Ekyn SJ, Phillips I. The aetiology of perirectal sepsis. Br J Surg 1982; 69:166–8.

17. Lunnis PJ, Phillips RKS. Surgical assessment of acute anorectal sepsis a better predictor of fistula than microbiological analysis. Br J Surg 1994; 81:368–9.

> Study by two highly experienced fistula surgeons highlighting that when fistula in ano occurs with an anorectal abscess there is always pus in the intersphincteric space. Criticised as a technique only safe in the hands of experienced anal surgeons.

18. Schouten WR, van Vroonhoven Th. Treatment of anorectal abscess with or without primary fistulectomy. Neth J Surg 1987; 392:43–5.

> Study showing a drastically reduced recurrence rate if fistula managed synchronously. Some concerns raised about changes in continence following surgery but also seen in 1 in 5 of the control group.

19. Tang C-L, Chew S-P, Seow-Choen F. Prospective randomised trial of drainage alone vs drainage and fistulotomy for acute perianal abscesses with proven internal opening. Dis Colon Rectum 1996; 39:1415–17.

20. Ho Y-H, Tan MRN, Chui C-H, Leong AM, Eu K-W, Seow-Choen F. Randomised trial of primary fistulotomy with drainage alone for perianal abscesses. Dis Colon Rectum 1997; 40:1435–8.

> Randomised trial that shows a significant reduction in recurrence rates of abscess or fistula in patients treated with synchronous fistulotomy without any disturbances in continence. All participating surgeons were experienced in coloproctology.

21. Macdonald A, Wilson-Storey D, Munro F. Treatment of perianal abscess and fistula in ano in children. Br J Surg 2003; 90:220–1.

22. Sondenaa K, Nesvik I, Anderson E, Natas O, Soreide JA. Bacteriology and complications of chronic pilonidal sinus treated with excision and primary suture. Int J Colorectal Dis 1995; 10:161–6.

23. Clothier PR, Haywood IR. The natural history of post anal (pilonidal) sinus. Ann R Coll Surg Engl 1984; 66:201–3.

24. Jensen SL, Harling H. Prognosis after simple incision and drainage for a first episode of acute pilonidal abscess. Br J Surg 1988; 75:60–1.

> A study of 73 patients with pilonidal abscess treated under local anaesthetic. Highlights that the technique is frequently all that is required to eradicate the disease.

25. Matter I, Kunin J, Schein M, Eldar S. Total excision versus non-resectional methods in the treatment of acute and chronic pilonidal disease. Br J Surg 1995; 82:752–3.

   Study with 29 patients in both arms revealed that undertaking any type of excisional surgery at the time of incision and drainage slows recovery and does not reduce recurrence rates.

26. Larpent JL, Dussaud F, Gorce D, Lunaund B, Pelissier E. The use of glycerine trinitrate in inexaminable patients with anal fissure. Int J Colorectal Dis 1996; 11:263.

27. Frezza EE, Sandie F, Leoni G, Biral M. Conservative and surgical treatment in acute and chronic anal fissure: a study on 308 patients. Int J Colorectal Dis 1992; 7:188–91.

   A sizeable study of acute and chronic fissures revealing that the condition is self-limiting in the vast majority of patients.

28. Lewis TH, Corman Ml, Prager ED, Robertson WG. Long term results of open and closed sphincterotomy for anal fissure. Dis Colon Rectum 1988; 31:368–71.

29. Walker WA, Rothenberger DA, Goldberg SM. Morbidity of internal sphincterotomy for anal fissure and stenosis. Dis Colon Rectum 1985; 28:832–5.

30. Loder PB, Kamm MA, Nicholls RJ, Phillips RKS. Reversible chemical sphincterotomy by local application of glyceryl trinitrate. Br J Surg 1994; 81:1386–9.

31. Carapeti EA, Kamm M, Evans B, Phillips R. Topical diltiazem and bethanechol decrease anal sphincter pressure without side effects. Gut 1999; 45:719–22.

32. Lund JN, Scholefield JH. A randomised, prospective, double-blind, placebo controlled trial of glyceryl trinitrate ointment in the treatment of anal fissure. Lancet 1997; 349:11–14.

33. Knight J, Birks M, Farouk R. Topical diltiazem ointment in the treatment of chronic anal fissure. Br J Surg 2001; 88:553–6.

34. Kocher H, Steward M, Leather AJ, Cullen P. Randomised clinical trial assessing the side-effects of glyceryl trinitrate and diltiazem ointment in the treatment of chronic anal fissure. Br J Surg 2002; 89:413–17.

35. Grace RH, Creed A. Prolapsing thrombosed haemorrhoids: outcome of conservative management. Br Med J 1975; 3:354.

   A follow-up study of 92 patients with an initial presentation of acute haemorrhoids. Subsequent symptoms of prolapse and bleeding are common and 10% of patients present with another acute attack.

36. Mazier WP. Emergency haemorrhoidectomy: a worthwhile procedure. Dis Colon Rectum 1973; 16:200.

37. Eu KW, Seow Choen F, Goh HS. Comparison of emergency and elective haemorrhoidectomy. Br J Surg 1994; 81:308–10.

   A well-powered case–control study undertaken by experienced coloproctologists that reveals that they can perform emergency haemorrhoidectomy as safely as in the routine setting. However, there is no suggestion that this technique should be undertaken without appropriate training in the technique in the emergency setting.

38. Boley SJ, DiBiase A, Brandt LJ, Samartano RJ. Lower intestinal bleeding in the elderly. Am J Surg 1979; 37:57–64.

39. Levine JH, Longo WE, Pruitt C, Mazuski JE, Shapiro MJ, Durham RM. Primary repair without diversion may be feasible in some rectal injuries. Am J Surg 1996; 172:575–9.

40. Vitale GC, Richardson JD, Flint LM. Successful management of injuries to the extraperitoneal rectum. Am Surg 1983; 49:159–62.

41. Sleep J, Grant A. West Berkshire Perianal Management Trial. Br Med J 1987: 295:749–51.

42. Sultan AH, Kamm MA, Hudson CN et al. Anal sphincter disruption during vaginal delivery. N Engl J Med 1993; 329:1905–11.

43. Sultan AH, Kamm MA, Hudson CN et al. Third degree obstetric anal sphincter tears. Br Med J 1994; 308:887–91.

44. Cohen JS, Sackier JM. Management of colorectal foreign bodies. J R Coll Surg Edinb 1996; 41:312–15.

Twelve

Paediatric surgical emergencies

Lewis Spitz and
Ian D. Sugarman

INTRODUCTION

Abdominal emergencies in children should be considered with regard to the age of the child. Three age periods are considered separately: (i) neonatal period (up to 44 weeks postgestational age), (ii) infancy (1 month to 2 years of age) and (iii) child (2 years of age and older).

NEONATAL PERIOD

Intestinal obstruction

Intestinal obstruction is the most common presentation of almost all abdominal emergencies in the neonatal period. The cardinal sign of intestinal obstruction is bile-stained vomiting. In high obstructions the vomitus is clear green in colour, whereas in obstructions affecting the lower intestine the vomitus is green initially but becoming more faeculent with increasing delay in establishing the diagnosis. Where the obstruction is above the ampulla of Vater, the vomitus will be non-bilious but will be persistent and forceful. The degree of abdominal distension (**Fig. 12.1**) will depend on the level of the obstruction, affecting only the upper abdomen in high obstruction. In low obstructions or where there has been a significant pneumoperitoneum, there will be gross abdominal distension, occasionally severe enough to cause respiratory embarrassment. In complete obstructions, the infant either fails to pass any meconium or may pass small quantities of mucus. A minority of infants with intestinal atresia may pass a small amount of normal meconium,

which entered the distal bowel prior to the development of the atresia. Oedema of the anterior abdominal wall and/or periumbilical erythema signifies the presence of perforation, peritonitis or impending or established intestinal necrosis.

A plain abdominal radiograph is often diagnostic and the only radiological investigation required. It may indicate the level of the obstruction as well as providing additional information, such as pneumoperitoneum in the event of perforation, calcification from antenatal perforation or pneumatosis intestinalis in necrotising enterocolitis.

In doubtful cases of incomplete high obstruction, such as malrotation, an upper gastrointestinal contrast study is the investigation of choice, whereas in suspected low obstructions a contrast enema will define whether the colorectum is involved or whether the obstruction involves the distal small intestine. It is impossible on a plain radiograph to distinguish between small and large intestine.

PRENATAL DIAGNOSIS

With the increasing sensitivity of antenatal ultrasonography, two factors are important. First, congenital abnormalities are being diagnosed with increasing frequency. Examples include the prenatal diagnosis of exomphalos or gastroschisis, the 'double-bubble' appearance of duodenal atresia and dilated multiple loops in small intestinal atresia. Second, radiologists are now describing findings of uncertain significance, such as 'hyperechogenic' bowel, which is reported to be associated with the diagnosis of meconium ileus and cystic fibrosis. However, the sensitivity and specificity of this association is low and a formal prospective study is

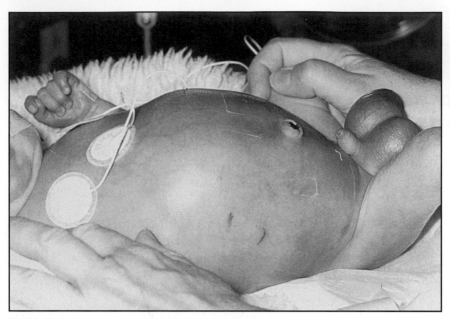

Figure 12.1 • Neonate with abdominal distension.

awaited.[1] Another example is the finding of intra-abdominal bowel dilatation in gastroschisis. This may imply that the size of the gastroschisis defect is narrowing, which could lead to infarction of the extra-abdominal bowel. Urgent delivery under these circumstances may prevent the loss of extensive lengths of intestine.[2] Antenatal counselling is a major and important commitment of the paediatric surgeon and close collaboration with obstetricians and neonatologists is vital.

GENERAL PRINCIPLES

Infants with suspected intestinal obstruction should be transferred in a portable incubator to a specialised paediatric surgical unit for definitive management. A large-calibre nasogastric tube (size 8–10 Fr) should be passed, aspirated at frequent intervals and kept on free drainage at all other times. Intravenous fluid resuscitation may be necessary in the base hospital prior to transfer. An initial bolus of 20 mL/kg human albumin solution, or normal saline, should be administered if hypovolaemia is present. In other circumstances, a maintenance solution of 0.18% sodium chloride in 10% glucose should be given at 4 mL/kg per hour, with nasogastric losses being replaced with an equal volume of normal saline containing 10 mmol potassium chloride per 500 mL saline (final concentration 20 mmol/L).

AETIOLOGY OF OBSTRUCTION

The cause of the intestinal obstruction may be broadly classified into two main categories: mechanical and paralytic (**Box 12.1**).

Box 12.1 • Classification of neonatal intestinal obstruction

MECHANICAL
Intraluminal
Meconium ileus
Intramural
Atresia/stenosis
Hirschsprung's disease
Anorectal anomalies
Extrinsic
Malrotation ± volvulus
Duplications
Inguinal hernia
PARALYTIC ILEUS
Septicaemia
Necrotising enterocolitis

Meconium ileus

Cystic fibrosis is the most common inherited defect affecting the Caucasian population. It is transmitted as an autosomal recessive condition affecting 1 in 2500 live births, with a carrier rate of 1 in 25. The gene for the cystic fibrosis transmembrane conductance regulator is located on the long arm of chromosome 7 and the ΔF508 mutation is mainly responsible. Around 10–15% of affected infants present at birth with meconium ileus, which may be uncomplicated or complicated by volvulus, atresia or perforation with meconium peritonitis.

In uncomplicated meconium ileus, the obstruction is caused by the thick, sticky, tenacious meconium occurring intraluminally in the distal ileum. The colon and terminal ileum are filled with greyish inspissated pellets. The diagnosis may be suspected on the plain abdominal radiograph, which shows dilated loops of intestine of varying calibre, an absence of air–fluid levels and a 'soap bubble' appearance in the right lower quadrant of the abdomen. A contrast enema will reveal a 'micro-colon' containing meconium pellets. In the absence of complicated meconium ileus, the obstruction may be relieved by a therapeutic enema using Gastrografin (diatrizoate meglumine), which is hyperosmolar and contains an emulsifying agent. The enema is performed by an experienced paed-iatric radiologist following satisfactory rehydration of the infant with intravenous fluids. The diluted Gastrografin is carefully infused into the colon under fluoroscopic control until the contrast is seen to enter the dilated loops of ileum. If the infant remains obstructed after the initial enema and is otherwise stable, the procedure can be repeated once or even twice. The success rate is around 55%; those for whom this is unsuccessful require simple enterotomy and mechanical washout of the obstructing meconium.[3]

Infants with complicated meconium ileus present at birth with gross abdominal distension. An abdominal mass may be palpable. The plain abdominal radio-graph shows clear evidence of intestinal obstruction while the presence of calcification denotes the presence of meconium peritonitis. These infants require vigorous resuscitation followed by prompt laparotomy. In the presence of a volvulus or atresia, the grossly affected bowel is resected, the proximal and distal intestine cleared of meconium and primary end-to-end anastomosis performed. Blood loss in meconium peritonitis may be considerable because of vascular adhesions. All necrotic intestine should be resected and the small and large bowel mobilised and inspected before a primary anasto-mosis is fashioned. Ileostomies (double-barrelled or Bishop–Koop) are reserved for the occasional unstable infant.

The definitive diagnosis of cystic fibrosis should be confirmed by gene probe (ΔF508) and sweat test (minimum 100 g sweat), showing sweat sodium and chloride levels in excess of 60 mmol/L (60 mEq/L).

Intestinal atresia/stenosis
Duodenum The occurrence of associated anomalies in over 50% of patients with duodenal atresia is an

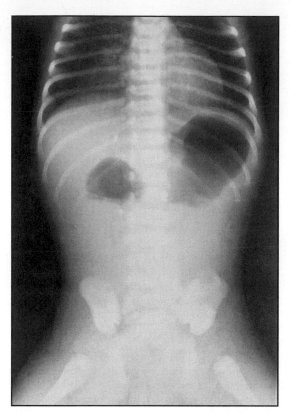

Figure 12.2 • Abdominal radiograph showing the typical 'double-bubble' appearance of duodenal atresia.

indication that the aetiology of the abnormality is developmental rather than acquired in utero. Down's syndrome and malrotation occur in 30%, congenital cardiac malformations in 20% and oesophageal atresia and anorectal anomalies in 8%. The diagnosis is confirmed by a 'double-bubble' appearance on abdominal radiograph (**Fig. 12.2**). Contrast studies are only required in incomplete obstruction, where it is important to differentiate intrinsic from extrinsic causes, such as malrotation with volvulus or duplications. Treatment is by side-to-side duodenoduodenostomy.

Small intestinal atresia Small intestinal atresias are usually isolated anomalies caused by intra-uterine interference with the blood supply to the affected segment. The lesions are classified into four types.

- Type I: membrane or web between the proximal and distal intestine, which is in continuity with an intact mesentery.
- Type II: blind ends joined by a band.
- Type IIIa: disconnected blind ends with a V-shaped gap in the mesentery.

- Type IIIb: 'Apple peel' or 'Christmas tree' deformity as in type IIIa but with an extensive mesenteric defect, the distal ileum receiving its blood supply from a collateral vessel from the ileocolic artery.
- Type IV: multiple atresias.

Types III and IV are associated with a shorter than normal length for the small intestine. The proximal bowel is grossly dilated and hypertrophied and displays defective peristalsis for some distance from its blind end. The diagnosis is generally made on plain abdominal radiograph (**Fig. 12.3**), with contrast enema being reserved for distinguishing large from small bowel obstruction. Treatment consists of resection of grossly distended proximal bowel (**Fig. 12.4**) and a limited length of distal intestine, with the fashioning of an end-to-end seromuscular anastomosis. In high jejunal atresias, the extent of proximal resection is restricted and a tapering jejunoplasty may be necessary in order to achieve an end-to-end anastomosis.

Hirschsprung's disease

Hirschsprung's disease results from an absence of ganglion cells within the wall of the intestine, commencing at the internal sphincter of the rectum and extending for a varying distance proximally. The disease is confined to the rectosigmoid in 75% and has total colonic involvement in 10%. The incidence is estimated to be 1 per 5000 live births. An autosomal dominant gene responsible for

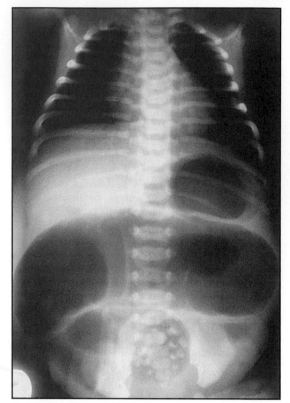

Figure 12.3 • Abdominal radiograph showing massively dilated small intestinal loops characteristic of a high small bowel atresia.

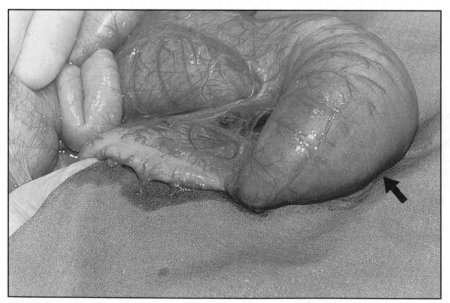

Figure 12.4 • Operative view of an intestinal atresia showing the proximally dilated and hypertrophied intestine and the collapsed distal bowel.

certain cases of Hirschsprung's disease has been mapped to chromosomes 10 and 13. The region concerned contains the *RET* proto-oncogene.

Over 80% of cases of Hirschsprung's disease present in the neonatal period with delayed passage of meconium, which is defined as failure to pass meconium during the first 24 hours after birth. A few progress to complete intestinal obstruction, but in the majority the passage of meconium is stimulated by a digital rectal examination or a saline rectal washout, only for the problem to recur within a few days. Around 25% of infants may present initially with enterocolitis: profuse diarrhoea often accompanied by blood in the stool, abdominal distension, bilious vomiting and dehydration. This is a life-threatening complication that demands vigorous resuscitation, gentle distal bowel washouts followed by the establishment of a proximal defunctioning stoma.

Confirmation of the diagnosis is achieved on rectal suction biopsy, which typically shows an absence of ganglion cells in the submucosa, the presence of large nerve trunks and an increase in acetylcholinesterase-stained nerve fibres in the muscularis mucosa and the lamina propria (**Fig. 12.5**). Rarely the diagnosis may be substantiated by a carefully performed barium enema and/or anorectal manometry. The barium may show a contracted rectum with cone-shaped transitional zone above before contrast enters a dilated colon proximally.

Definitive treatment consists of bypass (Duhamel, Soave) or excision (Swenson, Rehbein) of the aganglionic intestine and restoration of intestinal continuity in a one-, two- or three-stage procedure. The procedure may be performed laparoscopically but it is essential that expert histopathology is available at the time of the operation. More recently, a totally transanal procedure has been described in which the mobilization commences at the dentate line of the rectum with a submucosal dissection and entry into the peritoneal cavity at higher level. Thereafter, the dissection is carried close to the bowel wall until ganglionic bowel is reached. The proximal colon is pulled through and anastomosed as in a Soave procedure.

The outcome in terms of complications (such as enterocolitis) and long-term results (in respect of continence) for the single- or multiple-stage procedures is still under debate.[4]

Anorectal anomalies

Anorectal malformations cover a wide spectrum of abnormalities that occur in 1 in 5000 births. Of crucial importance is the precise determination of the level of the defect. A low anomaly can be diagnosed clinically by evidence of the passage of meconium on the perineum (**Fig. 12.6**). These lesions are amenable to immediate local reconstructive

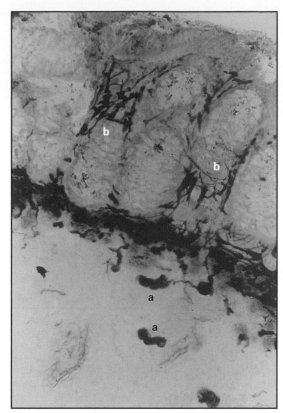

Figure 12.5 • Acetylcholinesterase stain of a rectal suction biopsy in Hirschsprung's disease showing an absence of ganglion cells, hypertrophied nerve trunks in the submucosa **(a)** and increased nerve fibres in the lamina propria **(b)**.

surgery in the expectation of the acquisition of reasonably normal continence. However, Rintala et al. showed that these patients were more prone to constipation than incontinence and that the incidence of normal continence was only 60%, with 7% being frankly incontinent.[5] All other anomalies (supralevator, high and intermediate lesions) require the fashioning of a defunctioning colostomy in the neonatal period, followed by meticulous reconstruction of the anorectal muscular complex after mobilising the distal end of the rectum and fashioning a new anal orifice (posterior sagittal anorectoplasty).

Malrotation

Failure to complete the normal process of intestinal rotation and fixation by week 12 of intrauterine development leads to the potentially lethal condition of malrotation. The duodenojejunal flexure lies to the right of the midline and the caecum and appendix are located in the right hypochondrium or upper midline of the abdomen. The result is a

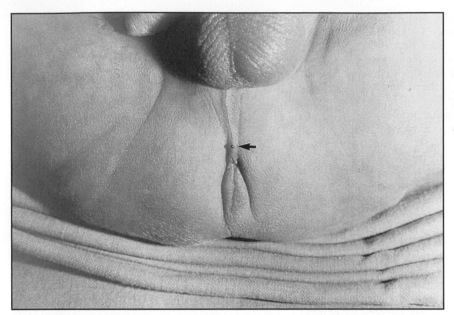

Figure 12.6 • Infant with a low anorectal anomaly. Note the spot of meconium (arrow) just anterior to the covered anus.

narrow-based mesentery of the midgut, which is prone to undergo volvulus.

The infant presents with intermittent bile-stained vomiting. This may be the only clinical indication of the presence of a malrotation until volvulus occurs, when the infant rapidly becomes shocked and passes blood per rectum and develops abdominal tenderness. In the older child, presentation varies from intermittent vomiting, failure to thrive and anorexia to colicky abdominal pain and malabsorption.

The plain abdominal radiograph in the infant with volvulus typically shows a 'gasless' appearance (**Fig. 12.7**). If time permits, an upper gastrointestinal contrast study is the investigation of choice. It will show an abnormally placed duodenojejunal flexure with small intestinal loops located on the right side of the abdomen in uncomplicated cases or a 'corkscrew' of 'twisted ribbon' appearance in the presence of a volvulus.

Treatment consists of urgent resuscitation and emergency laparotomy to untwist the volvulus and reposition the bowel after widening the mesentery of the midgut (Ladd's procedure).

Duplications

Duplications are rare anomalies that may be cystic or tubular and may affect any part of the alimentary tract. Cystic lesions present clinically with intestinal obstruction and a palpable or ultrasonographically detected mass, whereas tubular duplication causes intestinal bleeding through the presence of ectopic gastric mucosa within the duplication causing ulceration in the adjacent intestine.

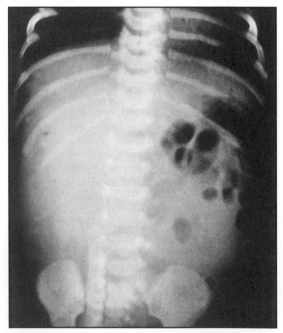

Figure 12.7 • Abdominal radiograph showing a relatively gasless abdomen suspicious of malrotation with midgut volvulus.

Inguinal hernia

Inguinal hernia is the most common condition treated by paediatric surgeons. It occurs in 2% of full-term infants and in 10% of preterm infants. There is a male preponderance of 5–10:1 and the

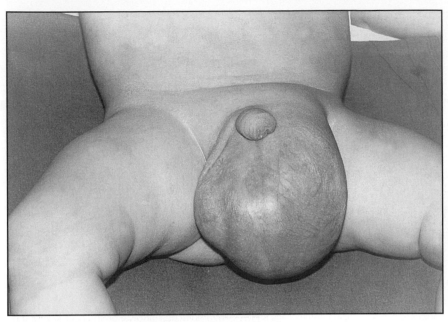

Figure 12.8 • Infant with an incarcerated left inguinal hernia.

right side is affected twice as often as the left. Bilateral hernia occurs in 10%. The hernias most commonly present with an intermittent bulge in the groin, which increases with crying and reduces spontaneously when the infant is relaxed. The hernia not infrequently presents initially with irreducibility. The vast majority of these irreducible hernias can be manually reduced by 'taxis' once the infant has been sedated. Treatment consists of simple herniotomy, which in infancy should be undertaken as soon as possible after diagnosis as the chances of incarceration (**Fig. 12.8**) are very high. There has been much debate as to whether a prophylactic contralateral herniotomy should be performed in certain cohorts of the neonate/infant presenting with a unilateral inguinal hernia.[6]

Necrotising enterocolitis

Necrotising enterocolitis predominantly affects preterm infants and is one of the most common surgical emergencies encountered in the neonatal period. The pathogenesis involves three processes: (i) intestinal ischaemia, (ii) bacterial colonisation and (iii) the presence of a substrate, milk formula, in the lumen of the intestine. It most commonly affects the terminal ileum and colon but no part of the intestine is immune.

The infant displays lethargy, abdominal distension, bilious vomiting or nasogastric bile-stained aspirate, refusal of feed and bleeding per rectum. Early signs may be indistinguishable from neonatal septicaemia. The pathognomonic radiological finding is the presence of pneumatosis intestinalis (**Fig. 12.9**),

while pneumoperitoneum indicates a perforation and portal venous gas indicates extensive, but not necessarily lethal, intestinal involvement.

Early institution of medical treatment, including nasogastric decompression, broad-spectrum antibiotics, fluid and electrolyte resuscitation and parenteral nutrition for 7–10 days, results in resolution of the process in 70–80% of patients. Indications for surgery include intestinal perforation and failure to respond to conservative treatment, indicating advanced intestinal disease.

At surgery, frankly necrotic bowel is resected and, as is common in UK practice, a primary anastomosis is fashioned or, as is common in the USA, stomas are constructed.[7]

About 10–15% of infants develop late postoperative strictures that require surgical resection.

INFANCY

Pyloric stenosis

Pyloric stenosis occurs most commonly at 4–6 weeks of age and presents with projectile non-bilious vomiting. In addition, the infant has failed to thrive, is constipated and may be frankly dehydrated. The incidence is approximately 1 in 200 with a 4:1 male to female ratio. The diagnosis is usually made by palpation of an 'olive-shaped' mass in the right hypochondrium, which can be palpated directly or

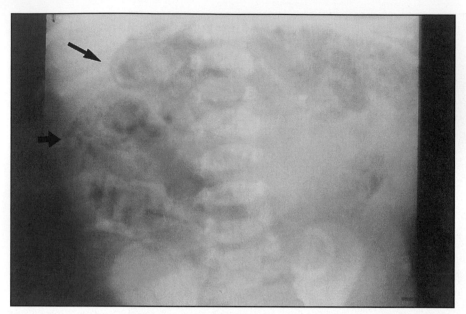

Figure 12.9 • Abdominal radiograph in necrotising enterocolitis showing intramural gas (arrows) on the right side of the abdomen (pneumatosis intestinalis).

during a test-feed. If this fails, ultrasonography is the investigation of choice, a barium meal being reserved for those infants where the diagnosis is still in doubt. Initial management is rehydration and correction of the electrolyte disturbance. This comprises a hypochloraemic metabolic alkalosis and correction is with 0.45% sodium chloride with added potassium. Surgery should not be undertaken until full correction of the electrolytes has been achieved as anaesthesia with a raised serum bicarbonate predisposes to an increased risk of respiratory depression. Surgery is classically a Ramstedt pyloromyotomy performed via a right upper quadrant incision; however, cosmesis is improved by a periumbilical incision as described by Tan and Bianchi[8] and some surgeons advocate that the procedure is best performed laparoscopically.[9]

Intussusception

Intussusception is the most common cause for an abdominal emergency in infants between the ages of 3 months and 2 years. The peak incidence is from 6 to 9 months and there appears to be a seasonal incidence, with the peaks in spring and midwinter. Most cases of intussusception at this age are 'idiopathic', with the leading point being an enlarged Peyer's patch that develops secondary to a viral infection. Only around 5% of intussusceptions in infants result from a recognisable lesion such as a polyp, Meckel's diverticulum, duplication or tumour. The site of intestine most frequently

involved is the ileocaecal region, although any part of the intestine may be affected.

The pathophysiology of the intussusception commences with the invagination of one part of the intestine (intussusceptum) into the adjacent part (intussuscipiens) causing a subacute incomplete intestinal obstruction and venous compression of the intussusceptum; if uncorrected, this will eventually result in arterial insufficiency and bowel necrosis.

The clinical features of an intussusception include colicky abdominal pain and vomiting secondary to the incomplete obstruction, and the passage of blood and mucus per rectum as a result of the venous engorgement. In addition, a sausage-shaped mass may be palpable on abdominal examination. The episodes of abdominal pain are classically intermittent, with recurrent attacks of screaming and of the infant drawing up its knees accompanied by pallor. The attacks last about 1–2 minutes and recur every 10–15 minutes.

The diagnosis may be made solely on the clinical findings. A plain abdominal radiograph may show air outlining the head of the intussusception, which appears as a soft tissue mass, and an absence of gas in the right iliac fossa (**Fig. 12.10**). Where the diagnosis remains doubtful, a contrast enema or an ultrasound scan will establish the pathology.

Treatment of an intussusception commences with initial resuscitation, with correction of any fluid and electrolyte imbalance and nasogastric decompression. In the uncomplicated case, the treatment of choice is reduction by means of either an air or a

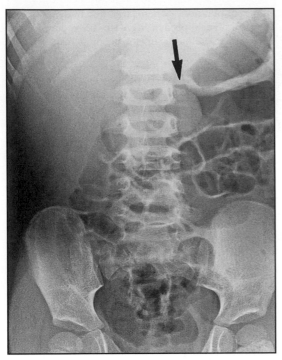

Figure 12.10 • Abdominal radiograph showing the soft tissue mass (arrow) of an intussusception in the upper abdomen.

contrast enema under fluoroscopic or ultrasound control.

 Reduction can be successful in up to 90% of infants for whom air reduction is attempted.[10]

Where complications have developed, such as perforation, or where there is clinical evidence for bowel necrosis and when reduction has failed, an operative approach is adopted. At surgery (Fig. 12.11) the intussusception is either reduced manually or a limited resection and primary anastomosis is undertaken if the intussusception is not viable or there is a recognised leading point.

CHILDREN

Appendicitis

The diagnosis of acute appendicitis should be considered at all ages (see also Chapter 9) but is most common between the ages of 5 and 15 years. The pathological process of appendicitis commences with intraluminal obstruction as a result of a faecolith or secondary to mucosal or submucosal lymphoid hyperplasia. The mucosa distal to the obstruction continues to secrete and peristalsis increases in an attempt to overcome the obstruction; as a result pressure within the lumen of the appendix increases. Bacteria within the lumen proliferate in the presence of stasis and, helped by the

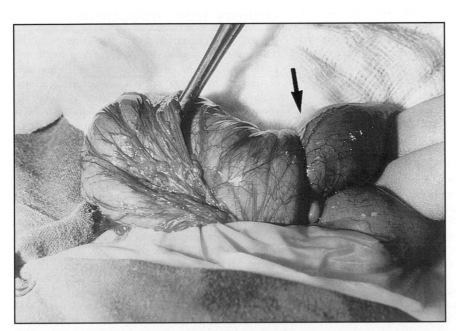

Figure 12.11 • Operative view of an ileocolic intussusception.

increased intraluminal pressure, invade the wall of the appendix. The process may progress to full-thickness necrosis with perforation and local or generalised peritonitis.

The classical presentation of acute appendicitis is of vague non-specific periumbilical pain that rapidly radiates and localises in the right iliac fossa. There is almost invariably loss of appetite and vomiting and a low-grade pyrexia of 38°C. Palpation of the abdomen reveals tenderness and guarding in the right iliac fossa, with rigidity when perforation has occurred. There is no need to attempt to elicit rebound pain, which is an unreliable sign in young children and only increases the distress and the discomfort. A rectal examination may be helpful in doubtful cases but is unnecessary if the diagnosis has already been made. The rectal examination may reveal a mass in the presence of perforated pelvic appendicitis.

The diagnosis of acute appendicitis is generally made on clinical findings. Laboratory investigations are less helpful, but a leucocytosis of 10×10^9 to 15×10^9 cells/L supports the diagnosis. Radiological investigations are not often required, but a plain abdominal radiograph may show a calcified faecolith; more recently, ultrasonography has been found to be useful in doubtful cases, particularly in teenage girls. The ultrasound may reveal other gynaecological causes such as an ovarian cyst or may be suggestive of the diagnosis of appendicitis when the diameter of the appendix is greater than 6 mm and there is surrounding fluid in the vicinity. Diagnostic laparoscopy has also been advocated and is again most helpful in the teenage girl.

The differential diagnosis of acute appendicitis is extensive. It is particularly difficult to establish the diagnosis in very young children, who usually present late with perforation and peritonitis, teenage girls, and children suffering from other medical conditions such as urinary tract infections, sickle cell disease, diabetes mellitus and leukaemia.

Treatment of appendicitis in children falls into four categories. In early uncomplicated appendicitis, the patients should undergo appendicectomy as soon as possible. Patients with perforated appendicitis with signs of peritonitis require intensive resuscitation and antibiotic administration prior to being subjected to appendicectomy. The presence of an abdominal mass indicates a localised perforation, which generally responds to antibiotic therapy with appendicectomy delayed electively for 6–8 weeks. In patients where the diagnosis is in doubt, a period of active observation in hospital is strongly recommended. It is extremely rare for such an appendix to rupture during observation and the diagnosis will usually become apparent within 12–24 hours.

The role of laparoscopic appendicectomy in paediatric surgery is perhaps less clear than in the adult population, where the advantages of the laparoscopic approach seem to be reduced post-operative pain and a shorter hospital stay.[11,12]

A recent randomised study of 61 children has now demonstrated similar advantages in the paediatric population,[13] and it will be interesting to see whether, with time, open surgery remains the most common procedure performed in children, which is certainly the case at present.

Torsion of the testis

There are two types of testicular torsion: extravaginal torsion, which occurs in the perinatal period; and intravaginal torsion related to an abnormal suspension of the testis ('bell-clapper' anomaly), which affects the older child. The onset of torsion is heralded by sudden severe scrotal pain. The testis is swollen and tender and lies within the upper scrotum. The diagnosis is made on clinical examination and the condition should be distinguished from torsion of a testicular appendage, which can be treated conservatively, and epididymo-orchitis. If there is any doubt, it is preferable to proceed to an emergency exploration of the scrotum. The testis is detorted and its viability assessed. If the testis is clearly necrotic, it should be removed; if viable, it should be fixed with three or four non-absorbable sutures to prevent a recurrence. It is mandatory to fix the contralateral testis in a similar fashion to protect it from torsion as the abnormal lie of the testis is commonly bilateral.

Urinary tract infections

Urinary tract infections can occur at any age and the symptoms produced vary according to the age period at which the infection occurs. In the neonatal period, the common presenting features are irritability, temperature instability, lethargy, anorexia, vomiting and jaundice. In infancy, failure to thrive is a common presentation. Screaming and irritability are frequent symptoms and may be associated with vomiting and diarrhoea. Malodorous or cloudy urine, haematuria and frequency are more specific features of urinary tract infections. Older children tend to present with frequency and dysuria associated with pyrexia and abdominal pain.

Confirmation of the diagnosis is obtained on urinalysis and culture. All patients with a documented urinary tract infection merit full investigation, which should include ultrasonography of the kidneys, ureters and bladder. In addition, a voiding cystourethrogram should be performed. The most common underlying abnormalities associated with urinary tract infections include vesicoureteric reflux and voiding dysfunction and pelviureteric junction obstruction, which classically presents with pain, a mass, haematuria, nausea and vomiting, and hypertension.

Key points

- Neonatal and complex surgery on children should ideally take place only in specialist paediatric surgical units.
- The cardinal sign of intestinal obstruction in neonates is *bile*-stained vomiting.
- Delayed passage (>24 hours) of meconium should arouse suspicion of Hirschsprung's disease.
- An inguinal hernia in an infant is a relative emergency.
- Resuscitation is an essential first step in treatment.

REFERENCES

1. Stringer MD, Thornton JG, Mason GC. Hyperechogenic fetal bowel. Arch Dis Child 1996; 76:F1–F2.

2. Omran W, Nicolaides K, Haugen S, Davenport M. Intrauterine closed gastroschisis. Unpublished presentation at the 46th Annual Congress of the British Association of Paediatric Surgeons, Liverpool, July 1999.

3. Murshed R, Spitz L, Kiely EM, Drake DP. Meconium ileus: a ten-year review of thirty-six patients. Eur J Pediatr Surg 1997; 7:257–77.

4. Stringer MD, Oldham KT, Mouriquand PDE, Howard ER. Pediatric surgery and urology: long term outcomes. London: WB Saunders, 1998; pp. 329–56.

5. Rintala R, Mildh L, Lindahl H. Fecal continence and quality of life in adult patients with an operated low anorectal malformation. J Pediatr Surg 1992; 27:902–5.

6. Tackett LD, Brewer CK, Luks FI et al. Incidence of contralateral inguinal hernia. J Pediatr Surg 1999; 34:684–7.

7. Fasching G, Hollworth ME, Schmidt B et al. Surgical strategies in very-low-birthweight neonates with necrotising enterocolitis. Acta Paediatr 1994; 396(Suppl.):62–4.

8. Tan KC, Bianchi A. Circumbilical incision for pyloromyotomy. Br J Surg 1986; 73:399.

9. Fujimoto T, Lane GS, Segawa O et al. Laparoscopic extramucosal pyloromyotomy versus open pyloromyotomy for infantile hypertrophic pyloric stenosis: which is better? J Pediatr Surg 1999; 34:370–2.

10. Hadidi AT, El Shah N. Childhood intussusception: a comparative study of non-surgical management. J Pediatr Surg 1999; 34:304–7.

11. McAnena OJ, Austin O, O'Connell BR et al. Laparoscopic versus open appendicectomy: a prospective evaluation. Br J Surg 1992; 79:818–20.

12. Garbutt JM, Soper NJ, Shannon WD et al. Meta-analysis of randomized controlled trials comparing laparoscopic and open appendectomy. Surg Laparosc Endosc Percutan Tech 1999; 9:17–26.

13. Lintula H, Kokki H, Vanamo K. Single blind randomised clinical trial of laparoscopic versus open appendicectomy in children. Br J Surg 2001; 88:510–14.

This randomised study of 61 children aged 4–15 years demonstrated significantly less pain and shorter hospital stay after the laparoscopic approach.

CHAPTER

Thirteen

Abdominal trauma

Kenneth D. Boffard

INTRODUCTION

There are few areas of trauma care where rapid detection and early intervention can affect outcome as dramatically as in patients with life-threatening intra-abdominal injuries. It is well recognised that, without organised trauma care, some 20–35% of patients who reach hospital alive in the UK will die unnecessarily.[1] In the now classic study of trauma centres versus non-trauma centres in California published in 1979, West et al. demonstrated that the majority of preventable deaths resulted from unrecognised, and therefore untreated, intra-abdominal haemorrhage.[2]

Approximately 6% of all patients with blunt abdominal trauma will require laparotomy, primarily for haemorrhage from solid organ injuries. The majority of these injuries will be from motor vehicle crashes. However, with the increasing use of seat belts, hollow viscus injuries are also possible and require considerable expertise in their early detection. In addition to motor vehicular trauma, falls and pedestrian crashes may cause significant abdominal injury.

Penetrating torso trauma poses its own decision-making problems, especially with regard to whether the peritoneal cavity has actually been penetrated and, if so, whether intra-abdominal injury has occurred.

RISK FACTORS

Mackersie et al.,[3] in an evaluation of 3223 patients with blunt trauma, found that the risk of abdominal injury was significantly increased in the presence of an arterial base deficit of 3 mmol/L or more, the presence of major chest trauma, the presence of pelvic fractures or the presence of hypotension. Taylor and Eichelberger[4] studied 482 paediatric patients and found that haematuria and objective abdominal findings (distension, abrasions, contusions, blood in the gastrointestinal tract) were associated with abdominal injury. Knudson et al.[5] investigated the association between haematuria and blunt abdominal injuries in a group of patients that included adults and children. In this study, the association between haematuria and significant intra-abdominal injuries not related to the kidney increased with the degree of haematuria. In patients with greater than 100 red blood cells per high-power field, 17% had an intra-abdominal injury; this increased to 24% in those with gross haematuria. When patients with a history of shock were evaluated, even microscopic haematuria (<100 red blood cells per high-power field) was associated with a 29% incidence of abdominal injury.[5]

Criteria that identify patients at significant risk for abdominal injury, and therefore requiring objective evaluation, include:

- unexplained haemodynamic instability;
- unexplained hypovolaemic shock;
- associated major chest injury;
- presence of pelvic fracture;
- impaired sensorium;
- significant base deficit;
- presence of haematuria;
- objective physical findings (e.g. tenderness);
- major mechanism of injury.

ASSESSMENT IN THE EMERGENCY DEPARTMENT

The entire philosophy of the abdominal injury can be summed up by answering the following questions.

- Is the abdomen involved in an injury process?
- Is a surgical procedure necessary to correct it?
- What additional support does the patient require?

In hypotensive patients, the goal is to stop the bleeding, and this includes the rapid determination of whether the abdomen is the cause of the hypotension. If intra-abdominal bleeding is the cause of the hypotension or haemodynamic instability, then emergency measures will be needed to control that bleeding. These include emergency transfusion in order to 'buy time', or emergency thoracotomy in the emergency room to control the descending aorta and thus bleeding distally. It should be emphasised that transfusion alone is only a means to an end, and for hypotensive patients with penetrating torso injuries, delay in aggressive fluid resuscitation until rapid operative intervention has occurred improves outcome.[6] Haemodynamically stable patients without signs of abdominal irritation may undergo a more extended assessment in order to answer the above questions.

Most conventional texts emphasise the need for a careful history and physical examination of the abdomen. While this is of undoubted importance, it is extremely difficult to assess the abdomen in the trauma situation as the history may not be available and all the existing physical signs are misleading. Fresh blood is not a peritoneal irritant.

The history of the mechanism of injury is critically important in assessing the potential for abdominal injury. This information may be obtained from the patient, relatives, police or emergency care personnel. When assessing the patient who has sustained a penetrating injury, pertinent historical information includes the time of injury, type of weapon, number and direction of (especially) bullet wounds (e.g. entrance and an exit wound, or two entry wounds with the bullets retained). If possible, the history also includes the magnitude and location of any abdominal pain, and whether this pain is referred to the shoulder.

It is unacceptable to withhold analgesia. Judicious use of intravenous opiates will not significantly affect the clarity of the history, nor will it 'mask' pain, depress cerebration or respiration, or alter the blood pressure. What it will do is make the injury more comfortable for the patient and allow the clinician a much more accurate picture of both the history and the clinical presentation.

DIAGNOSTIC MODALITIES IN BLUNT ABDOMINAL TRAUMA

Even with experience, the accuracy of physical examination of the abdomen in detecting intra-abdominal injuries is limited. There are many patient factors that contribute to the difficult physical examination, including the presence of other painful distracting injuries, especially if they occur both above and below the abdomen, and an altered level of consciousness as the result of drugs, alcohol or head injury. Recognising these limitations, most trauma surgeons advocate a more objective evaluation of the abdomen in patients at risk for intra-abdominal injury.

Routine screening radiographs

As laid down by the Advanced Trauma Life Support (ATLS) Programme of the American College of Surgeons, the routine radiographs include lateral cervical films, an anteroposterior (AP) chest film and a pelvic film.[7] Supine chest or erect abdominal films are not always useful. If possible (and if it is safe to do so), an erect chest radiograph will provide more information than an erect abdominal film when looking for infradiaphragmatic air (see also Chapter 5).

In all cases of penetrating trauma, it is important to appreciate that the radiograph is unlikely to influence management in the unstable patient, who requires an immediate laparotomy. However, in the stable patient, useful additional information regarding the track of the bullet can be obtained. It is essential in such a situation to make use of bullet markers to show the entry/exit wounds.[8] These can be simply paper clips taped onto the skin. After the clips are applied to all torso wounds, the radiographs are taken and will give an indication not only of the track of the bullet but also of the presence of other fragments.

Contrast studies

URETHROGRAPHY

It is unnecessary to perform emergency urethrography if a rupture of the urethra is suspected. A suprapubic cystostomy should be considered as an alternative.

CYSTOGRAPHY

Rupture of the bladder is diagnosed using transurethral cystography, via the Foley catheter. It is important to introduce 400–500 mL of contrast into the bladder to distend it adequately. AP, lateral and oblique films, as well as a post-micturition film, form essential components of the examination.

INTRAVENOUS UROGRAPHY

A high-dose rapid injection of contrast is used where visualisation of kidney function and anatomy is desired. It is essential to visualise both kidneys in the nephrogram phase, which occurs 2–5 minutes after injection of contrast. Non-function of a kidney on one side mandates further investigation, either by arteriogram or by contrast-enhanced computed tomography (CT).

GASTROINTESTINAL CONTRAST STUDIES

Where there is concern regarding a particular viscus as an isolated injury, or retroperitoneal injury, specific contrast studies may be useful.

Special diagnostic studies

The advantages and disadvantages of each of the objective methods of examining the abdomen for injuries are summarised in **Box 13.1**.

DIAGNOSTIC PERITONEAL LAVAGE

Root et al. introduced diagnostic peritoneal lavage (DPL) as a method of evaluation of the abdomen,[9] and while it has frequently been superseded by more sophisticated (and potentially more expensive) techniques, it remains the standard against which all other diagnostic examinations are judged. The main advantage of DPL is that it can be performed quickly and with few complications by relatively inexperienced clinicians. DPL is also highly sensitive and specific for the detection of abdominal blood (>97%) but does not identify the organ of injury. Injuries of the retroperitoneum will be missed by DPL, and the presence of pelvic fractures may lead to a false-positive result.

A DPL is generally considered positive if:

- red cell count is >100 000/mm^3;
- white cell count is >500/mm^3;
- there is amylase or bowel content in the lavage return.

In addition, if surgeons are committed to operating on all patients with positive DPL, the ability to manage patients non-operatively may be lost. The lavage is therefore regarded as an indicator of the presence of abdominal pathology, but not necessarily as an indication for surgery (see section on non-operative management below).

COMPUTED TOMOGRAPHY

With CT, it is possible both to recognise the organ that is injured and to grade the severity of the injury. Both intraperitoneal and retroperitoneal injuries can be detected with CT, and the amount of intra-abdominal blood loss can be estimated. Serial scanning can be used to follow the resolution (or progression) of an injury. The disadvantages of CT include the need to move the patient to the radiology suite and the time required to perform the scan, although with the introduction of helical and multislice scanners the latter factor has become less important. CT is expensive and there is the potential for allergic reactions to the injected contrast material, or for aspiration of oral contrast (a rare event).

Although CT is relatively insensitive in the detection of hollow viscus injuries, a bowel injury (and especially a duodenal injury) is suggested by finding a thickened bowel wall, extraluminal air and the presence of intraperitoneal fluid in the absence of a solid organ injury.[10,11] CT may also miss a pancreatic injury early in its course. The accuracy of CT is generally poor in the detection of diaphragmatic, hollow organ and mesenteric injuries, and there have been reports of a high incidence of false-negative results.[12] Despite these limitations, however,

Box 13.1 • Special techniques for diagnostic examination of abdominal injury

	Advantages	Disadvantages
Clinical examination	Quick, non-invasive	Unreliable
Diagnostic peritoneal lavage	Quick, inexpensive	Invasive, too sensitive, limited specificity
Ultrasound	Quick, non-invasive	User dependent, unhelpful for hollow viscus injury
Computed tomography	Organ-specific retroperitoneal information	Patient must be stable, expensive
Laparoscopy	Organ specific	Painful, anaesthesia required
Laparotomy	Highly specific	Complications, expensive

CT remains the method of choice for objective evaluation of the abdomen in stable trauma patients who are likely to have an intra-abdominal injury.

DIAGNOSTIC ULTRASOUND

Ultrasonography is a tool that has enjoyed widespread popularity in portions of Europe and China, especially for use with the obstetric patient. Until recently, ultrasonography was regarded as being of limited use in the trauma patient, but the attraction of being able to carry out a non-invasive, quick and relatively cheap examination at the bedside has changed this perception.

The sensitivity of ultrasound for the detection of free intraperitoneal fluid in blunt trauma has been shown to be 81–99%.[13] The disadvantages of ultrasound are its lack of sensitivity for injuries that do not produce blood or peritoneal fluid and the fact that its accuracy is directly related to the experience of the ultrasonographer. Nonetheless, surgeons can be taught to perform and interpret ultrasound examinations rapidly and accurately, with a sensitivity/specificity and accuracy each over 90%.[14–16] This diagnostic method has particular appeal in paediatric trauma patients and in the injured gravid patient.

In many centres, ultrasound has already replaced DPL for evaluation of the unstable patient following blunt trauma. However, since the examination will miss small amounts of intraperitoneal fluid, the role of ultrasound in the diagnosis of penetrating abdominal trauma is still controversial.

DIAGNOSTIC LAPAROSCOPY

Laparoscopy has been found to be of little use in the evaluation of the patient with blunt abdominal trauma.[17] With few exceptions, laparoscopy requires general anaesthesia, is expensive and has the potential to create a tension pneumothorax[18] or air embolus during insufflation. Close monitoring and prompt reaction to problems when they occur would seem to be satisfactory in anticipating these problems; isopneumonic (gasless) laparoscopy has been reported in an attempt to avoid air embolus.[19] The main advantages of this technique are the avoidance of problems associated with the pneumoperitoneum and the ability to use conventional surgical instruments. The main disadvantage is the cost of the abdominal wall retraction system. Its use in penetrating injury has been reported in the successful repair of injuries of the diaphragm and stomach.[20]

An additional drawback of diagnostic laparoscopy currently is the relative cost compared with other modalities, especially those performed at the bedside, such as ultrasound. The technique can only be used on relatively stable patients, and laparoscopy is still limited in its ability to detect intestinal injury.

Laparoscopy is most useful in the patient with penetrating abdominal trauma when there is a question of peritoneal penetration or diaphragmatic injury.[21] With regard to specific organs, it has been shown to be particularly helpful in the area of the diaphragm, where other diagnostic tests used in abdominal trauma are least sensitive. The diaphragm is also an area where delay or missed diagnosis dramatically increases the morbidity.[22] Laparoscopy can identify not only clinically unsuspected diaphragm injuries but also other injuries that have been 'missed' by other diagnostic tests.

Diagnostic laparoscopy does not confer any advantages or improvements over other techniques when it comes to investigation of retroperitoneal injuries to organs such as the duodenum and pancreas. However, it can be used to assess the spleen, although may still not be able to give adequate information, and CT remains more accurate in this regard.

LAPAROTOMY

Mandatory laparotomy

While laparotomy remains the most appropriate therapy for an unstable patient with obvious abdominal trauma, a non-therapeutic laparotomy is not necessarily benign. In a recent prospective study of unnecessary laparotomies performed in 254 trauma patients, complications occurred in 41% of patients, and included atelectasis, postoperative hypotension, pleural effusion, pneumothorax, prolonged ileus, pneumonia, surgical wound infection, small bowel obstruction and urinary infection.[23]

Nonetheless, many centres still practise a policy of mandatory laparotomy for abdominal gunshot wounds because of the higher morbidity associated with delayed diagnosis.[24,25] However, in one study a negative laparotomy rate (absence of injury) was observed in 12% of gunshots, 23% of stab wounds and 6% of blunt trauma, suggesting that there is a more accurate investigation of the abdomen in blunt trauma.[26] Overall, negative laparotomies are associated with a morbidity of 5–22%.[27]

Selective laparotomy (i.e. selective conservatism) in penetrating injury

Several studies have considered the possibilities of selectively treating certain patients by observation only, even when a laparotomy seems to be required. Two South African studies reviewed selective conservatism in the management of abdominal gunshot wounds. Muckart et al. reported no delayed laparotomies or morbidity, with only a 7% negative laparotomy rate,[25] while Demetriades et al. had a delayed laparotomy rate of 17%.[28]

It is obvious that the decision not to operate should be carefully considered; if taken, meticulous and repeated re-examination of the patient for changing abdominal signs should be performed. A general dictum should be that the more there is uncertainty in the assessment, and the more inexperienced the assessor, the more aggressive should be the tendency towards laparotomy.

OPERATIVE MANAGEMENT OF ABDOMINAL TRAUMA

Timing of laparotomy in patients with multisystem trauma

In patients who are judged, by any of the diagnostic criteria above, to need a laparotomy for control of their injuries, the timing of laparotomy in relation to the detection and/or repair of concomitant injuries requires input from an experienced trauma surgeon. Although open to debate, the following

scenarios are offered along with a suggested algorithm (**Fig. 13.1**).

THE UNSTABLE PATIENT WITH INTRA-ABDOMINAL BLEEDING

The unstable patient with obvious intra-abdominal haemorrhage should undergo immediate operative intervention. However, if other injuries are also pressing (e.g. severe closed head injury or associated pelvic haemorrhage), a 'damage control' procedure (abbreviated laparotomy) should be considered to allow management of the patient's physiology or other life-threatening injuries.

During the laparotomy, however brief, if the patient had an initial Glasgow Coma Scale (GCS) of less than 815, it is recommended that intracranial pressure monitoring be instituted. The most lethal secondary brain injury is induced by hypotension or hypoxia.

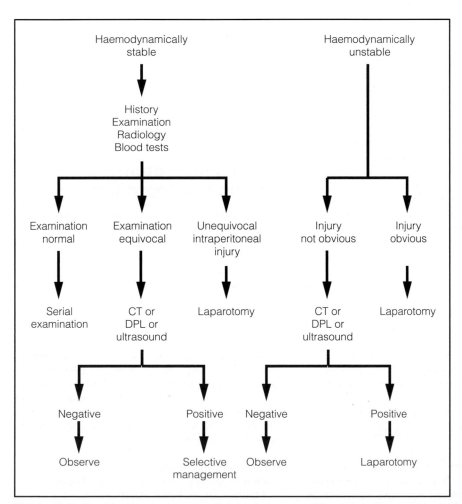

Figure 13.1 • Algorithm for management of abdominal trauma. CT, computed tomography; DPL, diagnostic peritoneal lavage.

If a widened mediastinum is present, the situation must be assessed and priorities of care selected. In the patient who is unstable because of intra-abdominal pathology, the diagnostic processes for the mediastinum may have to take place **after** the therapeutic laparotomy. Consideration should be given to the use of beta-blockade and hypotensive resuscitation until the aorta/great vessels can be properly evaluated.

There is considerable information available to support medical treatment of contained thoracic aortic injuries until other injuries are stabilised.[29,30]

THE UNSTABLE PATIENT WITH INTRA-ABDOMINAL AND PELVIC HAEMORRHAGE

In the unstable patient with both intra-abdominal haemorrhage and pelvic bleeding, the surgeon must decide which injury is causing the hypotension. If the DPL is grossly positive or ultrasound demonstrates a large amount of fluid in Morrison's pouch, laparotomy should be performed promptly. As most fractures of the pelvis bleed extraperitoneally, this bleeding is unlikely to originate in the pelvis. An unstable patient who has signs of bleeding from both pelvis and abdomen should have external stabilisation of the pelvis, with a knotted sheet, a pneumatic antishock garment (PASG) or external fixation applied immediately, followed by laparotomy or angiography of the pelvis and embolisation of bleeding vessels. Ultrasound is unreliable for quantifying injuries in such circumstances and, if the patient is stable enough, CT of both pelvis and abdomen should be carried out. Not only will CT provide significant information regarding the pelvic fractures, it will also give information as to possible injury to intra-abdominal organs. Furthermore, it may exclude a diaphragmatic rupture, which has a significant association with pelvic fractures. If the DPL is only mildly positive (red cell count <200 000/mm^3) or ultrasound demonstrates blood only in the pelvis and the major bleeding appears to be of pelvic origin, the patient will benefit from external fixation. Intrapelvic bleeding that is not controlled by external fixation is best dealt with by angiography and embolisation if the bleeding is arterial and by packing or PASG if it is venous.

THE STABLE PATIENT WITH COMBINED HEAD, CHEST AND ABDOMINAL INJURIES

In stable patients with combined head, chest and abdominal injuries, CT with contrast can rapidly identify injuries that need operative intervention. A study by Wisner et al. described 800 patients who were thought to have potentially correctable injuries to both the head and the abdomen.[31] Of these, only 52 had a head injury requiring craniotomy, 40 required laparotomy, and only three needed both craniotomy and therapeutic laparotomy. These results lend support to the concept that if patients with combined head and abdominal trauma are stable and have a negative ultrasound (or DPL), they can undergo CT of both the head and abdomen. Although it was previously thought that patients with the combination of neurological injury and solid abdominal organ injury were not candidates for observational treatment, this view has recently been challenged and many patients with head trauma and stable liver/spleen injuries are now being treated non-operatively.[32]

THE PATIENT WITH ABDOMINAL INJURIES AND LIMB FRACTURES

With the exception of pelvic fractures, fracture/dislocations and in the presence of vascular impairment, most fractures can be simply splinted during other surgical procedures. Open fractures should be irrigated and debrided within 6 hours of the injury, and antibiotics administered. Although there is still considerable debate about the timing of fracture fixation in multitrauma patients, those with head and/or pulmonary injuries still benefit from early fracture fixation, if hypotension and hypoxia can be avoided during the surgery.

Trauma laparotomy: a systematic approach

If it is decided that the injured patient would benefit from laparotomy, the operation should be approached in an orderly fashion. Although the detailed treatment of specific intra-abdominal injuries is beyond the scope of this chapter, it is important to recognise the components of the 'trauma laparotomy'. The vital initial goals are to **stop the bleeding** and **limit contamination**.

PREPARATION

An adequately stocked operating theatre is essential, and once the decision has been made to operate, rapid transport to the theatre must be initiated. Delay in surgery is the most common cause of unnecessary ongoing bleeding. In addition to routine equipment, the following should be considered as mandatory equipment:

- rapid infusion devices;
- blood warming equipment (Alton Deane, Mallincrodt, or Level One);
- patient warming blankets (e.g. Bair Hugger);
- autotransfusion if available.

INCISION

A long midline abdominal incision is used, one that can be extended inferiorly or superiorly as a sternotomy. The ideal incision is always 'too big rather than too small' and should extend from the xiphisternum to the symphysis pubis.

BLEEDING CONTROL

If upon opening the abdomen gross blood is encountered, as much as possible is scooped out, and the abdomen is packed using layered abdominal swabs:

- below the left hemidiaphragm;
- lateral to the descending colon;
- the pelvis;
- lateral to the ascending colon;
- below the liver;
- lateral to the liver;
- over the dome of the liver, under the right hemidiaphragm;
- central abdomen.

Additional packs are used to isolate bleeding areas as required.

With blunt injuries, the most likely sources of bleeding are the liver, spleen and mesentery. The solid organs are packed and bleeders in the mesentery are clamped using artery or mosquito forceps. No attempt is made to tie off individual vessels (which is time-consuming) until all major bleeding has been controlled with clamps. If necessary, a soft bowel clamp is used across the mesentery to control all mesenteric bleeding.

With penetrating injuries, the liver and retroperitoneal structures, vascular structures and mesentery are all examined.

If packing does not control the bleeding, the blood supply to the organ is isolated using proximal clamping or isolation techniques. If additional assistance is needed for blood pressure control, the abdominal aorta can be manually compressed at the hiatus. When the patient is reasonably stable, the packs are removed systematically, uncovering the most likely injury **last**. Any bleeding sites are then rapidly controlled by clamps, sutures or repacking as needed.

CONTAMINATION CONTROL

Gross contamination from the gastrointestinal tract is quickly controlled with sutures or staples.

PHYSIOLOGICAL CONTROL

No further surgery is performed until the anaesthesia team has the patient stabilised. This may require a period of resuscitation in the intensive care unit.

FULL INSPECTION FOR INJURY

Once there is control of haemorrhage and contamination, a systematic inspection is performed at a more leisurely pace.

In addition to inspecting the liver and spleen, a full trauma laparotomy includes exploration of the anterior/posterior stomach; the entire large and small bowel (including the duodenum); the diaphragm; the gastrohepatic ligament; the head, body and tail of the pancreas; and any central retroperitoneal haematomas. In order to achieve this, it will be necessary not only to perform a conventional reflection of the duodenum (Kocher manoeuvre) but also to reflect the right and left hemicolon to view the great vessels (Cattel–Braasch and Mattox manoeuvres).[33]

The abdomen is only closed when it is safe to do so (see sections Damage control laparotomy and Abdominal compartment syndrome below).

Damage control laparotomy

Since the mid-1980s, there has been a re-emergence of the concept of packing and closing for abdominal injuries with profuse haemorrhage. Further experience with this technique has resulted in its extension to patients with other vascular/intestinal injuries, and new terms such as 'damage control' surgery, 'abbreviated laparotomy', 'staged laparotomy' or 'planned reoperation' have emerged.[34]

The concept of damage control has as its objective the delay in imposition of additional surgical stress at a moment of physiological frailty. The concept is not new: livers were packed as many as 90 years ago, although failure to understand the underlying rationale or deal with the resulting disruption to physiological processes led to disastrous results.

In 1979, Elerding et al. analysed fatal hepatic haemorrhage after trauma and reported that 82% of deaths following liver trauma were caused by uncontrollable haemorrhage and a progressive coagulopathy, seemingly exacerbated by hypothermia and acidosis.[35] The concept of packing was re-examined, and the technique of initial abortion of laparotomy, establishment of intra-abdominal pack tamponade and then completion of the procedure once coagulation returned to an acceptable level proved to be life-saving. This approach was initially advocated for patients with severe liver injuries, especially those with retrohepatic venous injuries. When properly applied, packs above/below the liver can compress and control venous injuries long enough for the patient's coagulopathy, acidosis and temperature to be corrected.

Often, when the patient is returned to the operating room after packing for liver injuries, the bleeding has already stopped, and irrigation, debridement and formal closure are all that are required. The concept of staging applies to both routine and emergency procedures, and it can apply equally well in the chest, pelvis and neck as in the abdomen.

This approach has been used for patients with both penetrating and blunt injuries, and it generally includes clamping of major bleeding vessels, packing of bleeding solid organ injuries and stapling/dividing bowel injuries but without reconstruction. A variety of temporary methods of closure of the abdomen have been developed, including mesh and other synthetic material, plastic intravenous bags and towel clips. However, it must be remembered that the type of closure is much less important than the recognition of the need to terminate the operation and save the patient.

The settings for initiating damage control generally and the stages that are followed are described below.

PATIENT SELECTION FOR DAMAGE CONTROL

Patients are selected for a damage control approach if there is:

- inability to achieve haemostasis;
- inaccessible major venous injury, e.g. retrohepatic vena cava;
- anticipated need for a time-consuming procedure (>90 minutes);
- demand for non-operative control of other injuries, e.g. fractured pelvis;
- inability to approximate the abdominal incision;
- desire to reassess the intra-abdominal contents (directed relook).

Irrespective of setting, a coagulopathy in the presence of hypothermia is the single most common reason for abortion of a planned procedure or the curtailment of definitive surgery. It is important to abort the surgery before the coagulopathy becomes obvious.

Hirshberg and Mattox[36] described three distinct indications for planned reoperation in severely injured patients:

- avoidance of irreversible physiological insult in a hypothermic coagulopathic patient by rapid termination of the surgical procedure;
- inability to obtain direct haemostasis (by ligation, suture or vascular repair), necessitating indirect control of bleeding by packing or balloon tamponade;
- massive visceral oedema precluding formal closure of the abdomen or chest.

Garrison et al.[37] described criteria that predicted the need to pack early for severe intra-abdominal haemorrhage:

- Injury Severity Score (ISS) >35;
- coagulopathy (prothrombin time >19 seconds);
- hypotension (systolic blood pressure <70 mmHg) for longer than 70 minutes;
- pH <7.2;
- serum lactate >5 mmol/L;
- temperature <34°C.

The cumulative experience with packing/damage control operations has resulted in a survival rate of 48%. In their study of 46 patients with penetrating abdominal injury who required transfusion of more than 10 units of blood, Rotondo et al. identified a subset of patients they called their 'maximum injury' group, whose survival after damage control was markedly better than an equivalent group who underwent definitive laparotomy (10 of 13 survived, compared with 1 of 9).[34]

Damage control procedures can be considered under the following stages.

STAGE 1: DAMAGE CONTROL PROCEDURE

In damage control, the technical aspects of surgery are dictated by the injury pattern, with the primary objectives as follows.

Arrest bleeding and the resulting (causative) coagulopathy

Procedures for haemorrhage control include:

- repair or ligation of accessible blood vessels;
- occlusion of inflow into the bleeding organ (e.g. Pringle's manoeuvre for bleeding liver);
- tamponade using wraps or packs;
- intravascular shunting;
- intraoperative or postoperative embolisation;
- autotransfusion if available.

Limit contamination and the sequelae thereof

This is achieved by:

- ligation or stapling of bowel;
- isolation of pancreatic injury;
- adequate suction drainage (e.g. with a Blake's drain).

Temporary abdominal closure

The abdomen is closed to limit heat and fluid loss and to protect viscera. This depends on whether the abdomen can be approximated to achieve closure. If not, closure can be achieved using the following.

- Towel clips.
- OpSite 'sandwich' or 'Vacpac': a technique in which one side of an abdominal swab is covered with OpSite and the swab is placed with the OpSite in contact with the bowel; two

suction drains are placed in the abdominal wound, and a further sheet of OpSite is used to seal the abdomen.
- Bogota bag: temporary silo.

STAGE 2: TRANSFER TO THE INTENSIVE CARE UNIT FOR ONGOING RESUSCITATION

The timing of the transfer of the patient from the operating theatre to the intensive care unit is critical. Prompt transfer is cost-effective; premature transfer is counter-productive. In addition, once haemostasis has been properly achieved, it may not be necessary to abort the procedure and it may be possible to proceed to definitive surgery. Conversely, there are some patients with severe head injuries where the coagulopathy is induced by severe irreversible cerebral damage, and further surgical energy is futile.

In the operating theatre, efforts must be started to reverse all the associated adjuncts, such as acidosis, hypothermia and hypoxia, and it may be possible to improve the coagulation status through these methods alone. Adequate time should still be allowed for this, following which reassessment of the abdominal injuries should take place, as it is not infrequent to discover further injuries or ongoing bleeding.

STAGE 3: RESUSCITATION IN THE INTENSIVE CARE UNIT

Priorities on reaching intensive care are:

1. Restoration of body temperature:
   (a) passive rewarming with warming blankets, warmed fluids, etc.;
   (b) active rewarming using lavage of chest or abdomen.
2. Correction of clotting profiles by blood component repletion.
3. Optimisation of oxygen delivery:
   (a) volume loading to achieve optimum preload;
   (b) haemoglobin optimisation to a value of 9 g/dL;
   (c) temperature optimisation (>35°C);
   (d) measurement and correction of lactic acidosis.
4. Monitoring of intra-abdominal pressure (IAP), to prevent abdominal compartment syndrome (ACS), using Foley (bladder) catheter or intragastric catheter.

STAGE 4: RETURN TO THE OPERATING THEATRE FOR DEFINITIVE SURGERY.

The patient is returned to the operating theatre as soon as stage 3 is achieved. The timing is determined by:

- the indication for damage control in the first place;
- the injury pattern;
- the physiological response.

Patients with persistent bleeding despite correction of the other parameters merit early return to control the bleeding. Patients who develop major ACS must be re-opened early and any further underlying causes corrected.

Every effort must be made to return **all** patients to the operating theatre within 24 hours (or, at most, 48 hours) of their initial surgery. By leaving matters longer, other problems such as adult respiratory distress syndrome, systemic inflammatory response syndrome and sepsis may intervene (cause or effect) and may preclude further surgery.

STAGE 5: DEFINITIVE SURGERY AND ABDOMINAL WALL RECONSTRUCTION IF REQUIRED

Once the patient has received definitive surgery and no further operations are contemplated, then the abdominal wall can be closed. This is often difficult and methods include:

- primary closure;
- closure of the sheath, leaving the skin open;
- silo bag (Bogota bag), with subsequent gradual closure;
- grafts with Vicryl mesh, Gore-Tex sheets, or other synthetic sheets.

ABDOMINAL COMPARTMENT SYNDROME (ACS)

ACS may be defined as the adverse physiological consequences that occur as a result of an acute increase in IAP.[38] Clinically, the organ systems most affected include the cardiovascular, renal and pulmonary systems. Decreased cardiac output, increased peripheral resistance, oliguria, anuria, increased airway pressures, decreased compliance and hypoxia may all occur. If untreated, ACS leads to lethal organ failure. In contrast, decompression of the abdominal cavity immediately reverses the above pathophysiological changes. The most common cause of the syndrome is coagulopathy and postoperative haemorrhage.

Raised IAP is divided into:

- normal (<10 cmH$_2$O);
- mild (10–25 cmH$_2$O);
- moderate (25–40 cmH$_2$O);
- severe (>40 cmH$_2$O).

To make the diagnosis of IAP at least three of the following are needed:

- appropriate clinical scenario (liver packing or large pelvic haematoma);
- increased IAP (>25 cmH_2O);
- increase in P_aCO_2 to >45 mmHg;
- decrease in tidal volume and rise in airway pressure;
- sudden decrease in urinary output.

Pathophysiology

The incidence of increased IAP (taken as >25 mmHg or >30 cmH_2O) may be 30% of postoperative general surgery patients in intensive care; after emergency surgery the incidence is even higher. The causes of acutely increased IAP are usually multi-factorial. The first clinical reports of postoperative increased IAP were often after aortic surgery, with postoperative haemorrhage from the graft suture line. Peritonitis and intra-abdominal sepsis, tissue oedema and ileus are the predominant causes of increased IAP. Raised IAP in trauma patients is often caused by a combination of blood loss and tissue oedema. Patients with trauma and the surgery of trauma are one of the commonest subsets to develop increased IAP and ACS.

Causes of increased IAP include:

- tissue oedema secondary to insults such as ischaemia, trauma and sepsis;
- ileus;
- intraperitoneal or retroperitoneal haematoma;
- ascites;
- pneumoperitoneum.

Effect of raised IAP on organ function

RENAL FUNCTION

In 1945, Bradley, in a study of 17 volunteers, demonstrated that there was a reduction in renal plasma flow and glomerular filtration rate (GFR) in association with increased IAP.[39] In 1982, Harman et al. showed that an increase in IAP from 0 to 20 mmHg in dogs resulted in a decrease in GFR of 25%.[39] When IAP reached 40 mmHg, the dogs were resuscitated. Cardiac output returned to normal but GFR and renal blood flow did not improve, indicating a local effect on renal blood flow. However, the situation in seriously ill patients may be different and the exact cause of renal dysfunction in the intensive care situation is not clear because of the complexity of critically ill patients. In a recent study, it was found that of 20 patients with

increased IAP and renal impairment, 13 already had impairment before IAP increased.[40]

The most likely direct effect of increased IAP is an increase in renal vascular resistance, coupled with a moderate reduction in cardiac output. Pressure on the ureter has been ruled out as a cause, as investigators have placed ureteric stents with no improvement in function. Other factors that may contribute to renal dysfunction include hormonal factors and intraparenchymal renal pressures. The absolute value of IAP that is required to cause renal impairment is probably in the region of 20 mmHg. Maintaining adequate cardiovascular filling pressures in the presence of increased IAP also seems to be important.

CARDIAC FUNCTION

Increased IAP reduces cardiac output as well as increasing central venous pressure, systemic vascular resistance, pulmonary artery pressure and pulmonary artery wedge pressure. Cardiac output is affected mainly by a reduction in stroke volume, secondary to a reduction in preload and an increase in afterload. This is further aggravated by hypovolaemia. Paradoxically, in the presence of hypovolaemia, an increase in IAP can be temporarily associated with an increase in cardiac output. Venous stasis occurs in the legs of patients with IAP values above 12 cmH_2O. In addition, recent studies of patients undergoing laparoscopic cholecystectomy show up to a fourfold increase in renin and aldosterone levels.

RESPIRATORY FUNCTION

In association with increased IAP, there is diaphragmatic stenting, which exerts a restrictive effect on the lungs with reduction in ventilation, decreased lung compliance, increase in airway pressures and reduction in tidal volumes. The mechanism by which increased IAP impairs pulmonary function appears to be purely mechanical. As IAP increases, the diaphragm is forced higher into the chest, thereby compressing the lungs. Adequate ventilation can still be achieved, but only at the cost of increased airway pressures.

In critically ill, ventilated patients the effect on the respiratory system can be significant, resulting in reduced lung volumes, impaired gas exchange and high ventilatory pressures. Hypercarbia can occur and the resulting acidosis can be exacerbated by simultaneous cardiovascular depression as a result of the raised IAP. The effects of raised IAP on the respiratory system in the intensive care setting can sometimes be life-threatening, requiring urgent abdominal decompression. Patients with true ACS undergoing abdominal decompression demonstrate a remarkable change in their intraoperative vital signs.

VISCERAL PERFUSION

Interest in visceral perfusion has increased with increased awareness of gastric tonometry, and there is an association between IAP and visceral perfusion as measured by gastric pH. This has been confirmed recently in 18 patients undergoing laparoscopy, where a reduction in blood flow of 11 and 54% was seen in the duodenum and stomach, respectively, at an IAP of 15 cmH$_2$O. Animal studies suggest that reduction in visceral perfusion is selective, affecting intestinal blood flow before, for example, adrenal blood flow. In a study of 73 patients after laparotomy, it was shown that IAP and pH are strongly associated, suggesting that early decreases in visceral perfusion are related to IAP at levels as low as 15 cmH$_2$O.[40] Visceral reperfusion injury is a major consideration after a period of raised IAP, and may of itself have fatal consequences.

INTRACRANIAL CONTENTS

Raised IAP can have a marked effect on intracranial pathophysiology and cause severe rises in intracranial pressure.

Measurement of IAP

The most common method for measuring IAP uses a urinary catheter, as described by Kron et al.[41] The patient is positioned flat in the bed. A standard Foley catheter is used with a T-piece bladder pressure device attached between the urinary catheter and the drainage tubing. This piece is then connected to a pressure transducer. The pressure transducer is placed in the midaxillary line and the urinary tubing is clamped. Approximately 50 mL isotonic saline is inserted into the bladder via a three-way stopcock. After zeroing, the pressure on the monitor is recorded.

MEASUREMENT TECHNIQUES

The following factors are important in achieving effective IAP measurements.

- A strict protocol and staff education on the technique and interpretation of IAP is essential.
- Very high pressures (especially unexpected ones) are usually caused by a blocked urinary catheter.
- The size of the urinary catheter does not matter.
- The volume of saline instilled into the bladder is not critical, but it should be enough to overcome the resistance of the contracted bladder; 50–100 mL is adequate.
- A central venous pressure manometer system can be used but it is more cumbersome than online monitoring.
- Elevation of the catheter and measuring the urine column provides a rough guide and is simple to perform.

- If the patient is not lying flat, IAP can be measured from the pubic symphysis.

Treatment of raised IAP

GENERAL SUPPORT

In general, the best treatment is prevention, by minimising the causative agents and by early appreciation of the potential complications.

REVERSIBLE FACTORS

The second aspect of management is to correct any reversible cause of ACS, such as intra-abdominal bleeding. Massive retroperitoneal haemorrhage is often associated with a fractured pelvis, and consideration should be given to measures that would control haemorrhage, such as pelvic fixation or vessel embolisation. In some cases, severe gaseous distension or acute colonic pseudo-obstruction can occur in patients in intensive care. This may respond to drugs such as neostigmine but if it is severe, surgical decompression may be necessary (see also Chapter 10). Ileus is a common cause of raised IAP in patients in intensive care. There is little that can be actively done in these circumstances apart from optimising the patient's cardiorespiratory status and serum electrolytes.

It must be remembered that ACS is often only a symptom of an underlying problem. In a prospective review of 88 patients after laparotomy, Sugrue et al. found those with an IAP of 18 cmH$_2$O had an increased odds ratio for intra-abdominal sepsis of 3.9 (95% confidence interval 0.7–22.7).[40] Abdominal evaluation for sepsis is a priority and this obviously should include a rectal examination as well as investigations such as ultrasound and CT. Surgery is obviously the mainstay of treatment in patients whose rise in IAP is caused by postoperative bleeding.

Maxwell et al. reported on secondary ACS, which can occur without abdominal injury, and stated that, again, early recognition could improve outcome.[42]

SURGERY

As yet, there are few guidelines for exactly when surgical decompression is required in the presence of raised IAP. Some studies have stated that abdominal decompression is the only treatment and that it should be performed early in order to prevent ACS. This is an overstatement and not supported by strong evidence.

The indications for abdominal decompression are related to correcting pathophysiological abnormalities as much as achieving a precise and optimum IAP. The abdomen is decompressed and a temporary abdominal closure is achieved. A large number of different techniques have been used to facilitate temporary abdominal closure, including intravenous bags, Velcro, silicone and zips. Whatever technique, it is important that effective decompression be achieved with adequate incisions.

Tips for the surgical decompression of raised IAP include the following.

- Early investigation and correction of the cause of raised IAP.
- Ongoing abdominal bleeding with raised IAP requires urgent operative intervention.
- Reduction in urinary output is a late sign of renal impairment; gastric tonometry, or urinary bladder pressure monitoring, may provide earlier information on visceral perfusion.
- Abdominal decompression requires a full-length abdominal incision.

The surgical dressing should be closed using a sandwich technique with two suction drains placed laterally to facilitate fluid removal from the wound. If the abdomen is very tight, pre-closure with a silo should be considered.[43]

Unfortunately, clinical infection is common in the open abdomen and the infection is usually polymicrobial. It is desirable to close the abdominal

defect as soon as possible. This is often not possible because of persistent tissue oedema. There is no indication for prophylactic antibiotics.

Summary

The concept of IAP measurement and its significance is increasingly important in the intensive care unit and is rapidly becoming part of routine care. Patients with raised IAP require close and careful monitoring, aggressive resuscitation and a low index of suspicion for requirement of surgical abdominal decompression.

SCORING SYSTEMS FOR INJURIES

Penetrating Abdominal Trauma Index

Moore et al. facilitated identification of the high-risk patient when they developed the Penetrating Abdominal Trauma Index (PATI) scoring system (**Tables 13.1** and **13.2**).[44] In a group of 114 patients

Table 13.1 • Calculation of the Penetrating Abdominal Trauma Index (PATI)

Organ injured	Risk factor	Score	Injury
Duodenum	5	1	Single wall
		2	<25% wall
		3	>25% wall
		4	Duodenal wall and blood supply
		5	Requiring pancreaticoduodenectomy
Pancreas	5	1	Tangential
		2	Through-and-through (duct intact)
		3	Requiring major debridement or distal duct injury
		4	Proximal duct injury
		5	Requiring pancreaticoduodenectomy
Liver	4	1	Non-bleeding: peripheral
		2	Bleeding, central, or requiring minor debridement
		3	Requiring major debridement or hepatic vessels artery ligation
		4	Requiring lobectomy
		5	Requiring lobectomy with caval repair or extensive bilobar debridement
Large bowel	4	1	Serosa
		2	Single wall
		3	<25% wall
		4	>25% wall
		5	Colon wall and blood supply
Major vascular	4	1	<25% wall transected
		2	>25% wall transected
		3	Complete transection: primary repair
		4	Requiring interposition grafting or bypass
		5	Requiring ligation

Table 13.1 • (*Cont'd*) Calculation of the Penetrating Abdominal Trauma Index (PATI)

Organ injured	Risk factor	Score	Injury
Spleen	3	1 2 3 4 5	Non-bleeding Requiring cautery or haemostatic agent Requiring minor debridement or suturing Requiring partial resection Requiring splenectomy
Kidney	3	1 2 3 4 5	Non-bleeding Requiring minor debridement or suturing Requiring major debridement Pedicle or major caliceal injury Requiring nephrectomy
Extrahepatic biliary	3	1 2 3 4 5	Contusion Requiring cholecystectomy <25% common duct wall >25% common duct wall Requiring biliary enteric reconstruction
Small bowel	2	1 2 3 4 5	Single wall Through-and-through <25% wall or two to three injuries 25% wall or four to five injuries Wall or blood supply or more than five injuries
Stomach	2	1 2 3 4 5	Single wall Through-and-through Requiring minor debridement Requiring wedge resection Requiring >35% resection
Ureter	2	1 2 3 4 5	Contusion Laceration Requiring minor debridement Requiring segmental resection Requiring reconstruction
Bladder	1	1 2 3 4 5	Single wall Through-and-through Requiring debridement Requiring wedge resection Requiring reconstruction
Bone	1	1 2 3 4 5	Periosteum Cortex Through-and-through Intra-articular Major bone loss
Minor vascular	1	1 2 3 4 5	Non-bleeding small haematoma Non-bleeding large haematoma Requiring suturing Requiring ligation of isolated vessels Requiring ligation of named vessels

The PATI score is obtained for each organ by multiplying its risk factor by the injury estimate score, e.g. duodenum >25% wall injured would be 5 × 3 and liver non-bleeding peripheral injury would be 4 × 1. The final PATI score is the sum of the individual organs (in this example 15 + 4 = 19).

From Moore EE, Dunn EL, Moore JB, Thompson JS. Penetrating Abdominal Trauma Index. J Trauma 1981; 21:439–45, with permission.

Table 13.2 • Use of the Penetrating Abdominal Trauma Index (PATI) to assess the likelihood of postoperative complications

PATI score	Percentage of patients developing complications
1–5	0
6–15	6
16–25	12
26–35	44
36–45	47
46–55	50
>55	50

From Moore EE, Dunn EL, Moore JB, Thompson JS. Penetrating Abdominal Trauma Index. J Trauma 1981; 21:439–45, with permission.

with gunshot wounds to the abdomen, they showed that a PATI score greater than 25 dramatically increased the risk of postoperative complications (46% of patients with a PATI score of >25 developed serious postoperative complications compared with 7% of those with a PATI score of <25). Subsequent reports have confirmed the accuracy of a high PATI score in predicting postoperative complications and have also identified multiple blood transfusions and the presence of underlying medical illness as a further predictor of postoperative complications.[45]

Organ injury scaling systems

The American Association for the Surgery of Trauma (AAST) has developed an organ injury scaling system for all major injuries in the body.[45–52] The scores not only allow a clear anatomical language when dealing with organ injury but also, since surgical policies are often dictated by the injuries sustained, a degree of consistency in both treatment and prognosis. The scaling system can be accessed on the Internet at http://www.aast.org

SURGICAL DECISION-MAKING IN ABDOMINAL TRAUMA

Experience in dealing with injury clearly leads to a better outcome: good judgement comes from experience. Unfortunately, experience comes from bad judgement. There is limited evidence-based decision-making in trauma, although certain practice guidelines have been developed.[53]

Antibiotic prophylaxis in abdominal trauma

Guidelines for patient selection and specific antimicrobial regimens are based on good evidence, those regarding high-risk patients and duration of therapy less so (**Boxes 13.2–13.5**).[54,55] The trauma surgery setting is fundamentally different from that of elective surgery, especially with regard to prophylactic antibiotics. Antibiotics are given after the peritoneal insult and possible contamination has occurred.

Hepatic injury

Repair and resection for treatment of hepatic trauma demands a working knowledge of the anatomy of the liver, including the arterial supply, portal venous supply and hepatic venous drainage. Segmental anatomical resection has been well documented but usually is not applicable to injury. The three main hepatic veins divide the liver into four sections: right posterior lateral, right anterior medial, left anterior and left posterior. Each of these sectors receives a portal pedicle. The liver is practically divided into eight Couinaud's segments (**Fig 13.2**).

Understanding the anatomy also helps to explain some of the patterns of injury following blunt trauma. There are also differences in tissue elasticity, which determine injury patterns. The forces from

---

Box 13.2 • Evidence-based guidelines for prophylactic antibiotic administration: summary of recommendations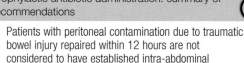

1. Patients with peritoneal contamination due to traumatic bowel injury repaired within 12 hours are not considered to have established intra-abdominal infections, and should be treated with prophylactic antimicrobials for 24 hours or less **(Evidence level, 1)**

2. Systemic antibiotics should be administered as soon as possible after injury for patients with penetrating trauma requiring surgical intervention **(Evidence level, 2)**

3. A single broad-spectrum agent is at least as safe and effective as a double or triple antibiotic therapeutic regimen **(Evidence level, 2)**

4. Patients with a fully removable focus of inflammation (e.g. bowel necrosis) should be treated with prophylactic antimicrobials for 24 hours or less **(Evidence level, 2)**

5. Patients with more extensive conditions should be treated as having more extensive infections, and given therapeutic antimicrobials for greater than 24 hours **(Evidence level, 3)**

Box 13.3 • Evidence-based guidelines for duration of antibiotic therapy: summary of recommendations

1. High postoperative septic complications can be expected in patients with gunshot injuries to the colon, high PATI scores, major blood loss, and common need for postoperative care. There is no evidence that extending prophylactic antibiotic therapy beyond 24 hours decreases that high risk (**Evidence level, 2**)

2. Antimicrobial therapy of most established intra-abdominal infections should be limited to no more than 5 days (**Evidence level, 2**)

3. Antimicrobial therapy can be discontinued in patients when they have no clinical evidence of infection such as fever or leucocytosis (**Evidence level, 2**)

4. Continued clinical evidence of infection at the end of the time period designated for antimicrobial therapy should prompt appropriate diagnostic investigations rather than prolongation of antimicrobial treatment (**Evidence level, 3**)

5. If adequate source control cannot be achieved, a longer duration of antimicrobial therapy may be warranted (**Evidence level, 3**)

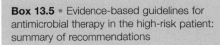

Box 13.5 • Evidence-based guidelines for antimicrobial therapy in the high-risk patient: summary of recommendations

1. In patients with intra-abdominal infections, treatment failure and death is associated with patient-related risk factors such as advanced age, poor nutritional status, low serum albumin concentration, and pre-existing medical disease. A higher APACHE II score is the most consistently recognised risk factor for both death and treatment failure (**Evidence level, 1**)

2. Disease and treatment-related risk factors, including nosocomial origin of infection, the presence of resistant pathogens and the lack of adequate source control, are associated with treatment failure and death (**Evidence level, 2**)

3. Routine addition of an aminoglycoside to other agents having broad-spectrum Gram-negative coverage provides no additional benefit (**Evidence level, 2**)

4. Addition of empiric antifungal therapy with fluconazole is reasonable for patients with postoperative intra-abdominal infections at high risk for candidiasis (**Evidence level, 2**)

5. Patients at higher risk for failure (e.g. damage control) should be treated with an antimicrobial regimen having a broader spectrum of coverage of Gram-negative aerobic/facultative anaerobic organisms (de-escalation therapy) (**Evidence level, 3**)

Box 13.4 • Evidence-based guidelines for antimicrobial regimens: summary of recommendations

1. Antimicrobial regimens for intra-abdominal infections should cover common aerobic and anaerobic enteric flora. No regimen has been demonstrated to be superior to another (**Evidence level, 1**)

2. Once-daily administration of aminoglycoside is the preferred dosing regimen for patients receiving these agents for intra-abdominal infections (**Evidence level, 2**)

3. Aminoglycosides should be avoided in the acute trauma patient due to difficulty in reaching adequate minimum inhibitory concentrations without toxicity (**Evidence level, 3**)

4. For less severely ill patients with community-acquired infections, antimicrobial agents having a narrower spectrum of activity, such as antianaerobic cephalosporins, are preferable to more costly agents having broader coverage of Gram-negative organisms and/or a greater risk of toxicity (**Evidence level, 3**)

5. The routine use of intraoperative cultures is controversial, and there is no evidence that altering the antimicrobial regimen on the basis of intraoperative culture results improves outcome (**Evidence level, 3**)

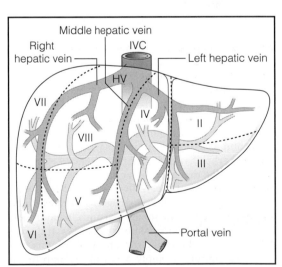

Figure 13.2 • Couinaud's segments of the liver. With permission from Garden OJ, Bismuth H. Anatomy of the liver. In: Carter DC, Russell RCG, Pitt HA, Bismuth H (eds) Operative surgery: hepatobiliary and pancreatic surgery. London: Chapman & Hall, 1996; pp. 1–4. Reproduced by permission of Edward Arnold.

blunt injury are usually direct compressive forces or shear forces. The elastic tissue within arterial blood vessels makes them less susceptible to tearing than any other structures within the liver. Venous and biliary ductal tissues are moderately resistant to shear forces, whereas the liver parenchyma is the least resistant of all. Therefore, fractures within the liver parenchyma tend to occur along segmental fissures or directly into the parenchyma. This causes shearing of lateral branches to the major hepatic and portal veins. With severe deceleration injury, the origin of the hepatic veins may be ripped from the inferior vena cava, causing devastating haemorrhage. Similarly, the small branches from the caudate lobe entering directly into the cava are at high risk for shearing, with linear tears on the caval surface.

Direct compressive forces usually cause tearing between segmental fissures in an anterior–posterior sagittal orientation. Horizontal fracture lines into the parenchyma give the characteristic burst pattern to such liver injuries. If the fracture lines are parallel, these have been dubbed 'bear-claw' type injuries and probably represent where the ribs have been compressed directly into the parenchyma. Occasionally, there will be a single fracture line across the horizontal plane of the liver, usually between the anterior and posterior segments. This can cause massive haemorrhage if there is direct extension or continuity with the peritoneal cavity.

The liver is at risk in any penetrating trauma to the right upper quadrant of the abdomen. Virtually all penetrating injuries to the abdomen should be explored promptly, especially when they occur in conjunction with hypotension. The surgeon should be aware that penetrating injuries to the right lower chest which present with haemothorax may have penetrated the diaphragm, with the bleeding originating from the liver.

The diagnosis of blunt injury can be difficult. Knowledge of the mechanism of injury, such as a history of rapid deceleration, may be helpful. Shoulder harnesses can cause blunt injuries to the liver, and fracture of underlying ribs can directly lacerate the liver. Contrast-enhanced CT has improved the diagnosis of significant liver injury.

The treatment of severe liver injuries begins with temporary control of haemorrhage. Most catastrophic bleeding from hepatic injury is venous in nature and can therefore be controlled by liver packs. If there is bright red blood pouring from the parenchyma, it is then appropriate to apply a vascular clamp to the porta hepatis (Pringle's manoeuvre) via the gastro-hepatic ligament. If this controls the bleeding, the surgeon should be suspicious of hepatic arterial or possible portal venous injury. While control is being obtained, it is important to establish more intravenous access lines and other monitoring devices as needed. Hypothermia should be anticipated and corrective measures taken.

After haemostasis and haemodynamic resuscitation have been achieved, any packs in the two lower abdominal quadrants are removed. If there is abdominal contamination, it is appropriate to control this as rapidly as possible. The packs in the left upper quadrant are then removed. If there is an associated spleen injury, a decision must be made either to remove it promptly or to clamp the hilum of the spleen temporarily with a vascular clamp to reduce further bleeding. Finally, the packs are removed in the right upper quadrant and the injury to the liver rapidly assessed.

If there is bleeding from the porta hepatis, careful exploration for a portal vein injury should be carried out, with repair or shunting. Traction on the dome of the liver which produces a sudden gush of retrohepatic blood should make the surgeon suspicious of injury to the posterior hepatic veins or inferior vena cava. The options for hepatic vein and cava injuries include direct compression (packing), extension of the laceration, atrial–caval shunt, non-shunt isolation (Heaney technique) and veno-veno bypass. Liver packs can also be definitive treatment, particularly when there is bilobar injury, or they can simply buy time if the patient develops coagulopathy or hypothermia or there are no blood resources.

Pancreatic trauma

Penetrating pancreatic trauma should be obvious since the patient will almost invariably have been explored for an obvious injury.[56] Once the retroperitoneum has been violated, it is imperative for the surgeon to perform a thorough exploration in the central region, including:

- an extended Kocher manoeuvre to examine the entire duodenum;
- a right medial visceral rotation (Cattel–Braasch manoeuvre) to examine the back of the head of the pancreas;
- division of the ligament of Treitz to examine the front of the pancreas;
- division of the gastrocolic omentum to examine the top of the pancreas;
- a left medial visceral rotation to examine the anterior and posterior surfaces of the tail of the pancreas as it extends towards the splenic hilum.

Any parenchymal haematoma of the pancreatic head should undergo thorough exploration, which should include irrigation of the haematoma and adequate drainage with a suction drain (e.g. a Blake's drain).

Blunt pancreatic trauma is much more of a problem since the pancreas is a retroperitoneal organ and there may be no anterior peritoneal signs.[56] History can be helpful, for example if there is a history of epigastric trauma. The physical examination is often misleading. Amylase and blood count are non-specific; water-soluble contrast swallow has fair sensitivity, CT is 85% accurate and endoscopic retrograde cholangiopancreatography can be helpful in selected stable patients.

Injuries to the tail and body of the pancreas can usually be drained or, if there is strong suspicion of major ductal injury, resection can be carried out with good results. However, the injuries that vex the surgeon most are those to the head of the gland, particularly those with juxtaposed injuries or also involving the duodenum. Resection (Whipple procedure) is usually reserved for those patients who have destructive injuries or those in whom the blood supply to the duodenum and pancreatic head has been embarrassed. This procedure should only be embarked upon in the stable patient, with consideration being given to appropriate damage control procedures in all others. The remainder are usually treated with variations of drainage and pyloric exclusion. This would include tube duodenostomy and extensive closed drainage around the injury site. Common duct drainage is not indicated.

Aorta and inferior vena cava

Aorta and caval injuries are primarily a problem of access (rapid) and control of haemorrhage. If the surgeon opens the abdomen and there is extensive retroperitoneal bleeding centrally, there are two options. If the bleeding is primarily venous in nature, the right colon should be mobilised to the midline, including the duodenum and head of the pancreas (Cattel–Braasch manoeuvre). This will expose the infrarenal cava and infrarenal aorta. It will also facilitate access to the portal vein.

If the bleeding is primarily arterial in nature, it is best to approach the injury from the left. Initial control can be obtained by direct pressure at the oesophageal hiatus, or via the lesser sac. Additional exposure can be obtained by simply dividing the left crus of the diaphragm. Exposure includes reflecting the left colon medially and mobilising the pancreas, kidney and spleen to the midline (Mattox manoeuvre). By approaching the aorta from the left lateral position it is possible to identify the plane of Leriche more rapidly than by approaching it through the lesser sac. The problem is the coeliac and superior mesenteric ganglia, both of which can be quite dense and hinder dissection around the origins of the coeliac and superior mesenteric arteries.

Treatment of aortic or caval injuries is usually straightforward, either by direct suture or occasionally grafting. Caval injuries below the renal vein, if extensive, can be ligated, although repair is preferred. Injuries above the renal veins in the cava should be repaired if at all possible. If there is injury to the posterior wall of the vein, it is preferable to isolate the segment and repair it from within the vein using an anterior approach.

Colonic injuries (Box 13.6)

The significant morbidity and financial costs associated with creation and reversal of colostomy, and the destructive effect of colostomy on the patient's quality of life, have been cited as evidence to support the primary repair of colonic wounds.[55,57–59]

Many studies have shown primary repair of colonic injuries to be safe in patients at low risk of postoperative complications; however, identification of the high-risk patient in whom avoidance of an intraperitoneal colonic suture line may be beneficial is still controversial. Stone and Fabian excluded patients from primary repair in the presence of shock, major blood loss, more than two organs injured, faecal contamination more than 'minimal', delay to repair of more than 8 hours and wounds of the colon or abdominal wall so destructive as to require resection.[60] Murray et al. reviewed 140 patients with colonic injuries that required resection.[61] They suggested that the majority of patients can safely undergo colonic resection with primary colo-colonic anastomosis, even for severe injuries; however, there is a subgroup of critically injured patients at higher risk of anastomotic leakage (indicated by high PATI score and preoperative hypotension) who may be best treated by colostomy.[61]

Cornwell et al. also postulate that there is a group of critically injured patients (reliably identified by high PATI scores, high blood transfusion requirements and/or premorbid cardiovascular compromise) in whom suboptimal gut perfusion and postoperative acidosis is likely to be prolonged and for whom colonic repair or anastomosis is unsafe.[62]

In the 'physiologically challenged' patient, hypoperfusion of splanchnic tissues leads to local tissue hypoxia, and repair or anastomosis under these circumstances is more likely to fail. This high-risk group should be treated by damage control techniques, with restoration of continuity of the bowel once the physiological insult has been corrected. Patients should be selected for damage control by the recognition of a severe injury pattern (i.e. high PATI score) plus a combination of physiological variables, the most important of which are hypothermia, lactic acidosis, hypotension and blood transfusion requirements.[45] These factors reflect the physiological status of the patient, for us the critical determinant of the choice and extent of surgery.[55]

Box 13.6 • Evidence-based guidelines for management of colon injuries: summary of recommendations

1. Primary repair is supported for **non-destructive** colon wounds (involvement of <50% of the bowel wall without devascularisation) in the absence of peritonitis. The risk is not obviated by colostomy, and intra-abdominal sepsis frequently occurs in the absence of suture line disruption. Accordingly, the majority of colon injuries in civilian practice may be managed by primary repair (**Evidence level, 1**)

2. Patients with penetrating colon wounds which are **destructive** can undergo resection and primary anastomosis if they are:
   (a) haemodynamically stable without evidence of shock
   (b) have no significant underlying disease
   (c) have minimal associated injuries (PATI <25, ISS <25)
   (d) have no peritonitis
   (**Evidence level, 2**)

3. Given the small number of patients in high-risk categories with destructive colon injuries requiring resection who were randomised to primary repair, there is still room to consider colostomy in the management of these patients (**Evidence level, 2**)

4. Patients with shock, underlying disease, significant associated injuries or peritonitis should have destructive wounds managed by resection and colostomy (**Evidence level, 2**)

5. Colostomies performed following colon and rectal trauma can be closed within 2 weeks if contrast enema is performed to confirm distal healing. This recommendation pertains to patients who do not have non-healing bowel injury or unresolved wound sepsis or who are unstable (**Evidence level, 2**)

6. A barium enema should not be performed to rule out colon cancer or polyps prior to colostomy closure for trauma in patients who otherwise have no indications for being at risk (**Evidence level, 2**)

7. Multiple blood transfusions, shock and a high PATI score reliably identify patients at high risk for septic complications following penetrating colon injuries (**Evidence level, 2**)

Box 13.7 • Evidence-based guidelines for management of haemorrhage in pelvic fracture: summary of recommendations

1. Patients with evidence of unstable fractures of the pelvis associated with hypotension should be considered for some form of pelvic stabilisation (**Evidence level, 2**)

2. Patients with evidence of unstable pelvic fractures who warrant laparotomy should receive external pelvic stabilisation prior to laparotomy incision (**Evidence level, 2**)

3. Patients with a major pelvic fracture who have signs of ongoing bleeding after non-pelvic sources of blood loss have been ruled out should be considered for pelvic angiography and possible embolisation (**Evidence level, 2**)

4. Patients with major pelvic fractures who are found to have bleeding in the pelvis, which cannot be adequately controlled at laparotomy, should be considered for pelvic angiography and possible embolisation (**Evidence level, 2**)

5. Patients with evidence of arterial extravasation of intravenous contrast in the pelvis by CT should be considered for pelvic angiography and possible embolisation (**Evidence level, 2**)

6. Patients with hypotension and gross blood in the abdomen as evidence of intestinal perforation warrant emergency laparotomy (**Evidence level, 2**)

7. The diagnostic peritoneal tap appears to be the most reliable diagnostic test for this purpose. Urgent laparotomy is warranted for patients who demonstrate signs of continued intra-abdominal bleeding after adequate resuscitation, or evidence of intestinal perforation (**Evidence level, 2**)

8. Patients with evidence of unstable fractures of the pelvis not associated with hypotension but who do require steady and ongoing resuscitation should be considered for some form of external pelvic stabilisation (**Evidence level, 3**)

Associated complex pelvic fracture (Box 13.7)

Complex pelvic fractures can be some of the most difficult injuries to treat. Initially, they can cause devastating haemorrhage and may subsequently be associated with overwhelming pelvic sepsis and distant multiple organ failure.

For those patients who present with complex pelvic fractures and who are haemodynamically stable, diagnostic studies should be carried out as rapidly as possible, including plain films of the pelvis, CT

Colostomy as the initial management of colonic injury may perhaps be abandoned in the knowledge that the majority of patients are best served by primary colonic repair or resection with primary anastomosis, by application of the evolving concepts of damage control, and with the awareness that 'outcome is determined by the patient's physiological envelope and not by anatomic integrity'.[63,64]

and occasionally arteriogram, particularly if the patient is initially unstable, resuscitated and there is a margin of time to do the arteriogram safely. All patients with such pelvic fractures should be taken to the operating theatre as soon as the necessary diagnostic studies have been carried out or, in the case of the patient who is haemodynamically unstable, to allow continuing resuscitation.[65]

The priorities facing the surgeon are to control the pelvic haemorrhage and rule out other intra-abdominal organ injuries with associated haemorrhage. Sometimes it is prudent to perform a rapid laparotomy to exclude additional haemorrhage, but if there is not a strong suspicion of abdominal bleeding, it is best to avoid laparotomy until the pelvic bleeding has been arrested. Stabilisation of pelvic bleeding can often be achieved by the application of an external fixation device. If this fails and laparotomy has not yet been carried out, arteriography and selective embolisation is the next option. If laparotomy has already been carried out, haemostasis should be temporarily achieved by packing the wound and then making the decision as to whether to obtain a pelvic arteriogram.

Stabilisation of the pelvis is initially by compression (using a PASG, knotted sheet or external fixation). External fixation is used for stabilisation of the anterior pelvis but will fail if the posterior pelvis is unstable. These patients may require plating of the sacroiliac joint and are best managed by stabilisation with a PASG, inflated to 25–40 mmHg, and then assessed by CT and arteriography. Based on location of the injury, colostomy may be required in order to prevent contamination of the perineal wound in the post-injury period. In general, all compound injuries involving the perineum and perianal area should have a diverting colostomy.

In patients with associated major perineal injuries, after initial fixation of the pelvis has been obtained, daily wound examination, debridement and gradual removal of packs should take place. A caveat of pack removal is that the longer they are left in, the greater the risk of pelvic sepsis.

NON-OPERATIVE APPROACH TO ABDOMINAL SOLID ORGAN INJURIES (Box 13.8)[66]

Liver

In 1990, it was suggested that a number of patients with blunt liver injuries might be candidates for expectant management.[67] The success of non-operative treatment was independent of the degree of injury but rather could be predicted by the stability of patient. In a multicentre study, it was

---

Box 13.8 • Evidence-based guidelines for the non-operative management of abdominal injury: summary of recommendations

1. Non-operative management of blunt hepatic and/or splenic injuries in a haemodynamically stable patient is reasonable (**Evidence level, 2**)

2. The severity of hepatic or splenic injury (as suggested by CT grade or degree of haemoperitoneum), neurological status and/or the presence of associated injuries are not contraindications to non-operative management (**Evidence level, 2**)

3. Abdominal CT is the most reliable method for identifying and assessing the severity of injury to the spleen or liver (**Evidence level, 2**)

4. The clinical status of the patient should dictate the frequency of follow-up scans (**Evidence level, 3**)

5. Initial CT of the abdomen should be performed with oral and intravenous contrast to facilitate the diagnosis of hollow viscus injuries (**Evidence level, 3**)

6. Medical clearance to resume normal activity status should be based on evidence of healing (**Evidence level, 3**)

7. Angiographic embolisation is an adjunct in the non-operative management of the haemodynamically stable patient with hepatic and splenic injuries and evidence of ongoing bleeding (**Evidence level, 3**)

---

found that, in the hands of experienced trauma surgeons, the success with the non-operative approach to liver injuries was greater than 98%.[68]

Currently, all patients with liver injuries following blunt trauma should be considered candidates for non-operative management, if haemodynamic stability can be assured. Unlike the spleen, delayed haemorhage from the liver is rare. The complications in those patients managed expectantly are frequently related to the biliary system and can usually be treated by endoscopic or interventional techniques. While non-operative management has most frequently been applied to patients with blunt injuries, a few stable patients with liver injuries as the result of penetrating trauma have also been managed expectantly.[69]

Spleen

In children, the success of non-operative management of the spleen is over 90%, but this has not been the experience in adults. Currently, most surgeons will attempt to manage non-operatively the injured adult spleen with an AAST grade I–III injury; the management of grade IV or V injuries remains controversial.

In a recent report of 190 consecutive patients with splenic injuries managed at a single institution,[70] 102 (54%) were initially treated without surgery, including 15 patients with intrinsic splenic pathology and six patients with isolated stab wounds. Only two of these patients failed non-operative management, and both survived. It was suggested that 65% of all blunt splenic injuries and selected stab wounds can be managed non-operatively, with minimal transfusions, morbidity or mortality and a success rate of 98%. In contrast, splenectomy, when necessary, is associated with excessive transfusion and an inordinately high postoperative sepsis rate.

• Key points

- In order to avoid missed injuries and preventable deaths, trauma patients who have any of the risk factors for abdominal injury should undergo objective evaluation of the abdomen.
- In patients who are unstable, the preferred objective study is bedside ultrasound. If an ultrasound examination is unavailable or equivocal, DPL should be performed.
- In stable patients, abdominal CT with oral and intravenous contrast is the preferred method of objective examination of the abdomen.
- When laparotomy is required, it should be approached in a systematic fashion and the treatment of injuries prioritised.
- In patients who are cold, coagulopathic and acidotic, a damage control operation should be accomplished promptly.

REFERENCES

1. Anderson ID, Woodford M, de Dombal T, Irving MH. A retrospective study of 1000 deaths from injury in England and Wales. Br Med J 1988; 296:1305–8.

2. West JC, Trunkey DD, Lim RC. System of trauma care: a study of two counties. Arch Surg 1979; 114:455–60.

3. Mackersie RC, Tiwary AD, Shackford SR, Hoyt DB. Intra-abdominal injury following blunt trauma: identifying the high-risk factors. Arch Surg 1989; 124:809–13.

4. Taylor GA, Eichelberger MR. Abdominal CT in children with neurologic impairment following blunt trauma. Ann Surg 1989; 210:229–33.

5. Knudson MM, McAninch JA, Gomez R, Lee P, Stubbs HA. Haematuria as a predictor of abdominal injury after blunt trauma. Am J Surg 1992; 164:482–6.

6. Bickell WH, Wall MJ, Pepe PE et al. Immediate versus delayed fluid resuscitation for hypotensive patients with penetrating torso injuries. N Engl J Med 1994; 331:1105–9.

7. American College of Surgeons. Advanced Trauma Life Support Programme: Abdominal trauma. Washington, DC: American College of Surgeons, 1997.

8 Brooks A, Bowley DM, Boffard KD. Bullet markers: a simple technique to assist in the evaluation of penetrating trauma. J R Army Med Corps 2002; 148:259–61.

9. Root HD, Hauser CW, McKinley CR, LaFave JW, Mendiola RP. Diagnostic peritoneal lavage. Surgery 1965; 57:633–7.

10. Donohue JH, Federle MP, Griffiths BG, Trunkey DD. Computed tomography in the diagnosis of blunt intestinal and mesenteric injuries. J Trauma 1987; 27:11–17.

11. Brasel KJ, Olson CH, Stafford R, Johnson TJ. Incidence and significance of free fluid on abdominal computed tomographic scan in blunt trauma. J Trauma 1998; 44:889–92.

12. Sherck JP, Oakes DD. Intestinal injuries missed by computed tomography. J Trauma 1990; 30:1–7.

13. McKenney MG, Martin L, Lopez C. 1000 consecutive ultrasounds for blunt abdominal trauma. J Trauma 1996; 40:607–12.

14. Rozycki GS, Ochsner MG, Schmidt JA et al. A prospective study of surgeon-performed ultrasound as the primary adjuvant modality for injured patient assessment. J Trauma 1995; 39:492–7.

15. Shackford SR. Focused ultrasound examinations by surgeons: the time is now. J Trauma 1993; 35:181–2.

16. Rozycki GS, Ballard RB, Feliciano DV, Schmidt JA, Pennington SD. Surgeon-performed ultrasound for the assessment of truncal injuries: lessons learned from 1540 patients. Ann Surg 1998; 229:557–67.

17. Brooks AJ, Boffard KD. Current technology: laparoscopic surgery in trauma. Trauma 1999; 1:53–60.

18. Fabian TC, McCord S. Therapeutic laparoscopy in trauma. Trauma Q 1993; 34:313–15.

19. Smith RS, Fry WR, Tsoi EKM. Gasless laparoscopy and conventional instruments. Arch Surg 1993; 70:632–7.

20. Zantut LF, Ivatury RR, Smith S. Diagnostic and therapeutic laparoscopy for penetrating abdominal trauma: a multicentre experience. J Trauma 1997; 42:825–31.

21. Fabian TC, Croce MA, Steward RM et al. A prospective analysis of diagnostic laparoscopy in trauma. Ann Surg 1993; 217:557.

22. Degiannis E, Levy R, Sofianos C, Potokar T, Florizoone M, Saadia R. Diaphragmatic herniation after penetrating trauma. Br J Surg 1996; 83:88–91.

23. Renz BM, Feliciano DV. Unnecessary laparotomies for trauma: a prospective study of morbidity. J Trauma 1995; 38:350–6.

24. Moore EE, Moore JB, van Duzer-Moore S, Thompson JS. Mandatory laparotomy for gunshot wounds penetrating the abdomen. Am J Surg 1980; 140:847–51.

25. Muckart DJ, Abdool-Carim AT, King B. Selective conservative management of abdominal gunshot wounds: a prospective study. Br J Surg 1990; 77:652–5.

26. Ross SE, Dragon GM, O'Malley KF, Rehm CG. Morbidity of negative celiotomy in trauma. Injury 1995; 26:393–4.

27. Weigelt JA, Kingman RG. Complications of negative laparotomy for trauma. Am J Surg 1988; 156:544–7.

28. Demetriades D, Charalambides D, Lakhoo M, Pantanowitz D. Gunshot wound of the abdomen: role of selective conservative management. Br J Surg 1991; 78:220–2.

29. Maggisano R, Nathens A, Alexandrova NA et al. Traumatic rupture of the thoracic aorta: should one always operate immediately? Ann Vasc Surg 1995; 9:44–6.

30. Camp PC, Shackford SR, Knudson MM et al. Outcome following blunt traumatic thoracic aortic laceration: identification of a high risk cohort. J Trauma 1997; 43:413–22.

31. Wisner DH, Victor NS, Holcroft JW. The priorities in the management of multiple trauma: intracranial versus intra-abdominal injury. J Trauma 1993; 35:271–8.

32. Archer LP, Rogers RB, Shackford SR. Selective non-operative management of liver and splenic injuries in neurologically impaired adult patients. Arch Surg 1996; 131:309–15.

33. Cattel RB, Braasch JW. A technique for the exposure of the third and fourth parts of the duodenum. Surg Gynecol Obstet 1960; 111:379–83.

34. Rotondo MF, Schwab CW, McGonigal MD et al. 'Damage control': an approach for improved survival in exsanguinating penetrating abdominal injury. J Trauma 1993; 35:375–82.

35. Elerding SC, Aragon GE, Moore EE. Fatal hepatic haemorrhage after trauma. Am J Surg 1979; 138:883–8.

36. Hirshberg A, Mattox KL. Planned re-operation for severe trauma. Ann Surg 1995; 222:3–8.

37. Garrison JR, Richardson JD, Hilakos A et al. Predicting the need to pack early for severe intra-abdominal haemorrhage. J Trauma 1996; 40:923–9.

38. Burch J, Moore E, Moore F, Franciose R. The abdominal compartment syndrome. Surg Clin North Am 1996; 76:833–42.

39. Harman PK, Kron IL, McLachlan HD. Elevated intra-abdominal pressure and renal function. Ann Surg 1982; 196:594–7.

40. Sugrue M, Buist MD, Hourihan F, Deane S, Bauman A, Hillman K. Prospective study of intra-abdominal hypertension and renal function after laparotomy. Br J Surg 1995; 82:235–8.

41. Kron IL, Harman PK, Nolan SP. The measurement of intra-abdominal pressure as a criterion for abdominal re-exploration. Ann Surg 1984; 199:28–30.

42. Maxwell RA, Fabian TC, Croce MA, Davius KA. Secondary abdominal compartment syndrome: an underappreciated manifestation of severe haemorrhagic shock. J Trauma 2000; 47:995–9.

43. Sugrue M, Jones F, Janjua J, Deane SA, Bristow P, Hillman K. Temporary abdominal closure. J Trauma 1998; 45:914–21.

44. Moore EE, Dunn EL, Moore JB, Thompson JS. Penetrating Abdominal Trauma Index. J Trauma 1981; 21:439–45.

45. Stewart RM, Fabian TC, Croce MA, Pritchard FE, Minard G, Kudsk KA. Is resection with primary anastomosis following destructive colon wounds always safe? Am J Surg 1994; 168:316–19.

46. Moore EE, Shackford SR, Pachter HL et al. Organ Injury Scaling: spleen, liver and kidney. J Trauma 1989; 29:1664–6.

47. Moore EE, Cogbill TH, Malangoni MA, Jurkovich GJ, Shackford SR, Champion HR. Organ Injury Scaling: pancreas, duodenum, small bowel, colon and rectum. J Trauma 1990; 30:1427–9.

48. Moore EE, Cogbill TH, Jurkovich GJ. Organ Injury Scaling III: chest wall, abdominal vascular, ureter, bladder and urethra. J Trauma 1992; 33:337–8.

49. Moore EE, Malangoni MA, Cogbill TH et al. Organ Injury Scaling IV: thoracic, vascular, lung, cardiac and diaphragm. J Trauma 1994; 36:299–300.

50. Moore EE, Cogbill TH, Jurkovich GJ, Shackford SR, Malangoni MA, Champion HR. Organ Injury Scaling: spleen and liver (1994 revision). J Trauma 1995; 38:323–4.

51. Moore EE, Jurkovich GJ, Knudson MM et al. Organ Injury Scaling VI: extrahepatic biliary, oesophagus, stomach, vulva, vagina, uterus (nonpregnant), uterus (pregnant), fallopian tube, and ovary. J Trauma 1995; 39:1069–70.

52. Moore EE, Malangoni MA, Cogbill TH et al. Organ Injury Scaling VII: cervical vascular, peripheral vascular, adrenal, penis, testis and scrotum. J Trauma 1996; 41:523–4.

53. Hoff WS, Holevar M, Nagy KK et al. Practice management guidelines for the evaluation of blunt abdominal trauma. EAST Practice Management Guidelines Work Group, 2001. Available online at http://www.east.org

54. Mazuski JE, Sawyer RG, Nathens AB et al. The Surgical Infection Society Guidelines on antimicrobial therapy for intra-abdominal infections: an executive summary. Surg Infect 2002; 3:161–73.

55. Cornwell EE III, Campbell KA. Trauma. In: Gordon TA, Cameron JL (eds) Evidence-based surgery. Hamilton, Ontario: BC Decker, 2000; pp. 415–28.

56. Boffard KD, Brooks AJ. Pancreatic trauma. Eur J Surg 2000; 166:4–12.

57. Brasel KJ, Borgstrom DC, Weigelt JA. Management of penetrating colon trauma: a cost utility analysis. Surgery 1999; 125:471–9.

58. Bern JD, Velmahos GC, Chan LS, Asenscio JA, Demetriades D. The high morbidity of colostomy closure after trauma: further support for the primary repair of colon injuries. Surgery 1998; 123:157–64.

59. Pachter HL, Hoballah JJ, Corcoran TA, Hofstetter SR. The morbidity and financial impact of colostomy closure in trauma patients. J Trauma 1990; 30:1510–14.

60. Stone HH, Fabian TC. Management of perforating colon trauma: randomisation between primary colon closure and exteriorisation. Ann Surg 1979; 190:430–6.

61. Murray JA, Demetriades D, Colson M et al. Colonic resection in trauma, colostomy versus anastomosis. J Trauma 1999; 46:250–4.

62. Cornwell EE, Velmahos GC, Berne TV et al. The fate of colonic suture lines in high risk patients: a prospective analysis. J Am Coll Surg 1998; 187:58–63.

63. Hirschberg A, Walden R. Damage control for abdominal trauma. Surg Clin North Am 1997; 77:813–21.

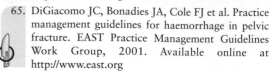

64. Cayten CG, Fabian TC, Garcia VF et al. Patient management guidelines for penetrating intraperitoneal injuries. EAST Practice Parameter Working Group, 1998. Available online at http://www.east.org

65. DiGiacomo JC, Bonadies JA, Cole FJ et al. Practice management guidelines for haemorrhage in pelvic fracture. EAST Practice Management Guidelines Work Group, 2001. Available online at http://www.east.org

66. Alonso M, Brathwaite C, Garcia V et al. Practice management guidelines for the nonoperative management of blunt injury to the liver and spleen. EAST Practice Management Guidelines Work Group, 2003. Available online at http://www.east.org

67. Knudson MM, Lim RC, Oakes DD, Jeffrey RB. Nonoperative management of blunt liver injuries in adults: the need for continued surveillance. J Trauma 1990; 30:1494–500.

68. Pachter HL, Knudson MM, Esrig B et al. Status of nonoperative management of blunt hepatic injuries in 1995: a multicenter experience with 404 patients. J Trauma 1996; 40:31–8.

69. Renz BM, Feliciano DV. Gunshot wounds to the right thoracoabdomen: a prospective study of nonoperative management. J Trauma 1994; 37:737–44.

70. Pachter HL, Guth AA, Hofstetter SR, Spencer FC. Changing patterns in the management of splenic trauma: the impact of nonoperative management. Ann Surg 1998; 227:708–19.

Fourteen

Prophylaxis and treatment of deep venous thrombosis

George Hamilton

INTRODUCTION

Throughout the Western world, thrombosis arising in the leg veins is a common occurrence. Often it is completely unsuspected and may result in considerable morbidity and mortality, especially when the proximal leg veins are involved. The two major complications are pulmonary embolism, still a major killer in hospital and community patients, and the post-thrombotic syndrome, which gives rise to considerable suffering and is a major burden to medical services everywhere. This is not a condition limited to the postsurgical patient but is just as common in the bedridden and elderly in hospitals, nursing homes and the community. In its varied forms, venous thromboembolic disease is therefore a common presentation.

EPIDEMIOLOGY

In the USA, deep venous thrombosis (DVT) and pulmonary embolism are estimated to afflict over 2 million people per year. A population-based study conducted in short-stay community hospitals in Massachussetts found an annual incidence of documented DVT of 56 per 100 000 and of pulmonary embolism of 23 per 100 000 inpatients, with a 12% mortality occurring in this group. Extrapolation of these findings to the whole population in the USA suggests an incidence of 260 000 cases per year of clinically diagnosed thromboembolic events in the acutely hospitalised population.[1] Pooled data from several similar studies indicate an incidence of between 50 and 150 venous thromboses per 100 000 population per year.[2] A high prevalence

of silent DVTs and pulmonary emboli, particularly in the severely ill, and a low rate of post-mortem examinations makes the true incidence much higher.

The incidence of venous thromboembolism rises exponentially with age, being negligible in children, about 30 per 100 000 cases in the third decade, and 300–500 per 100 000 cases in those over 70 years of age.[3] Despite the recognised increased risk of venous thromboembolism with the use of oral contraceptive and hormone replacement therapy, no significant difference in its incidence could be found in the relationship between male and female. Venous thromboembolism occurs mostly where there are pre-existent risk factors, such as malignancy, trauma or surgery. In treated patients the recurrence rate for DVT is approximately 7% at 6 months, with recurrence of pulmonary embolism more likely after a pulmonary embolism than after DVT.[3] Mortality at 30 days is 6% after DVT, rising to 12% after pulmonary embolism, with a strong association of risk of death with the presence of cancer, old age and cardiovascular disease. Primary or idiopathic venous thromboembolism has been estimated to occur in 25–50% of first-time cases. About 15–25% are associated with cancer and about 20% will occur within 3 months of surgery.

Geographical differences in the incidence of venous thromboembolism are exemplified by the much lower rates found in African and Asian populations.[4,5] In North America, death rates from pulmonary embolism are higher in men than in women and in non-whites than in white populations.[6] Many post-mortem studies confirm that, despite the widespread availability of diagnostic methods, antemortem diagnosis of pulmonary embolism contributing to death is made in the minority of cases.[7] Clearly, a high threshold of suspicion for diagnosis of DVT and pulmonary embolism must prevail to improve outcome.

The vast majority of the data relates to hospital inpatients. A study of all admissions to a single UK district general hospital found that 10% of all deaths (i.e. 0.9% of all admissions) were from pulmonary embolism.[8] Likewise, it has been found to be the cause of death in 3% of surgical inpatients,[9] and a finding in 24% of post-mortem examinations in a large series of surgical patients.[10] It has long been established that DVT is very common in hospitalised patients, with up to 30% having asymptomatic non-obstructive calf vein thrombosis, as shown by radioactive fibrinogen leg scanning.[11] The clinical importance of these localised thromboses is debated but patients with thrombus propagation and, in particular, involvement of the popliteal and more proximal venous segments have a high risk of developing pulmonary embolism.[12] In their original report of 1969, Kakkar et al. found a 10% incidence of pulmonary embolism in patients where propagation to the popliteal vein and more proximally had occurred.[10] Asymptomatic pulmonary embolism with a clinical diagnosis of DVT occurs in 50% of proximal DVTs and 30–50% of isolated calf vein thromboses.[13] Conversely, 36–45% of patients with pulmonary embolus confirmed on ventilation–perfusion scanning or pulmonary angiography will have asymptomatic DVT on duplex scanning.[14]

The post-thrombotic syndrome results mainly from valvular destruction, post-thrombotic scarring and stiffening of the venous wall. Progression to this syndrome probably occurs only when the popliteal or more proximal segments are involved in the thrombosis.[15] The complications of the post-thrombotic syndrome, particularly venous ulceration, are common in the elderly and form a major source of morbidity.

Finally, there is much emphasis on the incidence and risk of postoperative venous thromboembolism. It is well recognised that pulmonary embolism occurs most commonly within the first 10 days after surgery but it is becoming increasingly apparent that a significant proportion may occur late in the postoperative period and even after discharge from hospital.[10,16] Also it is salutary to remember that only one in four patients with fatal pulmonary embolism in hospital in the UK had undergone recent surgery. Venous thromboembolic disease affects a diverse group of patients, postoperative, non-surgical inpatient and outpatient alike (**Box 14.1**).

AETIOLOGY

No dissertation on venous thromboembolic disease is complete without mention of Virchow and his

Box 14.1 • Natural history of venous thromboembolism

Most deep vein thrombosis (DVT) starts in the calf veins

About half the episodes of DVT associated with surgery start intraoperatively and about half resolve spontaneously within 72 hours

The risk of progression of postoperative DVT is greatest in the presence of continuing risk factors and where the initial thrombosis is large

After orthopaedic surgery, 75% of episodes of DVT occur in the operated leg

Symptomatic risk of venous thromboembolic disease is highest within 2 weeks of surgery but is maintained for 2–3 months

Isolated calf DVT is rarely symptomatic and rarely results in clinically significant pulmonary embolism

Approximately 25% of episodes of untreated symptomatic calf DVT extend to the proximal veins within 1 week of presentation

Approximately 70% of patients with symptomatic pulmonary embolism have a DVT (approximately two-thirds involve the proximal veins)

Without treatment approximately 50% of patients with symptomatic proximal DVT or pulmonary embolism will have a recurrent thrombosis in 3 months. The greatest risk of fatal postoperative pulmonary embolism occurs 3–7 days after surgery and 10% of symptomatic DVTs are fatal within 1 hour of first symptoms

Between 5 and 10% of patients with pulmonary embolism present with shock.

Isolated calf DVT is associated with half the risk of recurrence of proximal DVT or pulmonary embolism

The risk of recurrence is similar following proximal DVT and pulmonary embolism

Recurrent DVT in the same leg predisposes to post-thrombotic syndrome

Approximately 50% resolution of perfusion defects occurs after 2–4 weeks of treatment for pulmonary embolism, with complete resolution in two-thirds of patients thereafter

Pulmonary hypertension will develop in approximately 5% of patients with pulmonary embolism

Adapted from Kearon C. Natural history of venous thromboembolism. Circulation 2003; 107:I-22–I-30, with permission.

celebrated triad. In 1858 at the age of 25 years, he had documented the pathological correlation of pulmonary embolism to venous thrombosis and proposed that thrombosis was primarily caused by the interplay of three classical factors: reduced or stagnant blood flow in the veins, injury to the vein wall and hypercoagulability of the blood. Although this provided a conveniently simple framework of explanation, the pathogenesis of venous thrombosis is rather more complex and indeed to an extent perplexing.

Thrombus formation can occur in any part of the venous system but the vast majority arise in the soleal veins of the calf, more specifically in the vein valve pockets.[18,19] The importance of stasis in generation of venous thrombosis is debated, but in the immobilised or immediately postsurgical patient it is obviously a major factor. Contrast medium is often seen to remain in the soleal veins of patients undergoing ascending venography for several minutes after injection, confirming that flow is often extremely sluggish in this portion of the venous tree in the supine position. It has long been observed, however, that blood in an isolated ligated vein will remain fluid for many hours. This is the result of several natural antithrombotic mechanisms, including local production of prostacyclin, nitric oxide and tissue plasminogen activator (tPA), cell surface glycosaminoglycans such as heparin sulphate and the physiological inhibitors of clotting, namely antithrombin, protein C and protein S.

Animal studies of venous stasis induced by ligation showed evidence of thrombosis occurring only after 24–72 hours.[20] Leucocyte adhesion to endothelium and migration across the cells to the subendothelial layers is an early response to stasis but does not seem to be causative of thrombosis.[21] Hypoxaemia is a rapid development after induction of stasis, particularly in the valve sinuses, and hypoxic endothelial cell damage has been suggested as a causative factor in thrombosis.[22] However, post-mortem studies fail to show significant endothelial cell damage even at the valve pockets in patients with DVT.[23] Some form of vessel wall or endothelial damage has been proposed as an essential feature in the development of venous thrombosis. However, experimental studies of injury to veins caused by clamping or crushing failed to show significant thrombus formation after exposure to low-velocity blood flow or even stagnant blood.[24] Consequently, a combination of stasis and vessel wall injury alone cannot explain the development of the initiating thrombus.

The importance of hypercoagulability in producing thrombosis has been demonstrated both experimentally and clinically. In the presence of stasis, activation of the intrinsic clotting system by several means results in clotting that can develop in as little as 10 minutes. In the experimental situation, the combination of stasis and activated clotting factors provides the most potent scenario for initiating thrombosis.[25] In the clinical situation, this combination may arise because of local or systemic changes in coagulability and most often it is a combination of both.

There is a great deal of clinical evidence based on studies using radiolabelled fibrinogen or ascending venography showing that almost all thrombi (over 90%) develop in the calf either in isolation or in continuity with more proximal veins.[18,19] These findings, together with the histological studies by Sevitt,[25] suggest that the probable mechanism of thrombosis formation is from a nidus of thrombus in a valve pocket. Flow studies have revealed a stagnant region deep in the valve pocket with extremely low velocities precisely where the earliest thrombus nidus is found in histological studies.[22] Therefore, in this area, a combination of stasis, accumulation of activated clotting factors, possible hypoxaemic endothelial cell damage and release of thromboxane and thrombin would result in generation of a nidus of thrombus.

Close to the vein wall, the valve pocket thrombus is rich in red blood cells and fibrin and is described as red thrombus. Further away from the vein wall, the thrombus becomes white and is formed from platelets and fibrin-rich propagated growth.[23,26] The thrombus then either propagates proximally to form a free-floating non-occlusive clot or extends to attach to the vein's wall just beyond the valve pocket and thus often occludes the vein (Fig. 14.1).[27]

The fibrinolytic system

Local fibrinolytic activity will to a large extent determine whether an initial nidus of thrombus will propagate to a full-blown thrombosis or dissolve by a process of lysis. Fibrinolysis is activated by the generation of the serine protease enzyme thrombin and is a function of the balance between plasma levels of tPA and plasminogen activator inhibitor (PAI)-1, both produced by endothelial cells.[28] By using non-specific assays, it can be shown that blood fibrinolytic activity in venous stasis is lower in patients with thrombosis than in controls.[29] Studies using specific and sensitive assays of tPA and PAI-1 in plasma have consistently shown that 30–40% of patients with DVT have impaired thrombolysis. This is mainly a consequence of increased levels of PAI-1 but often these occur in combination with decreased tPA production after venous occlusion.[28,29] However, inflammation stimulates production of PAI-1, and the observed high levels in patients could be explained as part of the inflammatory response to the DVT. Transgenic mice with an extra human PAI-1 gene have increased PAI-1 levels in plasma and tissues and suffer from venous thrombosis shortly after birth;[30] by comparison mice with a tPA gene knock-out do not have thrombotic complications.[31] Therefore, although as yet there is no conclusive clinical evidence, it seems highly

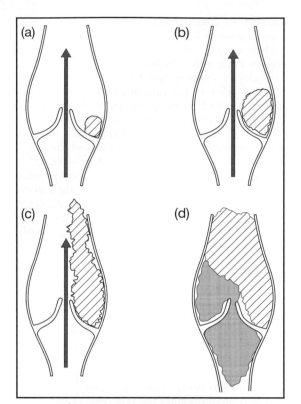

Figure 14.1 • Clot formation and propagation:
(a) nidus of clot forming in recess of the valve pocket;
(b) propagation of clot to fill the pocket; **(c)** propagation of free-floating thrombus without vein occlusion;
(d) thrombus extension and attachment to opposite vein wall causing occlusion and secondary thrombus propagation both proximal and distal. With permission from Hamilton G, Platt SA. Deep vein thrombosis. In: Beard JD, Gaines PA (eds) Vascular and endovascular surgery. London: WB Saunders, 1998; pp. 351–96.

probable that deficient fibrinolytic activity is a factor in the aetiology of idiopathic DVT. A study in patients with DVT demonstrated abnormal fibrinolysis in 86% of patients with recurrent idiopathic DVT but only in 29% of those with secondary DVT.[32] This would suggest that deficient fibrinolysis may be a less important factor in the aetiology of DVT secondary to other causes.

Trauma and major surgery cause a temporary increase in PAI-1 as part of an acute-phase reaction, resulting in deficient fibrinolytic activity over the first 7–10 days. Preoperative plasma PAI-1 levels in patients undergoing hip replacement correlate significantly with postoperative DVT risk[33] but such a relationship has not been shown in major abdominal surgery.[34] Elevated PAI-1 levels associated with genotypic abnormalities have been aetiologically associated with risk of coronary heart disease and myocardial infarction.[35] Further studies

of the role of PAI-1 activity in venous thromboembolism are required.

Hypercoagulability

In the hypercoagulable state, there is an increased risk of thrombosis in situations where there would be no risk in a normal individual. There are clearly many predisposing factors affecting local interactions between thrombin, tPA, tissue factor pathway inhibitor, proteins C and S and antithrombin such that thrombosis results. These may be inherited thrombophilias, such as deficiency of naturally occurring protein C, protein S or antithrombin, or genetic mutations such as factor V Leiden or prothrombin 20210A variant. Alternatively, hypercoagulability may be acquired, such as in malignancy, after major surgery, in immobilisation, when taking the oral contraceptive pill or in the antiphospholipid syndrome. Whereas the mechanisms of thrombosis in secondary hypercoagulable states remain poorly understood, thrombophilia is known to result from specific coagulation abnormalities. These have developed mainly from prothrombotic mutations and, to date, over 60% of all cases of thrombophilia have such an identifiable genetic defect.

Primary causes of hypercoagulability

There are four main natural anticoagulant mechanisms occurring in the coagulation cascade that maintain blood flow and limit the process of thrombosis to sites of vascular injury: antithrombin, protein C and protein S, the tissue factor pathway inhibitor and the fibrinolytic system (**Fig. 14.2**). These four factors act at strategic points across the coagulation pathway to quench and control the cascade. Deficiencies of each of these pathways can cause a prothrombotic state, but abnormalities of tissue factor pathway inhibitor causing thrombophilia have not as yet been identified. These deficiencies result from many different types of genetic mutation, mostly substitution of one nucleotide or deletions or insertions of less than ten nucleotides. Furthermore, patients can be heterozygous or homozygous for a single mutation or compound heterozygous for two different mutations.[36]

ANTITHROMBIN

Because antithrombin inactivates thrombin and other clotting factors (factors XIIa, XIa, IXa and Xa) and its action is catalysed by heparin-like glycosaminoglycans on the endothelial cell surface, it is the most centrally acting of the anticoagulant proteins. However, antithrombin deficiency is a rare

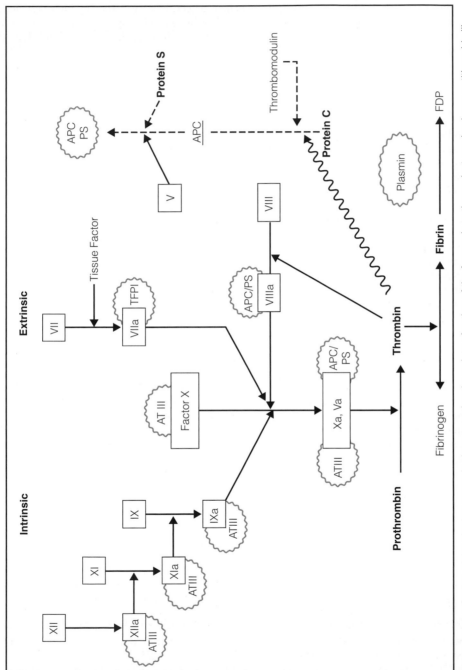

Figure 14.2 • Outline of the clotting cascade demonstrating the points of action of the four main anticoagulant mechanisms: antithrombin III (ATIII), plasmin, proteins C and S (APC/PS) and tissue factor pathway inhibitor (TFPI). FDP, fibrin degradation products. With permission from Hamilton G, Platt SA. Deep vein thrombosis. In: Beard JD, Gaines PA (eds) Vascular and endovascular surgery. London: WB Saunders, 1998; pp. 351–96.

autosomal dominant condition, with an estimated incidence of 0.2–0.4%; its true prevalence in the general population may be as high as 1 in 250–500 as measured by functional assay of antithrombin–heparin cofactor activity.[36–38] There are two types of antithrombin deficiency, type 1 and type 2 (type 2 has lesser risk of venous thrombosis), with a wide range of prevalence of thrombotic disease in affected families, ranging from 15 to 100%.[37] The annual incidence is about 1% in carriers, conferring a 10.6 times relative risk of thrombosis compared with non-carriers.[39]

PROTEIN C AND PROTEIN S

Protein C is produced by the liver and, like protein S (produced not only by the liver but also by endothelial cells, megakaryocytes and testicular Leydig cells), its synthesis is vitamin K dependent. This means that diagnosis of protein C and protein S deficiency is complicated in patients taking warfarin. Protein C is activated by thrombin, a process accelerated by the binding of thrombin to thrombomodulin on the endothelial membrane surface. The released activated protein C binds with its circulating cofactor protein S to form the protein C/S complex, which inactivates coagulation factors Va and VIIIa. Activated protein C is further supported and potentiated by factor V and has a long half-life in the circulation, acting as a circulating anticoagulant.[40]

Protein C and protein S deficiencies are autosomally inherited genetic abnormalities. Protein C deficiency is rare, with a prevalence of 0.1–0.5% of the general population,[41] and is a risk factor for thrombosis in 2–5% of patients.[42] Protein S deficiency is as commonly found in patients with venous thrombosis as protein C deficiency but its prevalence within the general population is unknown.[40] There are two types of protein C deficiency and three types of protein S deficiency.[43] In common with antithrombin deficiency, both qualitative and quantitative abnormalities of proteins C and S can be present, thus making functional rather than immunological assays preferable in the diagnosis and risk assessment of patients with thromboembolic disease.

ACTIVATED PROTEIN C RESISTANCE/FACTOR V LEIDEN

In 1993, Dahlbäck et al. reported a laboratory finding of resistance to the anticoagulant effect of activated protein C in the plasma of three families with histories of venous thrombosis.[44] This abnormality was then found in 20% of patients presenting with venous thrombosis to the University Hospital, Leiden, indicating the clinical importance of this disorder.[45] Many subsequent studies have confirmed the frequency of resistance to activated protein C in venous thrombosis and that this occurs in the vast majority of patients as a result of a single point mutation in the gene for factor V.[46] This genetic abnormality, most often called the factor V Leiden defect, has a remarkably high prevalence of 3–7% or higher in Europe and the USA but is lower elsewhere, such as in Africa and South-East Asia, where it is less than 1%.[47,48] The prevalence of resistance to activated protein C in patients with venous thrombosis is much higher, ranging from 17.5 to 64% in different studies.[49] Homozygous patients are more likely to present at an earlier age (median 31 years) than heterozygous patients (median 44 years), who in turn present at a younger age than those who do not have Leiden factor V (median 46 years).[48] The annual incidence of venous thromboembolism is 0.28% in carriers, conferring a relative risk of 2.8 compared with non-carriers.[42]

In common with deficiencies in antithrombin, protein C and protein S, resistance to activated protein C as a result of factor V Leiden is usually inherited as an autosomal dominant disorder. Recently, the hypothesis that hypercoagulability might be a multiple gene disorder has been gaining ground. Thrombotic events have been found to be much higher in carriers of both protein C deficiency and factor V Leiden mutations (71%) than in carriers of the single gene defect (36% and 10% respectively).[50] Furthermore, there is an increase in the risk of venous thrombosis when these defects are found in combination with hyperhomocysteinaemia or in patients taking the oral contraceptive pill.[48] Resistance to activated protein C is ten times more prevalent than all the other identified genetic abnormalities put together and it is obviously a major risk factor in venous thrombosis, particularly in conjunction with other genetic defects and in the presence of secondary prothrombotic disorders.

Resistance to activated protein C that does not result from factor V Leiden is probably of mixed genetic and acquired origin. A genetic basis has been inferred and may include an arginine to threonine mutation at the 306 cleavage site (factor V Cambridge). The oral contraceptive pill and pregnancy confer acquired resistance to activated protein C.[51]

MUTATION 20210A IN PROTHROMBIN

In 1996, Poort et al. described a sequence variation at the 3′-untranslated region of the prothrombin gene resulting in a glutamine to arginine substitution at position 20210.[52] Patients with this 20210A allele have elevated prothrombin levels, which is a risk factor for thrombosis. The prevalence in the normal population is 0.7–2.6% and in patients with DVT is 5–6.2%.[52–54] Thrombotic events are also more likely if this mutation is coinherited with factor V Leiden or deficiency of antithrombin or protein C or S. This recently identified abnormality is significant as, in Europe, it may be responsible for more thrombotic events than factor V Leiden.[51]

FACTOR VIII ELEVATION

Raised factor VIII levels are implicated in increased risk for a single episode of DVT and for recurrent DVT. As the levels rise, so does the risk of venous thromboembolism.[55] Raised factor VIII is not just part of an acute-phase reaction related to the DVT but can be persistently and independently raised in the absence of venous thromboembolic disease.[56] In fact, elevated factor VIII levels seem to be almost as common a risk factor for DVT as raised factor V Leiden. A recent study of 615 patients with a first spontaneous DVT found a higher rate of subsequent superficial thrombophlebitis and DVT in patients with increased factor VIII, which was identified as an independent risk factor.[57]

DISORDERS OF THE FIBRINOLYTIC SYSTEM

The importance of the fibrinolytic system has been discussed earlier with a description of abnormal fibrinolysis in patients having recurrent DVT. In addition to decreased tPA production and increased PAI-1 production, other abnormalities have been defined. Abnormalities of plasminogen have been implicated in the post-thrombotic state associated with increased risk of arterial and venous thrombosis; this is termed a dysplasminogenaemia. This condition may occur in up to 10% of normal patients, with a thrombotic event occurring only if another risk factor for thrombosis is superimposed.[58] Elevated levels of fibrinogen in the serum are associated strongly with risk of coronary thrombosis and peripheral vascular disease. However, there is no strong evidence directly implicating the elevated levels of fibrinogen with a probable thrombotic tendency. Other rarer causes of fibrinolytic disorders are hypoplasminogenaemia and increased histidine-rich glycoprotein. Probably the most important of these disorders of the fibrinolytic system is increased PAI-1 production.

Acquired or secondary causes of hypercoagulability

ANTIPHOSPHOLIPID SYNDROME

The antiphospholipid syndrome may involve every organ system, with protean clinical presentations to various medical disciplines. Acute arterial or venous thrombosis occurring in young, mostly female,

patients with no other prothrombotic risk factors is the usual presentation of this condition to the vascular specialist. The classical antiphospholipid protein syndrome was first described in 1983 as an association between arterial and venous thrombosis, recurrent spontaneous abortion, thrombocytopenia, neurological disorders and positive tests for lupus anticoagulant (LA) and/or anticardiolipin antibody (ACA).[59] The syndrome may occur in the setting of systemic lupus erythematosus (SLE) or systemic sclerosis. However, in many the diagnostic criteria for SLE are not present and the condition is called primary antiphospholipid syndrome; some of these patients may progress later in life to develop full-blown SLE.

LA and ACA are the two most important members of a family of immunoglobulins known as the antiphospholipid protein antibodies. LA is paradoxically associated with increased thrombotic and not haemorrhagic complications and is detected using a phospholipid-dependent test of coagulation (activated partial thromboplastin time (APTT), kaolin clotting time or dilute Russell viper venom time). ACA is detected by radioimmunoassay or enzyme-linked immunosorbent assay (Elisa). Until recently, ACA and LA were thought to be the same antibody but it is now accepted that they are different antibodies, making it important that both are measured. Both LA and ACA are associated with thromboembolic disease, with over 70% of thromboembolisms being venous and the remainder arterial.[60] Both LA and ACA are detected in 60% of patients with thromboembolic disease. Most commonly, arterial events present as stroke, with involvement of the cerebral circulation in younger patients.[61] Both antibodies will be raised in association with drugs, infection and malignancy. Because of this, the diagnosis of antiphospholipid syndrome is made by the presence of at least one clinical finding of arterial thrombosis, recurrent abortion or thrombocytopenia, plus tests for antiphospholipid protein antibodies that are positive on at least two occasions more than 8 weeks apart. Based on prospective clinical studies and in vivo measurement of markers of coagulation, there is evidence that the antibodies have a causative role.[62] In one prospective study, an association was found between initial positivity of ACA and subsequent venous thromboembolic disease.[63]

The major event in this syndrome is clearly thrombosis, with an increased risk of recurrence of approximately 50% over 5 years in patients who remain persistently positive for either LA or ACA.[64] Furthermore, the standard anticoagulant regimen, maintaining the International Normalised Ratio (INR) between 2.0 and 3.0, does not prevent recurrence, and these patients require more intensive anticoagulation with an INR maintained between

3.0 and 4.0. Antiphospholipid syndrome is clearly a complex disease in terms of clinical presentation, pathophysiology and management and is probably the most common cause of acquired thrombophilia. A recent study of 1000 patients with antiphospholipid syndrome reported the most common presentations as follows: DVT (31.7%), thrombocytopenia (21.9%), livedo reticularis (20.4%), stroke (13.1%), superficial thrombophlebitis (9.1%), pulmonary embolism (9%) and fetal loss (8.3%).[65] Screening for LA and ACA must be part of the diagnostic work-up of younger, particularly female, patients with no coexisting risk factors but who develop thromboembolic disease.

HEPARIN-INDUCED THROMBOCYTOPENIA

Since the 1970s, an association between heparin anticoagulation, thrombocytopenia and thrombosis has been recognised. Two patterns of presentation are found. The most common presents within 1–5 days of starting heparin therapy and is associated with a transient fall in platelets to lower than $100–150 \times 10^9/L$. There is rarely any clinical complication and the platelet count returns to normal despite continued heparin administration. Although common, the benign nature of this condition means that it is rarely diagnosed. Known as type I heparin-induced thrombocytopenia (HIT), this is an acute non-immune response probably caused by heparin binding directly to platelet membrane.

Type II HIT is a much more serious condition, characterised by severe thrombocytopenia with platelet counts often less than $50 \times 10^9/L$. This form of HIT develops after 6 days or more of heparin therapy in more than 90% of affected patients; however, on re-exposure, thrombocytopenia may develop within hours.[66,67] Inability to maintain adequate anticoagulation, as measured by prolongation of APTT despite increasing doses of heparin, may occur and is known as heparin resistance. If heparin is stopped, the platelet count may recover within a week, but full recovery may be more prolonged. The condition can occur in any age group, with an incidence of 5–15% found in prospective studies.[67] The source of the heparin used is important, with a greater incidence of HIT with bovine lung rather than porcine mucosal heparin preparations, even in highly purified preparations (5% vs. 1%).[66] Although HIT occurs with both therapeutic and prophylactic dosage, the risk is significantly lower with subcutaneous rather than intravenous heparin therapy.[68] Generally, the risk of HIT and complications is less with lower doses, but type II HIT has been reported with even the tiny quantities of heparin used with heparin flushes or heparin-coated pulmonary artery catheters.[69]

Paradoxically, in type II HIT, thromboembolic complications are more common than haemorrhagic complications, with approximately 10–20% developing the former (**Fig 14.3**). Lower platelet counts ($40–60 \times 10^9/L$) are associated with a high risk of thromboembolic complications, although haemorrhagic complications become more common when the platelet count is lower than $40–50 \times 10^9/L$. All patients receiving heparin therapy or prophylaxis for more than 1 week should have their platelet count monitored weekly.

As soon as the clinical diagnosis is made, treatment involves stopping heparin in all its forms, including heparin flushes, and establishing alternative anticoagulant methods. If the INR is in the therapeutic range, continuation of warfarin is all that is required. If the thrombocytopenia is not severe (i.e. $<100 \times 10^9/L$), it is reasonable to continue heparin therapy with rigorous monitoring of the platelet count until warfarin anticoagulation is established. However, in the presence of severe thrombocytopenia (i.e. $<50 \times 10^9/L$), other forms of anticoagulation may be needed. Platelet transfusion should be given only if the count falls significantly below $50 \times 10^9/L$ and where the clinical risk of haemorrhage is high. Platelets should not be given while there is still circulating heparin present.[70] If

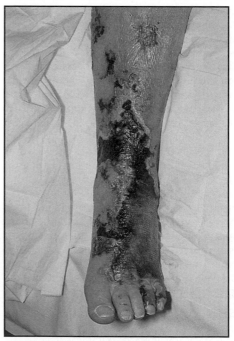

Figure 14.3 • Skin necrosis caused by heparin-induced thrombocytopenia. With permission from Hamilton G, Platt SA. Deep vein thrombosis. In: Beard JD, Gaines PA (eds) Vascular and endovascular surgery. London: WB Saunders, 1998; pp. 351–96.

urgent temporary anticoagulation is required, low-molecular-weight heparin (LMWH) can be used successfully, although cross-reactivity occurs with these agents that can also initiate sensitivity to heparin.[71]

HYPERHOMOCYSTEINAEMIA AND VENOUS THROMBOSIS

Mild hyperhomocysteinaemia, a disorder of methionine metabolism, is a known risk factor for vascular disease but until recently not for venous thrombotic disease.[72] The classical syndrome of homocysteinuria is associated with a high incidence of venous thrombosis, indicating that a link may well exist; indeed, a study from the Netherlands has shown that hyperhomocysteinaemia is a risk factor for venous thrombosis.[73] A direct relationship between increasing homocysteine levels and an increased odds ratio of recurrent venous thrombosis was found. Furthermore, the results suggested an increased risk at all ages. Another study found that 18% of patients below 40 years of age with recurrent thrombosis had hyperhomocysteinaemia.[74]

The mechanism of thrombosis in hyperhomocysteinaemia is not understood but it may result from endothelial cell damage caused by homocysteine or from an action of homocysteine on factor V activation and inhibition of thrombomodulin. There are few data to confirm an association between hyperhomocysteinaemia and venous thromboembolism.[75] The results of a prospective study of folic acid and vitamin B complex in the treatment of first venous thrombolic episodes in the Netherlands is awaited (VITRO study). Hyperhomocysteinaemia is clearly another significant primary cause of thrombosis that should take its place in the differential diagnosis of venous thromboembolic disease.

OTHER SECONDARY CAUSES OF HYPERCOAGULABILITY

A host of acquired disorders are recognised to predispose to thrombosis. The mechanisms of these secondary hypercoagulable states are multifactorial and poorly understood compared with the hypercoagulable states described above. These secondary states may involve increased venous stasis, activation of the coagulation pathways and increased platelet activation, acting either individually or in combination. The development of a secondary hypercoagulable state in an individual with an inherited or primary prothrombotic disorder not only provides the trigger for, but also dramatically compounds the risk of, venous thromboembolic episodes. The importance of venous stasis as an aetiological factor in venous thrombosis has been discussed and is implicated in the immobilised patient, particularly the elderly with heart failure, in obesity, after surgery and in paraparesis or paraplegia. The major acquired or secondary causes of thrombophilia, namely the antiphospholipid syndrome and HIT, have been discussed above.

Economy class syndrome/traveller's thrombosis

Flying as a risk factor for venous thromboembolism was first reported in the 1940s but has been the focus of much interest and study over recent years. There are several studies that support a link between travelling over 6 hours and risk of thrombosis but also others which do not support such an association.[76] Overall the evidence probably does support such an association but only for patients with additional risk factors. In such patients the risk of fatal pulmonary embolism is very low.[76] Two recent case–control and record linkage studies have helped to quantify these risks. An Italian study of 210 patients with proximal DVT found a risk of venous thromboembolism six times higher in the presence of thrombophilia, two times higher in the presence of air travel and 16 times higher when both risk factors were present. Further analysis of females in this group found a fourfold risk of venous thromboembolism in oral contraceptive users, a twofold higher risk in those who had flown and a 14 times higher risk in the presence of both risk factors.[77]

A record linkage study in Western Australia investigated the relationship between long-haul air travel and venous thromboembolism and found a 12% increased annual risk of venous thromboembolism after just one long-haul flight per year.[78]

Both of these studies found the average risk of death from pulmonary embolism to be small but greater in those patients with pre-existent risk factors.

Venous thromboembolism in the surgical patient

Although controversial, stasis is considered a major factor in the development of venous thromboembolism in the surgical patient, perhaps because it is the factor most amenable to treatment. Its importance has been discussed above but it must be emphasised that immobility is also a major factor in non-surgical patients. However, other important risk factors for thromboembolism in surgical patients, quite apart from the underlying illness or procedure to be performed, are now clearly recognised (**Box 14.2**).

The postoperative or post-trauma period is associated with an intrinsically increased state of coagulability that is poorly defined and understood. Systemic fibrinolytic activity is reduced for up to 10 days after surgery or trauma and antithrombin

Box 14.2 • Risk factors for thrombosis

Congenital

Antithrombin deficiency

Protein C deficiency

Protein S deficiency

Resistance to activated protein C

Increased factor VIII

Dysfibrinogenaemias

Increased plasma levels of tissue plasminogen activator inhibitor-1

Plasminogen deficiency

Factor VII deficiency

Factor XII deficiency

Tissue plasminogen activator deficiency

Thrombomodulin deficiency

Heparin cofactor II deficiency

Homocysteinaemia

Hypercholesterolaemia

Haemoglobinopathies

Disorders of histidine-rich glycoprotein

Acquired

Prolonged surgery and trauma

Immobilisation

Stroke, cardiac failure

Pregnancy, hormone replacement therapy, oral contraceptive

Increased factor VIII

Antiphospholipid syndrome

Hyperviscosity syndrome

Inflammatory bowel disease

Malignancy

Behçet's disease

Nephrotic syndrome

Paroxysmal nocturnal haemoglobinuria

Sepsis

Chronic inflammatory disorders

Diabetes

Haemolytic–uraemic syndrome

Thrombotic thrombocytopenic purpura

Heparin-induced thrombocytopenia

levels are said to be reduced. Reports of thromboembolic disease developing up to 6 weeks after surgery and after discharge from hospital suggest that the risk extends beyond the first 10 postoperative days.[14]

Age is an important risk factor, with many studies confirming increased risk in patients over the age of 40 years, with an exponentially increased risk in patients over the age of 70 years who have major illnesses, trauma or surgical intervention. Consequently, thromboembolic disease afflicts mainly the elderly and, to a lesser extent, the middle aged. Younger patients with thrombophilia or other risk factors undergoing major surgery will also be at increased risk and merit identification. Most important among these secondary risk factors are obesity, congestive cardiac failure, prolonged immobilisation, previous thromboembolic disease, pelvic, hip or knee surgery, and malignancy.[79]

The risk of DVT (as found on screening) in the absence of specific thromboprophylaxis varies with the type and duration of the surgical intervention. Major general surgery has an incidence overall of about 25%, with an incidence of fatal pulmonary embolism of 0.7%. Orthopaedic surgery (major hip or knee procedures) has the highest incidence: 40–80% DVT with fatal pulmonary embolism in 1–10%. Femoral and tibial plateau fractures have a DVT incidence of over 40%, with 22% in tibial shaft fractures. Gynaecological procedures for malignancy carry a higher risk (35%) than those for benign procedures such as abdominal hysterectomy (12%). Urological (including renal transplantation) and neurosurgical procedures have similar rates of thromboembolic disease to general abdominal procedures but because of concerns about intraoperative and postoperative haemorrhage, prophylaxis with heparin has classically been avoided, with mechanical methods of prophylaxis being preferred. Vascular procedures, including amputations, are associated with a higher incidence of venous thrombotic disease and pulmonary embolism, and this group of patients with its many other significant risk factors for venous disease should be considered at particularly high risk.

Surgery for varicose veins in the absence of other risk factors presents a particular medicolegal dilemma for the surgeon.[80] There is little evidence to support any association between the presence of varicose veins and thrombotic complications in patients who have no other risk factors. The original evidence supporting this association came from patients undergoing major abdominal and pelvic surgery. There is no association between risk of thromboembolic disease and the presence of varicose veins in a patient not otherwise at risk and not undergoing surgery. The presence of superficial thrombophlebitis of the lower limbs may be associated with an increased risk of DVT, although this remains controversial.[81] Therefore, the low-risk patient having varicose vein surgery is not significantly likely to develop DVT.[82] However, possibly because of its listing as an independent risk factor for thromboembolic disease, up to 62% of vascular surgeons in the UK selectively employ thromboprophylaxis, with 27% using it routinely.[80,83]

The oral contraceptive and hormone replacement therapy

Venous thrombosis in young people is rare, with an incidence in those aged 15–49 years estimated at 0.4–0.8 per 100 000 woman-years.[84] Carriers of the factor V Leiden mutation have an increased incidence of 5.7 per 100 000 woman-years. Women taking the oral contraceptive increase the risk to 3.0 per 100 000 woman-years and women who use the oral contraceptive and are carriers of the factor V Leiden mutation have an incidence of 28.5 per 100 000 woman-years, indicating the presence of a synergistic effect of these additional risk factors. Therefore, the use of the modern low-dose oral contraceptive results in a threefold increase in risk in normal women. Older users of the oral contraceptive (>30 years of age) have an increased risk, as do those using preparations with a higher oestrogen dose; a difference in risk is found even between two low-dose formulations, namely the 30 μg and the 50 μg oestrogen-containing pills.[86,87]

The use of third-generation oral contraceptives carries an increased risk of venous thromboembolism compared with second-generation preparations. This effect results from more pronounced acquired activated protein C resistance induced by the desogestrel contained in third-generation preparations compared with levonorgestrel, which is used in second-generation oral contraceptives.[88]

In addition, the prothrombotic effect of oral contraceptives is mediated by increased factor VII coagulant activity and raised fibrinogen levels, together with lowered antithrombin levels.[89] Reassuringly, these effects are not long term with no appreciable increase in pulmonary embolism found in past users.

Thus oral contraceptive use, even at the low-dose formulation of oestrogen, does increase venous thromboembolic disease. However, this must be seen in the context of a threefold increase of a very small risk of thrombosis in the normal woman. The risk of thromboembolism in oral contraceptive users undergoing surgery is also increased, but this is also a small absolute increase of 0.9% for users versus 0.5% for non-users. The question of whether the oral contraceptive should be stopped 4–6 weeks

before surgery remains controversial. A policy of routinely stopping the oral contraceptive pill does not seem to be justified unless there are additional risk factors present. In the emergency situation, the risk of thrombosis is greater and it is here that thromboprophylaxis is to be recommended.[79]

Until 1996, it was held that hormone replacement therapy (HRT) for perimenopausal and menopausal women carried little risk of venous thromboembolism. This feeling was largely based on the use of lower doses of oestrogen than in oral contraception and their smaller effect on haemostasis in comparison.

However, three studies published in 1996 confirmed that there is a twofold to fourfold increase in risk of venous thromboembolism with the use of HRT both in oestrogen only preparations and in combined oestrogen/progestogen preparations.[90–92]

Progestogen use may contribute to this effect, but it seems that even low levels of exogenous oestrogenic activity may increase thrombotic risk. These studies also suggest that the risk is greatest in the first year after starting HRT and in higher oestrogen formulations.

Once again, the relatively low risk of HRT must be emphasised, with estimates of annual totals of 5–16.5 cases of venous thromboembolism per 100 000 woman-years being attributable to HRT. The short- and long-term benefits of HRT on the relief of severe menopausal symptoms and in the reduction of the risk of osteoporosis and atherosclerotic disease remain important and must be taken into consideration. In the absence of other thromboembolic risk factors (recurrent thromboembolism, thrombophilia, obesity, immobilisation and lower limb venous insufficiency), the balance of benefits favours continuing use of HRT.

Malignant disease

The association between malignancy and venous thromboembolic disease has long been recognised, particularly in cancers of the stomach, lung, breast, pancreas and prostate. The underlying mechanism is activation of the coagulation cascade by production of tissue factor-like substances. Myeloproliferative disorders and haematological malignancies cause hypercoagulable states mainly by platelet activation and excess production of the cellular components of the blood. Immobility frequently accompanies these conditions, further compounding the risk factors for thrombosis. The high incidence of thromboembolic disease in this group of patients undergoing surgery is well recognised.

Screening for an underlying malignancy should be part of the investigation of older patients otherwise not at risk presenting with extensive DVT and pulmonary embolism. Treatment of the hyper-coagulability of malignancy can be extremely diffi-cult, particularly in disseminated malignant disease where massive anticoagulation is often required and very difficult to achieve. A severe prothrombotic state may also be precipitated by chemotherapy for disseminated malignant disease, presumably as a result of release of tissue factor by the malignant cells and activated inflammatory cells.

Summary of pathophysiology

There is now a clearer understanding of the patho-physiology of venous thromboembolism. Throm-bosis seems unlikely to develop in the presence of only one risk factor, with the exception of the more severe and rarer forms of primary thrombo-philia. Rather, thromboembolic disease will super-vene in the patient already primed with an underlying risk factor in whom other prothrombotic events or conditions, such as major surgery, are superimposed.

DIAGNOSIS OF VENOUS THROMBOSIS

Clinical features

The most common symptoms and signs of DVT are pain, swelling, mild rubor, tenderness along the thigh or calf, muscle induration and mild pyrexia. Many patients, however, will have no appreciable symptoms or signs in the affected limb, a common feature of studies using fibrinogen uptake where half the patients have 'silent' DVTs. Of these clinical features, unilateral pitting oedema is the most significant, indicating thrombosis in 70% of patients. Homan's sign of pain or discomfort on foot dorsiflexion is unreliable and castigated by most authorities, including Homan himself.

This uncertain presentation is most common when the thrombosis is localised to the calf veins. Once thrombosis involves the popliteal and femoral veins, the clinical features become more reliable. Distal iliac and femoral vein thromboses commonly present with a swollen painful leg, which is typically white. The pallor is probably a result of capillary compression in the skin caused by the oedema, which also causes difficulty in palpating the pedal pulses. This condition is known as phlegmasia alba dolens or white leg syndrome and is frequently confused with acute arterial insufficiency. Involve-ment of the whole iliac venous system produces a more dramatic oedema, with severe pain and cyanosis, known as phlegmasia caerulea dolens. Areas of patchy skin gangrene may develop in addition to gangrene of the peripheries, typically involving all of the toes of the affected limb. Venous gangrene can be differentiated from arterial by the marked oedema and cyanosis of the limb, in contra-distinction to the pallor and absence of swelling typical of acute arterial occlusion. Venous gangrene is caused partly by the extreme venous congestion resulting from total iliac vein occlusion but also by extension of thrombosis to the venules and capil-laries. There is invariably an underlying severe thrombophiliac condition in these patients.

Several other conditions have very similar presen-tations to venous thrombosis and must be excluded. Ruptured Baker's cyst presents with sudden onset of severe pain and swelling. The cyst is usually not palpable, the knee joint may not be obviously arthritic or abnormal and both conditions may be present at the same time. Duplex scanning will con-firm the diagnosis in most patients. Cellulitis is another common condition that will mimic venous thrombosis. There is often a history of lymphatic oedema or of local trauma and infection, such as an infected insect bite. Muscular problems such as a torn calf muscle or bleeding into the muscle in patients taking anticoagulants will be diagnosed by careful history-taking.

Superficial thrombophlebitis can be confused with DVT. Clinical examination will reveal the super-ficial, linear, often exquisitely painful thrombosed vein, typically in the presence of varicose veins. Recurrent superficial thrombophlebitis may indicate an underlying occult malignancy. The association between superficial thrombophlebitis and DVT is strong, reported to range from 17 to 40%, with superficial thrombophlebitis of the thigh recently associated with a 33% incidence of pulmonary embolism.[93] Because of these associations, venous duplex scanning is recommended to exclude the presence of DVT, particularly in the absence of varicose veins.

The clinical diagnosis of DVT can be both difficult and unreliable. However, clinical stratification of patients into levels of probability of thromboembolic disease is important. Initially, this is to allow reliable selection and interpretation of investigations and also to guide treatment. Wells et al. have shown that the use of a clinical model can stratify patients with suspected DVT into high, moderate or low probability groups (Box 14.3).[94] The use of such a model can simplify the diagnostic process by excluding patients with low probability of DVT and a normal duplex scan or venogram from further testing (Fig. 14.4).

D-dimer

D-dimer is a specific breakdown product of fibrin degeneration, measurement of which is highly sensi-tive and moderately specific for venous thrombo-embolic disease. The Simpli-RED D-dimer is a whole blood red cell agglutination assay that can be

Box 14.3 • Clinical diagnosis of deep vein thrombosis (DVT)

Major criteria
Active cancer
Paralysis or recent plaster immobilisation of leg
Recently bedridden (>3 days) or major surgery (<4 weeks)
Past history of DVT or strong family history
Thigh and calf swelling
Calf swelling to 3 cm more than on asymptomatic side

Minor criteria
History of recent leg trauma (<60 days)
Hospitalisation within the last 6 months
Unilateral pitting oedema
Unilateral erythema or dilated superficial veins

Clinical probability

High

More than three major points and no alternative diagnosis

More than two major points + more than two minor points + no alternative diagnosis

Low

One major point + more than two minor points + alternative diagnosis

One major point + more than one minor point + no alternative diagnosis

No major points + more than three minor points + alternative diagnosis

No major points + more than two minor points + no alternative diagnosis

Moderate

All other combinations

From Wells PS, Hirsh J, Anderson DR et al. Accuracy of clinical assessment of deep-vein thrombosis. Lancet 1995; 345:1326–30. Reprinted with permission of Elsevier.

rapidly performed by the bedside, with reported sensitivities of 85–95% and specificities of 65–68% in symptomatic patients. Alternatively, the newer Elisa for D-dimer can also be performed quickly in the laboratory without the need of the old assay method for batch-testing. In patients with thromboembolic disease, this assay has a high sensitivity of 90–100% but low specificity of 30–40%. Consequently, D-dimer testing has high false-positive rates. Its use with clinical risk group stratification and either compression ultrasound or impedance plethysmography has been clinically evaluated.[95]

Two large clinical studies have confirmed that the combination of a normal D-dimer concentration and a negative compression ultrasound or impedance plethysmograph at presentation excludes DVT. This finding safely allows anticoagulant therapy to be withheld, with less than 2% risk of thromboembolic complications.[96,97]

At present there seems to be a promising role for D-dimer in diagnosis of DVT based on its high negative predictive value in conjunction with other tests.

A recent randomised controlled study in 1096 patients has confirmed the value of D-dimer. Patients were categorised as likely or unlikely to have DVT and then randomised to either ultrasound alone or D-dimer testing. Ultrasound was performed in the D-dimer patients if the test was positive or if the patient was judged likely to have DVT. This study found that a low clinical probability for DVT combined with a negative D-dimer test excluded DVT, thus precluding the need for duplex scanning.[98]

Venography

Venography is regarded as the gold standard for diagnosis of lower-limb DVT but is invasive, uncomfortable and requires injection of contrast.

A positive diagnosis of DVT is made when filling defects are seen within the veins (**Fig. 14.5**). Even when the venous system is almost completely occluded by thrombus, contrast will normally pass between the outer surface of the thrombus and the vein wall to produce a ghost-like outline of the vein. When calf vein thrombosis is identified, it is vital to demonstrate the popliteal and proximal superficial femoral vein to show any propagated thrombus.

If the iliac vessels are not clearly shown, direct injection into the common femoral vein in the groin will produce full anatomical demonstration of the external and common iliac venous system, including any collaterals if there is occlusion. If direct venography demonstrates occlusion of the iliac system, then contralateral common femoral puncture or ascending venography should be performed to demonstrate the extent, if any, of propagation of thrombus into the inferior vena cava (**Fig. 14.6**).[99]

The specific advantages offered by venography are its almost universal availability, the ease of interpretation and relative safety of the procedure. The procedure itself often causes discomfort, particularly when the tourniquet is applied to an acutely swollen leg. There is now a very small risk of a serious contrast reaction and an almost negligible mortality. The theoretical possibility of displacing thrombus by the application of the thigh tourniquet also appears to be either an excessively rare occurrence

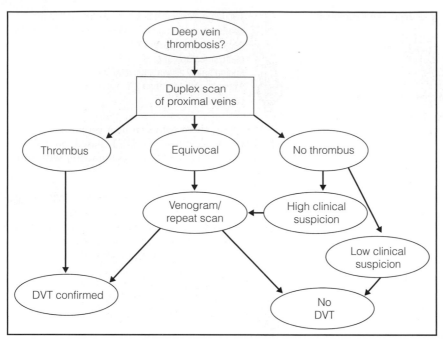

Figure 14.4 • Algorithm for the investigation of deep vein thrombosis (DVT) that largely relies on duplex scanning supplemented by clinical index of suspicion and venography or repeat scanning where doubt remains. With permission from Hamilton G, Platt SA. Deep vein thrombosis. In: Beard JD, Gaines PA (eds) Vascular and endovascular surgery. London: WB Saunders, 1998; pp. 351–96.

or without clinical consequence when it does occur. Venography does damage the endothelium of the veins and can cause venous thrombosis. This was not an uncommon occurrence when ionic contrast media were used, though it is considerably less likely when non-ionic contrast is employed.

Ultrasonography

B-mode ultrasound scanning is widely available, relatively inexpensive and is the non-invasive investigation of choice. The lumen of a patent vein is usually anechoic, appearing as a black area on the screen; unfortunately, thrombus within a vein is also anechoic. However, the clot is only slightly compressible, unlike the lumen of a patent vein, the walls of which are easily opposed by external compression by the ultrasound probe.[100] By using this simple technique, thrombus within the large veins of the thigh and popliteal region can be diagnosed with a sensitivity and specificity of 97% and 94% respectively (**Fig. 14.7**).[100–102] Colour flow does not add to the accuracy of the test, and it is not accurate in detecting calf vein thrombosis. Demonstration of pelvic veins, including the iliac veins, can often be difficult particularly when bowel gas obscures the retroperitoneum, as is often seen with patients who have been bed-bound. Also, the accuracy of ultra-

sonography is totally dependent on the operator.

Despite these limitations, compression ultrasonography is the first-line investigation in most clinical centres where reliable scanning is available. The major limitation is in diagnosis of a calf vein thrombus, but the safety of withholding anticoagulation in suspected DVT where normal sequential scans are found is well established. The risk of thromboembolic disease supervening in patients with two or three normal scans over a week is less than 2%.[100] Even where isolated calf vein thrombosis is present, up to 80% of these will not propagate but lyse spontaneously. The remaining 20–30% that will propagate into the popliteal segment will reliably be detected by serial scanning and can then be treated.[103] However, where there is a high clinical probability of DVT and a normal venous scan, venography should be obtained since in this scenario there is an 18% probability of thrombosis.[104]

Magnetic resonance studies

Magnetic resonance imaging (MRI) and magnetic resonance angiography (MRA) can be applied to both peripheral and central venous systems. Availability of MRI and MRA is not currently widespread, although this is likely to be where the future of

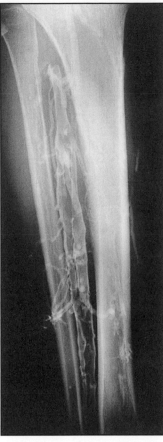

Figure 14.5 • Venogram demonstrating extensive thrombus within the calf veins. The contrast around the filling defects results in an appearance called tramlining. With permission from Hamilton G, Platt SA. Deep vein thrombosis. In: Beard JD, Gaines PA (eds) Vascular and endovascular surgery. London: WB Saunders, 1998; pp. 351–96.

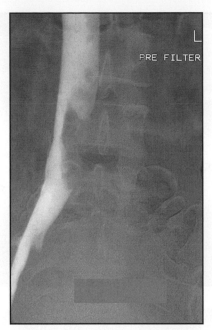

Figure 14.6 • Femoral venogram demonstrating complete occlusion of left iliac vein with thrombus extending into the inferior vena cava. With permission from Hamilton G, Platt SA. Deep vein thrombosis. In: Beard JD, Gaines PA (eds) Vascular and endovascular surgery. London: WB Saunders, 1998; pp. 351–96.

vascular imaging lies. MRI is used to demonstrate the presence of patent veins or the presence of thrombus within vessels. MRA is solely used to demonstrate the presence of patent vessels. These techniques are currently under investigation and offer the potential benefit of a totally non-invasive procedure. Intravascular contrast need not be administered and, like Doppler, MRA uses flow as the source of image contrast rather than any administered agent. This investigation is of particular value in suspected iliac vein thrombosis in the pregnant woman.

Computed tomography

Although not widely used in the imaging of peripheral venous occlusion, computed tomography (CT), particularly with intravenous contrast enhancement, can be very useful in the diagnosis of central venous occlusion. Both superior and inferior vena caval obstruction can be diagnosed on enhanced CT. Spiral or helical scanning is performed by moving the patient through the scanning detector while images are acquired. The main advantage of the technique is the speed of acquisition so that the study can normally be completed within a single breath-hold. This eliminates movement artefact and allows the acquisition of images timed to show dense vascular enhancement during its first pass rather than waiting for equilibrium of contrast opacification. Spiral CT pulmonary angiography is being increasingly used to diagnose pulmonary embolism.[105]

Plethysmography

Mercury strain gauge and impedance plethysmography demonstrate changes in the volume of the limb during occlusion of venous outflow by a pneumatic tourniquet and after release of the occlusion. They demonstrate the effect of venous obstruction proximal to the detector, and thus these methods cannot reliably demonstrate DVT that develops, and remains, below the knee. The sensitivity and specificity of this method are 83%

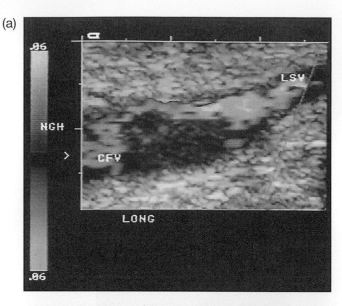

(a)

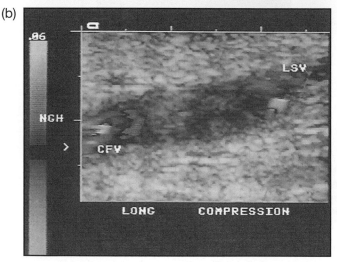

(b)

Figure 14.7 • Duplex scan of the common femoral vein: **(a)** a thrombus results in an area of no flow (black area); **(b)** the vein cannot be compressed because of the presence of the thrombus. With permission from Hamilton G, Platt SA. Deep vein thrombosis. In: Beard JD, Gaines PA (eds) Vascular and endovascular surgery. London: WB Saunders, 1998; pp. 351–96.

and 92% respectively. Direct comparison studies have confirmed the superiority of compression ultrasonography.

Radioisotope imaging

Isotope-labelled fibrinogen can demonstrate a calf thrombus that is being actively formed but it has been shown to be unreliable in demonstrating more proximal thrombus, particularly when causing complete occlusion. New agents that bind to fibrinogen receptors on activated platelets and labelled antibodies that bind to fibrin may have a major role in the investigation of venous thrombosis within the first decade of the 21st century.

Summary of diagnostic techniques

Ultrasonography in experienced and validated hands is the investigation of choice, with venography reserved for suspected calf vein or iliac vein thrombosis or where there is lack of concordance with the pretest clinical assessment of probability. This policy is putting increasing strain on vascular laboratories and ultrasound departments and the use of D-dimer assays may have a role in minimising this demand (**Fig. 14.8**). There remains a vital role for clinical assessment and stratification into low-, moderate- and high-risk groups before testing to maximise diagnostic accuracy and optimise treatment.

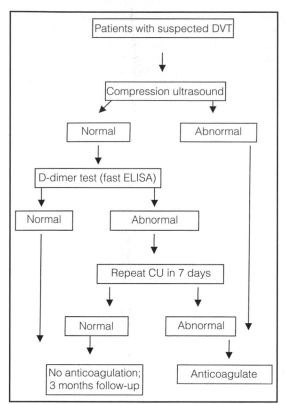

Figure 14.8 • Strategy for diagnosis of deep vein thrombosis (DVT) using D-dimer assay. ELISA, enzyme-linked immunosorbent assay; CU, compression ultrasound. Modified with permission from Chunilal SD, Ginsberg JS. Strategies for the diagnosis of deep vein thrombosis and pulmonary embolism. Thromb Res 2000; 97:V33–V48.

MANAGEMENT OF DEEP VENOUS THROMBOSIS

DVT can present with a spectrum of severity ranging from isolated thrombosis of the tibial veins detected with radiolabelled fibrinogen studies to the life- and limb-threatening phlegmasia caerulea dolens and venous gangrene. The severity of the clinical syndrome depends on the extent of thrombosis present combined with the various underlying prothrombotic factors driving this process. The major aims of treatment are initially to halt the prothrombotic process and thus clot propagation, to prevent or minimise the risk of pulmonary embolism, and to optimise resolution by fibrinolysis of the thrombus, thus reducing the likelihood of an eventual post-thrombotic syndrome. To achieve this, anticoagulation with heparin and warfarin remains the mainstay of modern treatment and has the further advantage of preventing recurrence.

Treatment of venous thromboembolism by anticoagulation

The importance of anticoagulation in the treatment of venous thromboembolic disease was first established by Barritt and Jordan in 1960, some 20 years after the introduction of both heparin and warfarin.[106] In a randomised trial in patients with suspected pulmonary embolism, a significant reduction in death and recurrent pulmonary embolism was shown in patients treated with warfarin.[106]

Because it establishes anticoagulation more rapidly, treatment is usually begun with heparin before warfarin is introduced several days later.

The clinical importance of this initial heparin therapy was confirmed by a double-blind randomised trial of oral anticoagulants alone versus oral anticoagulants and initial intravenous heparin. This showed a significantly higher incidence of recurrent venous thromboembolic events of 20% in the group receiving oral anticoagulants alone versus 6.7% in the group receiving initial intravenous heparin therapy.[107]

HEPARIN

Heparin is a heterogeneous mixture of sulphated polysaccharides of molecular mass 4000–40 000 Da. Its immediate anticoagulant effect is by catalytic acceleration of the reaction between thrombin and antithrombin III. This potentiates the inhibition of thrombin and the other active serine proteases (factors IXa, Xa, XIa and XII) by antithrombin III. The reaction between factor Xa and heparin–antithrombin III complex is particularly important, with inhibition of only one unit of factor Xa preventing generation of 50 units of thrombin. Heparin has a further catalytic effect on anticoagulation by directly binding with heparin cofactor II, an important selective inhibitor of thrombin. This effect is important in antithrombin deficiency, which can be inherited or may be induced by prolonged heparin therapy, where up to one-third of antithrombin will be complexed with serine proteases. Transfusion with fresh frozen plasma in these clinical situations will provide sufficient antithrombin to improve heparin anticoagulation.

Heparin is commercially obtained from bovine lung or porcine gut mucosa and formulated as either a sodium or calcium salt. It can be administered either intravenously or subcutaneously. Its anticoagulant effect is immediate when given intravenously, whereas the pharmacodynamics of subcutaneous absorption lead to peak effects after 4–6 hours but anticoagulation lasting 8–12 hours depending on the dose given. In comparison, intravenous heparin has a half-life of about 90 minutes. Because heparin is cleared by the reticuloendothelial system and not by the liver or kidney, failure of either of these organs will not affect heparin clearance.

Continuous intravenous infusion of heparin has been the preferred mode of administration because of its immediate effect, fewer haemorrhagic complications and requirement for smaller doses.[108] The standard regimen is an initial bolus injection of 100–200 units/kg followed by infusion of 1000–2000 units/hour. Because of individual variations in the pharmacokinetics of heparin, the rate of infusion must be defined by measurement of the APTT. A range of APTT between 1.5 and 2.5 times the normal control value is considered therapeutic, although bleeding complications are less common if the APTT is kept below 2.0.[109] Subcutaneous administration of heparin is also effective provided that APTT levels are monitored and maintained between 1.5 and 2.0.

Rapid attainment of therapeutic levels of heparin anticoagulation is of extreme clinical importance since there is a 15-fold higher incidence of recurrent thromboembolism in patients with APTT levels below 1.5 at 24 hours after initiation of treatment compared with those with APTT levels in the therapeutic range.[108,110] There is considerable evidence, however, that this goal is not achieved in the majority of patients.[111,112] Comparison of weight-based heparin dosage using a nomogram versus standard administration (as outlined above) has shown that more effective and rapid anticoagulation occurs with the former regimen (97% vs. 77%). Use of such a weight-based nomogram or of fixed-dose LMWH preparations would avoid the over-cautious approach to heparin administration that is widely prevalent, with its risk of subtherapeutic dosage and high recurrence rates.[113]

Two studies have compared a longer 10-day regimen of continuous intravenous heparin with the 5-day regimen, before oral anticoagulation.[114,115] Although relatively small numbers of patients were involved, the risk of thrombotic and haemorrhagic complications were similar in both regimens. Consequently, most centres now start oral anticoagulation with warfarin 24 hours after starting intravenous heparin. The heparin is discontinued when the warfarin dosage is therapeutic, usually at 5–10 days after starting.

LOW-MOLECULAR-WEIGHT HEPARIN

The LMWHs are derivatives of unfractionated heparin (UFH), with molecular masses in the range 3000–10 000 Da. Unlike UFH, these smaller mol-

ecules cannot bind simultaneously to antithrombin and thrombin, which is required for inhibition of thrombin to take place, but interact readily with factor Xa. This inhibition of factor Xa is the major antithrombotic effect of the LMWHs. Their inability to bind to antithrombin and thrombin decreases their anticoagulant activity and thus decreases bleeding complications. The bioavailability of subcutaneous LMWHs is much greater than standard heparin and they have longer biological half-lives. Because of these more predictable pharmacokinetics, a single daily dose that is fixed (but in most preparations related to the patient's weight) results in adequate anticoagulation without the need to monitor APTT levels.

Systematic review has shown that once-daily treatment with LMWH is as safe and effective as a twice-daily regimen.[116] A recent meta-analysis of trials comparing LMWHs with intravenous UFH in treatment of venous thromboembolic disease has confirmed the safety of initial treatment of DVT by LMWH, with a possible reduced bleeding risk.[117]

Two multicentre, prospective, randomised trials of proximal DVT compared initial treatment by LMWH, primarily as outpatient therapy, with UFH as inpatient treatment. Both groups followed this treatment with 3 months of oral anticoagulation. There was a trend to lower recurrent thromboembolism in the group treated with LMWH.[118,119] In both studies, up to half of all patients given LMWH had entirely outpatient treatment, with the remainder having a significantly shorter length of hospital stay (1–3 days vs. 6.5–8 days with heparin treatment).

Therefore, LMWH is not only as safe and efficacious as standard heparin but it also reduces inpatient stay and hospital cost. A review of eight studies of outpatient treatment for DVT with LMWH proved that this approach was safe, efficacious and cost-effective.[120] A review of the efficacy and safety of fixed-dose LMWH in comparison with adjusted-dose UFH for venous thromboembolism has been recently updated in the Cochrane Library. This exhaustive review was based on all truly randomised clinical trials of these therapies and represents the best clinical evidence currently available.[121]

In this review, LMWH was shown to be at least as safe and efficacious as UFH. There was a statistically significant reduction in occurrence of major bleeding during the initial treatment with LMWH: 1.1% (2158 patients) with LMWH and 2.0% (2196 patients) with UFH. Overall mortality at the end of the study was also significantly lower for LMWH: 5.2% (94 of 1803 patients) with LMWH and 6.9% (125 of 1816 patients) with UFH. Furthermore, a statistically significant reduction of thrombus size on venography was found for LMWH (reduction of 62% vs. 53%). Finally, in patients with proximal DVT, a significant reduction in recurrent thromboembolic disease was shown for LMWH (4.8% of 814 patients compared with 7.8% of 822 patients on UFH). The review concludes that LMWH can be safely adopted as standard therapy for DVT, and that comparison between the different LMWHs is now justified.

Meta-analysis of prospective randomised comparisons of UFH and LMWH confirms the effectiveness and safety of fixed-dose LMWH in the initial treatment of non-massive pulmonary embolism.[122]

WARFARIN

Warfarin acts by interfering with the production of vitamin K-dependent factors II, VII, IX and X in addition to protein C and protein S. Vitamin K is a cofactor in the production of the carboxyl glutamyl residues of clotting factors required to bind calcium. In the presence of warfarin, these factors are produced in active forms such that, in the fully anticoagulated state, the activity of factors II and IX is only 30–40% and that of factors VII and X is 10%. Prothrombin has a long circulating half-life of 36 hours and, consequently, anticoagulation with warfarin does not become effective until more than 48 hours from the starting dose, during which time, of course, heparin is required. The reduction in active vitamin K-dependent protein C and protein S concentrations caused by warfarin treatment also results in a prothrombotic state, which further supports the need for initial heparin therapy.

Warfarin is well absorbed from the gut, mainly bound to albumin, and has a circulating half-life of 36–40 hours; it is the unbound fraction (3%) that is the active component. There are different loading-dose regimens, but dosage should be reduced in liver failure, the elderly, patients having parenteral nutrition or those receiving broad-spectrum antibiotics. Regular monitoring by measurement of the prothrombin time is essential, with maintenance of the INR between 2.0 and 3.0. Warfarin crosses the placental barrier, causing fetal abnormalities, and cannot be used during pregnancy. LMWH should be used instead.

DURATION OF ANTICOAGULANT THERAPY

The accepted regimen of anticoagulant therapy for venous thromboembolism is 5–10 days of heparin followed by 3–6 months of oral anticoagulation with warfarin.

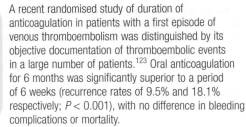

A recent randomised study of duration of anticoagulation in patients with a first episode of venous thromboembolism was distinguished by its objective documentation of thromboembolic events in a large number of patients.[123] Oral anticoagulation for 6 months was significantly superior to a period of 6 weeks (recurrence rates of 9.5% and 18.1% respectively; P < 0.001), with no difference in bleeding complications or mortality.

Interestingly, in both groups the INR was maintained at 2.0–2.85, with a similarly low major bleeding rate of 1.1% and 0.2% at 6 months and 6 weeks respectively. These studies support the need for anticoagulation for a minimum of 3 months after a first thromboembolic episode. In older patients with unexplained thrombosis, this should be extended to 6 months. Similarly, younger patients with secondary thrombosis should have 6 months on warfarin, while in those younger patients with unexplained thrombosis a 2-year period of anticoagulation is to be preferred.[124]

Longer periods of treatment, for example where there has been recurrent disease or major pulmonary embolism, is justified but will expose patients, particularly the elderly, to increased risk of major haemorrhage and death.

A recent meta-analysis of different durations of vitamin K antagonists confirmed reduced risk of recurrent venous thromboembolism for the duration of treatment. Over time there was reduction in the absolute risk of venous thromboembolism but no reduction in the risk of major haemorrhage.[125] There has been recent interest in the possibility that low-dose warfarin therapy might be as effective as full therapeutic doses but without the logistical disadvantage of monitoring. This question was addressed in a recent randomised double-blind comparison of conventional (INR 2.0–3.0) with low-intensity warfarin therapy (INR 1.5–1.9) which found that the conventional dose prevented recurrence more effectively without increased risk of bleeding. This well-conducted Canadian trial in 738 patients suggests that low-dose warfarin therapy is neither more efficacious nor safer than standard treatment.[126]

Management of patients with thrombophilia with venous thromboembolism

Patients with thrombophilia who have not had an episode of venous thromboembolism are best managed by counselling and advice regarding symptoms of thrombosis. Females should be counselled on the risk of taking the oral contraceptive or HRT. Careful evaluation of the risk of thrombosis should be made before any surgical or medical intervention, and appropriate prophylactic measures instituted. As has been previously discussed, the risks of haemorrhagic complications from long-term anticoagulant therapy probably outweigh those of developing thrombosis in a thrombophiliac who has not had a previous thrombotic event. Even in the thrombophiliac who has had one episode of thromboembolism, the balance of risks probably remains against long-term anticoagulation in the absence of other risk factors.[127] Clinical features, such as the site and severity of thrombosis (e.g. massive life-threatening pulmonary embolism), whether the thrombosis was spontaneous or related to predisposing risk factors, women of childbearing age, risk of haemorrhage in patient's occupation and family history, should all be taken into consideration when making decisions regarding long-term anticoagulation.

Other treatments

Several approaches to thrombolytic therapy have used plasmin, plasminogen and, most frequently, streptokinase, urokinase and recombinant t-PA. Therapy was initially given systemically and, more recently, by local catheter delivering to the affected area. Lysis of thrombus is undoubtedly achieved, but usually this is partial and there is no clinical evidence that this is of long-lasting benefit in terms of preservation of venous valvular function.[128] The best case for thrombolytic therapy is in patients with severe phlegmasia caerulea dolens, or with pulmonary embolism causing cardiorespiratory compromise.

Hirudin is an uncommonly used anticoagulant that is a direct thrombin inhibitor. Its use is recommended primarily in acute coronary syndromes and in the immunological type of HIT (type II). It may also be of value in breast-feeding women who do not wish to discontinue in order to be treated with warfarin. Hirudin has been shown to be safe in this scenario, with no detectable levels in breast milk in the presence of therapeutic serum levels in the mother.[129]

Novel anticoagulant agents

The LMWHs are a major therapeutic advance that have the bonus of not requiring dosage monitoring. However, most patients prefer oral rather than injected treatment and several oral agents which do not require monitoring are being clinically assessed.

Pentasaccharides are based on the smallest moiety of the heparin molecule with anticoagulant properties. These agents have the dual characteristics of high affinity for antithrombin and selective factor Xa inhibition.

Fondaparinux has been studied in trials of thromboprophylaxis in major orthopaedic surgery that all showed major benefit over enoxaparin (LMWH), with an overall risk reduction for venous thromboembolism greater than 50% without increased risk of bleeding.[130] However, these studies have been criticised for possible bias because of manufacturer sponsorship and the use of surrogate end points in analysis of outcomes.[131]

This oral anticoagulant shows promise but further clinical experience is required, in particular to exclude the possibility of increased risk compared with enoxaparin.

Oral direct thrombin inhibitors are another group of drugs that are promising.

One of these, ximelagatran, has been clinically assessed in several different trials of stroke prevention (SPORTIF III and V), thromboprophylaxis (METHRO II), secondary prophylaxis after myocardial infarction (ESTEEM) and secondary prevention of venous thromboembolism (THRIVE III).[132,133]

The trials show efficacy similar to or better than warfarin but with lower bleeding risk. The most frequently reported complication was of transient rises in aminotranferase in a small percentage of patients.

THROMBOPROPHYLAXIS

Pulmonary embolism remains the third most common cause of cardiovascular death. Untreated proximal DVT carries a significant risk of immediate pulmonary embolism and later post-thrombotic syndrome. For these reasons, it is incumbent on all doctors treating patients at risk of venous thromboembolism to be aware of these risks and also of the need to employ thromboprophylaxis to reduce this burden of disease. The main focus of thromboprophylaxis has been in the surgical disciplines, but there is a similarly strong need for prophylaxis in non-surgical patients. There is less clinical evidence available to make definitive recommendations in medical patients. In 1998, the Fifth Consensus Conference of the American College of Chest Physicians recommended the use of prophylaxis with low-dose UFH and LMWH in several categories of patients, particularly those with congestive cardiac failure and chest infections.[134] Several recently completed trials in medical patients suggest that the use of LMWH is recommended in higher-risk patients, particularly those with heart failure and ischaemic stroke.[135]

In all categories of patients, clinical stratification into categories of low, moderate or high risk has

Table 14.1 • Risk assessment protocol from the THRIFT Consensus Group

Risk level	Group	Suggested prophylaxis
Low	Minor surgery Major surgery <40 years Minor trauma Minor medical illness	Leg elevation and early mobilisation
Moderate	Major surgery >40 years Major trauma or burns Major medical illness Minor surgery and risks Inflammatory bowel disease	As low risk, plus antiembolism hosiery or subcutaneous heparin Mechanical calf compression
High	Hip, pelvis, knee fracture Major cancer surgery Surgery and thrombophilia Surgery and previous thrombosis Acute lower limb paralysis Illness and thrombophilia Illness and previous thrombosis	Both antiembolism hosiery and subcutaneous heparin Mechanical calf compression is highly effective

From Thromboembolic Risk Factors (THRIFT) Consensus Group. Risk of and prophylaxis for venous thromboembolism in hospital patients. Br Med J 1992; 305:567–74, with permission.

much to commend it (**Table 14.1**). Risk also varies according to the nature of the surgical procedure. In surgical patients, therefore, prophylaxis can be tailored according to risk giving the best risk–benefit ratio (**Table 14.2**).[80,136]

Mechanical methods

In the at-risk patient the most simple form of thromboprophylaxis is lower limb elevation. In a report from Ashby et al., the importance of elevation of the lower limbs was demonstrated with significantly increased blood velocity and decreased diameter of the deep veins when elevation of the leg up to 6° was maintained.[137] Alarmingly, diminished blood velocity with marked dilatation of the deep veins was found in patients with a leg-down posture. It would therefore seem that the classical posture of patients on the first postoperative day, who are forced to sit out of bed in an uncomfortable chair with their legs hanging down in order to avoid DVT, may in fact be achieving exactly the opposite.

Graduated compression stockings are a simple, safe and moderately effective form of thromboprophylaxis.[138] These stockings provide low-pressure compression of 18 mmHg at the ankle, 14 mmHg at calf level and 8 mmHg at knee level and probably work by increasing the velocity of venous blood flow. The major limitation in their use is in patients with severe peripheral vascular disease with ankle systolic pressure below 70 mmHg, where tissue necrosis may result.

In 1994, a comprehensive meta-analysis concluded that graduated compression stockings produced a highly significant risk reduction in postoperative venous thromboembolic disease of 68% in moderate-risk patients.[139] A recent review of stockings in both surgical and medical patients confirmed their effectiveness in reducing risk of venous thromboembolic disease, particularly when used on a background of other methods of prophylaxis.[140]

Intermittent pneumatic leg compression is provided by a single-chamber boot system, which gently applies intermittent, uniform, low-pressure compression on the entire lower leg. Typical compression pressures are 40–60 mmHg for 1 minute with a 90-second period of decompression. This increases the velocity of venous return and blood flow but may also enhance fibrinolytic activity.[141] A further possible effect is on inhibition of the tissue factor pathway.[142] There are limited data regarding the efficacy of this method, with two meta-analyses reporting DVT rates of 9.9 and 17.6% for intermittent pneumatic leg compression versus 20.3 and 27% for placebo, these differences being statistically significant. A newer variation of this method uses high-pressure, rapid-inflation, pneumatic compression, which can be delivered by devices using foot compression alone or a combination of foot and calf compression. This method significantly increases maximal velocities in the femoral and popliteal veins, particularly in postphlebitic limbs.[143]

Table 14.2 • Classification and incidence of level of risk for deep vein thrombosis (DVT) in the absence of prophylaxis

Risk category	Incidence of DVT (%)		Incidence of pulmonary embolism (%)	
	Calf	Proximal	Clinical	Fatal
Highest risk Major surgery in those >40 years old + prior venous thromboembolism, malignancy or hypercoagulable state Elective hip or knee surgery Hip fracture Stroke, multiple trauma, spinal cord injury	40–80	10–30	4–10	1–5
High risk Major surgery in those >60 years old + no additional risk factors Major surgery in those 40–60 years old + additional risk factors Myocardial infarction or medical patients + risk factors	20–40	4–8	2–4	0.4–1.0
Moderate risk Major or minor surgery in those 40–60 years old + no additional risk factors Major surgery in those <40 years old + no additional risk factors Minor surgery (any age) + risk factors	10–20	2–4	1–2	0.1–0.4
Low risk Minor or uncomplicated surgery in those <40 years old + no risk factors	2	0.4	0.2	0.002

Modified from Clagett GP, Anderson FA Jr, Geerts W et al. Prevention of venous thromboembolism. Chest 1998; 114:S531–S560, with permission.

Trials of the foot pump method have shown mixed results, with a large randomised comparison with LMWH in total knee replacement reporting a highly significant 30% difference in DVT rate in favour of LMWH prophylaxis (54% in foot pump group vs. 24% in the LMWH group).[144]

A Cochrane review in 2003 of the efficacy of mechanical pumping devices in hip fracture found that their use may protect against DVT and pulmonary embolism (7% with pumps vs. 22% without).[145] A randomised comparison of intermittent pneumatic compression and LMWH in 442 trauma patients showed similarly low rates of thromboembolic and bleeding complications, with the authors recommending use of intermittent pneumatic compression for thromboprophylaxis on the grounds of cost-effectiveness.[146]

Further assessment of these newer methods of mechanical prophylaxis is required but they certainly appear to lack efficacy if used alone in the higher-risk procedures.

Pharmacological methods

Several drugs have been used in the prophylaxis of DVT. It has been known since 1959 that warfarin anticoagulation reduces significantly the incidence of thromboembolic disease when it is used as prophylaxis.[147] This method has not been used by surgeons, however, mainly because of the considerable risk of haemorrhage either spontaneous or related to the surgery.

In the meta-analysis of the Antiplatelets Trialists' Collaboration, aspirin was found to reduce DVT significantly, although the poor quality of some studies included has led to many doubts regarding this finding. However, aspirin may have a role in prophylaxis of low-risk groups.[136] Other agents such as danaparoid, dermatan sulphate, hirudin and dextran have also been used but never adequately assessed or accepted.

Low-dose UFH (5000 units subcutaneously two or three times daily) has been used for more than 20 years. As early as 1988 a meta-analysis of 62 randomised placebo-controlled trials of UFH in

LOCAL INDUCTION

Trust policy requires that non-permanent staff receive a localised induction appropriate to their role. The Consultant/Business Manager is responsible for ensuring that all locums receive instruction in the following areas as a minimum:

Duties & responsibilities, introduction to key staff, an explanation of incident reporting, location of key areas and departments, and if appropriate informed of local protocols including prescription admin and care pathways, the bleep system and how to seek clinical help.

By signing the timesheet, both the Consultant/Business Manager and the Locum Doctor are confirming that this has been carried out. Locum doctors are expected to notify their supervisor or Senior Member of staff in the event they are unsure of any aspects of these duties or responsibilities, including the use of equipment.

Local induction paperwork is provided to the locum doctor by the Medical Staffing Department with their booking confirmation. Further copies of the Local induction document can be found on the intranet.

FALSE STATEMENT

By signing the declarations overleaf, the Locum and the Consultant/Business Manager understand that if they knowingly provide false information this may result in disciplinary action and they may be liable for prosecution and civil recovery proceedings. They also consent to the disclosure of information from this form to and by the Trust and the NHS Counter Fraud & Security Management Service for the purpose of verification of the claim and the investigation, detection and prosecution of fraud.

general, orthopaedic and urological surgery demonstrated a reduction in DVT and pulmonary embolism by two-thirds.[148] This was associated with a 2% increase in the incidence of minor bleeding events. Several large randomised trials have compared surgical prophylaxis using LMWH with UFH. These trials have shown LMWH to be at least as efficacious as UFH but with a small reduction in bleeding complications.[149] Two meta-analyses have shown superior results with LMWH after total hip replacement with regard to postoperative DVT (risk reduction of 17–32%) and pulmonary embolism (risk reduction of 50%).[150,151] A further interesting benefit of LMWH in hip arthroplasty is in the reduction in proximal venous thrombosis observed in several trials when compared with UFH or placebo (93.2% with LMWH, 54% with UFH and 57% with placebo).[152]

LMWH thromboprophylaxis has been shown to be cost-effective for moderate- and high-risk surgical patients.[153]

 A recent meta-analysis of LMWH compared with no treatment, placebo or UFH for thromboprophylaxis in general surgery confirmed its efficacy and safety.[154]

It is undoubtedly more convenient with its once-daily administration, and LMWH has largely replaced UFH as the pharmacological prophylactic agent.

A cautionary note has been struck, however, by a recently updated Cochrane review of relevant randomised controlled trials of heparin, LMWH and physical methods of prophylaxis in hip fracture surgery (a very high-risk group), which has found the evidence to support this swing to LMWH to be rather sparse. It found insufficient evidence to distinguish between UFH and LMWH, although the review did confirm the protective effect of injectable heparins against DVT.[145] Good-quality trials comparing mechanical methods as well as direct comparisons of heparin formulations were recommended by the reviewers.

Summary of prophylactic methods

The clinical evidence available shows effective prevention of DVT with LMWH and low-dose UFH but at the cost of a small but real risk of potentially clinically significant haemorrhage. Mechanical methods have no associated risks but are probably less effective in prevention. Combinations of LMWH and mechanical methods, particularly compression stockings, have shown superior efficacy in DVT prevention in several studies. Pending the results of ongoing trials, the following recommendations are generally agreed. In low-risk patients the use of heparins is best avoided because of the adverse risk–benefit ratio of the associated haemorrhagic risk (Table 14.3).[136] Moderate-risk patients will benefit from LMWH (unless there are major risks of haemorrhage, for example in neurosurgery; in these patients compression stockings are recommended), but the addition of compression stockings may not be cost-effective. In high-risk patients the additional protection expected from combined LMWH and mechanical methods justifies the costs.

Table 14.3 • Differential weighting of side effects of prophylaxis depending on risk of venous thromboembolic disease (VTE)

VTE risk category	Number of anticipated (preventable) events in absence of prophylaxis		Number of anticipated side effects of prophylaxis
	Proximal DVT	Fatal PE	Severe haemorrhage
High	200 (160)	30 (24)	3
Moderate	50 (40)	5 (4)	3
Low	5 (4)	<1 (<1)	3

DVT, deep vein thrombosis; PE, pulmonary embolism.
Data are based on a hypothetical cohort of 1000 patients undergoing surgery, assuming that the prophylactic tool has an efficiency of 80% and produces a severe bleeding side effect in 0.3% of patients.
From Bounameaux H. Integrating pharmacologic and mechanical prophylaxis of venous thromboembolism. Thromb Haemost 1999; 82:931–7, with permission.

• **Key points**

- Thromboembolic disease afflicts primarily the elderly, with involvement to a lesser extent of the middle-aged and young who more often have a background of primary or secondary thrombophilia.

- Thromboembolic disease is common, developing in about one-quarter of all general surgical patients and in over 40% of orthopaedic and major trauma patients. Pulmonary embolism is a common complication and a significant cause of perioperative morbidity and death.

- Venous thrombosis will develop in patients with well-described and categorised underlying risk factors in whom other prothrombotic conditions or events such as major surgery are superimposed. Prevention is possible in almost all surgical patients.

- Diagnosis is accurate and reliable using patient risk stratification, D-dimer measurement and venous compression ultrasonography. Spiral CT, pulmonary angiography and CT scanning is accurate in diagnosis of significant pulmonary embolism.

- Prompt anticoagulation (LMWH for 5 days and warfarin for 6 months) remains the mainstay of treatment for DVT extending above the calf veins.

- Thromboprophylaxis using graduated compression hosiery and LMWH is highly effective in surgical patients while intermittent pneumatic calf compression is also beneficial, particularly in hip and knee surgery and in trauma patients.

REFERENCES

1. Anderson FA Jr, Wheeler HB, Goldberg RJ et al. A population-based perspective of the hospital incidence and case-fatality rates of deep vein thrombosis and pulmonary embolism. The Worcester DVT Study. Arch Intern Med 1991; 151:933–8.

2. Carter CJ, Anderson FA, Wheeler HB. Epidemiology and pathophysiology of venous thromboembolism. In: Hull R (ed.) Venous thromboembolism. New York: Futura, 1996; pp. 3–26.

3. White RH. The epidemiology of venous thromboembolism. Circulation 2003; 107:I1–8.

4. Thomas WA, Davies JMP, O'Neal RM et al. Incidence of myocardial infarction correlated with venous and pulmonary thrombosis and pulmonary embolism. Am J Cardiol 1960; 5:41–7.

5. Woo KS, Tse LK, Tse CY et al. The prevalence and pattern of pulmonary thromboembolism in the Chinese in Hong Kong. Int J Cardiol 1988; 20:373–80.

6. Lilienfeld DE, Chan E, Ehland J et al. Mortality from pulmonary embolism in the United States: 1962 to 1984. Chest 1990; 98:1067–72.

7. Goldhaber SZ. Epidemiology of pulmonary embolism and deep vein thrombosis. In: Bloom AL, Forbes CD, Tuddenham EGD (eds) Haemostasis and thrombosis, 3rd edn. Edinburgh: Churchill Livingstone, 1994; pp. 1327–33.

8. Sandler DA, Martin JF. Autopsy proven pulmonary embolism in hospital patients: are we detecting enough deep vein thrombosis? J R Soc Med 1989; 82:203–5.

9. Flanc C, Kakkar VV, Clarke MB. The detection of venous thrombosis of the legs using 125-I-labelled fibrinogen. Br J Surg 1968; 55:742–7.

10. Kakkar VV, Howe CT, Flanc C, Clarke MB. Natural history of postoperative deep-vein thrombosis. Lancet 1969; ii:230–2.

11. Huisman MV, Buller HR, ten Cate JW et al. Unexpected high prevalence of silent pulmonary embolism in patients with deep venous thrombosis. Chest 1989; 95:498–502.

12. Doyle DJ, Turpie AG, Hirsh J et al. Adjusted subcutaneous heparin or continuous intravenous heparin in patients with acute deep vein thrombosis. A randomized trial. Ann Intern Med 1987; 107:441–5.

13. Lindhagen A, Bergqvist D, Hallbook T. Deep venous insufficiency after postoperative thrombosis diagnosed with 125I-labelled fibrinogen uptake test. Br J Surg 1984; 71:511–15.

14. Scurr JH, Coleridge-Smith PD, Hasty JH. Deep venous thrombosis: a continuing problem. Br Med J 1988; 297:28.

15. Nicolaides AN, Kakkar VV, Renney JT. Soleal sinuses and stasis. Br J Surg 1971; 58:307.

16. Rollins DL, Semrow CM, Friedell ML et al. Origin of deep vein thrombi in an ambulatory population. Am J Surg 1988; 156:122–5.

17. Kearon C. Natural history of venous thromboembolism. Circulation 2003; 107:I-22–I-30.

18. Schaub RG, Simmons CA, Koets MH et al. Early events in the formation of a venous thrombus following local trauma and stasis. Lab Invest 1984; 51:218–24.

19. Thomas DP, Merton RE, Hockley DJ. The effect of stasis on the venous endothelium: an ultrastructural study. Br J Haematol 1983; 55:113–22.

20. Hamer JD, Malone PC, Silver IA. The pO_2 in venous valve pockets: its possible bearing on thrombogenesis. Br J Surg 1981; 68:166–70.

21. Sevitt S. Pathology and pathogenesis of deep vein thrombi. In: Bergan JJ, Yao JST (eds) Venous problems. Chicago: Year Book, 1978; pp. 257–63.

22. Thomas DP, Merton RE, Wood RD, Hockley DJ. The relationship between vessel wall injury and venous thrombosis: an experimental study. Br J Haematol 1985; 59:449–57.

23. Thomas DP. Pathogenesis of venous thrombosis. In: Bloom AL, Forbes CD, Tuddenham EGD (eds) Haemostasis and thrombosis, 3rd edn. Edinburgh: Churchill Livingstone, 1994; pp. 1327–33.

24. Karino T, Motomiya M. Flow through a venous valve and its implication for thrombus formation. Thromb Res 1984; 36:245–57.

25. Sevitt S. The structure and growth of valve-pocket thrombi in femoral veins. J Clin Pathol 1974; 27:517–28.

26. Pandolfi M, Nilsson IM, Robertson B, Isacson S. Fibrinolytic activity of human veins. Lancet 1967; ii:127–8.

27. Hamilton G, Platt SA. Deep vein thrombosis. In: Beard JD, Gaines PA (eds) Vascular and endovascular surgery. London: WB Saunders, 1998; pp. 351–96.

28. Juhan-Vague I, Valadier J, Alessi MC et al. Deficient t-PA release and elevated PA inhibitor levels in patients with spontaneous or recurrent deep venous thrombosis. Thromb Haemost 1987; 57:67–72.

29. Wiman B, Hamsten A. Impaired fibrinolysis and risk of thromboembolism. Prog Cardiovasc Dis 1991; 34:179–92.

30. Erickson LA, Fici GJ, Lund JE et al. Development of venous occlusions in mice transgenic for the plasminogen activator inhibitor-1 gene. Nature 1990; 346:74–6.

31. Carmeliet P, Schoonjans L, Kieckens L et al. Physiological consequences of loss of plasminogen activator gene function in mice. Nature 1994; 368:419–24.

32. Harbourne T, O'Brien D, Nicolaides AN. Fibrinolytic activity in patients with idiopathic and secondary deep venous thrombosis. Thromb Res 1991; 64:543–50.

33. Eriksson BI, Eriksson E, Gyzander E et al. Thrombosis after hip replacement. Relationship to the fibrinolytic system. Acta Orthop Scand 1989; 60:159–63.

34. Mellbring G, Dahlgren S, Reiz S, Wiman B. Fibrinolytic activity in plasma and deep vein thrombosis after major abdominal surgery. Thromb Res 1983; 32:575–84.

35. Wiman B. Plasminogen activator inhibitor 1 (PAI-1) in plasma: its role in thrombotic disease. Thromb Haemost 1995; 74:71–6.

36. Aiach M, Gandrille S, Emmerich J. A review of mutations causing deficiencies of antithrombin, protein C and protein S. Thromb Haemost 1995; 74:81–9.

37. Meade TW, Dyer S, Howarth DJ et al. Antithrombin III and procoagulant activity: sex differences and effects of the menopause. Br J Haematol 1990; 74:77–81.

38. Tait RC, Walker ID, Davidson JF et al. Antithrombin III activity in healthy blood donors: age and sex related changes and prevalence of asymptomatic deficiency. Br J Haematol 1990; 75:141–2.

39. Dahlbäck B, Stenflo J. The protein C anticoagulant system. In: Stamatoyannopoulos G, Nienhuis AW, Majerus PW, Varmus H (eds) The molecular basis of blood diseases. Philadelphia: WB Saunders, 1994; pp. 599–628.

40. Griffin JH, Evatt B, Zimmerman TS et al. Deficiency of protein C in congenital thrombotic disease. J Clin Invest 1981; 68:1370–3.

41. Miletich J, Sherman L, Broze G Jr. Absence of thrombosis in subjects with heterozygous protein C deficiency. N Engl J Med 1987; 317:991–6.

42. Simioni P, Sanson BJ, Prandoni P et al. Incidence of venous thromboembolism in families with inherited thrombophilia. Thromb Haemost 1999; 81:198–202.

43. Marlar RA, Neumann A. Neonatal purpura fulminans due to homozygous protein C or protein S deficiencies. Semin Thromb Hemost 1990; 16:299–309.

44. Dahlbäck B, Carlsson M, Svensson PJ. Familial thrombophilia due to a previously unrecognized mechanism characterized by poor anticoagulant response to activated protein C: prediction of a cofactor to activated protein C. Proc Natl Acad Sci USA 1993; 90:1004–8.

45. Koster T, Rosendaal FR, de Ronde H et al. Venous thrombosis due to poor anticoagulant response to activated protein C: Leiden Thrombophilia Study. Lancet 1993; 342:1503–6.

46. Dahlbäck B. New molecular insights into the genetics of thrombophilia. Resistance to activated protein C caused by Arg506 to Gln mutation in factor V as a pathogenic risk factor for venous thrombosis. Thromb Haemost 1995; 74:139–48.

47. Rees DC, Cox M, Clegg JB. World distribution of factor V Leiden. Lancet 1995; 346:1133–4.

48. Price DT, Ridker PM. Factor V Leiden mutation and the risks for thromboembolic disease: a clinical perspective. Ann Intern Med 1997; 127:895–903.

49. Bertina RM, Reitsma PH, Rosendaal FR, Vandenbroucke JP. Resistance to activated protein C and factor V Leiden as risk factors for venous thrombosis. Thromb Haemost 1995; 74:449–53.

50. Koeleman BP, Reitsma PH, Allaart CF, Bertina RM. Activated protein C resistance as an additional risk factor for thrombosis in protein C-deficient families. Blood 1994; 84:1031–5.

51. Rosendaal FR. Risk factors for venous thrombotic disease. Thromb Haemost 1999; 82:610–19.

52. Poort SR, Rosendaal FR, Reitsma PH, Bertina RM. A common genetic variation in the 3′-untranslated region of the prothrombin gene is associated with elevated plasma prothrombin levels and an increase in venous thrombosis. Blood 1996; 88:3698–703.

53. Cumming AM, Keeney S, Salden A et al. The prothrombin gene G20210A variant: prevalence in a UK anticoagulant clinic population. Br J Haematol 1997; 98:353–5.

54. Brown K, Luddington R, Williamson D et al. Risk of venous thromboembolism associated with a G to A transition at position 20210 in the 3′-untranslated region of the prothrombin gene. Br J Haematol 1997; 98:907–9.

55. Kraaijenhagen R, Pieternella S, Koopman S et al. High plasma concentrations of factor VIII:C is a major risk of venous thromboembolism. Thromb Haemost 2000; 83:5–9.

56. O'Donnell J, Mumford A, Manning R et al. Elevation of factor VIII:C in venous thromboembolism is persistent and independent of the acute phase response. Thromb Haemost 2000; 83:10–13.

57. Schonauer E, Kyrle PA, Weltermann A et al. Superficial thrombophlebitis and risk for recurrent venous thromboembolism. J Vasc Surg 2003; 37:835–8.

58. Towne JB, Bandyk DF, Hussey CV, Tollack VT. Abnormal plasminogen: a genetically determined cause of hypercoagulability. J Vasc Surg 1984; 1:896–902.

59. Hughes GR. Thrombosis, abortion, cerebral disease, and the lupus anticoagulant. Br Med J 1983; 287:1088–9.

60. Alarcon-Segovia D. Clinical manifestations of the antiphospholipid syndrome. J Rheumatol 1992; 19:1778–81.

61. Nencini P, Baruffi MC, Abbate R et al. Lupus anticoagulant and anticardiolipin antibodies in young adults with cerebral ischemia. Stroke 1992; 23:189–93.

62. Triplett DA. Protean clinical presentation of antiphospholipid-protein antibodies (APA). Thromb Haemost 1995; 74:329–37.

63. Ginsburg KS, Liang MH, Newcomer L et al. Anticardiolipin antibodies and the risk for ischemic stroke and venous thrombosis. Ann Intern Med 1992; 117:997–1002.

64. Rosove MH, Brewer PM. Antiphospholipid thrombosis: clinical course after the first thrombotic event in 70 patients. Ann Intern Med 1992; 117:303–8.

65. Cervera R, Piette J, Font J et al. Antiphospholipid syndrome: clinical and immunologic manifestations and patterns of disease expression in a cohort of 1,000 people. Arthritis Rheum 2002; 46:1019–27.

66. Warkentin TE, Kelton JG. Heparin-induced thrombocytopenia. Prog Hemost Thromb 1991; 10:1–34.

67. King DJ, Kelton JG. Heparin-associated thrombocytopenia. Ann Intern Med 1984; 100:535–40.

68. Schmitt BP, Adelman B. Heparin-associated thrombocytopenia: a critical review and pooled analysis. Am J Med Sci 1993; 305:208–15.

69. Dryjski M, Dryjski H. Heparin induced thrombocytopenia. Eur J Vasc Endovasc Surg 1996; 11:260–9.

70. Sobel M, Adelman B, Szentpetery S et al. Surgical management of heparin-associated thrombocytopenia. Strategies in the treatment of venous and arterial thromboembolism. J Vasc Surg 1988; 8:395–401.

71. Sobel M. Heparin-induced thrombocytopenia. In: Goldstone J (ed.) Perspectives in vascular surgery. St Louis, MO: Quality Medical, 1992; pp. 1–27.

72. Currie IC, Wilson YG, Scott J et al. Homocysteine: an independent risk factor for the failure of vascular intervention. Br J Surg 1996; 83:1238–41.

73. den Heijer M, Blom HJ, Gerrits WB et al. Is hyperhomocysteinaemia a risk factor for recurrent venous thrombosis? Lancet 1995; 345:882–5.

74. Falcon CR, Cattaneo M, Panzeri D et al. High prevalence of hyperhomocysteinemia in patients with juvenile venous thrombosis. Arterioscler Thromb 1994; 14:1080–3.

75. Key NS, McGlennen RC. Hyperhomocyst(e)inaemia and thrombophilia. Arch Pathol Lab Med 2002; 126:1367–75.

76. O'Keefe D J, Baglin TP. Travellers thrombosis and economy class syndrome: incidence aetiology and prevention (review). Clin Lab Haematol 2003; 25:277–81.

77. Martinelli I, Taioli E, Battaglionli T et al. Risk of venous thromboembolism after air travel: interaction with thrombophilia and oral contraceptives. Arch Intern Med 2003; 163:271–4.

78. Kelman CW, Kortt MA, Becker NG et al. Deep vein thrombosis and air travel: a record link with linkage study. Br Med J 2003; 327:1072–5.

Important study based on linkage of hospital presentations of venous thromboembolic disease and recent long-haul air travel to a remote but civilised area with reliable electronic data gathering (Western Australia).

79. Thromboembolic Risk Factors (THRIFT) Consensus Group. Risk of and prophylaxis for venous thromboembolism in hospital patients. Br Med J 1992; 305:567–74.

Seminal consensus on risk stratification for venous thromboembolic disease in hospital populations.

80. Campbell B. Thrombosis, phlebitis, and varicose veins. Br Med J 1996; 312:198–9.

81. Jorgensen JO, Hanel KC, Morgan AM, Hunt JM. The incidence of deep venous thrombosis in patients with superficial thrombophlebitis of the lower limbs. J Vasc Surg 1993; 18:70–3.

82. Enoch S, Woon E, Blair S T. Thromboprophylaxis can be omitted in selected patients undergoing varicose vein surgery and hernia repair. Br J Surg 2003; 90:818–20.

83. Lees TA, Beard JD, Ridler BM, Szymanska T. A survey of the current management of varicose veins by members of the Vascular Surgical Society. Ann R Coll Surg Engl 1999; 81:407–17.

84. Vandenbroucke JP, Koster T, Briet E et al. Increased risk of venous thrombosis in oral-contraceptive users who are carriers of factor V Leiden mutation. Lancet 1994; 344:1453–7.

85. Bloemenkamp KW, Rosendaal FR, Helmerhorst FM et al. Enhancement by factor V Leiden mutation of risk of deep-vein thrombosis associated with oral contraceptives containing a third-generation progestagen. Lancet 1995; 346:1593–6.

86. Koster T, Small RA, Rosendaal FR, Helmerhorst FM. Oral contraceptives and venous thromboembolism: a quantitative discussion of the uncertainties. J Intern Med 1995; 238:31–7.

87. Gerstman BB, Piper JM, Tomita DK et al. Oral contraceptive estrogen dose and the risk of deep venous thromboembolic disease. Am J Epidemiol 1991; 133:32–7.

88. Rosing J, Middeldorp S, Curvers J et al. Low-dose oral contraceptives and acquired resistance to activated protein C: a randomised cross-over study. Lancet 1999; 354:2036–40.

Randomised crossover study of second- and third-generation oral contraceptives and their effect on activated protein C.

89. Meade TW. Risks and mechanisms of cardio-vascular events in users of oral contraceptives. Am J Obstet Gynecol 1988; 158:1646–52.

Case–control study that confirmed an association between use of HRT and risk of venous thromboembolic disease.

90. Daly E, Vessey MP, Hawkins MM et al. Risk of venous thromboembolism in users of hormone replacement therapy. Lancet 1996; 348:977–80.

91. Jick H, Derby LE, Myers MW et al. Risk of hospital admission for idiopathic venous thromboembolism among users of postmenopausal oestrogens. Lancet 1996; 348:981–3.

Case–control study that confirmed a threefold increased risk of venous thromboembolic disease in current HRT users.

92. Grodstein F, Stampfer MJ, Goldhaber SZ et al. Prospective study of exogenous hormones and risk of pulmonary embolism in women. Lancet 1996; 348:983–7.

93. Verlato F, Zucchetta P, Prandoni P et al. An unexpectedly high rate of pulmonary embolism in patients with superficial thrombophlebitis of the thigh. J Vasc Surg 1999; 30:1113–15.

94. Wells PS, Hirsh J, Anderson DR et al. Accuracy of clinical assessment of deep-vein thrombosis. Lancet 1995; 345:1326–30.

95. Chunilal SD, Ginsberg JS. Strategies for the diagnosis of deep vein thrombosis and pulmonary embolism. Thromb Res 2000; 97:V33–V48.

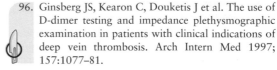

96. Ginsberg JS, Kearon C, Douketis J et al. The use of D-dimer testing and impedance plethysmographic examination in patients with clinical indications of deep vein thrombosis. Arch Intern Med 1997; 157:1077–81.

97. Bernardi E, Prandoni P, Lensing AW et al. D-dimer testing as an adjunct to ultrasonography in patients with clinically suspected deep vein thrombosis: prospective cohort study. The Multicentre Italian D-dimer Ultrasound Study Investigators Group. Br Med J 1998; 317:1037–40.

Prospective multicentre assessment of value of D-dimer in excluding DVT.

98. Wells PS, Anderson BR, Rodger N et al. Evaluation of D-dimer in the diagnosis of suspected deep vein thrombosis. N Engl J Med 2003; 349:1227–35.

Large prospective assessment of D-dimer in diagnosis of DVT in the outpatient setting; negative D-dimer and low clinical probability excludes DVT.

99. Thomas ML, MacDonald LM. The accuracy of bolus ascending phlebography in demonstrating the ilio-femoral segment. Clin Radiol 1977; 28:165–71.

100. Kearon C, Julian JA, Newman TE, Ginsberg JS. Noninvasive diagnosis of deep venous thrombosis. McMaster Diagnostic Imaging Practice Guidelines Initiative. Ann Intern Med 1998; 128:663–77.

101. Kearon C, Ginsberg JS, Hirsh J. The role of venous ultrasonography in the diagnosis of suspected deep venous thrombosis and pulmonary embolism. Ann Intern Med 1998; 129:1044–9.

102. Lensing AW, Prandoni P, Brandjes D et al. Detection of deep-vein thrombosis by real-time B-mode ultrasonography. N Engl J Med 1989; 320:342–5.

103. Huisman MV, Buller HR, ten Cate JW et al. Management of clinically suspected acute venous thrombosis in outpatients with serial impedance plethysmography in a community hospital setting. Arch Intern Med 1989; 149:511–13.

104. Wells PS, Anderson DR, Bormanis J et al. Value of assessment of pretest probability of deep-vein thrombosis in clinical management. Lancet 1997; 350:1795–8.

105. Mullins ND, Becker DM, Hagspiel KD, Philbrick JT. The role of spiral volumetric computed tomography in the diagnosis of pulmonary embolism. Arch Intern Med 2000; 160:293–8.

106. Barritt DW, Jordan SC. Anticoagulant drugs in the treatment of pulmonary embolism, a controlled study. Lancet 1960; i:1309–12.

Brandjes DP, Heijboer H, Buller HR et al. Acenocoumarol and heparin compared with acenocoumarol alone in the initial treatment of proximal-vein thrombosis. N Engl J Med 1992; 327:1485–9.

Prospective randomised study that confirmed the need for both heparin and oral anticoagulation in early treatment of venous thromboembolic disease.

108. Hull RD, Raskob GE, Hirsh J et al. Continuous intravenous heparin compared with intermittent subcutaneous heparin in the initial treatment of proximal-vein thrombosis. N Engl J Med 1986; 315:1109–14.

109. Hirsh J. Heparin. N Engl J Med 1991; 324:1565–74.

110. Hull RD, Raskob GE, Rosenbloom D et al. Optimal therapeutic level of heparin therapy in patients with venous thrombosis. Arch Intern Med 1992; 152:1589–95.

111. Fennerty AE, Thomas P, Backhouse G et al. Audit of control of heparin treatment. Br Med J 1985; 290:27–8.

112. Wheeler AP, Jaquiss RD, Newman JH. Physician practices in the treatment of pulmonary embolism and deep venous thrombosis. Arch Intern Med 1988; 148:1321–5.

113. Rubin BG, Reilly JM, Sicard GA, Botney MD. Care of patients with deep venous thrombosis in an academic medical center: limitations and lessons. J Vasc Surg 1994; 20:698–704.

114. Koopman MMW, Prandoni P, Piovella F et al. Treatment of venous thrombosis with intravenous unfractionated heparin administered in the hospital as compared with subcutaneous low-molecular-weight heparin administered at home. N Engl J Med 1996; 334:682–7.

Prospective randomised study that confirmed safety of outpatient treatment of proximal DVT with LMWH.

115. Hull RD, Raskob GE, Rosenbloom D et al. Heparin for 5 days as compared with 10 days in the initial treatment of proximal venous thrombosis. N Engl J Med 1990; 322:1260–4.

Treatment with 5 days of heparin is as effective and safe as 10 days.

116. van Dongen CJ, MacGillivray MR, Prins MH. Once versus twice daily LMWH for the initial treatment of venous thromboembolism (Cochrane review). Cochrane Library, issue 4, 2003.

No significant difference between once- or twice-daily LMWH.

117. Lensing AW, Prins MH, Davidson BL, Hirsh J. Treatment of deep venous thrombosis with low-molecular-weight heparins. A meta-analysis. Arch Intern Med 1995; 155:601–7.

Meta-analysis that confirms greater efficacy and safety of LMWH compared with UFH.

118. Levine M, Gent M, Hirsh J et al. A comparison of low-molecular-weight heparin administered primarily at home with unfractionated heparin administered in the hospital for proximal deep-vein thrombosis. N Engl J Med 1996; 334:677–81.

119. Gallus A, Jackaman J, Tillett J et al. Safety and efficacy of warfarin started early after submassive venous thrombosis or pulmonary embolism. Lancet 1986; ii:1293–6.

120. Segal JB, Bolgar DD, Jenckes NW et al. Outpatient therapy with low molecular weight heparin for the treatment of venous thromboembolism: a review of efficacy, safety and cost. Am J Med 2003; 115:324–5.

Efficacy, safety and cost-effectiveness of outpatient LMWH treatment of proximal DVT is confirmed by this review.

121. van den Belt AGM, Prins MH, Lensing AW et al. Fixed dose subcutaneous low molecular weight heparins versus adjusted dose unfractionated heparin for venous thromboembolism (Cochrane review). Cochrane Library, issue 4, 2003.

Cochrane review confirms safety and efficacy of LMWH in prevention of recurrent venous thromboembolic disease and with reduced risk of haemorrhage.

122. Quinlan DJ, McQuillan A, Eikelboom JW. Low-molecular-weight heparin compared with intravenous unfractionated heparin for the treatment of pulmonary embolism: meta-analysis of randomized controlled trials. Ann Intern Med 2004; 140:175–83.

Treatment of pulmonary embolism with LMWH is as effective and safe as UFH.

123. Schulman S, Rhedin AS, Lindmarker P et al. A comparison of six weeks with six months of oral anticoagulant therapy after a first episode of venous thromboembolism. Duration of Anticoagulation Trial Study Group. N Engl J Med 1995; 332:1661–5.

Lower recurrent venous thromboembolic disease rate with 6 months of anticoagulation compared with 6 weeks.

124. Prins MH, Hutten BA, Koopman MM, Buller HR. Long-term treatment of venous thromboembolic disease. Thromb Haemost 1999; 82:892–8.

125. Hutton BA, Prins MH. Duration of treatment with vitamin K antagonists in symptomatic venous thromboembolism (Cochrane review). Cochrane Library, issue 4, 2003.

Recurrent venous thromboembolic disease is prevented for the duration of anticoagulation, the absolute risk of recurrence declines with time, while the risk of haemorrhage does not.

126. Kearon C, Ginsberg JS, Kovacs MJ et al. Comparison of low intensity warfarin therapy with conventional-intensity warfarin therapy for long-term prevention of recurrent venous thromboembolism. N Engl J Med 2003; 349:631–9.

Conventional-dose oral anticoagulation is superior to low dosage in prevention of recurrence of venous thromboembolic disease.

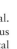
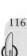

127. Bauer KA. Management of patients with hereditary defects predisposing to thrombosis including pregnant women. Thromb Haemost 1995; 74:94–100.

128. Gallus AS. Thrombolytic therapy for venous thrombosis and pulmonary embolism. Baillières Clin Haematol 1998; 11:663–73.

129. Lindhoff-Last E, Willeke A, Thalhammer C et al. Hirudin in a breastfeeding woman. Lancet 2000; 355:467–8.

130. Turpie AGG, Eriksson BI, Lassen MR for the Steering Committee of the Pentasaccharide Orthopaedic Prophylaxis Studies. Fondaparinux versus enoxaparin for the prevention of venous thromboembolism in major orthopaedic surgery. Arch Intern Med 2002; 162:1833–40.

   Meta-analysis suggesting that fondaparinux is superior to enoxaparin in prevention of venous thromboembolic disease, with lower bleeding risk in major orthopaedic surgery.

131. Lowe GDO, Sandercock PAG, Rosendaal FR. Prevention of venous thromboembolism after major orthopaedic surgery: is fondaparinux an advance! Lancet 2003; 362:504–5.

   Critical commentary on the fondaparinux meta-analysis which highlights the potential dangers of using surrogate rather than clinical end points and the potential bias inherent in a manufacturer-sponsored trial.

132. Verheugt FW. Can we pull the plug on warfarin in atrial fibrillation? Lancet 2003; 362:1686–7.

133. Schulman S, Wahlander K, Lundstrom T, Clason SB, Eriksson H for the THRIVE III Investigators. Secondary prevention of venous thromboembolism with the oral direct thrombin inhibitor ximelagatran. N Engl J Med 2003; 349:1713–21.

   Ximelagatran is superior to placebo in secondary prevention of venous thromboembolic disease.

134. Clagett GP, Anderson FA Jr, Geerts W et al. Prevention of venous thromboembolism. Chest 1998; 114:S531–S560.

135. Haas S. Low molecular weight heparins in the prevention of venous thromboembolism in nonsurgical patients. Semin Thromb Hemost 1999; 25(Suppl. 3): 101–5.

136. Bounameaux H. Intergrating pharmacologic and mechanical prophylaxis of venous thromboembolism. Thromb Haemost 1999; 82:931–7.

137. Ashby EC, Ashford NS, Campbell MJ. Posture, blood velocity in common femoral vein, and prophylaxis of venous thromboembolism. Lancet 1995; 345:419–21.

138. Agu O, Hamilton G, Baker D. Graduated compression stockings in the prevention of venous thromboembolism. Br J Surg 1999; 86:992–1004.

139. Wells PS, Lensing AW, Hirsh J. Graduated compression stockings in the prevention of postoperative venous thromboembolism. A meta-analysis. Arch Intern Med 1994; 154:67–72.

   Graduated compression stockings significantly reduce venous thromboembolic disease in moderate-risk patients (insufficient evidence in high-risk orthopaedic surgery).

140. Amaragiri SV, Lees TA. Elastic compression stockings for prevention of deep vein thrombosis (Cochrane review). Cochrane Library, issue 1, 2004.

   Review of randomised controlled trials that confirms the efficacy of stockings in prevention of venous thromboembolic disease in hospitalised patients.

141. Comerota AJ, Chouhan V, Harada RN et al. The fibrinolytic effects of intermittent pneumatic compression: mechanism of enhanced fibrinolysis. Ann Surg 1997; 226:306–13.

142. Chouhan VD, Comerota AJ, Sun L et al. Inhibition of tissue factor pathway during intermittent pneumatic compression: a possible mechanism for antithrombotic effect. Arterioscler Thromb Vasc Biol 1999; 19:2812–17.

143. Malone MD, Cisek PL, Comerota AJ Jr et al. High-pressure, rapid-inflation pneumatic compression improves venous hemodynamics in healthy volunteers and patients who are post-thrombotic. J Vasc Surg 1999; 29:593–9.

144. Blanchard J, Meuwly JY, Leyvraz PF et al. Prevention of deep-vein thrombosis after total knee replacement. Randomised comparison between a low-molecular-weight heparin (Nadroparin) and mechanical prophylaxis with a foot-pump system. J Bone Joint Surg Br 1999; 81:654–9.

145. Handoll HHG, Farrar MJ, McBirnie J, Tytherleigh-Strong G, Milne AA, Gillespie WJ. Heparin, low molecular weight heparin and physical methods for preventing deep vein thrombosis and pulmonary embolism following surgery for hip fractures (Cochrane review). Cochrane Library, issue 4, 2003.

   Updated Cochrane review that confirms the efficacy of both LMWH and UFH in DVT prevention but finds insufficient evidence for pulmonary embolism; calf and foot pumps appear to prevent DVT.

146. Ginzburg E, Cohn SM, Lopez J et al. Randomized clinical trial of intermittent pneumatic compression and low molecular weight heparin in trauma. Br J Surg 2003; 90:1338–44.

   Calf compression is as effective as LMWH in trauma patients.

147. Browse NL, Burnand KG, Irvine AT, Wilson NM. Deep vein thrombosis: prevention. In: Browse NL, Burnand KG, Irvine AT, Wilson, NM (eds) Diseases of the veins, 2nd edn. London: Arnold, 1999; pp. 359–83.

148. Collins R, Scrimgeour A, Yusuf S, Peto R. Reduction in fatal pulmonary embolism and venous thrombosis by perioperative administration of subcutaneous heparin. Overview of results of

randomized trials in general, orthopedic, and urologic surgery. N Engl J Med 1988; 318:1162–73.

149. Kakkar VV, Cohen AT, Edmonson RA et al. Low molecular weight versus standard heparin for prevention of venous thromboembolism after major abdominal surgery. The Thromboprophylaxis Collaborative Group. Lancet 1993; 341:259–65.

150. Leizorovicz A, Haugh MC, Chapuis FR et al. Low molecular weight heparin in prevention of perioperative thrombosis. Br Med J 1992; 305:913–20.

151. Nurmohamed MT, Rosendaal FR, Buller HR et al. Low-molecular-weight heparin versus standard heparin in general and orthopaedic surgery: a meta-analysis. Lancet 1992; 340:152–6.

152. Huber O, Bounameaux H, Borst F, Rohner A. Postoperative pulmonary embolism after hospital discharge. An underestimated risk. Arch Surg 1992; 127:310–13.

153. Bergqvist D, Lowe GD, Berstad A et al. Prevention of venous thromboembolism after surgery: a review of enoxaparin. Br J Surg 1992; 79:495–8.

154. Mismetti P, Laporte S, Darmon JY, Buchmuller A, Decousus H. Meta-analysis of low molecular weight heparin in the prevention of venous thromboembolism in general surgery. Br J Surg 2001; 88:913–30.

Efficacy and safety of LMWH in prevention of venous thromboembolic disease in general surgical patients is confirmed; optimal dosage of LMWH needs further study.

CHAPTER Fifteen

Patient assessment and surgical risk

Linda de Cossart

INTRODUCTION

Risk is a topic that continues to stimulate much discussion and debate in the 21st century. In medical practice an industry has been created producing data, guidelines and protocols with the aim of reducing risk to patients and to medical organisations. Newspapers regularly report the risks of medical and surgical care, often with little supporting evidence or scrutiny of their claims. There is considerable danger that all of these data will result in confusion and a failure to think deeply about what risk is and how it varies in different contexts. There is little evidence that the data produced actually aid patients' understanding on the subject and there is no evidence that such processes have eliminated risk.

Careful patient assessment by a competent surgeon with the knowledge and experience to understand and communicate the risks and benefits of surgical treatment is the mainstay of good patient care. However, there is a growing belief among health-care professionals that using numerical data to communicate the risk is the right way to inform patients. The development of professional judgement is sidelined despite the fact that investigation has shown that doctors often choose to give patients the most sensational numbers without either contextualising them or even fully understanding them.[1] If surgeons are to deal with this important aspect of surgical practice well, they must understand their responsibilities when communicating risk not only to their patients but also to their colleagues, both medical and managerial.

The aim of this chapter is to demonstrate the wide range of knowledge and understanding that is necessary in order for a surgeon to assess and communicate risk. It concludes with an example of a strategy for the collection, consideration and deployment of information relevant to both surgeons and their patients in establishing a dialogue for planning patient care. A strategy rather than a protocol is recommended, because good decision-making is complex and in surgical practice (and health care generally) individuals rarely, if ever, fit guidelines and rules.

BACKGROUND

Currently, there is a widespread belief by medical practitioners that a 'risk industry' has emerged, aimed not only at minimising the cost of medical negligence claims but also at regulating the profession. There may be some truth in this but it is an essential part of our professional responsibilities to ensure that patients subjected to surgical treatment have been helped to understand the risks and benefits of such action. The trust and respect that a surgeon receives from patients will indicate how well this is done. Understanding how to achieve this well is a great challenge for those learning and practising the art and craft of surgery.

Patients attending hospital for surgical treatment are vulnerable. They trust their surgeons and expect to receive a clear and sympathetic explanation.[2,3] However, there is a widespread feeling by the public that doctors in general and surgeons in particular have not mastered the art of good communication of the risks related to surgical operations and treatments. With public demand for more openness and accountability, surgeons are being driven to investigate their practice as never before.[4,5] This must go hand in hand with understanding how best to use this information to advise patients.

The last decade has seen much activity in attempting to produce meaningful information for surgeons about their performance, but it is not a simple task and may be confounded by the expectation that outcomes should be similar in quite different environments.[6] Although many studies are being published that involve manipulation of figures (e.g. length of stay, number of procedures performed, raw data on death rates), there is little evidence that these do anything to help the patient. There is a risk that they will deflect the focus away from understanding the patient's perspective of risk and may even mitigate against good communication between surgeon and patient.

How risk is communicated, both numerically and linguistically, and the values that individuals place on the benefits and risks of a particular course of action will affect their choice of treatment.[1,7] Quoting the risk as simply 'above average' is meaningless; discussing 'percentage risk' is also unsatisfactory. More complex statistics using relative and absolute risk are usually only appropriate if in discussion with someone knowledgeable about statistics. Even such patients are likely to say that, unless you know precisely who will fall in the 'bad' cohort, these too are meaningless and likely to be overridden by more personal considerations. Indeed, the use of numbers is only a small part of the range of knowledge needed for good communication of risk. Surprisingly, patients may not want it discussed in such terms.

The values and expectations of individuals significantly affect how they see a problem, and these values and expectations may differ from those of the surgeon.

Patients value highly the opportunity to be taken seriously in the decision-making process for their care.[8]

This creates an imperative for surgeons to learn about risk communication and the language that this may require.[9] The emphasis for a particular course of action will be influenced by each side's rational and irrational feelings, other quite separate influences on their lives, and considerations they may prioritise quite differently from their treatment or their illness. Surgeons must therefore be prepared to explore and understand the patient's perspective on this. The use of statistics is meant to help but, as Gigerenzer has pointed out, doctors can fall very short of understanding these and therefore further

compromise their usefulness.[1] Furthermore, surgeons tend to concentrate their discussions only on the specific operation to be performed.[10]

It is a myth that life is risk free. Everyday we face risks of one sort or another and are barely aware of them. Many continue to take risks despite the clear knowledge that danger exists (e.g. smoking and the 50% risk of death when climbing K2). In the event of a medical illness, however, the perception of risk is brought more sharply into focus because of a very real and immediate possibility of a life-harming event. This, coupled with the fact that individuals have to relinquish control over their fate, creates a vulnerable human being and none of us is exempt from this possibility.

A worried patient will just want the problem to go away and may expect the surgeon to offer such a solution. The surgeon, now in a position of power and influence over the patient, must exercise wisdom and knowledge with the aim of striving for the **best** care of the individual patient and communicating this effectively. This may only be achieved by understanding the demands that this makes on the surgeon, who will have formed his or her own opinions but who must now take serious account of the patient's wishes. What is best for the patient may not at first be best decided by the surgeon.

PATIENT-CENTRED DISCUSSION

The surgeon must be prepared to assess individual patients from their own perspective, while considering their range of knowledge and the condition from which they suffer. The treatment options must be considered in the light of this information. The range of factors that a surgeon needs to consider are shown in **Box 15.1**.

Creating an understanding of the clinical process that will be best for the patient is a very important first step. A salient history and clinical examination are essential and the ways of doing this have been very well described.[11–14] Careful recording of the findings and a plan of action must be made. It may be helpful to share this with the patient and some surgeons do this regularly by including patients in the distribution of letters concerning their management. Departments should consider this option when distributing letters about patients.

At the first consultation it may not be possible to give a full opinion of the options available, and the need for time and further investigation must be clearly communicated to the patient. On the other hand, straightforward cases such as hernias, skin lesions and other non-life-threatening conditions may lead the surgeon to believe that management of the patient is simple. However, what is simple in the

Box 15.1 • What a surgeon needs to know to discuss risk with a patient

The patient's expectations
The surgical condition and the findings of clinical examination
The results of investigations
The alternative options
Theoretical knowledge of the condition and its treatment options
Local and national guidelines
Information on the subject in the public domain
The option of a second opinion
The facilities available in the local trust
Trust consent policy, including information for patients
Their personal competence on the subject

mind of the surgeon is unlikely to be simple in the mind of the patient. The management of the condition therefore needs to be examined from the patient's perspective.

Patients want to know what will happen to them and how the treatment will affect their life in both the short and long term. It is sobering to remember that surgeons are more likely to face litigation if they raise patient expectations excessively, minimise the risks of surgery or embellish the benefits of the operation. The prime example of this is varicose vein surgery, the branch of surgery where there is the largest group of patients suing general surgeons. An apparently simple case (to the surgeon's way of thinking) is more likely to result in patient dissatisfaction than a life-threatening case. It is about expectations.

When patients consult a surgeon about their illness, their focus is on themselves. What exactly is wrong with them; can it be cured (as distinct sometimes from treated); how will the treatment affect them; will they die? They are at best nervous and at worst very scared about what the surgeon will say, especially if they have preconceived ideas of the likely outcome of their condition.

The patient's reaction will vary depending on the disease or condition. A 28-year-old patient who has a hernia is more likely to be worried about time off work and when it can be repaired than a 56-year-old man who has cancer of the colon that will require radiotherapy and surgery. The latter will be focused on his risk of death due to cancer. However, both see the surgeon as the answer to the problem, by being knowledgeable and in control of the situation. The surgeon is therefore set on a pedestal

before the consultation has even begun. The range of knowledge and 'know-how' required to satisfy both patients is considerable. The recognition of this exalted position becomes tempered with surgical experience but it is still difficult to regulate the feeling of power that it gives. It influences the surgeon's attitude to the patient.

It is interesting to note that research has demonstrated that patients value having a choice of treatment or investigation because this removes the subsequent regret they may feel without such choice. Their choices do not always follow scientifically proven outcomes. For example, the reasons men give for accepting prostate-specific antigen testing for prostate cancer include right to access and equitability,[15] despite the lack of evidence that this procedure saves more lives. Similarly, notwithstanding the fact that many women overestimate the risk of breast cancer and of dying from it,[16] some still choose to take hormone replacement therapy, even in the light of newspaper headlines that report the heightened risk associated with it.[17] These examples go some way to demonstrating the human ability to ignore risk in certain circumstances and surgeons must understand this.

Traditional medical teaching enables the surgeon to implement a strategy of examination, diagnosis and treatment, so as to be able to offer an operation. Young surgeons are full of facts and are focused on finding a surgical operation that may be applied to a particular patient's problem. In the past, surgeons have been accused of a paternalistic approach to their patients, working on the theory that 'doctor knows best'. In today's society this is no longer an acceptable relationship. Many patients are more informed than ever before, having access to facts about medical diseases to an unprecedented extent; consequently they are self-assured. Others have greater knowledge than the doctor they consult because they have surfed the Internet and have read the latest update on their diagnosis. They are seeking something more from their surgeon than just the facts.

Patients expect, and should get, an honest and empathetic response from an expert on their condition. They want to be given time, treated with dignity and as a fellow human being with a role in the decision-making process about their care. Most patients recognise that miracles are not possible, but managing those with excessive expectations and gaining their respect is an ability developed by surgeons by experience and increasing understanding.

The success of the consultation between patient and surgeon depends on what the surgeon has offered and whether this matches what the patient wanted to know. The relationship is based on understanding the values that each places on the consultation and each one's expectations of the outcome. It is therefore essential not to manipulate the response of the patient by presenting the treatment options in a surgeon-centred way.

RISK TO THE SURGEON

Surgeons like to be thought of as hard-working and doing a good job. In the past they built their reputations locally on the way they managed their patients and the respect that this generated. This is still a potent discriminator but their reputations are now also subject to scrutiny by the public as a result of the publication of outcomes (in particular death and complications) by independent groups. The risk to surgeons is therefore how they arm themselves to cope with this new way of scrutiny.

SURGEONS MUST LEARN TO UNDERSTAND THE COMMUNICATION OF RISK

When trainee surgeons begin the process of communicating the risk of surgery, it is likely that they will do so by imparting to the patient what they know and the clinical findings. This is encouraged by the current trend to tell the patient everything during the consent process and to include a percentage risk of complications. Such communication fails to personalise the risks to the patient and takes no account of what the patient expects and wants.

The use of percentage risk as a single statistic is unhelpful to patients and this is exemplified by the following example. A figure of 5% is often quoted by vascular surgeons as the risk of death related to aortic aneurysm surgery. In any unit offering aortic surgery there will be a range of percentage outcomes related to the physiological condition of the individual patient. In our unit this varies between 2 and 15% depending on the comorbidity of the patient. Moreover, to some a 5% risk may seem small, whereas to others it is high.

Gigerenzer argues that the use of frequency figures is a more acceptable form of words and that doctors should learn to understand and use this form of communication.[1]

Applying this argument to the example above, a patient would be told that of 100 patients undergoing aortic aneurysm surgery, five would die. The question that remains is, who are those five?

Percentage figures are only accrued from published data, although these are probably biased because only those data thought worthy of publication are used for computing such figures. The figures quoted from our unit demonstrate that a single figure could be misleading to individuals: it would be quite unfair to advise patients with poor comorbidity that they have only a 5% risk of death when it is more likely to be 15%. The risk in such a case may well be higher than the risk of death related to the natural history of the patient's condition. In the author's experience, patients still rely heavily on the surgeon's professional judgement to contextualise their surgical care.

Good surgeons use far more than the objective facts and figures when they agree a course of surgical care with their patient. It requires that they use discretion, empathy, up-to-date theoretical knowledge, expertise, commitment and professional judgement. What means do they use to do this? Experience and a well-developed understanding of clinical practice and patients probably contributes to this, although a humanistic approach helps. They are more likely to give the highest priority to spending time with the patient and his or her family and answering questions. Without recognising the latter and developing ways of distilling the salient features of a case and relating them to the patient, trainee surgeons will not develop mature judgement and good communication. However, the educational process necessary to achieve this requires that surgeons understand how they are learning and develop themselves in this complex surgical environment.

ACTING WITHIN THE PARAMETERS SET BY THE PROFESSION

It is a fundamental principle that surgeons take responsibility for the care of their patients and are acting within the standards set by being a member of a profession. Membership of a profession confers specific responsibilities on its members and sets standards for practice. Such standards have common values across professions and examples of these are listed in **Box 15.2**.[18]

The conduct of members of a profession evolves over time. The traditions developed bind members together and have a strong influence on how people work and relate to society. They have a moral and ethical basis and are valued by their members, who will use them to determine the standards of conduct for those in practice and for regulating those who fall short of this standard.

The professional standards expected of all doctors are set out by the General Medical Council in *Maintaining good clinical practice*[19] and specifically for surgeons in *The surgeon's duty of care* published by the Senate of Surgery[20] and *Good surgical practice*

It is complex, so in the public interest practitioners need to be educated and assessed by members of their profession in order to enter that profession. To continue within it, they must now be prepared to engage in lifelong development

Professional practitioners identify closely with their work, such that they develop intellectual interests in it

The work of a member of a profession takes place in practical settings, which require the use of esoteric theoretical knowledge, a researched base, and high-level skill (none of which a lay-person can entirely obtain, totally comprehend or fully evaluate)

It involves working with people who are vulnerable, and thus demands the professional practitioner's acknowledgement of moral and ethical considerations

The human situations in which professionals work involve some unpredictability, and so not every element of the work of a professional can be predetermined

Because every person for whom professionals work is particular and individual, professionals must use their judgement. Thus the work of a professional is discretionary in nature

This in turn requires that practitioners have self-knowledge and are aware of their own personal and professional values and the values of their profession

'Confidentiality', 'etiquette' and 'collegiality' are important concepts in the work of a professional practitioner

Their work requires practitioners to operate within the bounds and traditions of the profession through which they are licensed to practice. Such traditions have been developed over a long period in response to the demands and values of society

Professional bodies are the guardians of these standards, and as such are regulatory

From de Cossart L, Fish D. Membership of a profession: what it means and why it is important. Educational update issue 13:1, Mersey Deanery PGMDE, April 2002, with permission.

published by the Royal College of Surgeons of England in 2000.[21] In the tradition of developing standards these will be regularly reviewed and updated.

Surgeons also have responsibilities as employees of the trust or other health-care organisation to which they are contracted. It assumes that surgeons are prepared and willing to enter into a mutually respectful and trusting relationship with their patients. It recognises trust as being a function of both the care and competence of a doctor.[22]

RISK STRATIFICATION IN RELATION TO THE PATIENT AND THE DISEASE

In the last 20 years a number of prognostic scoring systems have been developed and many are still in the process of refinement.[14] They have been developed to meet the need to establish an objective measure of outcome for several purposes: (i) to evaluate a patient's condition and ensure appropriate care;[23] (ii) to provide a platform for comparative audit;[24] and (iii) to allow more useful discussion with individual patients and to optimise their care.[25] No one system has universal application and it is likely that with constantly changing clinical practice, refinement of them will be endless. However, they do provide a useful research tool but must never be seen as a replacement for sound clinical judgement.

Understanding risk stratification tools is essential for practising surgeons. It at least encourages the quest to collect accurate data. Having accrued data, subsequent analysis and reflection on the processes and outcomes will further increase the understanding of the surgeon, so hopefully improving surgical care.

 A well-designed multicentre audit of the treatment of acute pancreatitis demonstrated clearly that failure to risk stratify patients resulted in worse treatment.[25]

Although a significant change in the practice of surgeons has now resulted,[23] it remains unclear whether health institutions are able to offer adequate critical care facilities to match surgeons' commitment to change and improved care of patients.

In May 1998, following the General Medical Council's judgement of the Bristol cardiac surgeons,[26] the then Secretary of State for Health declared that patients had a right to know a surgeon's previous results. This has fuelled the release of death rates and league tables for hospitals. If the intention is to publish individual surgeon's results as raw data, as distinct from risk-stratified data, then not only will the data be misleading but the public will not be in a position to correctly interpret them.

Research into the best risk-stratification model therefore continues to challenge. However, the process poses more questions than it answers. At its heart is better understanding of clinical practice. All surgeons must embrace the understanding of these processes and contribute to the research to make them appropriate and valid for their speciality. The responsibility for specialty data collection must lie in the hands of the specialist surgeons supported by their colleges. This is not easy: 60% of vascular surgeons failed to submit data to the Vascular Surgical Society of Great Britain and Ireland annual registry, which provides risk-adjusted reports,[5] despite enthusiastic support for the endeavour by the society. However, the benefits of this process must be seen to not only improve patient care but also protect surgeons against newspaper humiliation. A willingness to be audited and scrutinised by our professional colleagues is a part of our professional responsibility. We fail our patients and ourselves if we do not aim to achieve this.

PRACTISING WITHIN THE PARAMETERS SET BY THE ORGANISATION

Consultants and trainee surgeons are both employees of the hospital in which they work and learn. Each is subject to the regulation related to their employment contract and this regulation has been extended in the light of new clinical governance arrangements designed to ensure safe patient care through a safe organisational environment (**Box 15.3**).[27] The Clinical Negligence Scheme for Hospitals is the contributory indemnity insurance scheme that covers negligence liability costs.[28] Incentives exist to reduce individual hospital's financial contribution to this scheme, including a demonstration, at least on paper, that the hospital is ensuring patient safety and minimising risk to patients and staff in its everyday activities. The resulting effect has yet to be seen.

Consultant surgeons and surgeons in training will be subject to risk assessment processes regulated by these new systems. The process of appraisal will take account of the different areas of surgical activity and will scrutinise such activity. Professional accountability, such as might be demonstrated through data contribution for national registry purposes, would assist surgeons in this process and is another good reason for surgeons' compliance with their professional bodies on these matters. Similarly for trainees, adherence to good educational practice with the maintenance of an educational portfolio, including evidence of learning surgical practice and surgical operations leading to meaningful assessment, will also support the trainee in these processes.

Patient consent is high on the local and national agenda. Understanding the processes of patient assessment and surgical risk is essential in performing this process well, and increasingly there is a multidisciplinary approach to obtaining consent. Doctors must maintain a lead in this area but will only do so if they see consent from the patients' perspective as well as their own.

Box 15.3 • Clinical governance: a quality organisation will ensure the following

Quality improvement processes (e.g. clinical audit) are in place and integrated with the quality programme for the organisation as a whole

Leadership skills are developed at clinical team level

Evidence-based practice is in day-to-day use with the infrastructure to support it

Good practice, ideas and innovations (which have been evaluated) are systematically disseminated within and outside the organisation

Clinical risk reduction programmes of a high standard are in place

Adverse events are detected, and openly investigated, and the lessons learned promptly applied

Lessons for clinical practice are systematically learned from complaints made by patients

Problems of poor clinical performance are recognised at an early stage and dealt with to prevent harm to patients

All professional development programmes reflect the principles of clinical governance

The quality of data collected to monitor clinical care is itself of a high standard

From Department of Health. The new NHS: modern, dependable. London: The Stationery Office, 1997, with permission.

AN EXAMPLE OF A STRATEGY TO SUPPORT A PROCESS OF COMMUNICATION OF RISK

There are three points to the strategy that may be applied to any new situation or at any time in a planned course of action: (i) do something actively new and list the pros and cons; (ii) continue the same course and list the pros and cons; and (iii) review all decisions (**Fig. 15.1**). The following case study illustrates the use of this strategy, which is

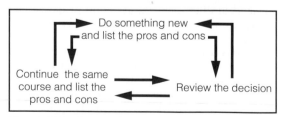

Figure 15.1 • Strategy for action in surgical decision and the balance of risks.

implicit in the practice of the author. The process helps to ensure consistency of approach and that all aspects of the case are regularly and appropriately reviewed. A written record of the process aids review and decision-making and provides a reflective record of why things were done, as well as providing information for audit.

CASE STUDY

A patient, aged 83 years, attends the vascular outpatient clinic for a second opinion about his 7.5-cm infrarenal abdominal aortic aneurysm and the prospects of surgical intervention. He is in remission from lymphoma. He is a retired scientist who worked in the chemical industry. He has a rather diffident manner but is aware of the 10–20% risk of rupture per year and has been told that endovascular aortic repair is experimental and dangerous. He has also been led to believe that there is a 5–7% risk of death related to open aortic surgery. He brings the results of computed tomography and chest radiography investigations.

First interview

- Ask the patient what he wishes to gain from the interview.
- Establish a rapport with the patient. **Allow the patient to reiterate his knowledge and understanding of his case and the pros and cons of surgical intervention for him.**
- Discuss in more detail the risks of open surgery and express the opinion that the risk of death may be higher than he has been quoted because he is immunocompromised, but there are no reliable statistics to back this up. Indicate that the facilities and back-up in the vascular unit would be of the standard appropriate to undertake his operation and that the clinicians would be prepared to proceed if he so wished. **Ask for his thoughts.**
- Revisit the endovascular repair option and explain that it is experimental but that there are short-term gains with respect to mortality. Express a preference for this and indicate that he would be part of a national trial if he wished to proceed. **Ask for his thoughts on this.**
- Undertake an examination of the patient, which reveals a thin man with no previous abdominal operations. **Record the salient features of the examination.**
- Offer a period of reflection before making a decision. Agreement to arrange a follow-up appointment in a month. **Arrange a follow-up date.**

STRATEGY: DO SOMETHING NEW

This interview took approximately 30 minutes but seemed to have gone well. A letter was dictated at the time and stored in the notes and on computer, supplemented with written notes at the time of consultation. The new activity was that a new relationship had been set and needed consolidation. More information had been given. The patient's wishes had been sought and recorded.

First follow-up interview

- Patient asked to reiterate his wishes with respect to the previous consultation.
- Surgeon listens as he expresses his concern about the possible increased risks of open surgery and the fear he has of the resurgence of his lymphoma. He is not keen to consider experimental endovascular surgery.
- Agree together that for now he should continue a conservative approach and that we should monitor his aneurysm with ultrasound scan. Arrange a repeat scan in 2 months and further follow-up.

STRATEGY: CONTINUE THE SAME COURSE

This consultation took 20 minutes and a summary of the processes and decision-making was recorded in the notes and sent to the GP. It is quite useful to send a copy of these deliberations to the patient; it is not our routine practice to do this but we have no hesitation in doing so if the patient requests it or if it seems to be an appropriate course of action.

Second follow-up interview

- Patient given the information that the aneurysm has not changed in size since the previous scan.
- Patient asked by the surgeon to review the previous deliberations.
- Patient asked by the surgeon to tell how he feels about his course of action and what further he would like to know and how we should proceed.
- Agree together to continue the conservative approach.
- Arrange 3-month follow up.
- Review the decisions.

STRATEGY: CONTINUE THE SAME COURSE

This interview took 15 minutes and ended cordially. Two months later the surgeon receives a letter from the patient's GP which states that the patient died at home from a ruptured aneurysm. Post mortem showed that there was no evidence of recurrent lymphoma. His family expressed their thanks for our care and consideration.

Lessons from this case

1. The patient's wishes were taken into account at every step.
2. The surgeon's implicit desire for endovascular intervention was resisted.
3. There was no guarantee that the patient would have survived aortic surgery but there will always be the unanswered question of whether he would have survived longer if he had undergone an operation. Unanswered questions are part of the uncertainty of professional life and surgeons must learn to cope with them.
4. There is a clear record of the process of discussion between surgeon and patient on the course of action.
5. There is no right or wrong action if time, thought and respect have been given to the patient's wishes.
6. The action taken conflicts with the statistical odds.
7. The patient's family bore no grudges and in fact were grateful for the care and attention that had been offered.
8. The process is what is respected and not necessarily the heroic acts of a surgeon. With another patient the decisions may be the reverse.
9. Surgeons need to understand and contribute their specialty's attempts to develop risk-adjusted data.

CONCLUSION

Being a good surgeon is more than knowing the facts. As surgeons we are on a steep learning curve with respect to discussing our reasons for action and operative intervention with patients. Our respect from patients must be earned and will depend on how we treat them as human beings in need of surgical intervention. Taking a patient-centred approach is essential as well as recognising that dependence on statistics is only part of the story.

• Key points

- Surgeons have responsibilities as members of the profession of surgery.
- Being a good surgeon is more than knowing the facts and reciting statistics.
- Patients are vulnerable and need to be at the centre of the decision-making process for their surgical care.
- Risk stratification needs to be understood by surgeons as a way of understanding best treatment and for comparative audit. All surgeons should take part in comparative audit.
- Clinical care is helped by surgeons having a strategy for managing patients.
- The use of single statistics to inform patients of risk is unhelpful.

REFERENCES

1. Gigerenzer G. Reckoning with risk. Learning to live with uncertainty. London: Penguin Books, 2002.

   Gigerenzer describes examples of how different ways of expressing statistics can both mislead and confuse patients. He emphasises too that some may use statistics to support an argument rather than to indicate the magnitude of risk that there may be to an individual.

2. Mehta SS, Powell L, Cooper JC. What your patients want to know about their surgery. Ann R Coll Surg Engl 2002; 84:141–3.

3. Mehta SS, Powell L, Cooper JC. What your patients want to know about their surgery. Ann R Coll Surg Engl 2003; 85:360–3.

4. Keogh BE, Kinsman R. National Adult Cardiac Surgical Database Report 1999–2000. London: Society of Cardiothoracic Surgeons of Great Britain and Ireland, 2000.

5. Ashley S, Ridler B, Kinsman R. National Vascular Database Report. London: Surgical Society of Great Britain and Ireland, 2002.

6. Bennett-Guerrero, Hyam JA, Shaefi S et al. Comparison of P-POSSUM risk adjusted mortality rates

after surgery between patients in the USA and the UK. Br J Surg 2003; 90:1593–8.

7. Gigerenzer G, Edwards A. Simple tools for understanding risks: from innumeracy to insight. Br Med J 2003; 327:741–4.

8. Thornton H, Edwards A, Elwyn G. Evolving the multiple roles of 'patients' in health-care research: reflections after involvement in a trial of shared decision making. Health Expectation 2003; 6:189–97. Available at http:\\www.healthpartnership.org/ studies/edwards.html

The authors use a qualitative research method to look at this topic from the patients' perspective. 'Being taken seriously', as the patients see it, is being given time for face-to-face contact with their medical practitioner to be informed and to ask questions about the options involved in their care. This paper is perhaps most pertinent as 2004 sees the start of 'choice agenda', where patients will be able to choose their hospital consultant and time of appointment. It bears little relationship to the findings in this study.

9. Calman KC. Cancer: science and society and the communication of risk. Br Med J 1996; 313:799–802.

10. Vincent C, Taylor-Adams S, Stanhope N. Framework for analyzing risk and safety in clinical medicine. Br Med J 1998; 316:1154–7.

11. de Cossart L. Patient assessment and risk stratification. In: Paterson-Brown S (ed.) Core topics in general and emergency surgery, 2nd edn. London: WB Saunders, 2001; pp. 389–407.

12. Kirk RM, Ribbans WJ (eds) Patient assessment, clinical surgery in general, 4th edn. Edinburgh: Churchill Livingstone, 2003; Section 2.

13. Cushieri A. Preoperative, operative and postoperative care. In: Cushieri A, Giles G, Moosa B (eds) Essential surgical practice. London: Butterworth, 1995; pp. 372–98.

14. Jones HJS, de Cossart L. Risk scoring in surgical patients. Br J Surg 1999; 86:149–57.

15. Chapple A, Ziebland S, Shepperd S, Miller R, Herxheimer A, McPherson A. Why men with prostate cancer want wider access to prostate specific antigen testing: qualitative study. Br Med J 2002; 325:737–9.

16. Rakovitch E, Franssen E, Kim J et al. A comparison of risk perception and psychological morbidity in women with ductal carcinoma in situ and early breast cancer. Breast Cancer Res Treat 2003; 77:2855–93.

17. Million Women Study Collaborators. Breast cancer and hormone replacement therapy in the million women study. Lancet 2003; 362:419–27.

18. de Cossart L, Fish D. Membership of a profession: what it means and why it is important. Educational update issue 13:1, Mersey Deanery PGMDE, April 2002. Available at http:\\www.Merseydeanery.ac.uk

19. Maintaining good medical practice. London: General Medical Council, 1999.

20. The surgeon's duty of care. London: Senate of Surgery of Great Britain and Ireland, 1998.

21. Good surgical practice. London: Royal College of Surgeons of England, 2000.

22. Paling J. Strategies to help patients to understand risks. Br Med J 2003; 327:745–8.

23. Glazer G, Mann DV, on behalf of the working party of the British Society of Gastroenterology. United Kingdom guidelines for the management of acute pancreatitis. Gut 1998; 42(Suppl. 2):S1–S13.

24. Copeland GP, Jones D, Walters M. POSSUM: a risk scoring system for surgical audit. Br J Surg 1991; 78:355–60.

25. Mann D, Hershman M, Hittinger R et al Multicentre acute audit of death from acute pancreatitis. Br J Surg 1994; 81:890–3.

The authors showed clearly that using only clinical assessment without multiple risk factor adjustment may result in less aggressive treatment and more deaths than necessary. Clinical evaluation alone without risk stratification is not as accurate and allows room for error and underscoring of patients.

26. A serious departure from safe professional standards. General Medical Council News 1998; 1:8–10.

27. Department of Health. The new NHS: modern, dependable. London: The Stationary Office, 1997.

28. The Clinical Negligence Scheme for Trust. Available at http:\\www.doh.org

Sixteen

Perioperative management of the surgical patient

Michael R. Grounds

INTRODUCTION

Over the last 25–50 years there has been evidence that the incidence of death directly attributable to anaesthesia has fallen but despite this the overall incidence of death following surgery has remained almost unchanged. In the mid-1950s a number of studies demonstrated that the postoperative mortality solely associated with anaesthesia was approximately 1 in 2500.[1-3] In 1987, Buck et al.[4] showed in their *Report of a confidential enquiry into perioperative deaths* that the cause of postoperative death solely attributable to anaesthesia had fallen significantly to approximately 1 in 185 000, while that following surgery had hardly changed. It would appear therefore that there are a significant number of patients undergoing surgery who do not have sufficient underlying physiological reserve to withstand the stress of the surgical procedure to which they are subjected. Some are easy to identify prior to surgery and are clearly moribund and unlikely to survive with or without surgery, but most of the patients who die following surgery are not so easily identified. In England and Wales, approximately 2 600 000 surgical operations are carried out each year and the report of the National Confidential Enquiry into Postoperative Deaths (NCEPOD) suggested that at least 20 000 of these patients will die in the first 28 days following surgery.[5] Shoemaker and colleagues[6,7] have studied the physiological patterns of patients surviving or not surviving similar surgical procedures in the USA. They collected a large number of surgical data and showed that patients who had evidence of one or more criteria suggesting poor physiological reserve had a hospital mortality rate in excess of 30% following major surgery (see below). Based on these data, it is estimated that perhaps as many as two million or more patients per year in the USA are at such risk and well over 200 000 patients are dying within the first 28 days of surgery.

Examination of four major intensive care databases (Scottish Intensive Care Society Audit Group database, South West Thames Intensive Care database, Intensive Care National Audit and Research Center Case Mix database and Riyadh Intensive Care Program) between 1990 and 1999, containing between them over 6000 patients admitted to intensive care following surgery, demonstrates an overall hospital mortality in excess of 20%. Elective and emergency patients had a mortality of approximately 11 and 33% respectively.

RISK FACTORS

For the general surgical population, the risk of death within 30 days of an operation is less than 1%; even more complex surgery, such as cardiac surgery, has an elective mortality of only 2–4%. However, when patients with poor preoperative physiological reserve undergo major surgery then the mortality is considerably higher. In a study of all colorectal cancer surgery in one region in the UK, Mella et al.[8] showed that of the 3520 patients studied, the overall 30-day postoperative mortality was 7.6% but rose to 21% for those who underwent emergency/urgent surgery. Furthermore, they were able to categorise their patients into their preoperative American Society of Anesthesiologists

(ASA) groups and show that although the 30-day mortality for those in ASA I was 4% for both elective and emergency surgery, the 30-day mortality for those in ASA IV (the patients with the poorest physiological reserve) was 22% for elective patients but over 55% for emergency patients. It seems clear, therefore, that there are a substantial number of patients undergoing major surgery who are at real risk of either dying within 30 days of surgery or developing a major complication that will lengthen their hospital stay. Furthermore, analysis by NCEPOD has shown that about 50% of these high-risk patients never received any form of intensive or high-dependency care during their hospital admission. There is also some evidence to suggest that there are complications occurring in patients undergoing less severe surgery, which again significantly increase the period of hospitalisation.[9]

Criteria for identification of perioperative risk

Although such data have been available for some years, in general relatively few workers have paid attention to the implications. The exception has been Shoemaker and his colleagues, who have published a series of papers that have examined the issue in some considerable detail.[6,7,10] Observational data acquired from several thousand patients undergoing major surgery indicated that up to 10% of such patients had a hospital mortality of 30–40%, and even those surviving had a high probability of developing a major complication that would significantly increase their hospital stay. From this database, Shoemaker et al.[11] identified a list of criteria, any one of which when present in patients undergoing major abdominal or vascular surgery placed the patient in the high-risk category (**Box 16.1**).

For example, a history of myocardial infarction or stroke within the previous 6 months, evidence of significant obstructive airways disease, evidence of impaired organ function, and so on all placed the patient in the high-risk group. This list had a total of 17 criteria, which were given equal weighting in terms of prognosis.

Variables for survival

Following the identification of these preoperative risk factors, Shoemaker and colleagues asked the question whether there were perioperative variables that separated the survivors from the non-survivors within this high-risk group. They examined 37 such criteria, including most of the commonly measured variables such as heart rate, blood pressure, temperature and urine output. They concluded that most of the variables measured in the perioperative

Box 16.1 • Criteria for identifying high-risk surgical patients developed by Shoemaker

Previous severe cardiorespiratory illness

Late-stage vascular disease

Age >70 years with limited physiological reserve

Extensive surgery for carcinoma: oesophagectomy, gastrectomy, cystectomy

Acute abdominal catastrophe with haemodynamic instability: peritonitis, perforated viscus, pancreatitis

Acute massive blood loss >8 units

Septicaemia: positive blood culture or septic focus

Respiratory failure: P_aO_2 <8.0 kPa or F_iO_2 >0.4 or mechanical ventilation >48 hours

Acute renal failure: urea >20 mmol/L or creatinine >260 mmol/L

period do not differ significantly between survivors and non-survivors until shortly before the death of the patient. Importantly, however, they showed that those variables that were directly or indirectly related to blood flow, and especially to the delivery of oxygen to the tissues, were more evident in patients who survived major surgery. In particular, they demonstrated that a tissue oxygen delivery greater than 600 mL/min per m² or a cardiac index of greater than 4.5 L/min per m² were both fundamentally associated with survival. Interestingly, these data confirmed the early work of Boyd et al.[12] and Clowes and Del Guercio,[13] who in the late 1950s and early 1960s had clearly demonstrated that patients undergoing major thoracic and abdominal surgery had a very high postoperative mortality if the patients were unable to mount a satisfactory cardiovascular response to supply adequate oxygen to the tissue in response to the surgery that was being undertaken.

TISSUE HYPOXIA

These findings suggested that a likely cause of the high mortality seen in this group of surgical patients was the development of tissue hypoxia during and immediately after surgery. Shoemaker and colleagues postulated that major surgery was associated with significant metabolic stress, leading to an increased oxygen demand from the tissues. If this demand could not be met, then tissue hypoxia developed. This led to an amplification of the inflammatory response occurring as a result of the surgery and this, in turn, resulted in important organ damage, with the subsequent development of multiorgan failure and a high mortality rate. This sequence of hypoxia, organ dysfunction and organ failure is exactly what is seen in clinical practice. Such organ failure will inevitably lead to a high rate for both postoperative complications and death. This of course mirrors clinical practice where we find that patients do not often die postoperatively from a single cause but develop a number of complications over a period of days and then finally die of multi-organ failure at some later date, often termed 'multiple organ dysfunction syndrome'. The NECPOD reports have consistently shown that perioperative deaths are still occurring 30 days after surgery, with the median day of postoperative death being the sixth day after surgery.

OXYGEN DEBT

In a later publication, Shoemaker and colleagues calculated the apparent oxygen debt developing during and after surgery in this cohort of patients.[14] They made the calculations based on the known changes in metabolic rate associated with surgery, anaesthesia and changes in temperature. They compared the calculated oxygen demand with the oxygen supply and concluded that in a substantial number of patients demand exceeded supply during surgery and in some for a prolonged period. These data showed that patients who repaid the acquired oxygen debt within 2 hours of returning from the operation all survived with no complications, while those who were only able to repay the debt by 24 hours all survived but had significant complications. In marked contrast, those patients whose oxygen debt increased with time and who were never able to repay it had major complications and all died. This work serves to emphasise the critical role that tissue perfusion and hence oxygen delivery play in determining outcome in patients undergoing major surgery.

RESULTS OF IMPROVING OXYGEN DELIVERY AND TISSUE PERFUSION

Clearly, if the development of tissue hypoxia at the time of surgery is the fundamental problem to be overcome to ensure survival following major surgery, then it will be appropriate to measure oxygen delivery in these high-risk patients. Where the target oxygen delivery of greater than 600 mL/min per m^2 or a cardiac index of greater than 4.5 L/min per m^2 is not achieved by the patient, then the clinicians will intervene to assist the patient to achieve these targets for survival. In 1988, Shoemaker et al.[11] published an important study which demonstrated that raising cardiac index and oxygen delivery to these goals resulted in a major reduction in mortality. This study of 57 patients was undertaken on a group of high-risk surgical patients. The control group was treated conventionally whereas the protocol-treated patients had pulmonary artery catheters inserted either preoperatively or immediately after surgery. In this group, fluids were given to increase pulmonary capillary wedge pressure to the higher end of the normal range, and if this did not achieve the goal for cardiac index and oxygen delivery, then inotropes were added. The mortality in the control group was 33% but fell to 3% in the protocol group; this was accompanied by a 50% reduction in the postoperative complication rate. Although the result seemed impressive, the study was criticised mainly because of the rather small sample size but also because it was felt that the patient groups were not well matched and the precise protocol used in the group was not clear.

In a larger double-blind, randomised, controlled study involving 107 patients having both elective and emergency surgery, Boyd et al.[15] again showed a significant reduction in mortality from 23% to 5.7% and a halving of the complication rate by targeting an oxygen delivery of 600 mL/min per m^2. In this study most patients were admitted to the intensive care unit prior to surgery, with oxygen delivery being increased in the preoperative period and maintained during the intraoperative and post-operative period, until the patient's serum lactate and base deficit returned to within the normal range. More recently, Lobo et al.[16] in Brazil adopted this goal-directed therapy approach for the care of their high-risk surgical (general surgical and vascular) patients and showed a mortality of 50% in the control group but a mortality of only 15.7% in the protocol-treated group.

All the studies described so far required the insertion of a pulmonary artery catheter in order to measure cardiac output. This has some disadvantages in that it is a time-consuming procedure requiring considerable skill and not without some risk. In addition, the patients have to be admitted to the intensive care unit preoperatively, which can clearly cause logistical problems. However, a less invasive method of monitoring using intra-oesophageal Doppler to monitor cardiac output from the descending aorta was used in a group of 60 patients undergoing cardiac surgery.[17] A significant reduction in major complication rate and both intensive care and overall hospital stay was seen in the protocol group. Using a similar protocol, Sinclair et al.[18] achieved a significant reduction in hospital stay of 40% in a group of elderly patients having surgery for fractured neck of femur.

Some studies have investigated the application of goal-directed therapy to the at-risk patient in the immediate postoperative period. One such study has been carried out in over 140 young trauma patients with severe penetrating injuries with the aim of achieving an oxygen delivery of 600 mL/min per m^2

immediately after the patient returned from the operating theatre.[19] This reduced the incidence of major organ failure by 50% and reduced mortality from 37% to 18%. Others have since confirmed the benefits of this approach in a group of 138 patients undergoing major elective surgery.[20] This study had a control limb of patients who only came to the intensive care unit if the clinician in charge of the case felt that such care was necessary. The two protocol groups were both admitted to the intensive care unit preoperatively, where arterial and pulmonary artery catheters were inserted and intravenous fluids administered. If goal-directed therapy did not produce an oxygen delivery of greater than 600 mL/min per m^2 by use of additional intravenous fluids and supplemental oxygen, then the patients were assigned to receive either adrenaline (epinephrine) or dopexamine to achieve the desired goal. This treatment was then continued both during and after surgery. The mortality fell from 17% in the control group to 3% in the combined treatment groups. Of added interest was the finding that the group which received dopexamine had a significantly lower complication rate and intensive care and hospital stay than both the control group and those receiving adrenaline. Furthermore, the total hospital stay for the 43 patients in the group receiving dopexamine was 41% less than the control group and 32% less than those receiving adrenaline.

The studies so far described have, in the main, been undertaken in the preoperative and intraoperative periods, although some of the patients in the studies of Shoemaker et al.,[11] Boyd et al.[15] and Bishop et al.[19] were entered postoperatively. In addition, all these studies monitored and manipulated cardiac output in an effort to improve perfusion and prevent the development of tissue hypoxia and an oxygen debt.

Using a different approach, Polonen et al.[21] studied over 400 patients undergoing cardiac surgery. All patients in this study had a pulmonary artery catheter inserted preoperatively. After return from the operating theatre, the control group was treated conventionally. In the protocol group, the circulation was manipulated with fluids and inotropes to maintain mixed venous saturation above 70% and blood lactate below 2.0 mmol/L. Both these variables are markers of tissue perfusion; mixed venous saturation is dependent on the relationship between cardiac output and tissue oxygen extraction, while a raised lactate is a marker of anaerobic tissue metabolism. The results were similar to those in the other studies so far described, with significant reductions in complications and readmission to the intensive care unit.

All the studies detailed here have shown significant improvements in one or more markers of outcome, which seems to confirm Shoemaker's hypothesis that prevention of tissue hypoxia is the crucial element in reducing mortality and morbidity in high-risk patients. This brief overview of the literature relating to the high-risk surgical patient leads to some inevitable conclusions:

1. There is good evidence to suggest that patients with poor cardiorespiratory reserve have a higher mortality and complication rate when undergoing major surgery. Most of these patients can be identified by simple clinical methods before surgery.

2. It is likely that there are significant numbers of patients undergoing different types of surgery who may be at substantial risk of developing major complications or death. The precise numbers are uncertain but it is clear there are probably 25 000 deaths occurring within 30 days of surgery, and only about 50% of these patients receive intensive or high-dependency care.

3. A number of randomised controlled clinical studies have consistently demonstrated the improvement in outcome that can be achieved in these patients by the use of goal-directed therapy aimed at temporarily improving the cardiovascular performance of high-risk patients so that non-survivors have the same cardiorespiratory performance as survivors.

4. Studies have shown that benefit may be obtained in a wide range of surgery, including vascular surgery, colorectal surgery, trauma, orthopaedics, major cancer surgery and cardiac surgery. The benefit is greatest when the surgery is performed as an emergency.

5. From the work by Shoemaker and colleagues it would seem that about 8% of the surgical population would fulfil his definition of being at high risk of complications or death following major surgery. It would appear that these patients have a postoperative 30-day mortality of 20–30%, representing 90–95% of all surgical deaths. This number is likely to increase with an ageing population on whom increasingly complex surgery is being performed.

6. Although optimising the circulation produces significant reductions in mortality and postoperative complications in the higher-risk patient, it is now clear that important reductions in complications can be achieved in patients who have a lower mortality but for whom a significant complication risk exists.

7. It is also apparent that optimising the circulation can be carried out using several different techniques and at different times (i.e. preoperatively, intraoperatively and postoperatively).

Box 16.2 • Clinical guidelines for the implementation of goal-directed therapy in high-risk surgical patients

Identify the high-risk patient

See Box 16.1 for Shoemaker criteria

Particularly identify elderly patients with poor cardiorespiratory reserve, ischaemic heart disease with evidence of heart failure

Identify the operation

Operations likely to last longer than 1.5 hours

Lack of postoperative critical care facilities

Emergency surgery, particularly abdominal surgery

Perioperative goal-directed therapy

1. Assess the patient preoperatively: where possible perform cardiovascular measurements to assess cardiac performance. Measure cardiac output and oxygen delivery

2. If cardiac index >4.5 L/min per m^2 and/or oxygen delivery >600 mL/min per m^2 (body surface area), then no further goal-directed therapy will be necessary. Patient can proceed to anaesthesia and surgery

3. If cardiac index <4.5 L/min per m^2 and/or oxygen delivery <600 mL/min per m^2 (body surface area), then further goal-directed therapy may be indicated either prior to surgery or, if this is not possible, then immediately following surgery in a dedicated critical care area

4. If cardiac index <4.5 L/min per m^2 and/or oxygen delivery <600 mL/min per m^2 (body surface area):

   (a) Increase intravenous fluids: direct therapy using flow-directed monitoring equipment to maximize intravascular filling pressure
   (b) Maintain adequate haemoglobin concentration with blood transfusion if necessary
   (c) Maintain blood oxygen saturation at 95% or greater with supplemental oxygenation or artificial ventilation

5. If despite these measures cardiac index is <4.5 L/min per m^2 and/or oxygen delivery <600 mL/min per m^2 (body surface area), then consider the use of inotrope therapy. Although a number of different inotropes have been used (including adrenaline and dobutamine), the best results seem to have been achieved using dopexamine. Start dopexamine at 0.5 µg/kg per min and increase the rate of infusion incrementally every 10–15 minutes until either the target oxygen delivery has been achieved or there is an increase in heart rate 20% greater than the patient's resting rate or there are signs of ischaemia on the ECG. (If the patient is very tachycardic prior to starting inotropes, it is important to recognize this and not try to increase cardiac output at the expense of increasing the already raised heart rate.) Maintain intravascular filling pressure during this period of inotrope therapy

Maintain this goal-directed therapy into the postoperative period until there is evidence that the intraoperative oxygen debt is repaid (return of base deficit to normal, blood lactate concentration within normal range)

Box 16.2 lists the clinical guidelines for the implementation of goal-directed therapy in high-risk surgical patients.

CLINICAL IMPLICATIONS

There is now a reasonable literature relating to the effects of optimising the circulation in the high-risk surgical patient. An important question, therefore, is whether, with the current state of knowledge, clinicians would be justified in applying these techniques to routine clinical practice. Unfortunately, there is as yet no clear definitive answer. However, the results do raise some important issues: when does a research finding become accepted clinical practice and, indeed, when is it actually unethical not to adopt the new technique? There seem to be several reasons why the surgical and anaesthetic communities have not generally adopted these techniques. It is clear that there is a general air of scepticism as to the existence of the high-risk surgical patient as a real clinical entity. Even if clinicians accept the concept of the high-risk patient, they may feel there is insufficient scientific evidence to justify embarking on a policy that will involve a major change in the clinical management of these patients. However, there are clinicians who do accept that increasing cardiac output in these patients is of proven benefit but feel that the resources are not yet available to introduce a protocol as part of routine clinical practice. They justifiably claim that there are too few intensive care beds to admit patients preoperatively and too little time in the anaesthetic room to undertake the appropriate instrumentation of the patients.

Lastly, there is renewed interest in early manipulation of the circulation in the immediate postoperative period. There is some evidence to suggest that the first few, perhaps up to 8, postoperative hours represent a golden window where increasing cardiac output to a target value may result in very considerable benefit. This option has obvious attractions in that many of the patients who might benefit from such an approach would have been admitted to the intensive care unit as a matter of routine because of the severity of the surgery and, furthermore, pulmonary artery catheters may well have been inserted as part of standard clinical care. The disadvantage is that significant numbers of high-risk patients will not, at this stage at least, be admitted to intensive care, either because beds are not available or because the clinician has failed to recognise that the patient is at high risk.

It is clear therefore that more work is required, using a variety of techniques in a variety of patient groups, before unequivocal evidence is available that will convince the medical community at large that significant benefits in clinical outcome can be produced by aggressive manipulation of the circulation in a relatively small number of surgical patients.

Key points

- Patients with poor cardiorespiratory reserve undergoing major operations have a high postoperative complication and mortality rate. The mortality rate is much higher if these patients have emergency operations.
- These patients can be identified preoperatively by simple clinical history and examination.
- This high postoperative complication and mortality rate can be significantly reduced by goal-directed therapy aimed at enhancing the cardiorespiratory performance of these patients with poor physiological reserve during the perioperative period.
- Goal-directed therapy aims to ensure that tissue oxygen delivery is enhanced to levels shown to confer survival without postoperative complications.

REFERENCES

1. Beecher HK, Todd DP. A study of the deaths associated with anaesthesia and surgery. Ann Surg 1954; 140:2–5.

2. Edwards G, Morton HJV, Pask EA et al. Deaths associated with anaesthesia. Anaesthesia 1956; 11:194–220.

3. Dornette WHL, Orth OS. Death in the operating room. Anesth Analg 1956; 3:545–69.

4. Buck N, Devlin HB, Lunn JN. The report of a confidential enquiry into perioperative deaths. London: Nuffield Provincial Hospitals Trust and the King Edward's Hospital Fund for London, 1987.

5. Campling EA, Devlin HB, Hoile RW, Lunn JN. National Confidential Enquiry into peri-operative deaths. London: Royal College of Surgeons, 1992.

6. Shoemaker WC. Cardiorespiratory patterns of surviving and non-surviving postoperative patients. Surg Gynecol Obstet 1972; 134:810–14.

7. Shoemaker WC, Montgomery ES, Kaplan E et al. Physiologic patterns in surviving and nonsurviving shock patients. Use of sequential cardiorespiratory variables in defining criteria for therapeutic goals and early warning of death. Arch Surg 1973; 106:630–6.

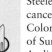

8. Mella J, Biffin A, Radcliff AG, Stamatakis JD, Steele RJ. Population-based audit of colorectal cancer management in two UK health regions. Colorectal Cancer Working Group, Royal College of Surgeons of England, Clinical Epidemiology and Audit Unit. Br J Surg 1997; 84:1731–6.

> This paper is important because it shows that for a group of patients in the UK the outcome following major surgery is the same as had been predicted by Shoemaker following his work on patients in the USA. The study shows conclusively that the iller the patient (with the worse physiological reserve), the worse they will do postoperatively. It also debunks the myth that UK surgeons do not have a high mortality rate for certain types of surgery. It shows clearly that if the patient is ASA IV and has an emergency operation for bowel cancer, then the postoperative mortality rate is over 50%.

9. Bennett-Guerrero E, Welsby I, Dunn TJ et al. The use of postoperative morbidity survey to evaluate patients with prolonged hospital stay after routine, moderate risk, elective surgery. Anesth Analg 1999; 89:514–19.

10. Shoemaker WC, Czer LS. Evaluation of biological importance of various hemodynamic and oxygen transport variables: which variables should be monitored in postoperative shock? Crit Care Med 1979; 7:424–31.

11. Shoemaker WC, Appel PC, Cram HB et al. Prospective trial of supranormal values of survivors as therapeutic goals in high risk surgical patients. Chest 1988; 94:1176–86.

12. Boyd AD, Tremblay RE, Spencer FC, Bahnson HT. Estimation of cardiac output soon after intracardiac surgery with cardiopulmonary bypass. Ann Surg 1959; 150:613–26.

13. Clowes GHAJ, Del Guercio LRM. Circulatory response to trauma of surgical operations. Metabolism 1960; 9:67–81.

14. Shoemaker WC, Appel PL, Kram HB. Role of oxygen debt in the development of organ failure, sepsis and death in high-risk surgical patients. Chest 1992; 102:208–15.

   This study is the culmination of much of Shoemaker's work in which he seeks to suggest that the problem with these patients is their inability to repay an oxygen debt produced during surgery, thus leading to subsequent organ deterioration, multiorgan failure and ultimately death.

15. Boyd O, Grounds RM, Bennett ED. A randomized clinical trial of the effect of deliberate perioperative increase of oxygen delivery on mortality in high risk surgical patients. JAMA 1993; 270:2699–708.

   This was the first full well-conducted, randomised, controlled study of goal-directed therapy for perioperative enhancement of the cardiovascular systems of these high-risk surgical patients. It was stopped before it was completed by the local hospital research ethics committee because the surgeons felt that it was obvious which group their patients were in and felt it was unethical to continue when the benefits were so obvious.

16. Lobo SM, Salgado PF, Castillo VG et al. Effects of maximizing oxygen delivery on morbidity and mortality in high-risk surgical patients. Crit Care Med 2000; 28:3396–404.

17. Mythen M, Webb AR. Perioperative plasma volume expansion reduces the incidence of gut mucosal hypoperfusion during cardiac surgery. Arch Surg 1995; 130:423–9.

18. Sinclair S, James S, Singer M. Intraoperative intravascular volume optimisation and length of hospital stay after repair of proximal femoral fracture: randomised controlled trial. Br Med J 1997; 315:909–12.

19. Bishop MH, Shoemaker WC, Appel PL et al. Prospective, randomized trial of survivor values of cardiac index, oxygen delivery, and oxygen consumption as resuscitation end points in severe trauma. J Trauma 1995; 38:780–7.

20. Wilson J, Woods I, Fawcett J et al. Reducing the risk of major elective surgery: randomized controlled trial of preoperative optimisation of oxygen delivery. Br Med J 1999; 318:1099–103.

   This study is important because not only did it have a control group where clinicians not involved with the study were able to decide on the postoperative treatment and send patients back to the ward postoperatively (which is common practice in many hospitals in the UK due to lack of critical care facilities) but it also divided the group admitted to intensive care into two groups for therapeutic intervention and thus showed that there could be a difference in outcome if different drugs were used for goal-directed therapy.

21. Polonen P, Rukonen E, Hippelainen M et al. A prospective, randomized study of goal-orientated hemodynamic therapy in cardiac surgical patients. Anesth Analg 2000; 90:1052–9.

Seventeen
Surgical nutrition

Steven D. Heys and
John Broom

INTRODUCTION

As we have embarked upon the new millennium, malnutrition is still a significant problem in clinical practice in the Western world, with up to 40% of hospitalised patients classified as being malnourished. For example, in patients undergoing gastrointestinal surgery, the prevalence of 'mild' and 'moderate' malnutrition has been estimated to be approximately 50% and 30% respectively. This is important because the consequences of malnutrition are a disturbance of cellular and organ function. The following can occur, which are of clinical importance in patients undergoing surgery:

- muscle wasting and impairment of skeletal muscle function;
- impaired respiratory muscle function;
- impaired cardiac muscle function;
- atrophy of smooth muscle in the gastrointestinal tract;
- impaired immune function;
- impaired healing, e.g. wounds and anastomoses.

The clinical importance of these malnutrition-induced changes is that they result in an increased risk of postoperative morbidity and mortality. Furthermore, patients who undergo surgery may also be fasted for varying periods of time (preoperatively and/or postoperatively), which may result in an exacerbation of the above disturbances of cellular and organ function. Moreover, if postoperative complications ensue (e.g. sepsis), these effects may be further potentiated.

It is important to consider first the metabolic and biochemical changes, termed the metabolic response to trauma and sepsis, which occur when a patient undergoes surgery, as these have clear implications for understanding the basis of nutritional support in critically ill patients.

METABOLIC RESPONSE TO TRAUMA AND SEPSIS

Trauma

Following trauma, a complex series of changes in tissue metabolism occurs. A major advance in the understanding of these changes took place more than 50 years ago when Sir David Cuthbertson described the loss of nitrogen from skeletal muscle that occurred following trauma.[1] Cuthbertson concluded that the response to injury could be considered as occurring in two phases (**Fig. 17.1**):

1. the 'ebb' phase, which is a short-lived response associated with hypovolaemic shock, increased sympathetic nervous system activity and reduced metabolic rate;
2. the 'flow' phase, which is associated with a loss of body nitrogen and resultant negative nitrogen balance.

These changes result in an increased resting energy expenditure, increased heat production, pyrexia, increased muscle catabolism and wasting and loss of body nitrogen, increased glucose production, glucose intolerance, increased breakdown of fat and

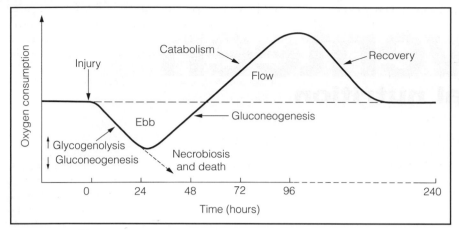

Figure 17.1 • Diagrammatic representation of the ebb and flow phases in the metabolic response to injury. With permission from Broom J. Sepsis and trauma. In: Garrow JS, James WPT (eds) Human nutrition and dietetics, 9th edn. Edinburgh: Churchill Livingstone, 1993; pp. 456–64.

reduced fat synthesis. If these changes continue as part of the 'ebb phase', then despite advances in anaesthetic and surgical technique, death is an inevitable outcome.

The central nervous system and the neuro-hypophyseal axis play key roles in mediating these metabolic changes following trauma, with a range of hormones and cytokines being key regulators. Afferent nerve impulses also stimulate the hypothalamus to secrete hypothalamic releasing factors that, in turn, stimulate the pituitary gland to release prolactin, vasopressin, growth hormone and adrenocorticotrophic hormone (ACTH). The changes in hormone levels in plasma following trauma are outlined in **Box 17.1**, with the so-called stress hormones (adrenaline, cortisol and glucagon) playing a pivotal role in these responses.

CHANGES IN PROTEIN METABOLISM

The increased loss of nitrogen following trauma is due to protein breakdown occurring at a rate in excess of synthesis,[2] whether the patient is fed or fasted. The magnitude of the nitrogen loss is proportional to the degree of operative trauma. A major site of protein breakdown is in the skeletal muscle, which contains 80% of the body's free amino acid pool, of which 60% is glutamine.[3]

The amino acids released can be used for:

1. fuel by muscle;
2. synthesis of proteins necessary for structural repair in the traumatised area;
3. hepatic production of proteins with immunological or tissue repair functions;
4. hepatic production of glucose from alanine (the latter being produced by a series of

transamination reactions from other amino acids);
5. energy substrates for the gut, lymphocytes and other rapidly proliferating tissues.

CHANGES IN CARBOHYDRATE METABOLISM

Glucose is the main fuel used for many different tissues and is obtained by absorption from the gastrointestinal tract, endogenous production from glycogen (glycogenolysis) or from other precursors such as amino acids. Glucose can be utilised for energy transduction or converted into glycogen or fat. Following trauma, there is an increase in hepatic glycogen breakdown (caused by increased sympathetic activity).[4] These stores are substantially, but not completely, depleted within 24 hours.[5] There is also an associated reduction in the peripheral utilisation of glucose. Insulin antagonists are also involved in the metabolic response to trauma (see **Box 17.1**).

Resistance to insulin occurs in patients who have been injured. The circulating concentrations of glucose and insulin are both elevated following injury, but there is a more marked rise in insulin concentrations. The circulating insulin level usually reaches a maximum several days after the injury, before returning towards normal basal levels.

In general, the carbohydrate response is to produce hyperglycaemia both in the immediate 'shock' and later 'flow' phase of the metabolic response. The origin of the increased glucose differs between these two phases. In the critically ill patient, as a direct result of sepsis and trauma, the advent of hypoglycaemia is a premorbid phenomenon.

Box 17.1 • Changes in hormone levels in plasma following trauma

Catecholamines

Rapid increases in concentrations of adrenaline and noradrenaline within a few minutes of injury due to increased activity of sympathetic nervous system. Levels return to normal within 24 hours

Glucagon

Rises within a few hours; maximal levels 12–48 hours post trauma

Insulin

Initially plasma levels are low following trauma, but rise to above normal levels and reach a maximum several days after the injury

Cortisol

Rapid increase in cortisol (due to stimulation by ACTH), returning to normal 24–48 hours later; may remain elevated for up to several days. Has 'permissive' effects with other hormones such as catecholamines

Growth hormone

Levels increased following trauma; usually return to normal levels within 24 hours

Thyroid hormones

Following trauma, systemic thyroxine level is normal but triiodothyronine is low and reverse triiodothyronine is high

Renin, aldosterone

Aldosterone levels increased after trauma, returning to normal within 12 hours. Its secretion is stimulated by renin, which in turn is produced in response to reduced renal perfusion

Testosterone

Plasma levels fall after trauma and may remain low for up to 7 days

Vasopressin

Plasma levels rise following trauma and may remain elevated for several days

Prolactin

Secretion increased following trauma but function in trauma is unknown

Cytokines

Increased secretion of interleukin (IL)-2, IL-6, tumour necrosis factor, etc.; interrelationship between these changes leads to differential responses seen in trauma and sepsis

CHANGES IN FAT METABOLISM

After trauma, there is an increase in the turnover of fatty acids and glycerol. Lipolysis of triacylglycerols is increased, with the production of free fatty acids and glycerol. The glycerol can be used by the liver for gluconeogenesis and the fatty acids can also be used as a fuel source.[6]

Sepsis

The metabolic response to sepsis is also characterised by alterations in protein, carbohydrate and fat metabolism. However, the changes occurring in patients with sepsis have definite differences from those occurring in response to trauma.[7] In patients with sepsis, the following occur.

- Septic patients experience a breakdown of skeletal muscle. The nitrogen losses can be substantial (more than 15–20 g of nitrogen per day). The amino acids released from muscle are utilised by the liver for the production of both acute-phase and visceral proteins and as substrates for the increase in gluconeogenesis that is required.
- Increased production of glucose by the liver (e.g. both gluconeogenesis and glycogenolysis), resulting in an elevated plasma glucose concentration.
- Increased rate of glucose uptake and oxidation by the peripheral tissues.
- Circulating levels of free fatty acids may increase or decrease in patients with sepsis.[8] The reasons for these differences may possibly be explained by the differing times during the septic episode at which concentrations have been measured.
- Increase in breakdown of fat stores in adipose tissue by lipolysis and hypertriglyceridaemia.
- Decrease in the peripheral uptake of these triacylglycerols and defective ketogenesis in the presence of sepsis (in contrast to the situation occurring after trauma).

A significant abnormality in the septic patient is the disruption of the microstructure of the hepatocyte mitochondria, particularly of the inner membrane. There is a block in the energy transduction pathways, with consequent reduction in the aerobic metabolism of both glucose and fatty acids. The body therefore depends on the anaerobic metabolism of glucose, with a resultant increase in lactate production. It is essential therefore that there is an adequate supply of glucose from gluconeogenic pathways. If this is impaired or inadequate, then hypoglycaemia (and death) may ensue. The development of hypoglycaemia during sepsis is an indicator of an extremely poor prognosis and is usually associated with inevitable mortality.

NUTRITIONAL REQUIREMENTS

Proteins and amino acids

Ingestion of protein is required for the maintenance of normal health and cellular function. Proteins have many functions, for example they are essential components of cellular structure and are required for the synthesis of a variety of secretory proteins produced by many organs. The average daily intake of protein is approximately 80 g in the UK, with a recommended daily intake of 0.8 g/kg body weight, with nitrogen comprising approximately 16% of its weight. However, it is of some interest to note that more than 50% of the world's population exist on less.

Conventionally, amino acids have been classified as either 'essential' or 'non-essential'. The essential amino acids cannot be synthesised endogenously and are required in the diet, whereas the non-essential amino acids can be synthesised by the human body. Both groups of amino acids, however, are necessary for normal tissue growth and metabolism. Dietary intake and endogenous synthesis of amino acids in the body maintain the relevant pool of amino acids, replacing those that have been lost as a result of excretion in the urine, losses from the skin and gastrointestinal tract, utilisation as precursors for non-protein synthetic pathways, irreversible modification and irreducible oxidation.

It has become recognised that under certain circumstances (e.g. sepsis, trauma, growth) the endogenous synthesis of some of the amino acids normally considered to be 'non-essential' is inadequate for the body's nitrogen fluxes. Therefore, unless these amino acids are present in the diet abnormal tissue protein metabolism may occur. These amino acids are described as being 'conditionally essential'. It seems likely that only three amino acids are actually non-essential: L-alanine, L-glutamate and L-aspartate, which are produced by a simple transamination reaction.

Energy requirements

Energy transduction is accomplished by the breakdown of carbohydrate, fat and proteins. The energy available from various common nutrients is as follows:

- fat 9.3 kcal/g (38.9 kJ/g);
- glucose 4.1 kcal/g (17.1 kJ/g);
- protein 4.1 kcal/g (17.1 kJ/g);
- alcohol 7.1 kcal/g (29.7 kJ/g).

The principal carbohydrates in the diet are polysaccharides (starch and dietary fibre), dextrins and free sugars (monosaccharides), disaccharides, oligosaccharides and sugar alcohols. Dietary fat includes triacylglycerol, containing long-chain fatty acids (C_{16} to C_{18} triacylglycerols) and medium-chain fatty acids (C_6 to C_{12} triacylglycerols) and cholesterol.

If the energy intake of an individual is greater than energy expenditure, extra carbohydrate intake will be channelled into glycogen synthesis; when glycogen stores are replete, glucose is metabolised to fatty acids and fat synthesis occurs. Additional fat intake will be stored in adipose tissue as triacylglycerol. In contrast, if there is a negative energy balance, then fat, glycogen and protein will be broken down to provide the required energy.

The total daily energy expenditure (TEE) is composed of the following components.

- the resting metabolic expenditure or RME (defined as the energy required for cardiorespiratory function plus that required for synthesis and maintenance of electrochemical gradients across cell membranes);
- activity energy expenditure (depends on physical work);
- diet-induced energy expenditure.

Under normal circumstances, approximately 25–30 kcal/kg (105–125 kJ/g) are required every day and the changes in requirements in some common conditions are shown in **Box 17.2**.

Micronutrients

VITAMINS

Vitamins are organic compounds that are essential for normal growth and maintenance of body functions, playing key roles in many different metabolic processes in both health and disease. In general, vitamins are classified into those that are fat soluble (A, D, E and K) and those that are water soluble, i.e. C and the B vitamins (folic acid, B_{12}, B_1, B_2, B_3, pantothenic acid, biotin and B_6). Details of these

Box 17.2 • Additional energy requirements in disease states

Trauma: $0.3 \times$ RME
Elective surgery: $0.1 \times$ RME
Sepsis: up to $0.5 \times$ RME
Severe sepsis: up to $0.6 \times$ RME
Massive burns: $1 \times$ RME

Box 17.3 • Functions of some vitamins important in surgical practice

Vitamin A
Stabilises epithelial cell membranes; necessary for fibroblast differentiation and collagen secretion
Vitamin D
Role in calcium and phosphate regulation
Vitamin E
Immunostimulant and free radical scavenger
Vitamin K
Required for liver synthesis of clotting factors
Vitamin B_{12}
Important in synthesis of proteins and nucleic acids
Ascorbic acid
Important in hydroxylation (e.g. collagen synthesis) and energy transduction
Thiamine
Necessary for carbohydrate metabolism and ATP synthesis

can be found in standard texts but some examples and their importance in surgical practice are shown in **Box 17.3**.

The exact requirement for vitamins during trauma and sepsis is still unclear and may alter depending on the type of metabolic support provided.

TRACE ELEMENTS

Trace elements are inorganic elements that are also important in the regulation of many metabolic processes.[5] For example, zinc is necessary for wound healing, being a cofactor in enzymes for protein and nucleic acid synthesis. Others of importance in the patient undergoing surgery include iron (involved in energy transfer), copper (necessary for collagen synthesis) and selenium (important in synthesis of antioxidant enzyme systems, which protect against peroxidation). A detailed description of other trace elements, their requirements and structure can be found in standard texts.[9]

However, it should be remembered that micronutrients, if given at high doses, could be toxic to tissues and organs. In particular, toxicity can be a problem with excess vitamins A and D, iron, selenium, zinc and copper. Care must be taken when these micronutrients are provided for a prolonged period to patients.

IDENTIFICATION OF PATIENTS WHO ARE MALNOURISHED

It is important to determine the nutritional status in all patients undergoing surgery and identify those who are malnourished. However, a reliable and reproducible assessment of nutritional status has proved difficult and, as yet, there is no definitive test for 'malnutrition'. However, assessments that have been used previously in clinical practice can be considered as falling into several categories:

- anthropometric measures;
- biochemical assessments and body composition measurements;
- evaluation of body function (skeletal and respiratory muscle function, immune responses).

Anthropometric measures

HEIGHT AND WEIGHT

Height and weight are two of the most commonly used indices of nutritional status. A body weight value for a particular patient can be compared with a series of standard values in order to assess the degree of leanness or adiposity.[10] However, these tables take no account of frame size of the individual. Therefore, the body mass index (BMI), defined as weight divided by the square of the height, has been suggested to be the best anthropometric indicator of total body fat in adults.

Loss of body weight has been used as an indicator of nutritional status. This is usually determined by subtracting the current weight from the recall weight when the patient was 'well' or from the 'ideal' weight, which is obtained from published tables. Although a patient's recall weight can be inaccurate, the loss of more than 10% of body weight, or more than 4.5 kg of recall weight, is associated with a significant increase in postoperative mortality in patients undergoing surgery. Furthermore, the shorter the period of time over which weight is lost, the more significant this is in predicting an increased risk of postoperative complications. By combining weight loss and the rate of weight loss, it has been suggested that malnutrition can be defined as a BMI of less than the 10th percentile with a weight loss of 5% or more.[11]

SUBCUTANEOUS FAT THICKNESS

Clinically, the most commonly used index of total body fat is skinfold thickness, as approximately 50% of total body fat is in the subcutaneous layer (depending on age, sex and which particular fat pad is measured). Triceps skinfold thickness is most commonly measured but assessment of skinfolds at multiple sites is better and has good correlation with total body fat content. Regression equations for the estimation of total body fat from these measurements have been developed and can be used in clinical practice.[12] However, measurements of skinfold thickness are susceptible to intraobserver and interobserver variability, which limits their use clinically.

Biochemical measures

SERUM PROTEINS

Albumin is the major protein in serum and the relationship between serum protein concentration and protein-energy malnutrition was first recognised over 150 years ago.[13] Subsequently, studies have shown that low serum albumin levels are associated with an increased risk of complications in patients undergoing surgery.[14]

In experimental starvation, however, serum albumin levels may not fall for several weeks[15] because although synthesis decreases, only 30% of the total exchangeable albumin is in the intravascular space, with the remainder being in the extravascular compartment. In addition, albumin has a relatively long half-life of approximately 21 days. It has been suggested that the extravascular compartment replenishes the intravascular pool, which then only falls when this can no longer occur. In fact, it has been estimated that the flux of albumin between the intravascular and extravascular compartments is about ten times the rate of albumin synthesis.[16] However, previous studies have shown that a 30% loss of body weight with long periods of semi-starvation was associated with an increase in serum albumin concentration, thus confirming that albumin bears no relationship to nutritional status. Furthermore, serum albumin is lowered in malignancy, trauma and sepsis, despite an adequate intake, and hence it should not be used as an assessment of nutritional state.

Alternatives to using albumin as a marker of nutritional status by measuring other serum protein concentrations have been evaluated, including transferrin (half-life 7 days), retinol-binding protein (half-life 1–2 hours) and pre-albumin (half-life 2 days). The changes in their serum concentrations should therefore more accurately reflect acute changes in nutritional state than does albumin. The serum levels of these proteins are also altered in stress, sepsis and cancer.

NITROGEN BALANCE

Most of the nitrogen lost from the body is excreted in urine, mainly as urea (approximately 80% of total urinary nitrogen). Urea alone may be measured as an approximate indicator of losses, or total urinary nitrogen may be measured, although this latter technique is less widely available. In addition, there are also losses of nitrogen from the skin and in stool of approximately 2–4 g per day. One equation used for balance studies is:

$$\text{Nitrogen balance} = (\text{dietary protein} \times 0.16) - (\text{urea nitrogen (urine)} + 2\,\text{g stool} + 2\,\text{g skin})$$

(where urine urea nitrogen (g) = urine urea (mmol) × 28)

Although nitrogen balance has not been shown to be a prognostic indicator, it is still an important way of assessing a patient's nutritional requirements and of assessing the response to the provision of nutritional support.

Body composition

More complicated techniques for assessing the body's different compartments (e.g. fat, fat-free mass, total body nitrogen and total body mineral contents) have become available but these often require specialised equipment and may not be readily applicable to clinical practice. Relatively simple techniques, such as bioelectrical impedance, can be used in clinical practice.

BIOELECTRICAL IMPEDANCE

This entails the passage of an alternating electrical current between electrodes attached to the hand and foot. The current passes through the water and electrolyte compartment of lean tissues and the drop in voltage between the two electrodes is measured.[17] This change in voltage gives an estimation of total body resistance, which depends principally on total body water and electrolyte content (i.e. lean body mass). The passage of current through the intra-cellular fluid compartment is impeded by the non-conductive cell membrane. This gives rise to a 'phase-shift' and a decrease in current at low (<1 kHz) frequencies. At higher frequencies (>50 kHz), current will be less impeded. Although bioelectrical impedance is an accurate measure of body composition in stable subjects, it becomes less reliable in patients with oedema and electrolyte shifts, and its value in critically ill patients is unclear.[13]

Tests of function

IMMUNE COMPETENCE

In malnutrition there is a reduction in the total circulating lymphocyte count and impairment in a wide variety of immune functions, e.g. decreased skin reactivity to mumps, *Candida* and tuberculin (these should be antigens to which the individual has been previously exposed) and reduced lymphocyte responsiveness to mitogens in vitro.[18,19]

A correlation between depressed immune function and postoperative morbidity and mortality has been demonstrated, and depression of total circulating lymphocyte count is also associated with a poorer prognosis in patients undergoing surgery.[20] However, these alterations in immune function are non-specific and can be affected by trauma, surgery, anaesthetic and sedative drugs, pain and psychological stress (all important in the surgical patient[21]) and therefore are not generally applicable to clinical practice.

MUSCLE FUNCTION

Skeletal muscle

Various aspects of skeletal muscle structure and function are deranged in the presence of malnutrition. Skeletal muscle fibres become atrophic and there are impairments in muscle function. In patients undergoing surgery, measurements of handgrip strength (which are cheap and easy to perform) may predict those patients who develop postoperative complications (with a sensitivity >90%). However, grip strength may be influenced by other factors such as the patient's motivation and cooperation. Furthermore, such tests may be difficult to apply to patients who are critically ill. Alternatively, stimulation of the ulnar nerve at the wrist, with a variable electrical stimulus, results in contraction of the adductor pollicis muscle, the force of which reflects nutritional intake.[22]

Respiratory muscle

The function of the respiratory muscles is also impaired by malnutrition and this can be detected by deterioration in various indices of standard respiratory function tests, in particular vital capacity.[23] Measurements of inspiratory muscle strength have the advantage that they can be performed even in patients who are intubated and who are affected by intercurrent illnesses.

NUTRITION RISK INDEX

A nutrition risk index is an index of nutritional status, based on a combination of variables. Although several indices exist, one that is commonly used depends on serum albumin, current weight and the patient's usual weight. These variables are used to calculate the index as follows:

$$\text{Nutrition risk index} = 1.519 \times \text{serum albumin (g/L)} + 0.417 \times (\text{current weight/usual weight}) \times 100$$

The score obtained is used to categorise the patient's nutritional state: <83.5, 'severely' malnourished; 83.5–97.5, 'mildly' malnourished; 97.5–100,

'borderline' malnourished. However, such an index bears no relationship to the patient's nutritional status but is purely a prognostic index.

How should nutritional status be assessed in clinical practice?

The various techniques for assessing nutritional status have been outlined above. Although they can predict the risks of complications in some (but not all) patients, there is at present no reliable technique for assessing nutritional status. Hill and Windsor[24] have suggested useful indicators for the bedside assessment of nutritional status that are readily applicable to clinical practice, including estimation of protein and energy balance, assessment of body composition and, most importantly, evaluation of physiological function.

PROTEIN AND ENERGY BALANCE

Protein and energy balance can be assessed either by a dietician or by the clinician, who determines the frequency and size of meals eaten by the patient. This information is compared with the patient's rate of loss of body weight and BMI.

ASSESSMENT OF BODY COMPOSITION

Loss of body fat can be determined by observing the physical appearance of the patient (loss of body contours) and feeling the patient's skinfolds between finger and thumb. In particular, if the dermis can be felt on pinching the biceps and triceps skinfolds, then considerable weight loss has occurred.

The stores of protein in the body can be assessed by examining various muscle groups. Those to be examined include the temporalis, deltoid, supra-scapular, infrascapular, biceps and triceps and the interossei of the hands. When the tendons of the muscles are prominent and the bony protruberances of the scapula are obvious, greater than 30% of the total body protein stores have been lost.

ASSESSMENT OF PHYSIOLOGICAL FUNCTION

Assessments of function are made by observing the patient's activities. Grip strength can be determined by asking the patient to squeeze the clinician's index and middle fingers for at least 10 seconds, and respiratory function by asking the patient to blow hard on a strip of paper held approximately 10 cm from the patient's lips. The measurement of metabolic expenditure requires specialised equipment, but additional metabolic stresses on the patient can also be determined from clinical examination. Extra metabolic stresses will be occurring if trauma or surgery has taken place recently or if there is evidence of significant sepsis (elevated temperature and/or white blood cell counts, tachycardia, tachypnoea, positive blood cultures) or active inflammatory bowel disease. In addition, patients should be asked about their ability to heal wounds (scratches, etc), changes in exercise tolerance and their 'tiredness'.

NUTRITIONAL SUPPORT IN SURGICAL PRACTICE

Route of nutritional support

The route of administration of nutritional support may be through either the gastrointestinal tract (enteral) or the intravenous (parenteral) route. In general, the enteral route is the preferred method of nutrient delivery whenever possible and the parenteral route is used for patients with primary intestinal failure.

Enteral nutritional support

If there is an intact and functioning gastrointestinal tract, then enteral feeding is the route of choice. Enteral feeding is contraindicated in patients with intestinal obstruction, paralytic ileus, with vomiting and diarrhoea, with high-output intestinal fistulas or in the presence of major intra-abdominal sepsis.

Experimental studies in animals have shown that in the absence of the provision of nutrients into the intestinal lumen, changes occur in the intestinal mucosa. There is a loss of height of the villi, a reduction in cellular proliferation and the mucosa becomes atrophic.[25,26] In addition, stimulation of the intestinal tract by nutrients is important for the release of the many gut-related hormones, including those responsible for gut motility and stimulation of production of secretions, which are necessary for normal maintenance of the mucosa. The activities of the enzymes found in association with the mucosa are also reduced and the permeability of the mucosa to macromolecules is increased.[27]

The gut also acts as a barrier to bacteria, both physically and by the release of chemical and immunological substances. There is evidence from experimental studies to suggest that atrophy of the intestinal mucosa is associated with loss of intercellular adhesion and the opening of intercellular channels. This is believed to predispose to increased translocation of bacteria and endotoxin from the gut lumen into the portal venous and lymphatic systems.[28] Loss of gut integrity is therefore believed to account for a substantial proportion of septicaemic events in severely ill patients. However, whether this does occur and the extent to which it contributes to sepsis in patients is far from clear at the present time.

The gut also serves the function of altering its nutrient intake and transport and is not simply an organ of digestion and absorption. Glucose arriving at the enterocyte via the luminal surface is transported intact through the hepatic portal system to the liver. In contrast, glucose arriving via the mesenteric arterial supply is metabolised to lactate and transported as such to the liver. Similarly, glutamine arriving at the enterocyte via the luminal surface is used by this cell as an energy substrate. The same is not the case for the arterial supply of glutamine to the enterocyte.

ROUTES OF ACCESS FOR ENTERAL NUTRITIONAL SUPPORT

Nasoenteric tubes

Nasogastric feeding via fine-bore tubes (made of polyvinylchloride or polyurethane) may be used in patients who require nutritional support for a short period of time. There has been considerable debate as to whether positioning of the feeding tube beyond the pylorus into the duodenum will result in a reduction in the risks of regurgitation of gastric contents and pulmonary aspiration (which occurs up to 30% of patients). This is most likely to occur in those patients with impaired gastric motility. In the latter, the fine-bore tube can be manipulated through the pylorus into the duodenum, reducing the risk of gastric aspiration. Other complications associated with the use of nasoenteric tubes include pulmonary atelectasis, oesophageal necrosis and stricture formation, tracheo-oesophageal fistulas, sinusitis and post-cricoid ulceration.

Gastrostomy techniques

Gastrostomy has been performed for more than 100 years in clinical practice. A gastrostomy tube is placed into the stomach at the time of laparotomy, although percutaneous endoscopic or percutaneous fluoroscopic techniques are the preferred methods. Details of how these are performed can be found in standard texts and are not discussed further in this chapter.

The establishment and use of a gastrostomy do have certain disadvantages and a recognised morbidity. It is an invasive procedure and may be associated with infection of the skin at the puncture site, necrotising fasciitis or deeper-sited sepsis, damage to adjacent intra-abdominal viscera, leakage of gastric contents into the peritoneal cavity (resulting in peritonitis), haemorrhage from the stomach and persistent gastrocutaneous fistula following removal of the feeding tube. The overall mortality rate for a gastrostomy is approximately 1–2%, with major and minor complications occurring in up to 15% of patients. Mechanical complications associated with the tube itself include tube blockage, fracture and displacement. Also, complications such as 'dumping' and diarrhoea are more common when the tip of the tube lies in the duodenum or jejunum.[29]

Jejunostomy

A feeding jejunostomy is usually carried out at the time of laparotomy if it is envisaged that a patient will need nutritional support for a longer period. Details of the operative technique used to fashion a jejunostomy are to be found in standard texts. The advantages of a feeding jejunostomy compared with a gastrostomy are:

- less stomal leakage with a jejunostomy;
- gastric and pancreatic secretions are reduced because the stomach is bypassed;
- less nausea, vomiting or bloating;
- the risk of pulmonary aspiration is reduced.

NUTRIENT SOLUTIONS AVAILABLE FOR ENTERAL NUTRITION

A range of nutrient solutions are currently available for use in enteral nutritional support and examples can be found in specialised texts. However, there are four main categories of enteral diet.

Polymeric diets

Polymeric diets are 'nutritionally complete' diets and are provided to patients whose gastrointestinal function is good. They contain whole protein as the source of nitrogen, and energy is provided as complex carbohydrates and fat. They also contain vitamins, trace elements and electrolytes in the standard amounts.

Elemental diets

Elemental diets are required if the patient is unable to produce an adequate amount of digestive enzymes or has a reduced area for absorption (e.g. severe pancreatic insufficiency or short bowel syndrome). Elemental diets contain the nitrogen source as oligopeptides. It is recognised that free amino acids are not as easily absorbed as dipeptide and tripeptide mixtures. The energy source is provided as glucose polymers and as medium-chain triacylglycerols.

Special formulations

Special formulations have been developed for patients with particular diseases. Examples of such diets include (i) those which have increased concentrations of branched-chain amino acids and are low in aromatic amino acids for use in patients with hepatic encephalopathy; (ii) those with a higher fat but lower glucose energy content for use in patients who are artificially ventilated; and (iii) diets containing key nutrients that modulate the immune response (see later sections).

Modular diets

Modular diets are not commonly used but allow the provision of a diet rich in a particular nutrient for use in an individual patient. For example, the diet may be enriched in protein if the patient is hypoproteinaemic, or in sodium if hyponatraemic. These modular diets can be used to supplement other enteral regimens or oral intake if required.

ENTERAL NUTRITION DELIVERY AND COMPLICATIONS

Previously, it was accepted that when starting an enteral nutrition feeding regimen, patients should receive either a reduced rate of infusion or a lower strength formula for the first 2 or 3 days in an attempt to reduce gastrointestinal complications. However, recent studies have demonstrated that this is not required and that nutritional support can commence using full-strength feeds and at the desired rate. Recent studies have indicated that cyclical feeding (e.g. 16 hours feeding with a post-absorptive period of 8 hours) is optimal and more closely mimics the natural feeding cycle than do the other types of feeding regimens.[30]

The enteral nutrition is administered through either a volumetric pump or, if this is not available, by drip flow via gravity. In patients whose conscious level is impaired and in patients confined to bed, it is recommended that the head should be elevated by approximately 25° so as to reduce their risks of pulmonary aspiration. Some clinicians prefer patients to be sitting upright when receiving enteral nutrition. The stomach contents should be aspirated every 4 hours during feeding and if there is a residual volume of more than 100 mL, enteral nutrition should be temporarily discontinued.

The aspirate can be checked again after 2 hours, and when satisfactory volumes are aspirated (<100 mL) feeding can be instituted again. If more than 400 mL per 24 hours is aspirated from the stomach, then feeding should be discontinued. Gastric emptying may be improved by the administration of either cisapride or erythromycin, which may allow feeding to be continued.

Metabolic disturbances are less likely with enteral than parenteral feeding, although they do occur. The other complications of enteral nutrition are those associated with the route of access to the gastrointestinal tract (**Box 17.4**).

Parenteral nutritional support

Patients who require nutritional support but in whom enteral feeding is contraindicated will require the provision of parenteral nutrition. These include:

- patients with a non-functioning or inaccessible gastrointestinal tract;

Box 17.4 • Complications of enteral nutrition

Gastrointestinal
Diarrhoea, nausea, vomiting, abdominal discomfort and bloating, regurgitation and aspiration of feed/stomach contents
Mechanical
Dislodgement of the feeding tube, blockage of the tube, leakage of stomach/small intestine contents onto the skin with the use of jejunostomies or gastrostomies
Metabolic
Hyperkalaemia, hyperglycaemia, hyperphosphataemia, hypomagnesaemia, hypozincaemia, hypophosphataemia
Infective
Local effects (e.g. diarrhoea, vomiting) or systemic effects (e.g. pyrexia, malaise)

- those with high-output enteric fistulas (enteral nutrition may stimulate gastrointestinal secretion);
- those for whom it is not possible to provide sufficient intake of nutrients enterally (e.g. because of a short segment of residual bowel or malabsorption, severe burns, major trauma).

Detailed guidance for the administration of total parenteral nutrition (TPN) to hospitalised patients has been published by the ASPEN Board of Directors and can be referred to for more details.[31]

PARENTERAL ROUTES OF ACCESS

Central venous access

Central venous access is obtained by positioning a catheter into the superior vena cava through the subclavian or internal jugular vein. The catheter either emerges through the skin (usually after being tunnelled in the subcutaneous fat for a short distance) or is connected to a port placed in the subcutaneous fat of the anterior chest wall. A variety of techniques for insertion of central venous lines are currently used in clinical practice. For example, catheters may be introduced into the subclavian vein either directly by 'blind' percutaneous puncture or by 'cut-down' techniques that utilise the cephalic vein to gain access to the subclavian vein. Alternatively, radiologists can insert these lines under fluoroscopic control. Details of these techniques can be found in standard texts. The advantages and disadvantages of these techniques are well recognised and have been described in detail elsewhere.[32–34] However, it is important that the individual who inserts a central venous line is expert at this technique.

Technical aspects of feeding lines Central lines are commonly manufactured from either polyurethane or silicone. Both of these materials are tolerated well in the body and have low thrombogenic potential. However, polyurethane does have advantages:

- it is stiffer than silicone at room temperature but at body temperature it becomes very pliable;
- it has a higher tensile strength than silicone and is therefore less likely to fracture;
- polyurethane catheters have a smaller outside diameter thus making cannulation easier, as well as a greater resistance to the development of thrombus on their surfaces.

Some catheter manufacturers have also attempted to reduce the risks of bacterial colonisation of the line by bonding antiseptics (e.g. chlorhexidene) and antibiotics (e.g. silver sulphadiazine) into the fabric of the catheter. Some catheters also have an antimicrobial cuff, usually made of Dacron, around their external surface. This is believed to act as a barrier to microorganisms, which may otherwise migrate from the subcutaneous tissues along the external aspect of the catheter to its tip. Although some studies have suggested that the risks of septicaemia are reduced by using a cuff around the catheter, this does make positioning of the catheter more difficult technically. The complications of central venous catheters are shown in **Box 17.5**.

Catheter care Appropriate dressings of the catheter are essential. For example, the dressing should normally be changed weekly; the skin exit site should be cleaned weekly with chlorhexidene using a sterile technique. A variety of dressings have also been used at the skin exit site, but sterile gauze and a transparent adherent type of dressing (e.g. Tegaderm) are used most commonly.

Box 17.5 • Complications of central venous catheter placement and incidence of occurrence

Catheter-related sepsis: variable, but reported in up to 40% of catheters
Thrombosis of central vein: variable, but reported in up to 20% of catheters
Pleural space damage: pneumothorax (5–10%), haemothorax (2%)
Major arterial damage: subclavian artery (1–2%)
Catheter problems: thrombosis (1–2%), embolism (<1%), air embolism (<1%)
Miscellaneous problems: brachial plexus (<1%), thoracic duct damage (<1%)

Infection of the catheter tip is the most serious type of infection that can occur. The patient usually has a pyrexia and may have systemic signs of sepsis. This may be diagnosed by taking blood cultures (at least three cultures 1 hour apart) and catheter cultures.[35] Antibiotic therapy may result in eradication of the organism, but in some cases the feeding line may have to be removed to eradicate the infection. However, less serious infection may occur in the skin at the exit site of the catheter. This is recognised by erythema of the surrounding skin, possibly associated with fluid exudate and pus.

Peripheral venous access

Peripheral venous cannulation, using a sterile technique, may be used to supply nutrients intravenously and avoids the hazards and complications associated with insertion of central venous catheters. Peripheral intravenous nutrition is likely to be used in patients who do not require nutritional support for long enough to justify the risks and complications of central vein cannulation or in whom central vein cannulation is contraindicated (e.g. central line insertion sites are traumatised, there are increased risks of infective complications, if there is thrombosis of the central veins, or in the presence of significant clotting defects).

Problems associated with the delivery of intravenous nutrition using the peripheral route include the following.

- There is a limit to the amount of nutrients that can be delivered and peripheral feeding should not be provided if there is a high requirement for protein, energy or electrolytes.
- There is a high incidence of complications, particularly phlebitis (which occurs in up to 45% of patients), and it is essential to ensure that there is good peripheral venous access, otherwise repeated episodes of phlebitis necessitating frequent cannula changes will ensue.

The lifespan of a peripheral intravenous cannula can be prolonged by treating it as one would a central line with regard to asepsis, and also by using a narrow-gauge cannula, which gives better mixing and flow characteristics of the nutrient solution. The risks of phlebitis can also be reduced by using frequent changes of the infusion site, ultrafine-bore catheters, by adding heparin and a small dose of hydrocortisone to the infusion solution, or by using a vasodilator (e.g. transdermal glyceryl trinitrate). Furthermore, peripheral intravenous nutrition can only be used where fat emulsion is part of the single-phase administration of nutrients to avoid thrombophlebitis.

NUTRIENTS USED IN PARENTERAL FEEDING SOLUTIONS

Some commercially available nutrient solutions (and their properties) commonly used in the provision of parenteral nutrition are listed in **Table 17.1**. A more complete list can be found in the *British National Formulary*.

Nitrogen sources

The nitrogen sources used are solutions of crystalline L-amino acids that contain all the essential and a balanced mixture of the non-essential amino acids required for protein synthesis. However, amino acids that are relatively insoluble (e.g. L-glutamine, L-arginine, L-taurine, L-tyrosine, L-methionine) may be absent or present in inadequate amounts.

Attention has focused on the provision of L-glutamine because of its key roles in metabolism. It can be supplied as N-acetylglutamine (hydrolysed in the renal tubule to release free L-glutamine, which is then reabsorbed into the systemic circulation) or as L-glutamine dipeptides such as alanylglutamine (which are also broken down to release free L-glutamine).[36] An alternative approach has been to supplement parenteral nutrition solutions with

Table 17.1 • Nutrient solutions available for use in patients receiving parenteral nutrition

	Volume (mL)	Energy (kcal)	Nitrogen (g)	Glucose (g)	Fat (g)	Na$^+$ (mmol)	K$^+$ (mmol)	Ca^{2+} (mmol)	Mg^{2+} (mmol)	Cl$^-$ (mmol)
Vamin 9	1000	250	9.4			50	20	2.5	1.5	50
Vamin 14	1000	350	13.5			100	50	5	8	100
Vamin 9 Glucose	1000	650	9.4	150		50	20	2.5	1.5	50
Vamin 18 EF	1000	460	18							
Intralipid 10%	1000	1100			100					
Intralipid 20%	1000	2000			200					

EF, electrolyte free.

ornithine α-ketoglutarate. The results from studies evaluating these substances have been promising but further investigation is necessary to clarify their role before their routine introduction into parenteral nutrition solutions.

Energy sources

Energy is supplied as a balanced combination of dextrose and fat. Glucose is the primary carbohydrate source and the main form of energy supply to the majority of the body tissues. During critical illness the body's preferred calorie source is fat, both in the fasted state and during glucose feeding.[37,38] However, there are current controversies as to the utilisation of fat in sepsis because of known defects in energy substrate metabolism at the oxidative level.

Glucose utilisation may be impaired in certain patients and glucose is then metabolised through other metabolic pathways. This results in increased production of fatty acids (causing fatty infiltration of the liver, if excessive) and increased oxidation of fatty acids, resulting in an increased amount of carbon dioxide (which has to be excreted through the lungs). In addition, if glucose is the only energy source, then patients may develop an essential fatty acid (linolenic, linoleic) deficiency.

Fat (e.g. soyabean oil emulsions) is also given as an energy source. Usually, for most clinical circumstances, approximately 30–50% of the total calories are given as fat and the non-protein calorie to nitrogen ratio varies from 150:1 to 200:1 (this may be lower in hypercatabolic conditions). However, the provision of exogenous lipids has also been associated with certain problems. Intravenous fat emulsions have been shown to impair lung function, inhibit the reticuloendothelial system and modulate neutrophil function.[39,40]

Other nutrients

Commercially available preparations of trace elements (e.g. Addamel or Additrace) and water-soluble vitamins (e.g. Solivito) can be used to supply the daily requirements of these micronutrients. In addition, the total fluid volume and the amounts of electrolytes can be modified on a daily basis to meet the particular needs of any patient.

DELIVERY AND ADMINISTRATION OF TPN

In clinical practice, the commercially available solutions for parenteral infusion are mixed under sterile conditions in a laminar flow facility. The feeding regimen is made up in a 3-L bag (made of ethyl vinyl acetate) and comprises all nutrients and can be stored for up to 1 week prior to use, although compatibility between all the different constituents

must be ensured. Under current legislation, no additions of drugs can be made to these bags at any time. The advantages of the 3-L bags include:

- cost-effectiveness;
- reduced risks of infection;
- a more uniform administration of a balanced solution over a prolonged period;
- decreased lipid toxicity as a result of the greater dilution of the lipid emulsion and the longer duration of its infusion;
- ease of delivery and storage and reduced long-term accumulation of triacylgycerols (which can occur with glucose-based TPN).

More recently, prepared bags have become available where the fat emulsion is stored separately from the aqueous solution and is mixed by bag rupture immediately prior to administration. Such bags should be used for short-term support only as the overall nutrient composition may not be appropriate.

COMPLICATIONS OF PARENTERAL NUTRITIONAL SUPPORT

The instant availability of nutrients provided by the intravenous route can lead to metabolic complications if the composition or flow rate is inappropriate. Rapid infusion of high concentrations of glucose can precipitate hyperglycaemia, which may be further complicated by lactic acidosis. Electrolyte disturbances may present problems, not least because the intravenous feeding regimen is usually prescribed in advance for a 24-hour period. Prediction of the patient's nutrient requirements must be complemented by frequent monitoring, as described above. The provision of nutrients may lead to further electrolyte abnormalities when potassium, magnesium and phosphate enter the intracellular compartment. This is particularly noticeable in patients whose previous nutrient intake was especially poor. Others complications of TPN are shown in **Box 17.6**.

Monitoring patients receiving nutritional support

ENTERAL NUTRITION

Patients receiving nutritional support should be monitored by keeping an accurate recording of their fluid balance, and by daily weighing. The daily intake of calories and nitrogen should be documented. Biochemical assessments may include twice-weekly measurements of renal and liver function, and regular checks of phosphate, calcium, magnesium,

Box 17.6 • Metabolic complications of parenteral nutrition

Glucose disturbances

Hyperglycaemia: excessive administration of glucose, inadequate insulin, sepsis

Hypoglycaemia: rebound hypoglycaemia occurs if glucose is stopped abruptly but insulin levels remain high

Lipid disturbances

Hyperlipidaemia: excess administration of lipid, reduced metabolism (e.g. renal failure, liver failure)

Fatty acid deficiency: essential fatty acid deficiency leads to hair loss, dry skin, impaired wound healing

Nitrogen disturbances

Hyperammonaemia: occurs if deficiency of L-arginine, L-ornithine, L-aspartate or L-glutamate in infusion. Also occurs in liver diseases

Metabolic acidosis: caused by excessive amounts of chloride and monochloride amino acids

Electrolyte disturbances

Hyperkalaemia: excessive potassium administration or reduced losses

Hypokalaemia: inadequate potassium administration or excessive loss

Hypocalcaemia: inadequate calcium replacement, losses in pancreatitis, hypoalbuminaemia

Hypophosphataemia: inadequate phosphorus supplementation, also tissue compartment fluxes

Liver disturbances

Elevations in aspartate aminotransferase, alkaline phosphatase and gamma-glutamyl transferase may occur because of enzyme induction secondary to amino acid imbalances or deposition of fat and/or glycogen in liver

Ventilatory problems

If excessive amounts of glucose are given, the increased production of CO_2 may precipitate ventilatory failure in non-ventilated patients

albumin and protein levels and haematological indices, until the patient is stabilised. After stabilisation, weekly or fortnightly measurements only are necessary. Other methods of assessment may be used at regular intervals to ascertain patient progress (see nutritional assessment, p. 315). In addition, the routes of access should be regularly examined to ensure that the catheter is in the correct position and is mechanically satisfactory.

PARENTERAL NUTRITION

Patients receiving parenteral nutrition require careful monitoring, both clinically and by using laboratory indices. The patient's clinical condition should be evaluated daily (daily weighing, signs of fluid depletion or overload). Various biochemical indices should be monitored; serum electrolytes, urea, creatinine and glucose are checked daily, while serum albumin, protein, calcium, magnesium, phosphate and liver function are checked twice per week. Haematological indices (haemoglobin, white blood cell count, haematocrit) are checked twice weekly. The circulating glucose level should be monitored four times daily, initially in case the patient becomes hyperglycaemic.

Other assessments, for example muscle function, nitrogen balance, measurement of trace elements and vitamins, may also be performed if required. In addition, the catheter, its site of access and the equipment infusing the feeding solution must also be carefully examined for any possible complications or dysfunction.

Nutritional support teams

It has become clear that for the optimal provision of nutritional support, a multidisciplinary nutritional support team is required. This may comprise a clinician with a special interest in the provision of nutrition and understanding of metabolic pathways, a biochemist, pharmacist, dietician and nursing specialist. It has been demonstrated that the provision of nutritional support by such a team results in the most cost-effective use of nutritional support and is associated with the least risk of infective, metabolic and feeding line complications.[41]

NUTRITIONAL SUPPORT IN DEFINED CLINICAL SITUATIONS

Nutritional support in the perioperative period

There is still much debate as to which patients require preoperative and/or postoperative nutritional support. Although many studies have evaluated the effects of nutritional support in the perioperative period, clinical benefit with supplemental nutrition has not been a consistent finding. This may have been because these were often small studies, with many different end points (e.g. morbidity, mortality), frequently without proper randomisation or allowance and stratification for malnutrition prior to commencing the study.

However, given the limitations of many of these trials and in this era of evidence-based medicine, can meta-analyses answer some of the more important questions regarding nutritional support in the perioperative period? A meta-analysis that addressed many important questions examined 27 randomised controlled trials (more than 2907 patients) of nutritional support in the perioperative period.[42] The results of this analysis are important and provide us with some basis for the rational use of nutritional support in the perioperative period. The overall results and the key findings are detailed in **Table 17.2**.

When TPN was given in the preoperative period there was a reduction in complication rates (relative risk 0.52, 95% confidence interval 0.30–0.91) in malnourished patients but not in patients whose nutritional state was judged to be adequate. However, there was no difference in mortality in these patients. Analysis of studies of patients in the postoperative period indicated that there are no reductions in complications (relative risk 1.08, 95% confidence interval 0.81–1.43) or mortality in patients receiving TPN. In addition, subgroup analyses were also carried out which indicated that nutritional support in the preoperative period should be considered for:

- those with a serum albumin of less than 30–32 g/L;
- patients with a weight loss of 15% or more that is associated with impairment of physiological function;
- patients with a nutrition (prognostic) risk index of less than 83.5.

Nutritional support should be given for at least 7–10 days preoperatively if the reduction in post-operative morbidity is to be achieved. However, post-operative mortality is not affected.

Nutritional support in the postoperative period should be considered for:

- patients in whom it is anticipated that normal oral intake is unlikely for 7 days or more after surgery;
- those with severe sepsis or burns;
- those with enterocutaneous fistulas (particularly if high output);
- patients who have lost 15% or more of their usual weight prior to surgery being undertaken.

Nutritional support in patients with acute pancreatitis

Severe pancreatitis produces a major catabolic stress, with rapid loss of muscle proteins. The daily nitrogen requirements of such patients are higher than normal, reaching 1.2–2.0 g/kg of protein (0.2–0.3 g/kg of nitrogen). Daily energy require-ments also increase with disease severity and are

Table 17.2 • Effect of perioperative nutritional support on morbidity and mortality in surgical patients

	Complications (RR and 95% CI)	Mortality (RR and 95% CI)
Malnourished patients	0.53 (0.30–1.91)	1.13 (0.78–71)
Adequate nutrition	0.95 (0.75–1.21)	0.90 (0.66–1.2)
Preoperative TPN	0.70 (0.52–0.95)	0.85 (0.6–1.20)
Postoperative TPN	1.01 (0.70–1.96)	1.08 (0.73–1.58)
Overall effects	0.81 (0.65–1.01)	0.97 (0.76–1.24)

CI, confidence interval; RR, relative risk; TPN, total parenteral nutrition.
From Heyland DK, Montalvo M, MacDonald S, Keefe L, Sy XY, Drover JW. Total parenteral nutrition in the surgical patient: a meta-analysis. Can J Surg 2001; 44:102–11, with permission.

in the range of 28–35 kcal/kg. Previous recommen-dations suggested that patients with pancreatitis should be fasted in order to avoid stimulation of the pancreas. In severe and/or complicated cases of pancreatitis, patients were fed by the parenteral route.

Recent randomised controlled clinical trials have demonstrated that if patients with pancreatitis are fed by the oral route immediately, there is a reduction in the risk of developing major complications.[43,44]

These initial studies are promising but further well-designed clinical trials are needed to confirm these results.

Nutritional supplementation in inflammatory bowel disease

A significant number of patients with Crohn's disease and ulcerative colitis can become mal-nourished. The reasons for this include decreased nutrient intake, malabsorption by the small intestine (decreased length, bacterial overgrowth, protein-losing enteropathy) and possibly increased calorie and nitrogen requirements in those with coexistent sepsis. Furthermore, there may also be deficiencies of specific vitamins and trace elements in these patients.

Nutritional support in such patients may have two roles: (i) to provide the nutritional require-ments and correct any nutritional deficiencies that the patient may have; and (ii) the possibility that the provision of TPN with bowel rest in Crohn's disease may itself be therapeutically beneficial.

The results of studies that have addressed this latter point have been disappointing,[45,46] suggesting that parenteral nutrition itself does not have a therapeutic effect in patients with inflammatory bowel disease. Furthermore, there is evidence to show that enteral nutritional support is as effective as TPN in these patients.[47] This has the added benefits of maintaining the integrity of the gut mucosa and stimulating the production of gut hormones necessary for gut function.

Nutritional support in enterocutaneous fistulas

Nutritional support has an important role to play in the management of patients with enterocutaneous fistulas. It has been shown that up to 50% of patients with fistulas are malnourished. The importance of adequate nutritional support in these patients was demonstrated by Chapman et al.[48] They found that if patients with fistulas received nutritional support with TPN and enteral feeding [>3000 kcal (12.6 MJ) daily], then spontaneous fistula healing with a reduced mortality occurred compared with patients with fistulas who received less than 1000 kcal (4.1 MJ) daily. The management of patients with fistulas commences with correction of any fluid and electrolyte deficits and elimination of foci of sepsis. TPN is required to correct any nutritional deficits and to provide maintenance requirements when the patient is stabilised. However, if the fistula output is low, then enteral nutritional support should be considered because of the benefits outlined.

Nutritional support in patients with burns

Major burns induce severe hypermetabolic and hypercatabolic states. There is increased skeletal muscle breakdown, with nitrogen losses of 15 g daily or more, and up to a doubling of the metabolic rate. In patients with burns of greater than 20% of their body surface area, nutritional support is required, either orally or by nasoenteric feeding. If these routes are not possible, for example in the presence of gastric stasis, ileus or other coexistent injuries, then parenteral nutrition is required.

Several formulae exist for calculating the protein and calorie requirements of the individual patient (see Chiarelli et al.[49] for summary). However, up to 20–25 g of nitrogen per day may be required initially, with a non-protein calorie to nitrogen ratio of 100–200 being advocated. Energy is provided as carbohydrate and lipids, with the calorie requirement being 35–50% as lipid (minimising the problems associated with a high glucose load).

NUTRITIONAL SUPPLEMENTATION WITH KEY NUTRIENTS: APPLICATION TO CLINICAL PRACTICE

Certain nutrients can have marked effects on the function of normal cells and tissues, as well as on tissues involved in various pathological processes. Furthermore, some of these nutrients can also modulate immune and inflammatory responses if given in excess of normal intake or requirements. The use of nutrients in this way has been termed 'nutritional pharmacology'. Examples include the following.

- L-Arginine: stimulates various aspects of immune function, improves nitrogen retention after surgery and enhances wound healing.[50,51]
- L-Glutamine: stimulates immune function, reduces nitrogen loss postoperatively and may be important in maintaining gut-barrier function.[52]
- Branched-chain amino acids: may control protein synthesis in muscle and stimulate whole body protein synthesis, especially in severely traumatised patients.[53]
- Essential fatty acids: originally thought to stimulate the immune system but more recent evidence suggests that they may actually inhibit immune function.[54,55]
- Polyribonucleotides and ribonucleic acid: stimulate immune function.

The clinical benefits of supplementation with one of these key nutrients have been difficult to demonstrate but interest has focused on L-glutamine supplementation (e.g. 30 g daily) (**Table 17.3**).

In a recent analysis of randomised controlled clinical trials of patients who have undergone bone marrow transplantation, surgery for cancer, or trauma (11 trials of over 1000 patients), there was a suggestion that there may be reductions in infectious complications, hospital stay and mortality.[59]

However, further well-designed studies are required to confirm the place of L-glutamine in clinical practice.

Nutrient combinations in clinical practice

Several studies have evaluated the use of combinations of key nutrients in clinical practice in patients with a range of critical illnesses (trauma, surgery for

Table 17.3 • Glutamine supplementation in surgical practice

	Patients	Results
Morlion et al.[56]	28 patients undergoing colorectal resection received either glutamine-supplemented TPN or control TPN	Reduction in hospital stay in glutamine-supplemented TPN patients
Houdijk et al.[57]	72 patients with ISS 20 or more received either glutamine-supplemented diet or control diet	Reduction in pneumonia and sepsis in patients receiving glutamine supplementation
Griffiths et al.[58]	ITU patients with multiple organ failure received either glutamine supplementation or control diet	Reduced mortality rate 6 months later in patients receiving glutamine supplementation

TPN, total parenteral nutrition; ISS, International Society of Surgery index; ITU, intensive therapy unit.

malignant disease, burns), but particularly in patients with upper gastrointestinal cancer. A combination of L-arginine, *n*-3 essential fatty acids and ribonucleic acid is commercially available (Impact; Sandoz Nutrition, Minneapolis, MN, USA) and has been used in many of these clinical trials.

The supplemented nutrition has been given in the postoperative period (by nasoenteric tube or feeding jejunostomy), starting within 12–48 hours of the critical events and continued for several days.

A recent meta-analysis of the studies that have compared supplemented nutritional versus standard nutritional diets (**Figs 17.2** and **17.3**) has shown that supplemented nutrition does have clinical benefits:[60]

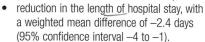

- reduction in infectious complications (wound infections, intra-abdominal abscesses, septicaemia), with an odds ratio of 0.47 (95% confidence interval 0.32–0.70);
- reduction in the length of hospital stay, with a weighted mean difference of −2.4 days (95% confidence interval −4 to −1).

However, there was no significant difference in mortality between the patients receiving either diet. A subsequent meta-analysis of 17 trials has confirmed this clinical benefit.[61]

While this is very encouraging, further studies are evaluating more precisely the role of nutritional supplementation with key nutrients in clinical practice.

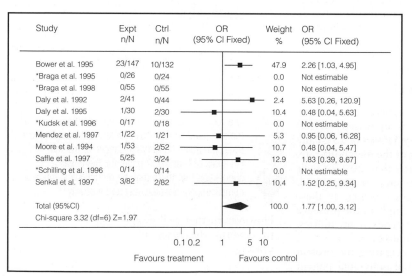

Study	Expt n/N	Ctrl n/N	OR (95% CI Fixed)	Weight %	OR (95% CI Fixed)
Bower et al. 1995	23/147	10/132		47.9	2.26 [1.03, 4.95]
*Braga et al. 1995	0/26	0/24		0.0	Not estimable
*Braga et al. 1998	0/55	0/55		0.0	Not estimable
Daly et al. 1992	2/41	0/44		2.4	5.63 [0.26, 120.9]
Daly et al. 1995	1/30	2/30		10.4	0.48 [0.04, 5.63]
*Kudsk et al. 1996	0/17	0/18		0.0	Not estimable
Mendez et al. 1997	1/22	1/21		5.3	0.95 [0.06, 16.28]
Moore et al. 1994	1/53	2/52		10.7	0.48 [0.04, 5.47]
Saffle et al. 1997	5/25	3/24		12.9	1.83 [0.39, 8.67]
*Schilling et al. 1996	0/14	0/14		0.0	Not estimable
Senkal et al. 1997	3/82	2/82		10.4	1.52 [0.25, 9.34]
Total (95%CI)				100.0	1.77 [1.00, 3.12]
Chi-square 3.32 (df=6) Z=1.97					

0.1 0.2   1   5 10

Favours treatment   Favours control

Figure 17.2 • Effect of immuno-enhancing diets on the incidence of major infective complications (wound infections, intra-abdominal abscesses, pneumonia, septicaemia). Expt, patients receiving immuno-enhancing diets; Ctrl, patients receiving standard nutrition; n, number of events; N, number of patients in each group on an intention-to-treat basis; OR, odds ratio; CI, confidence interval. (Study sources are given in Heys et al.[60]) With permission from Heys SD, Walker LG, Smith IC, Eremin O. Enteral nutritional supplementation with key nutrients in patients with critical illness and cancer. A meta-analysis of randomised controlled clinical trials. Ann Surg 1999; 229:467–77.

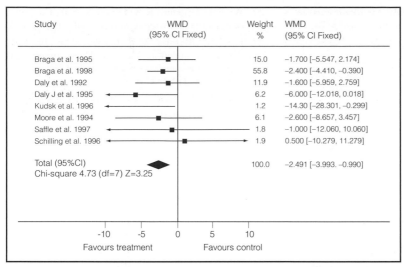

Figure 17.3 • Effect of immuno-enhancing diets on the length of hospital stay. WMD, weighted mean difference; CI, confidence interval. (Study sources are given in Heys et al.[60]) With permission from Heys SD, Walker LG, Smith IC, Eremin O. Enteral nutritional supplementation with key nutrients in patients with critical illness and cancer. A meta-analysis of randomised controlled clinical trials. Ann Surg 1999; 229:467–77.

Key points

- Malnutrition is associated with loss of body weight and impairments in organ function.
- The metabolic changes that occur in patients undergoing surgery or in those who have experienced trauma and sepsis can be compounded by inadequate nutritional support.
- Nutritional requirements must take into consideration the underlying pathophysiological changes.
- An assessment of nutritional status should be made in all patients.
- If nutritional support is considered necessary, the route and composition of this support should be considered carefully.
- The role of certain key nutrients and their effects, either individually or in combination, on aspects of organ and immune function should be taken into consideration when planning nutritional interventions.
- Careful monitoring of patients receiving nutritional support and the role of the multi-disciplinary team is essential for all patients.

REFERENCES

1. Cuthbertson DP. Observations on the disturbances of metabolism produced by injury to the limbs. Q J Med 1932; 1:233–46.

2. O'Keefe SJD, Sender PM, James WPT. Catabolic loss of body nitrogen in response to surgery. Lancet 1974; ii:1035–8.

3. Bergstrom J, Furst P, Noree L-O et al. Intracellular free amino acid concentration in human muscle tissue. J Appl Physiol 1973; 36:693–8.

4. Stoner HB. Studies on the mechanism of shock. The quantitative aspects of glycogen metabolism after limb ischaemia in the rat. Br J Exp Pathol 1958; 39:635–51.

5. Allsop JR, Wolfe RR, Burke JF. Glucose kinetics and responsiveness to insulin in the rat injured by burn. Surg Gynecol Obstet 1978; 147:565–73.

6. Nordenstrom J, Carpentier YA, Askanazi J et al. Free fatty acid mobilisation and oxidation during total parenteral nutrition in trauma and infection. Ann Surg 1983; 198:725–35.

7. Broom J. Sepsis and trauma. In: Garrow JS, James WPT (eds) Human nutrition and dietetics, 9th edn. Edinburgh: Churchill Livingstone, 1993; pp. 456–64.

8. Rich AJ, Wright PD. Ketosis and nitrogen excretion in undernourished surgical patients. J Parenteral Enteral Nutr 1979; 3:350–4.

9. Demling RH, DeBiasse MA. Micronutrients in critical illness. Crit Care Clin 1995; 11:651–73.

10. Metropolitan Life Assurance Company. Statistical Bulletin 1959; 40:1.

11. Pettigrew RA. Assessment of malnourished patients. In: Burns HG (ed.) Clinical gastroenterology. London: Baillière Tindall, 1988; pp. 729–49.

12. Durnin JVGA, Womersley J. Body-fat assessed from total body density and its estimation from skin-fold thickness: measurements on 481 men and women aged from 16 to 72 years. Br J Nutr 1987; 32:77–97.

13. Kushner RE, Kunigk A, Alspaugh M et al. Validation of bioelectrical-impedance analysis as a measurement of change in body composition in obesity. Am J Clin Nutr 1990; 52:219–23.

14. Ryan JA, Taft DA. Preoperative nutritional assessment does not predict morbidity and mortality in abdominal operations. Surg Forum 1980; 31:96–8.

15. Rothschild MA, Oratz M, Schreiber SS. Albumin metabolism. Gastroenterology 1973; 64:324–37.

16. Fleck A, Raines G, Hawker F et al. Increased vascular permeability: a major cause of hypoalbuminaemia in disease and injury. Lancet 1985; i:781–4.

17. Lukaski HC. Methods for the assessment of human body composition. Am J Clin Nutr 1987; 46:537–56.

18. Eremin O, Broom J. Nutrition and the immune response. In: Eremin O, Sewell HF (eds) The immunological basis of surgical science and practice. Oxford: Oxford University Press, 1992; pp. 133–44.

19. Bistrian BR, Blackburn GL, Scrimshaw NJ et al. Cellular immunity in semistarved hospitalized adults. Am J Clin Nutr 1975; 28:1148–55.

20. Seltzer MH, Bastidas JA, Cooper DM et al. Instant nutritional assessment. J Parenteral Enteral Nutr 1979; 3:157–9.

21. Heys SD, Khan AL, Eremin O. Immune suppression in surgery. Postgrad Surg 1995; 5:62–7.

22. Lopes J, Russke DM, Whitwell J et al. Skeletal muscle function in malnutrition. Am J Clin Nutr 1982; 36:602–10.

23. Daley BJ, Bistrian BR. Nutritional assessment. In: Zaloga GP (ed.) Nutrition in critical care. St Louis: Mosby Year Book, 1994; p. 28.

24. Hill G, Windsor JA. Nutritional assessment in clinical practice. Nutrition 1995; 11(suppl.):198–201.

25. Johnson LR, Copeland EM, Dudrick SJ et al. Structural and hormonal alterations in the gastro-intestinal tract of parenterally fed rats. Gastroenterology 1975; 68:1177–83.

26. Levine GM, Deren JJ, Steiger E et al. Role of oral intake in maintenance of gut mass and disaccharide activity. Gastroenterology 1974; 67:975–82.

27. Wilmore D, Smith R, O'Dwyer S et al. The gut: a central organ after sepsis. Surgery 1988; 104:917–23.

28. Fong Y, Marano MA, Barber A et al. Total parenteral nutrition and bowel rest modify the metabolic response to endotoxin in humans. Ann Surg 1989; 210:449–56.

29. Grimble GK, Payne-James JJ, Rees RGP, Silk DBA. Nutrition support. London: Medical Tribune UK, 1989; pp. 32–51.

30. Gayle D, Pinchcofsky-Devlin RD, Kaminski MV. Visceral protein increase associated with inter-rupted versus continuous enteral hyperalimentation. J Parenteral Enteral Nutr 1985; 9:474–6.

31. ASPEN Board of Directors. Guidelines for the use of total parenteral nutrition in the hospitalised adult patient. J Parenteral Enteral Nutr 1987; 10:441–5.

32. Adam A. Insertion of long term central venous catheters: time for a new look. Br Med J 1995; 311:341–2.

33. Robertson LJ, Mauro MA, Jaques PF. Radiologic placement of Hickman catheters. Radiology 1989; 170:1007.

34. Lameris JS, Post PJM, Zonderland HM, Gerritsen PG, Kappers-Klunne MC, Schutte HE. Percutaneous placement of Hickman catheters: comparison of sonographically guided and blinded techniques. Am J Roentgenol 1990; 155:1097–9.

35. Maki DG, Ringer M. Evaluation of dressing regimens for prevention of infection with peripheral intravenous catheters. JAMA 1987; 258:2396–403.

36. Furst P, Albers D, Stehle P. Stress-induced intra-cellular glutamine depletion. The potential use of glutamine containing peptides in parenteral nutrition. In: Adibi SA, Fekl W, Oehmke M (eds) Dipeptides as new substrates in nutrition therapy. Munich: Karger, 1987; pp. 117–36.

37. Levinson MR, Groeger JS, Jeevanandam M et al. Free fatty acid turnover and lipolysis in septic mechanically ventilated cancer-bearing humans. Metabolism 1988; 37:618–25.

38. Shaw JHF, Woolfe RR. Energy and protein metabolism in sepsis and trauma. Aust NZ J Surg 1987; 57:41–7.

39. Venus B, Patel CB, Mathru M et al. Pulmonary effects of lipid infusion in patients with acute respiratory failure (abstract). Crit Care Med 1984; 12:293.

40. Seidner DL, Mascioli EA, Istfan NW et al. Effects of long chain triacylglycerol emulsions on reticulo-endothelial system function in humans. J Parenteral Enteral Nutr 1989; 13:614–19.

41. Meguid MM, Campos ACL. Peri-operative feeding. In: Heatley RV, Green JH, Losowsky MS (eds) Consensus in clinical nutrition. Cambridge, UK: Cambridge University Press, 1994; p. 286.

42. Heyland DK, Montalvo M, MacDonald S, Keefe L, Sy XY, Drover JW. Total parenteral nutrition in the surgical patient: a meta-analysis. Can J Surg 2001; 44:102–11.

   A meta-analysis of randomised controlled trials of parenteral nutritional support which attempts to draw together the evidence as to which patients benefit from TPN.

43. Croad NR. The management of acute severe pancreatitis. Br J Intensive Care 1999; 2:38–45.

44. Kanwar A, Windsor ACJ, Li A et al. Benefits of early enteral nutrition in acute pancreatitis. Br J Surg 1997; 84:875.

45. Dickinson RJ, Ashton MG, Axon ATR, Smith RC, Yeung CK, Hill GL. Controlled trial of intravenous hyperalimentation as an adjunct to the routine therapy of acute colitis. Gastroenterology 1980; 79:1199–204.

46. Muller JM, Keller HW, Erasmi H, Pichlmaier H. Total parenteral nutrition as sole therapy in Crohn's disease: a prospective study. Br J Surg 1983; 70:40–3.

47. Jones VA. Comparison of total parenteral nutrition and enteral diet in induction of remission in Crohn's disease: long term maintenance of remission by personalised food exclusion. Dig Dis Sci 1987; 32(Suppl.):1005–75.

48. Chapman R, Foran R, Dunphey JE. Management of intestinal fistulas. Am J Surg 1964; 108:157–64.

49. Chiarelli A, Siliprandi L. Burns. In: Zagola GP (ed.) Nutrition in critical care. St Louis: Mosby Year Book, 1994; pp. 587–97.

50. Brittenden J, Park KGM, Heys SD et al. L-Arginine stimulates host defences in patients with breast cancer. Surgery 1994; 115:205–12.

51. Brittenden J, Heys SD, Ross JA, Park KGM, Eremin O. Nutritional pharmacology: effects of L-arginine on host defences, responses to trauma and tumour growth. Clin Sci 1994; 86:123–32.

52. Heys SD, Park KGM, Garlick PJ, Eremin O. Nutrition and malignancy: implications for surgical practice. Br J Surg 1992; 79:614–23.

53. Heys SD, Gough DB, Kahn AL, Eremin O. Nutritional pharmacology and malignant disease: a therapeutic modality in patients with cancer? Br J Surg 1996; 83:608–19.

54. Purasiri P, Murray A, Richardson S, Heys SD, Horrobin D, Eremin O. Modulation of cytokine production in vivo by dietary essential fatty acids in patients with colorectal cancer. Clin Sci 1994; 87:711–17.

55. Purasiri P, McKechnie A, Heys SD, Eremin O. Modulation in vitro of human natural cytotoxicity, lymphocyte proliferative response to mitogens and cytokine production by essential fatty acids. Immunology 1997; 92:166–72.

56. Morlion BJ, Stehle P, Wachtler P et al. Total parenteral nutrition with glutamine dipeptide after major abdominal surgery. Ann Surg 1998; 227:302–8.

57. Houdijk AP, Rijnsburger ER, Jansen J et al. Randomised trial of glutamine-enriched enteral nutrition on infectious morbidity in patients with multiple trauma. Lancet 1998; 352:772–6.

58. Griffiths R, Jones C, Palmer TE. Six-month outcome of critically ill patients given glutamine supplemented nutrition. Nutrition 1997; 13:295–302.

59. Heys SD, Ashkanani F. Glutamine. Br J Surg 1999; 86:289–90.

60. Heys SD, Walker LG, Smith IC, Eremin O. Enteral nutritional supplementation with key nutrients in patients with critical illness and cancer. A meta-analysis of randomised controlled clinical trials. Ann Surg 1999; 229:467–77.

   This is the first meta-analysis which indicated that immunonutrition could result in clinically important benefits for patients in terms of reduction in infectious complications postoperatively.

61. Heyland DK, Novak F, Drover JW, Jain M, Su X, Suchner U. Should immunonutrition become routine in critically ill patients? JAMA 2001; 286:944–53.

   This is an updated meta-analysis of randomised controlled trials that confirms the previous meta-analysis and extends it further by examining different subgroups of patients in an attempt to try to understand further which patients are the most likely to benefit from immunonutrition.

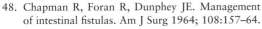

Eighteen

Sepsis and intensive care management

Nick Everitt and
Brian J. Rowlands

INTRODUCTION

Morbidity increases with the complexity of surgical treatment and many of today's patients are elderly with multiple chronic health problems. The modern surgeon should be able to recognise not only the consequences of disease but also of their own actions and manage them appropriately.

Severe sepsis has become increasingly common in recent decades with little change in mortality.[1] In the UK, the incidence of sepsis among hospital admissions has steadily risen from 1.8% in 1985 to 8.0% in 1996.[2] Sepsis is reported to account for 9% of all deaths in the USA, an incidence of 3 per 1000 people, with a mortality from sepsis of 28.6%.[3] Sepsis is a significant problem; its presence substantially increases mortality in patients admitted to the intensive care unit (ICU).[4]

In the first part of this chapter, the definitions and pathophysiology of sepsis and related conditions are outlined and the management of septic patients discussed. In the second part, the management of specific problems encountered in the critically ill is considered, with particular reference to the importance of tissue oxygenation.

THE SYSTEMIC INFLAMMATORY RESPONSE, SEPSIS AND THEIR SEQUELAE

The term 'sepsis' derives from the Greek *sépein*, meaning putrefaction.[5] It has been used as a synonym for infection and, more recently, the term 'septic' has been used to describe the physiological response elaborated by patients harbouring Gram-negative infections. In the 1970s, it was recognised that when death followed severe infection it was preceded by progressive deterioration of organ function.[6] However, not all patients who displayed these signs had an identifiable focus of infection,[7] yet all were at risk of multiple organ failure and death; furthermore, specific treatment of an infective focus did not guarantee recovery.[8] In 1991, consensus definitions relating to the inflammatory response were produced (**Box 18.1**).[9] These criteria form the basis of the following discussion.

Systemic inflammatory response syndrome

The systemic inflammatory response syndrome (SIRS) is a common initial non-specific response (**Box 18.1**) to a variety of insults (**Box 18.2**) and it is evident that almost all critically ill patients will exhibit SIRS. Approximately 70% of patients referred for tertiary care in the USA have SIRS and 30% develop sepsis.[10] Sepsis is defined as SIRS in the presence of a focus of infection. Septic shock is a subset of severe sepsis and, for the purpose of the definition in **Box 18.1**, hypoperfusion includes acidosis, oliguria and acute alteration of mental state.

The onset of SIRS does not accurately predict development of sepsis[11] or the multiple organ dysfunction syndrome (MODS),[12] yet the progression from SIRS to severe sepsis is associated with increasing risk of organ failure.[10] Therefore, timely

Box 18.1 • Definitions of the systemic inflammatory response syndrome (SIRS) and its sequelae

SIRS

The diagnosis of SIRS requires the presence of two or more of:

- temperature >38°C or <36°C
- pulse >90 beats/min
- respiratory rate >20/min or P_aCO_2 <4.3 kPa
- white cell count >12 × 10^9/L (>12 000/mL) or <4 × 10^9/L (<4000/mL) or >10% immature cell forms

Infection

An inflammatory response to microorganisms or their invasion of normal sterile host tissue

Sepsis

SIRS + confirmed infective process

Severe sepsis

SIRS + organ dysfunction, hypoperfusion or hypotension

Septic shock

Sepsis with hypotension and hypoperfusion despite adequate fluid resuscitation

Multiple organ dysfunction syndrome (MODS)

Alteration of organ function in acute illness such that homeostasis cannot be maintained without intervention

---

Box 18.2 • Precipitants of the systemic inflammatory response syndrome

Infection

Endotoxin

Hypovolaemia including haemorrhage

Ischaemia

Reperfusion injury

Major trauma

Pancreatitis

Inflammatory bowel disease

---

recognition of SIRS alerts the clinician to a potentially deteriorating situation at a time when prompt intervention may yet avert catastrophe. Development of shock increases the mortality attributable to SIRS from less than 10% to greater than 50%,[9] and approximately 30% of septic patients develop at least one organ dysfunction.[13] The mortality

from MODS ranges between 20 and 80% and, in general, increases with the number of organ systems affected[14] and with the severity of physiological disturbance at onset.[15] The respiratory system often deteriorates first, but the organs involved and the sequence of their dysfunction are also determined by the site of the original insult and the underlying comorbidity.

PATHOGENESIS: 'MEDIATOR DISEASE'

The development of SIRS involves activation of host humoral and cellular components (**Box 18.3**). These mediators are subject to amplification cascades and control mechanisms. They down-regulate their own release, stimulate antagonist release and

---

Box 18.3 • Factors implicated in the pathogenesis of inflammation

Cells

Macrophages

Neutrophils

Vascular endothelial cells

Platelets

Endogenous mediators

Cytokines: interleukin (IL)-1, IL-2 and IL-6; tumour necrosis factor (TNF)-α, interferon-α

Eicosanoids: thromboxanes, prostaglandins, leukotrienes

Complement products: C3a, C5a, C567 complex

Chemokines

Coagulation factors: factors VIIa and XIIa, von Willebrand factor

Fibrinolytic factors: tissue plasminogen activator, plasminogen

Platelet-activating factor

Reactive oxygen species: superoxide and hydroxyl radicals, hypochlorous acid, hydrogen peroxide

Cellular adhesion molecules: endothelial leucocyte adhesion molecule 1, intercellular adhesion molecule 1

Growth factors: granulocyte and granulocyte–macrophage colony-stimulating factors

Endothelial vasoactive compounds: nitric oxide, endothelins

Endogenous anti-inflammatory mediators

Cytokines: IL-4, IL-10, IL-11 and IL-14

Growth factors: TNF-β, colony-stimulating factors

Receptor antagonists: soluble receptor for TNF-α, IL-1 receptor antibody

inhibit their own function depending on local concentrations and interactions. It must be assumed that the inflammatory response is designed to protect the individual from injury. When specific components are congenitally absent, repeated infection is a constant threat to life.[16,17] However, uncontrolled proinflammatory mediator activity is harmful and the well-being of the individual in health and disease depends on the responsiveness and intrinsic modulation of the inflammatory response.[18]

The macrophage is the pivotal cell in the development of inflammation. It releases priming mediators, principally tumour necrosis factor (TNF)-α and interleukin (IL)-1 and IL-6, which initiate other mediator cascades and activate neutrophils, vascular endothelial cells and platelets.

Activation of vascular endothelial cells is associated with expression of leucocyte adhesion molecules. Endothelial cells themselves produce various inflammatory mediators that include cytokines and nitric oxide. Vasodilatation occurs and microvascular permeability increases as a consequence of endothelial activation,[19] leading to the formation of an inflammatory exudate. The endothelium changes from being antithrombotic to prothrombotic: tissue factor and plasminogen inhibitor are released. The microvascular coagulation that occurs probably serves to localise the process and its cause. In addition to its thrombogenic properties, thrombin has an intrinsic proinflammatory action that amplifies the systemic response.

Endothelial cells are also activated directly by local hypoxia or ischaemia–reperfusion injury. Release of chemotactic mediators attracts neutrophils that adhere to and subsequently penetrate the endothelium to enter the interstitium. Both neutrophils and macrophages participate in destruction and phagocytosis of infecting organisms. As the precipitating cause is cleared, counter-regulatory mechanisms take control. Macrophages coordinate tissue repair, by facilitating fibrosis and angiogenesis, and remove apoptotic neutrophils by ingesting them.

Pyrexia is common and neuroendocrine activation increases heart rate and stroke volume. Tissue oxygen consumption escalates and, unless oxygen delivery keeps pace, anaerobic metabolism follows. These physiological events are seen in sick patients and in healthy volunteers receiving experimental infusions of the initiators of sepsis.[20–22]

The development of SIRS is triphasic.[18] Initially, the precipitant causes local proinflammatory mediator activation only. In the second stage, mediators 'spill over' from the site of injury into the general circulation and promote hepatic synthesis of acute-phase proteins. Counter-inflammatory mechanisms[23] contain the response. In the third stage, control mechanisms fail and a vicious cycle of uncontrolled proinflammatory mediator amplification emerges. Deleterious physiological consequences develop, including loss of myocardial contractility and systemic vascular resistance (SVR), and the interstitial accumulation of fluid and protein ('third space loss'). Hypotension may follow, with tissue hypoperfusion and hypoxia leading to subsequent organ dysfunction. The 'two-hit' hypothesis suggests that successive insults are required for SIRS to progress to MODS.[24] The first challenge primes the inflammatory response, then the second tips the balance towards overwhelming proinflammatory activation and organ damage. Studies confirm that a minimal stimulus is required to activate inflammatory cells previously primed by a larger dose of the same mediator.[25]

METABOLIC CHANGES

The development of SIRS is associated with hypermetabolism.[26] Catabolism is accelerated and resting energy expenditure and oxygen consumption increase. The respiratory quotient increases, indicating mixed fuel oxidation, and the majority of energy is derived from amino acids and fat, with a consequent rapid reduction in lean body mass. Much of the increased energy expenditure occurs through futile cycling of metabolic intermediaries. These changes are not suppressed by feeding until the underlying cause has resolved. Sepsis is associated with insulin resistance that, together with increases in catecholamines, growth hormone and cortisol, leads to hyperglycaemia. The metabolic consequences of sepsis are covered in greater detail in Chapter 17.

Biochemical indicators

Hypoalbuminaemia is common in sepsis but does not indicate impaired nutritional status.[27] Albumin concentration is influenced not only by the total body protein pool but also, and more importantly, by plasma volume and capillary permeability. Therefore, hypoalbuminaemia is most likely to represent plasma dilution and capillary leakage. It is an indicator of adverse outcome[28] and it is possible that hypoalbuminaemia and malnutrition may coexist. Nutritional support may be indicated for other reasons, but normal plasma albumin levels are unlikely to return while sepsis remains unresolved. Cytokine activation is associated with an acute-phase response,[29] and measurement of plasma albumin and C-reactive protein may provide valuable information with regard to the progress of the septic patient.

THERAPEUTIC MODULATION OF THE METABOLIC RESPONSE TO SEPSIS

Hyperglycaemia predisposes to sepsis, myopathy and neuropathy, each of which may impede recovery.

A recent study investigated the benefits of rigorous glycaemic control in adult ventilated patients.[30] They were randomised to intensive insulin therapy, which controlled blood glucose between 4.4 and 6.1 mmol/L, or to receive insulin only when blood glucose exceeded 11.9 mmol/L with the aim of maintaining it between 10 and 11.1 mmol/L. Intensive insulin therapy was associated with significantly reduced mortality in patients who remained on intensive care for more than 5 days. The greatest effect applied to deaths due to multiple organ failure with sepsis. Intensive insulin therapy was also associated with less prolonged ventilation, shorter intensive care stay and reduced haemofiltration requirements.

Multiple organ dysfunction syndrome

The term 'multiple organ dysfunction syndrome' is preferred to 'multiple organ failure' because it recognises that organ dysfunction is progressive rather than an 'all or none' phenomenon. It acknowledges the potentially reversible situation in which an organ that functions normally in health can no longer maintain homeostasis under the challenge of major illness. It follows that comorbid disease predisposes to MODS (**Box 18.4**). The manifestations of organ dysfunction in critical illness are described in **Box 18.5**. Specific conditions, such as acute respiratory distress syndrome (ARDS),[26,31] have accepted definitions but there is no consensus definition of

Box 18.4 • Comorbid conditions that may predispose to development of the systemic inflammatory response and its sequelae

Extremes of age
Malnutrition
Underlying malignancy
Intercurrent disease
Hepatic impairment or jaundice
Renal impairment
Respiratory impairment
Diabetes mellitus
Immunosuppressive conditions
Post splenectomy
Organ transplant recipient
HIV infection
Primary immunodeficiency disease
Immunosuppressive therapy
Corticosteroids and azothioprine
Cytotoxic chemotherapy
Radiotherapy

Box 18.5 • Clinical manifestations of multiple organ dysfunction

Pulmonary
Hypoxia
Hypercapnia
Acid–base disturbance
Cardiovascular hypotension
Dysrhythmia
Fluid overload
Metabolic acidosis
Renal
Loss of renal concentrating power
Oliguria
Fluid overload
Electrolyte and acid–base disturbance
Hepatic
Jaundice
Coagulopathy
Hypoglycaemia
Metabolic acidosis
Encephalopathy
Gastrointestinal
Ileus
Pancreatitis
Cholecystitis
Gastrointestinal haemorrhage
Malabsorption
Metabolic
Hyperglycaemia
Haematological
Coagulopathy
Anaemia
Leucopenia
Neurological
Altered level of consciousness
Convulsions
Neuropathy
Myopathy

dysfunction of various organ systems, although several have been proposed.[24] Primary MODS is a direct consequence of a specific insult that causes early dysfunction of the organs involved. Secondary MODS occurs when organ dysfunction is a consequence of the host response itself. Typically, in secondary MODS, organ dysfunction develops some time after the initial insult and SIRS is more pronounced.

MANAGEMENT OF THE PATIENT WITH SEPSIS

Although effective management of patients with severe sepsis may entail complex investigations and procedures, the results of these manoeuvres are often suboptimal or even lethal, without adequate prior resuscitation. A systematic approach has much to recommend it and the authors advocate the techniques described in the *Care of the Critically Ill Surgical Patient* course.[32] **Immediate assessment** follows the principle of assessment with correction of life-threatening conditions taught by the advanced trauma life support (ATLS) course.[33] **Definitive assessment** determines the cause of any problem identified and excludes other conditions that would prove deleterious if untreated. It includes a thorough appraisal of the patient's notes and charts. A high index of clinical suspicion, combined with anticipation of potential complications, is essential when dealing with the critically ill patient. Patients should improve after clinical interventions and failure to progress, or deterioration, suggests a new problem.

Antimicrobial therapy in sepsis

Definitive management of sepsis requires identification of the source of infection. The history and examination provide clues, and the nature and timing of any interventions will suggest potential complications. When sepsis is suspected, blood cultures, urine, wound swabs and sputum should be submitted for urgent Gram staining and culture. If intravascular catheters are removed, their tips should be cultured. Appropriate antibiotics should be started and their spectrum should cover the expected range of infecting organisms. The route of administration must ensure adequate plasma levels and the drugs should penetrate adequately into the tissues. Intravenous infusion is usually necessary, but under certain circumstances other routes are preferable, for example intrathecal infusion in central nervous system infection. In critical illness, renal or hepatic impairment may require adjust-

ment of drug dosage. In most instances, pathogens will be bacteria, but antifungal agents may be required. Whenever there is doubt concerning the optimal choice of antibiotics, the advice of a medical microbiologist is a priority.

Antibiotic resistance is a significant problem, with multiresistant organisms evolving.[34] Resistance usually develops after recent antibiotic therapy and is most common where antimicrobial use is heaviest and patients are subject to multiple invasive procedures (e.g. in the ICU). It appears less common when antibiotic use is restricted, with strict infection control protocols and high nurse to patient ratios.[35] The importance of cross-infection through attendant staff cannot be underestimated. In the UK, microbial resistance is most common in ventilated patients and in teaching hospitals.[36] It has been recommended that empirical therapy be started only when infection poses a sufficient risk to warrant treatment before microbiological diagnosis,[36] but many critically ill patients fulfil this criterion. Broad-spectrum prescription is more likely to induce resistance than specific therapy, but there may be no alternative. Once started, antibiotics should be continued for sufficient time to prevent resistance developing in the target organism. Prescriptions should be reviewed regularly, because longer courses increase the risk of resistance emerging in nosocomial commensals.

Imaging in the septic patient

Various imaging techniques may be employed to localise an infective focus. Most patients will be fit enough to have a chest radiograph. Computed tomography (CT) or magnetic resonance imaging (MRI) can provide excellent information in thoracic, abdominal and pelvic sepsis provided that the patient can be transferred safely to the scanner and imaged without encumbrance from infusions, drains and metallic prostheses. Bedside ultrasound may be a valuable option and is the investigation of choice when endocarditis is suspected.[37] When a focus of sepsis cannot be identified radiologically, isotopic methods may help.[38] White cell scanning using indium-111 label has good sensitivity for identification of occult abscesses but may be positive in sterile inflammation, and hence specificity is lower.[39]

Laparotomy and drainage in sepsis

When sepsis develops after blunt abdominal trauma or abdominal and pelvic surgery, exploratory laparotomy may be the most expeditious means to exclude and treat an abdominal or pelvic cause.[40]

Blind laparotomy for all-comers is unlikely to reveal a cause in many,[41] but occult abdominal pathology should be suspected when MODS develops rapidly or when haemodynamic and renal compromise precede pulmonary dysfunction.[13] Moreover, unstable patients are often safer in the operating theatre than in the radiology department.

Infected collections require drainage, either percutaneously or at open surgery, and specimens should be sent for prompt Gram staining. Coagulopathy must be excluded or corrected beforehand and blood for transfusion should be available. Although drainage may be an essential prerequisite to resolution of sepsis, it is not infrequent for bacteraemia, as a consequence of the intervention, to cause a temporary deterioration in the patient's condition. Indeed, a bacteraemia may represent the 'second hit' that precipitates MODS. Such circumstances should be anticipated, and an appropriate level of post-procedure care arranged beforehand. Percutaneous procedures may be less invasive than open surgery but will only be effective if good drainage is achieved. Most percutaneous drains are narrow and inadequate when infected fluid is viscid or contains necrotic tissue. When open surgery is performed for sepsis, the procedure will vary according to the underlying pathology. Nonetheless, general principles apply and the most straightforward procedure is often preferable to a complex time-consuming operation. The aim is to improve the patient's condition without risking further complication. Non-viable tissue must be excised, but even when extensive debridement is required, tissues must always be handled gently to avoid further compromise to tissue perfusion. Generous lavage is recommended on completion of the procedure and, when soiling is gross, continuous irrigation or reinspection under anaesthesia should be considered. Delayed wound closure may be preferable to primary suture, or wounds may be left to close by secondary intention if sepsis is substantial. On occasion, delayed skin grafting and plastic reconstruction will be necessary. Both patient and relatives should be informed from the onset that definitive surgery may only be possible once the patient has recovered and that this may be some time later.

Therapeutic modulation of inflammatory mediators in sepsis

Identification of proinflammatory mediators has led to the development of specific antagonists. Some are antibodies against microbial components (e.g. endotoxin[42]), host mediators (e.g. TNF-α[43]) or mediator receptors (e.g. IL-1 receptor[44]). Others have pharmaceutical actions, for example platelet-

activating factor antagonists,[45] ibuprofen[46] and corticosteroids (see below). Despite encouraging results in animals, few clinical studies have shown evidence of overall outcome benefit when mediator antagonists are used in sepsis.

There are a number of potential explanations for this. It is possible that the underlying hypothesis is incomplete. Although increased mediator concentrations correlate with severity and poor outcome,[14] it does not follow that they cause sepsis. The mediators identified to date may be markers of some more fundamental event that triggers the inflammatory process. If so, then the antagonists proposed may be attempting to stem the mediator cascade when it is already in full force. The clinician certainly lacks control regarding the onset and magnitude of the insult that leads to sepsis and it must be remembered that, in practice, the causes of sepsis are often multiple. Few clinical studies have focused on a single causative pathology; indeed aetiology is frequently not obvious at presentation. Although mediator–antagonist interactions can be determined in vitro, there is no guarantee that similar relationships pertain in vivo. A mediator may have different actions[47-49] depending on its local concentration. One mediator's action might be influenced by those of others, the timing of its appearance in the inflammatory milieu, or the action of the compensatory anti-inflammatory response system.[50] Clinical studies are complicated by patient and treatment heterogeneity, and the effects of other therapeutic interventions cannot be discounted. Few studies agree on definitions of complications and, in some, there is no a priori definition at all. Such problems assume greater relevance when multicentre studies or meta-analyses are considered. Ideally studies should address specific patient groups that are comparable for the cause and severity of their sepsis. Consensus must be reached over the definition of end points. Only in this way are we likely to determine whether mediator antagonists influence outcome. The same criticisms can be applied to studies of other interventions in sepsis.

Therapeutic modulation of the prothrombotic response in sepsis

Whereas inflammatory mediator antagonists have yet to prove efficacious, evidence is emerging that modulation of the coagulation and fibrinolytic pathways may influence outcome. Sepsis is associated with deficiencies of activated protein C and antithrombin III that predispose to microcirculatory failure and subsequent organ dysfunction.[51] Protein C inhibits fibrin synthesis and promotes fibrinolysis. Independent of its antithrombotic actions, protein C antagonises the proinflammatory response and may protect the endothelium from endotoxin-induced apoptosis. Antithrombin III inhibits fibrin synthesis and also, via prostacyclin induction, inhibits many of the proinflammatory actions of platelets, neutrophils and endothelial cells.

In a randomised, controlled, multicentre study of adults with severe sepsis (PROWESS study), mortality at 28 days was significantly reduced in patients who received recombinant activated protein C (rAPC), irrespective of protein C deficiency on entry to the study. Approximately 25% of patients underwent surgery in each group and the lungs or abdomen were the most common sources of infection. Treatment was associated with an increased risk of haemorrhage and, overall, bleeding was most common in patients with peptic ulceration, haemorrhagic trauma or coagulopathy.[52] However, in a separate randomised, controlled, multicentre study (KyberSept trial) no significant reduction in mortality was associated with antithrombin III administration to adult patients with severe sepsis.[53] The explanation for these disparate results is almost certainly multifactorial.[54] The actions of rAPC and antithrombin III differ and dosage was adjusted for body weight in the PROWESS study but was fixed in the KyberSept trial. Patients could be recruited to the PROWESS study with less severe organ dysfunction and at an earlier stage in their illness. Moreover, control group mortality was higher in the KyberSept trial, suggesting that these patients were more unwell at enrolment. More patients in the KyberSept trial had undergone surgery and this may have contributed to the higher incidence of haemorrhagic complications reported. Nevertheless, the apparent benefits of rAPC therapy are encouraging.

Therapeutic modulation of the endocrine response in sepsis

Adrenal insufficiency may complicate sepsis and a blunted cortisol response to administered corticotrophin is associated with increased mortality.[55] Hypoaldosteronism in association with high plasma renin levels may also occur.[56] In septic shock, hydrocortisone administration improves vascular responsiveness to catecholamines.[57] Nevertheless, systematic reviews have suggested that use of high-dose corticosteroids in severe infection is of no benefit[58] or possibly even hazardous.[59]

However, a randomised controlled study demonstrated significantly reduced 28-day mortality and no excess morbidity when adult ventilated patients with septic shock received physiological doses of hydrocortisone

and fludrocortisone for 7 days.[60] Patients so treated could be weaned from vasopressor therapy sooner. The benefits of steroid therapy were more obvious in patients with an abnormal cortisol response to corticotropin.

The clinical features of adrenal insufficiency in the critically ill are subtle and therefore it has been suggested that it may now be appropriate to start empirical short-term low-dose steroid therapy in all such patients.[61]

Admission to the high-dependency or intensive care unit

A high-dependency unit (HDU) commonly has a nurse to patient ratio of 1:2 and patients are normally under the responsibility of the surgical team, but advice should be sought from intensivists when required. An HDU should allow automated monitoring of pulse, oxygen saturation, systemic arterial pressure and central venous pressure (CVP). Patients who need HDU care have single organ failure or require closer monitoring or nursing care than is possible on the general ward.[62]

An ICU provides a higher level of care, with a nurse to patient ratio of 1:1, 24-hour consultant intensivist cover and continuous supervision by dedicated residents with appropriate skills.[62] An ICU offers facilities for ventilation, cardiac output monitoring and invasive renal support. Patients who need ICU support typically require mechanical ventilation, have organ dysfunction in two or more systems or have acute dysfunction of a single organ against a background of chronic impairment of other systems. Although intensivists assume primary responsibility for ICU care, surgeons should participate in assessment and decision-making for their patients. Multidisciplinary care enables optimal management and smooth transition to a lower level of care.

If a patient deteriorates, transfer to higher level care should be considered before decompensation occurs, and preoperative admission to HDU or ICU may facilitate optimal resuscitation before surgery in the critically ill. Whatever the indication, transfer should only occur when immediate threats to life have been stabilised and after discussion with senior surgical and anaesthetic staff. Evidence suggests that many patients receive suboptimal basic care before an ICU opinion is sought and that referral is often delayed to the patient's detriment. Mortality is higher in patients admitted to ICU from the general ward than in those admitted from theatre or the emergency department,[63] and more timely and appropriate intervention by ward staff might

Box 18.6 • Indications for seeking an opinion from an intensivist

Airway
Threatened airway
Breathing
Respiratory arrest
Respiratory rate >40 or <8 breaths/min
S_aO_2 <90% on 50% oxygen
Rising P_aCO_2 with acidosis
Circulation
Cardiac arrest
Pulse rate <40 or >140 beats/min
Systolic blood pressure <90 mmHg
Metabolic acidosis
Disability
Sudden fall in level of consciousness (fall in Glasgow Coma Score >2 points)
Repeated or prolonged seizures
Any other area giving acute cause for concern

Adapted from Smith GJ, Nielsen N. ABC of intensive care. Criteria for admission. Br Med J 1999; 318:1544–7, with permission.

Box 18.7 • Patient requirements that indicate the need for intensive or high-dependency care*

Advanced respiratory support
Oral endotracheal intubation and/or mechanical ventilation (ICU)
Potential sudden airway compromise (ICU)
Basic respiratory support
Need for >50% oxygen (HDU)
Potential deterioration in breathing, e.g. fatigue (HDU)
Need for regular clearance of airway secretions (HDU)
Continuous positive pressure ventilation by mask or other non-invasive ventilation (HDU)
Cardiovascular support
Intra-aortic balloon pump (ICU)
Need for vasoactive drugs to support circulation (HDU†)
Hypovolaemia unresponsive to modest volume replacement (HDU)
Major operative or gastrointestinal haemorrhage (HDU)
Coagulopathy with haemorrhage (HDU)
Post resuscitation from cardiopulmonary arrest (HDU)
Renal support
Need for acute haemofiltration or acute haemodialysis (ICU)
Neurological support
Altered consciousness compromising the airway or its reflexes (ICU)
Monitoring
Pulmonary artery catheter (ICU)
Transoesophageal Doppler (ICU)
Intracranial pressure transducer (ICU)
Arterial catheter (HDU)
Central venous catheter (HDU)
Gastric tonometry (HDU)

HDU, high-dependency unit; ICU, intensive care unit.
*Suggested minimal level of care is indicated in parentheses.
†If one agent only required; otherwise ICU.
Adapted from Department of Health guidelines on admission to and discharge from intensive care and high dependency units. London: Department of Health, 1996, with permission.

reduce the number of patients requiring higher level care.[64,65] Common problems encountered include management of the airway, breathing and circulation, together with poor communication and a failure to appreciate clinical urgency. Indications for seeking an intensivist opinion and for ICU and HDU care are shown in **Boxes 18.6**[66] and **18.7**.

The use of early warning scores and illness severity scoring systems[67–69] (see also Chapter 15) may be valuable in identifying patients who might benefit from a higher level of care at a stage when catastrophic deterioration in their condition might still be averted. However, such tools are usually validated for specific populations and may be unreliable when used in different case mixes. They rarely predict individual outcome with sufficient accuracy to discriminate when higher level care might be withheld on the grounds of futility.

When ICU discharge is contemplated, an adequate level of receiving care must be ensured. The mortality after transfer may be as high as 15%,[70] but can be reduced if an HDU is used as an intermediary to general ward care.[71]

INTENSIVE CARE MANAGEMENT

In MODS, organ dysfunction usually indicates other underlying pathology and a holistic approach to management is required. In severe illness, tissue hypoxia contributes to the development of MODS, and the consequent organ dysfunction may lead to worsening hypoxia. This section begins with consideration of tissue oxygenation and a brief review of goal-directed therapy (see also Chapter 16). An overview of the management of common respiratory, cardiovascular and renal problems encountered in critically ill surgical patients follows and the relationship between critical illness and abdominal pathology is also discussed.

Assessment of tissue oxygenation and perfusion in critical illness

There is no substitute for basic clinical skill supplemented by regular measurement of pulse, blood pressure and urine output; however, in critical illness, additional monitoring is required.

PULSE OXIMETRY

Pulse oximetry enables continuous assessment of pulse rate and arterial oxygen saturation (S_aO_2) in the peripheries. Poor perfusion, jaundice, shivering or convulsions may render readings unreliable. Anaemia or carboxyhaemoglobin can cause over-estimation of S_aO_2 and oximetry yields no information regarding arterial carbon dioxide tension (P_aCO_2); nonetheless, the pulse oximeter is a valuable tool that enables detection of subtle changes in S_aO_2.

ARTERIAL BLOOD GAS ANALYSIS

Arterial blood gas analysis provides information regarding gas exchange and acid–base status. For patients receiving oxygen, the minimum expected arterial oxygen tension (P_aO_2) can be calculated from the fractional inspired oxygen (F_iO_2):

$$P_aO_2 = F_iO_2 \times 500 \text{ (mmHg)}$$
or
$$PO_2 = F_iO_2 \times 65 \text{ (kPa)}$$

If the observed P_aO_2 is less, then the patient would be hypoxic when breathing air.[72]

Metabolic acidosis represents systemic acidosis and is a poor prognostic indicator.[73] The underlying pathology may be local (e.g. bowel ischaemia) or generalised (e.g. shock). Metabolic acidosis often reflects tissue hypoxia, but other conditions, including diabetic ketoacidosis and renal tubular disease, cause acidosis independent of hypoxia. Acidosis secondary to hypoperfusion often responds to restoration of the circulation, and unless there is continued bicarbonate loss (e.g. from a pancreatic fistula), bicarbonate replacement is rarely required.

INVASIVE ARTERIAL BLOOD PRESSURE

A non-compliant peripheral arterial catheter connected to a damped transducer allows continuous measurement of pulse rate and systemic blood pressure. Mean arterial pressure (MAP) is calculated as

Mean arterial pressure = diastolic pressure + pulse pressure/3 (mmHg)

Analysis of the pulse waveform may yield information with regard to volume status and arterial catheterisation provides access for repeated arterial blood gas sampling.

CENTRAL VENOUS PRESSURE

CVP measurement enables estimation of left ventricular end-diastolic pressure (LVEDP), or systemic preload, provided that there is no abnormality in the tone of the great veins, the right heart or the pulmonary circulation. However, CVP catheters are not without complication.[74] Multiple-lumen catheters provide access for venous blood sampling or infusion but are also a significant source of infection.[75] The relationship between CVP and venous filling is not linear and, unless CVP is extremely high or low, the change in pressure in response to a fluid challenge is more informative than an absolute value.[76] CVP can be measured with a manometer or a transducer. The latter displays the CVP waveform and dramatic variation with breathing may indicate hypovolaemia.

PULMONARY ARTERY FLOTATION CATHETER

A pulmonary artery flotation catheter (PAFC; Swan–Ganz catheter), inserted via the jugular or subclavian vein, enables measurement of pulmonary artery wedge pressure (PAWP). A temperature transducer in the catheter enables calculation of cardiac output (CO) by thermodilution. PAWP is a more direct reflection of LVEDP than CVP and is not influenced by central venous tone or right heart disease. It is still influenced by pulmonary vascular resistance and mitral valve function. The PAWP response to a fluid challenge is similar to that for CVP. If systemic blood pressure is known, SVR and derived variables relating to tissue oxygenation can be calculated. The oxygen content of arterial blood (C_aO_2) is found from

$$C_aO_2 = (S_aO_2 \times Hb \times 1.34) + (0.023 \times P_aO_2) \text{ (mL/dL)}$$

The first term represents oxygen bound to haemoglobin (Hb) and the second (less significant) the oxygen dissolved in plasma. Oxygen delivery (DO_2) is calculated as

$$DO_2 = 10 \times CO \times C_aO_2 \text{ (mL/min)}$$

A DO_2 of 300 mL/min is required to maintain life at rest.[77] Oxygen uptake (VO_2) is

$$VO_2 = 10 \times CO \times (C_aO_2 - C_vO_2) \text{ (mL/min)}$$

where C_vO_2 is mixed venous oxygen content. These variables may each be divided by body surface area to provide 'indexed' values corrected for patient size. Reference values are given in **Table 18.1**.

PAFCs are associated with significant complications[78] in up to 20% of patients and technical errors in PAWP measurement occur in 20%.[79] Studies have demonstrated increased mortality associated with PAFC use.[80] The precise explanation is uncertain[81] but could be related to case mix differences, catheter-related morbidity, poor interpretation of derived data[82] or complications of consequent therapy. Results of prospective studies are awaited and it is possible that innovative less-invasive techniques may prove more efficacious.

TRANSOESOPHAGEAL DOPPLER

Transoesophageal Doppler enables assessment of left ventricular stroke volume with 85–90% accuracy[83] and thus cardiac output and myocardial contractility can be calculated. Waveform analysis can assess preload, contractile force and afterload.[84] A study performed in adults undergoing elective coronary

artery bypass indicated that Doppler measurement of cardiac output compared favourably with assessment measurement by thermodilution.[85]

LITHIUM DILUTION CARDIAC OUTPUT MEASUREMENT

The lithium dilution technique enables near-continuous measurement of cardiac output without the need for a PAFC. Lithium chloride is injected intravenously, either peripherally or centrally, and a dilution curve is constructed via a lithium-sensitive transducer in an arterial catheter.[86] Initial clinical studies have demonstrated the reliability of the method, including immediately after cardiac surgery when significant changes in body temperature are common.[87]

GASTRIC MUCOSAL TONOMETRY

Mucosal hypoxia results in anaerobic metabolism and hence decreased intramucosal pH (pH_i). Tonometry enables pH_i calculation from gastrointestinal mucosal carbon dioxide tension by means of a nasogastric tube that includes a gas-permeable balloon. In critically ill patients, low pH_i was found to correlate with poor outcome[88] and prompt correction of pH_i after trauma was associated with improved outcome.[89] Nevertheless, it is still unclear whether tonometry is a valuable management aid, or if abnormal pH_i is merely a surrogate marker of severe illness.[90]

PHYSIOLOGY OF TISSUE OXYGENATION

In health, DO_2 greatly exceeds VO_2 and oxygen consumption is termed 'supply independent'. Below a critical point, VO_2 decreases in proportion to DO_2; therefore, oxygen consumption is dependent on supply and anaerobic metabolism ensues. Anaerobic metabolism also occurs when oxygen demand exceeds maximal extraction or when mitochondria are unable to utilise available oxygen. The latter occurs in carbon monoxide toxicity and possibly in sepsis. Anaerobic energy production is inefficient, and accumulation of intracellular lactate leads to acidosis.

A P_aO_2 of 8 kPa corresponds to an S_aO_2 of 90%, but owing to the steep slope of the oxygen dissociation curve, further small reductions in P_aO_2 lead to marked reduction in S_aO_2. Conversely, increasing P_aO_2 with supplemental oxygen leads to dramatic increases in S_aO_2 and hence DO_2.

The combination of low S_aO_2 and anaemia dramatically reduces oxygen delivery. Tissue oxygenation is further influenced by cardiac output and regional blood flow. In the lung, discrepancy between ventilation and perfusion ($\dot{V}/\dot{Q}$ mismatch) reduces oxygenation while local arteriolar tone will

Table 18.1 • Reference values for physiological variables

Variable	Symbol	Reference value
Cardiac output	CO	4.0–7.0 L/min
Cardiac index		2.8–4.2 L/min per m²
Systemic vascular resistance (afterload)	SVR	770–1500 dyne s cm⁻⁵
Oxygen delivery	DO_2	640–1200 mL/min
Oxygen delivery index		500–600 mL/min per m²
Oxygen uptake	VO_2	100–180 mL/min
Oxygen uptake index		120–160 mL/min per m²

influence oxygen supply to the tissues. Shunting impairs oxygen loading in acute lung disease, but $\dot{V}/\dot{Q}$ mismatch is of greater significance in chronic lung disease[91] and is exacerbated by low or high cardiac output. Under hyperdynamic conditions, reduced circulation time may impair diffusion of oxygen to and from erythrocytes. Reduction in DO_2 is associated with redistribution of blood flow away from organs able to increase oxygen extraction (e.g. gut) in order to maintain oxygenation of supply-limited organs (e.g. brain).[92]

Respiratory support

RESPIRATORY FAILURE

Two patterns of respiratory failure are described but, in practice, elements of both may coexist. In hypoxaemic (type I) failure, P_aO_2 is reduced but P_aCO_2 is normal or reduced because of hyperventilation. In ventilatory (type II) failure, gas exchange is impaired, P_aO_2 is reduced and P_aCO_2 elevated.

Hypoxia Hypoxaemic failure is caused by shunting, $\dot{V}/\dot{Q}$ mismatch, diffusion impairment and altered oxygen binding by haemoglobin. Clinical causes of shunting include atelectasis, consolidation and ARDS as well as cyanotic heart disease, whereas $\dot{V}/\dot{Q}$ mismatch is commonly caused by chronic lung disease or pulmonary oedema. Pulmonary embolism can cause both shunting and $\dot{V}/\dot{Q}$ mismatch.

Ventilatory failure Ventilatory failure results from defective control or mechanics of breathing. Central control of ventilation may be impaired by head injury or drugs such as opiates. High cervical spine injuries may paralyse respiratory muscles, and thoracic wall disruption will also impair ventilation. Chest movement is hampered by pain and diaphragmatic splinting caused by gastrointestinal distension or intraperitoneal fluid. Effective lung volume is reduced by intrapleural air or fluid, or atelectasis or consolidation: when combined with fatigue, hypoventilation may ensue. Gas exchange is further impaired by pulmonary oedema and by increased airway resistance, as in asthma.

AIRWAY MANAGEMENT

Critically ill patients frequently require airway support. Tracheobronchial suction may be necessary to clear secretions while nebulisers can reverse bronchoconstriction and aid mucolysis. Physiotherapy can facilitate airway clearance and bronchoscopy may aid removal of mucous plugs. A definitive airway is usually required for mechanical ventilation or when there is risk of aspiration of gastric content. Usually a cuffed endotracheal tube will be employed in the first instance, but acute upper airway obstruction may necessitate a cricothyroidotomy.

Indications for tracheostomy Prolonged endotracheal intubation is uncomfortable, often entails sedation and may cause subglottic stenosis. A tracheostomy should be considered if protracted endotracheal intubation is anticipated. Patients who require regular airway toilet may benefit from tracheostomy; a minitracheostomy is an alternative for short-term use. Permanent tracheostomy is an inevitable consequence of laryngeal or pharyngeal resection or when a sentient patient cannot protect the airway. Temporary tracheostomy may be required after head and neck trauma, and before radiotherapy to the neck.

SUPPLEMENTAL OXYGEN DELIVERY

Most critically ill surgical patients benefit from supplementary oxygen and few will rely on hypoxic drive to breathe. Administered oxygen should be humidified whenever possible.

Mask delivery F_iO_2 depends on oxygen flow and the patient's pattern of ventilation. At an oxygen flow of 4 L/min, nasal cannulae and simple masks provide an F_iO_2 of 0.3–0.4. High-flow air-entrainment masks provide a fixed F_iO_2 that is independent of the pattern of ventilation. Depending on the mask type and oxygen flow, a constant F_iO_2 of between 0.28 and 0.60 can be provided; to achieve a higher F_iO_2 requires a reservoir.

Continuous positive airway pressure Continuous positive airway pressure (CPAP)[93] is provided via a tight-fitting facial or nasal mask and can recruit collapsed alveoli or disperse pulmonary oedema. It may improve left heart function in cardiac failure and reduce the work of breathing. Judicious CPAP may avoid the need for mechanical ventilation or facilitate its weaning. Airway pressure release ventilation allows two levels of CPAP; in one variant, bilevel positive airway pressure (BiPAP), there is a background of CPAP that is intermittently reduced to aid expiration.[94]

Non-invasive positive pressure ventilation Non-invasive positive pressure ventilation (NIPPV) has been associated with reduced morbidity and shorter ICU stay compared with mechanical ventilation.[95] It may be particularly useful in chronic lung disease and can facilitate weaning from mechanical ventilation. Avoidance of an endotracheal tube may reduce life-threatening infection in the immunocompromised. NIPPV is suitable for awake patients who can coordinate breathing with the ventilator-derived flow pattern.[96]

MECHANICAL VENTILATION

Indications for ventilation Ventilation is indicated for hypoxia that cannot be corrected by more conservative means. It is also indicated when carbon dioxide retention develops acutely and when normalisation of P_aCO_2 is required to reduce intracranial pressure. Elective ventilation may be beneficial in critical illness, particularly when fatigue is likely. Some patients require multiple surgical procedures within a short period of time and continued ventilation is often desirable. Patients with open laparostomy will require ventilation with paralysis until evisceration is no longer a risk.

Ventilator modes Mechanical ventilation may be volume or pressure controlled.[97] **Volume control** ensures gas flow at the expense of variable pressure. When lung compliance is heterogeneous it may lead to overdistension of compliant areas while non-compliant areas remain hypoventilated. Over-distension may produce lung injury and hence **pressure control** has been suggested as an alternative.

Positive end-expiratory pressure Addition of positive end-expiratory pressure (PEEP)[93] produces similar effects to CPAP. Increased tidal volumes are generated by increasing inspiratory time in relation to the expiratory time (reversed I:E ratio). This manoeuvre also improves gas distribution through recruitment of slow-opening alveoli[98] and produces an element of PEEP. The abnormal breathing pattern is uncomfortable, and sedation and paralysis are often necessary.

Intermittent positive pressure ventilation Intermittent positive pressure ventilation (IPPV) provides total respiratory support and is not influenced by patient effort; consequently, sedation and paralysis are normally necessary.

Assist-control ventilation In assist-control ventilation the patient's inspiratory effort triggers a complete machine breath, while pressure-support ventilation (PSV) delivers pressure assistance each time the patient attempts inspiration. PSV reduces the work of breathing[99] and causes less haemodynamic disturbance than conventional ventilation. It may be of use in chronic lung disease and in weaning patients from mechanical ventilation.

Synchronised intermittent mandatory ventilation Ventilation protocols can be combined to match patient requirements. For example, a number of mandatory breaths can be preset to guarantee adequate ventilation (synchronised intermittent mandatory ventilation) or the machine can be set to intervene if patient-generated breaths prove inadequate (mandatory minute ventilation).

COMPLICATIONS OF POSITIVE PRESSURE TECHNIQUES

Pulmonary complications Increased airway distension in PEEP can cause interstitial emphysema[100] and possible tension pneumothorax or gas embolism. Repeated shear stresses may lead to development of hyaline membranes and surfactant activity may be impaired,[101] precipitating acute lung injury. Ventilation itself may result in release of proinflammatory

mediators.[102] Theoretically, reduction of ventilation rate, pressures and tidal volumes should minimise the risk of barotrauma, but the patient's condition may preclude these manoeuvres.

Haemodynamic complications Increasing lung volume increases pulmonary vascular resistance, except possibly when pre-existing pulmonary hypertension is secondary to hypoxic vasoconstriction. Increased intrathoracic pressure reduces preload, and in most cases cardiac output falls. However, reduction of venous return may improve output in cardiac failure. Increased intrathoracic pressure reduces systemic afterload and, providing that intravascular volume is normal, reduces cardiac work. Both hepatic and mesenteric blood flow are reduced by PEEP.

Renal complications Urine output and sodium excretion are compromised by PEEP. In addition to reduced renal perfusion pressure, ventilation alters baroreceptor activity and increases secretion of vasopressin and renin while reducing release of atrial natriuretic factor.[103]

General complications Prolonged use of tight-fitting masks can cause facial pressure necrosis, and gastric distension is not uncommon when CPAP or NIPPV is used.

OTHER STRATEGIES FOR RESPIRATORY SUPPORT

Prone ventilation Pulmonary oedema leads to compression and atelectasis of dependent parts of the lungs. These dependent portions remain perfused but their ventilation is impaired and $\dot{V}/\dot{Q}$ mismatch results.[104] The lung is triangular in section, with the greater part posteriorly, and non-dependent alveoli receive proportionally more ventilation. Prone positioning may improve P_aO_2 in acute respiratory failure[105] but whether outcome is improved is uncertain.

High-frequency jet ventilation High-frequency jet ventilation (HFJV) delivers oxygen in pulses of 60–600/min and, in adults, may be indicated in the management of air leakage (e.g. bronchopleural fistula or tracheal laceration[106]) or in patients prone to pneumothorax. Low pressures are used and gas distribution depends on airway resistance rather than compliance. In this way, adequate alveolar ventilation can be maintained while a leak closes. HFJV has also been suggested as a means to minimise lung injury in acute lung injury. Initial results are encouraging[107] but firm evidence has not been produced.

Inhaled nitric oxide In normal circumstances inhaled nitric oxide has no effect, but when there is pulmonary vasoconstriction, it reduces pulmonary vascular resistance without systemic effects.[108] The effects are limited to ventilated alveoli and hence

$\dot{V}/\dot{Q}$ matching is improved. While low nitric oxide concentrations may be beneficial, higher doses are less so,[109] probably because they induce $\dot{V}/\dot{Q}$ mismatch in underventilated alveoli. Inhaled nitric oxide improves P_aO_2/F_iO_2 ratios in acute respiratory failure[110] but may not be beneficial against a background of chronic obstructive pulmonary disease,[111] again because $\dot{V}/\dot{Q}$ mismatch worsens. However, a meta-analysis of randomised controlled trials that compared inhaled nitric oxide with maximal conventional therapy and inhaled placebo failed to demonstrate any significant effect on mortality in adults and children treated for acute hypoxaemic respiratory failure.[112]

Extracorporeal membrane oxygenation The mortality from severe neonatal respiratory failure may be substantially reduced with extracorporeal membrane oxygenation,[113] although improved survival in adults has not been demonstrated in controlled studies.[114]

Liquid ventilation Liquid ventilation is performed through lungs filled with perfluorocarbon solutions, which dissolve oxygen and carbon dioxide.[115] Recruitment of dependent lung and improved compliance have been reported, but the method is experimental and there is limited experience in adults.[116]

ACUTE LUNG INJURY

Acute lung injury (ALI), also known as ARDS, develops in 25% of septic patients.[31,117] Interstitial oedema causes hypoxaemia and reduces pulmonary compliance while reduced recoil leads to air entrapment and renders the lung more prone to barotrauma. Moreover, the inflammatory component of ALI may be exacerbated by repeated stress and shear forces that are a consequence of alveolar overdistension and repeated opening and closing caused by mechanical ventilation. The earliest sign of ALI may be hypoxaemia alone, and the classical radiological pulmonary infiltrates occur relatively late.

General treatment of ALI Management is predominantly supportive; oxygenation and circulating volume must be maintained, without fluid overload. CPAP may be beneficial, although mechanical ventilation is usually necessary. A randomised controlled study suggested that prolonged administration of methylprednisolone may aid recovery and reduce mortality in unresolving ALI, but patient numbers were very small.[118]

Ventilation strategies in ALI In ALI, collapse and consolidation of alveoli leads to a loss of functional lung capacity. Ventilation strategies should aim to recruit as many alveolar units as possible without causing further lung damage. Collapsed lung is more amenable to recruitment than consolidated

tissue and hence the potential to recruit the lung may be greater when the cause of ALI is other than primary pulmonary disease.[119]

Ventilation to maintain an 'open lung' has been proposed; the method has three components. Firstly, a ventilation pressure exceeding the opening pressure of the collapsed lung units is required. This pressure is influenced by the elastance of the chest wall which, in turn, may be impaired by abdominal pressure.[120] Secondly, end-expiratory pressure sufficient to prevent subsequent re-collapse is applied. Finally, the ratio between alveolar gas flow and perfusion must be adequate to prevent atelectasis secondary to gas resorption: low-rate high tidal volume 'sigh' ventilation may be efficacious. Overall, titration of ventilator settings is probably preferable to rigid implementation of empirical parameters and the general advice is to treat the lung gently'.[121]

Mortality and duration of ventilation were significantly reduced in a randomised study when adult patients with ALI were ventilated with lower tidal volumes and inspiratory pressures.[122] Although other studies have failed to confirm these findings, a recent meta-analysis suggests that the pooled data were in favour of a volume- and pressure-limited approach.[123]

Pressure-control ventilation, inverse I:E ratio and BiPAP have also been advocated for ALI;[124] others recommend the use of prone ventilation. It is possible that HFJV, extracorporeal membrane oxygenation and liquid ventilation may prove efficacious but definitive evidence is still awaited.

Cardiovascular support

If respiratory function is satisfactory, tissue oxygenation is dependent on cardiac output and an adequate circulation.

Cardiac output = heart rate × stroke volume

Systemic blood pressure = cardiac output × SVR

Stroke volume is determined by the amount of blood returning to the heart (preload), myocardial contractility and SVR (afterload). Heart rate and stroke volume are interrelated; tachycardia or other dysrhythmias impair left atrial filling and reduce cardiac output, even though the heart rate has increased. Moreover, myocardial ischaemia reduces contractile force. Ischaemia is more likely as cardiac work increases and the duration of diastole, when the coronary arteries fill, is reduced. The physiological response to stress has developed to maintain brain oxygenation, but at the potential expense of other systems, not least the gut. Cardiovascular support should optimise circulation to all tissues, but many agents used to improve cardiac function potentially compromise the splanchnic circulation.

SHOCK

Shock exists when the circulation is unable to maintain tissue perfusion and oxygenation. Various types of shock are described and all may be seen in the critically ill.

Hypovolaemic shock Hypovolaemic shock is a consequence of fluid loss. It is usually caused by haemorrhage or extensive burns but other causes include profuse gastrointestinal losses, particularly in the frail and at the extremes of age. In the early stages of hypovolaemic shock, hypotension is not manifest.[33] Management comprises fluid replacement with prompt arrest of haemorrhage.

Sepsis In septic shock, inflammatory mediator activation causes systemic vasodilatation, interstitial fluid sequestration and myocardial suppression. Ventricular dilatation occurs and ejection fraction is reduced. Septic shock is characterised by a hyperdynamic circulation and fever, although in the later stages it may be indistinguishable from hypovolaemic shock. The underlying cause must be addressed in addition to maintenance of the circulation.

Neurogenic shock Neurogenic shock results from loss of sympathetic tone and is usually associated with spinal cord injury. Diastolic blood pressure is low, often with relative or absolute bradycardia secondary to cervical sympathetic denervation. Fluid replacement and possibly pressor agents are required and, after trauma, a hypovolaemic element may coexist.

Anaphylactic shock Anaphylactic shock represents an overwhelming immune response to a foreign substance. Histamine and kinin release is associated with massive fluid redistribution and myocardial suppression. Airway oedema and bronchospasm are common. Immediate management comprises cessation of any precipitating cause with administration of oxygen, adrenaline (epinephrine) and rapid fluid replacement.[125]

Cardiac shock Cardiogenic shock occurs when there is acute heart failure. It is characterised by failing cardiac output in the presence of normal or elevated CVP or PAWP. Fluid replacement is contraindicated once concomitant hypovolaemia is excluded. Both tension pneumothorax and cardiac tamponade cause cardiogenic shock by impairment of venous return, and either may be associated with hypovolaemia after trauma. Immediate thoracocentesis or pericardiocentesis, respectively, are indicated.

Critically ill patients are at risk of myocardial infarction, dysrhythmia and pulmonary embolism, all of which can cause cardiogenic shock. Fluid overload caused by overzealous fluid replacement or renal failure may also cause cardiac failure. Patients with pre-existing cardiac impairment will be more at risk. Treatment of cardiogenic shock after myocardial infarction can be complex; there may be pulmonary oedema and afterload may be high or low.[126] Optimal therapy is determined by the balance between pulmonary congestion and peripheral hypotension. Measurement of cardiac output and preload may facilitate management. In cardiac failure, the neuroendocrine response to falling cardiac output increases venous tone and SVR to maintain cardiac filling and systemic blood pressure. However, a vicious cycle may develop in which myocardial work and pulmonary oedema increase; in this situation vasodilator therapy is necessary.

FLUID RESUSCITATION

There is much debate regarding the ideal fluid for volume resuscitation in critical illness.

Two meta-analyses by epidemiologists reported increased mortality associated with use of colloids[127] and albumin[128] rather than crystalloids. In each there was wide variability in the fluids used and the clinical assumptions and conclusions are debatable. In contrast, a meta-analysis conducted by intensivists suggested no difference between colloids and crystalloids.[129] Certainly, neither colloids in general nor albumin seem to improve survival substantially compared with crystalloids. Albumin is expensive and is a potential vector for prion infection. It does not raise colloid oncotic pressure effectively,[130] is not retained in the vascular compartment in sepsis and possibly leads to salt and water overload.[131] These arguments militate against its use. However, the conclusion that other colloid solutions should not be used for resuscitation outside of clinical trials[127] cannot be supported at present.

In general, the fluid used should reflect that which was lost and the value of blood in major haemorrhage must not be ignored. Haemoglobin solutions may soon be available for clinical use.[132]

BLOOD TRANSFUSION IN CRITICAL CARE

The balance between risk and benefit from blood transfusion in the critically ill is unclear. It has been reported that anaemia increases mortality.[133] However, it is also possible that blood transfusion may cause immunosuppression and impair flow in the microcirculation.

A Canadian controlled study was conducted in normovolaemic adult ICU patients who were randomised to either restrictive or liberal blood transfusion policies.[134] In the former, the trigger for transfusion was a haemoglobin below 7.0 g/dL, in the latter a haemoglobin below 10 g/dL. Overall mortality was similar in each group but was significantly lower in the restrictive group when the young and less severely ill were considered as subsets. The study was terminated early because of failure to recruit; nevertheless, the authors maintained that the findings could be extrapolated to 'most critically ill patients'. However, most of the patients studied suffered primary cardiorespiratory disease and relatively few were septic or had undergone surgery. Contrary to UK practice, leucocyte-depleted blood was not used.

INOTROPIC AND PRESSOR SUPPORT

Inotropes increase myocardial contractile force and thus improve stroke volume, although this often increases myocardial oxygen demand. Pressor agents increase SVR and are used to maintain systemic blood pressure but also increase afterload and cardiac work. Most drugs used to support the circulation mimic catecholamines and have mixed agonist activity. Consequently, their actions with respect to cardiac output, SVR and regional blood supply vary. Increased contractile force and tachycardia are mediated by β_1-adrenergic agonists. Vasodilatation is mediated by β_2-adrenoceptors while vasoconstriction is mediated by α_1-adrenoceptors. Dopaminergic D_{1A} activity causes splanchnic and renal vasodilatation. The effects of inotropes in health and in vitro differ from the effects in sepsis. Inflammatory mediators promote vasodilatation and possibly directly antagonise some inotropic effects, and the interrelating effects of comorbid disease and MODS confuse the results of clinical studies. In sepsis, the critical DO_2 of the intestine is greater than that of the body as a whole.[135] Splanchnic perfusion increases with cardiac output, but splanchnic VO_2 increases more than global VO_2.[136] Consequently, the gut may continue to be oxygen dependent even when global DO_2 appears satisfactory. Furthermore, inotropes may interact directly with the inflammatory[137] and neuroendocrine responses to stress.

Dobutamine Dobutamine is principally a β_1-agonist; its positive inotropic and chronotropic actions make it a popular choice when an inotrope is required. Provided that intravascular volume is satisfactory, dobutamine leads to improved cardiac output and DO_2 compared with that achieved with dopamine.[138]

Noradrenaline (norepinephrine) Noradrenaline is an α_1-agonist with minor β_1 and β_2 effects. It is often employed when increased SVR is required to maintain MAP after fluid replacement has proved inadequate. In health, noradrenaline increases splanchnic vascular resistance, but animal evidence suggests that this does not occur in sepsis.[139] In hypotensive patients with septic shock, noradrenaline infusion is associated with increased urine output, probably through elevation of MAP rather than through a direct renal effect.[140]

Adrenaline Adrenaline is principally an agonist at β_1- and β_2-adrenoceptors at low dose, but at higher doses effects at α_1-adrenoceptors predominate. In sepsis, adrenaline increases MAP, cardiac output, and global DO_2 and VO_2,[141] but at the potential expense of splanchnic perfusion.[142]

Dopamine Dopamine, at low dose, is predominantly a D_{1A} agonist; at intermediate doses β_1-adrenoceptor effects appear and α_1-adrenoceptor effects dominate at high doses. Although dopamine has been recommended as a first-choice drug to restore MAP in sepsis,[143] its vasoconstrictor activity is concerning. In one large study, dobutamine was more effective than dopamine when improvements in DO_2 and VO_2 were considered.[144] Moreover, shocked patients resuscitated with dopamine had lower pH_i than those in whom dobutamine was used.[145] The renal effects of dopamine are discussed below.

Dopexamine Dopexamine is predominantly a β_2-agonist with D_{1A} activity and seems directly inotropic in low-output cardiac failure.[146] Dopexamine may increase splanchnic blood flow and pH_i in patients with SIRS[147] and the drug has been used in several studies of goal-directed therapy (see below). However, a randomised controlled study of adult general intensive care patients failed to demonstrate significant changes in gastrointestinal mucosal permeability or creatinine clearance in those who received a 7-day intravenous infusion of dopexamine, intended to improve splanchnic blood flow.[148] Hence it is not clear that dopexamine has a genuine gut-protective action.

Enoximone and amrinone Enoximone and amrinone are phosphodiesterase III inhibitors that increase intracellular cyclic AMP. They are positive inotropes and reduce SVR ('inodilatation') and are effective in cardiogenic shock.[149] Addition of dobutamine may be synergistic.[150] Prophylactic enoximone administration to patients over the age of 80 years who underwent cardiac surgery, a group prone to SIRS and MODS, was associated with reduced levels of postoperative inflammatory markers, less alteration in liver enzymes and less renal tubular damage compared with placebo.[151] Enoximone and milrinone administered before aortic cross-clamping in cardiac surgery were associated with improved postoperative cardiac function and oxygen transport.[152] Whether inodilators actually influence outcome or have a role to play in septic shock is undetermined.

MECHANICAL ASSIST DEVICES

Intra-aortic balloon counterpulsation can improve cardiac output and myocardial oxygenation and is principally used as an adjunct to cardiac surgery. A balloon is directed into the thoracic aorta via the femoral artery and is inflated and deflated in synchrony with the electrocardiogram trace. Inflation during diastole increases LVEDP and coronary artery flow while forward flow is improved as blood is displaced from the aorta. Deflation during systole allows blood to circulate, and the sudden increase in aortic volume reduces myocardial work and oxygen consumption.[153]

VASODILATOR THERAPY

Glyceryl trinitrate (nitroglycerin) and nitroprusside infusions cause vasodilatation, reducing preload and afterload. They have short half-lives and can be titrated against the cardiovascular response. Vasodilators are used with inotropes in cardiogenic shock and are also used in conservative management of aortic dissection.

MANAGEMENT OF DYSRHYTHMIA

Cardiac rhythm changes may represent primary cardiac disease but other causes, including hypoxia, hypovolaemia, anaemia, sepsis, and acid–base and electrolyte disorders, must be considered. Conditions such as heart failure and pulmonary embolus should be excluded, and medication reviewed. Hypokalaemia, hypocalcaemia or hypomagnesaemia may cause dysrhythmia; moreover, they may coexist and only resolve when all are corrected. They may occur, together with hypophosphataemia and thiamine deficiency, in the 'refeeding syndrome' seen in severely ill patients during nutritional support.[154] Pain, fever or anxiety alone may cause sinus tachycardia. Management of dysrhythmia entails assessment of haemodynamic stability and correction of the underlying aetiology. It should be noted that many antiarrhythmic drugs have a negative inotropic effect.

Tachyarrhythmias

Significant haemodynamic compromise is an indication for immediate cardioversion. Many supraventricular tachycardias are abolished by either carotid sinus massage or adenosine. Even if the tachyarrhythmia is not reversed, it may slow to allow a more precise diagnosis to be made. Significant atrial fibrillation or flutter can be treated with either digoxin or amiodarone. Treatment is not mandatory for short runs of ventricular tachycardia but sustained or symptomatic ventricular tachycardia can be treated with lidocaine (lignocaine) or amiodarone, or by cardioversion if refractory. Ventricular fibrillation always requires cardioversion and subsequent lidocaine infusion.

Bradyarrhythmias

Asymptomatic sinus bradycardia requires no treatment but if there is hypotension, atropine or a β-agonist can be used. Pacing is indicated for refractory symptomatic bradycardia and when lesser degrees of block may progress to complete heart block.

Goal-directed therapy

Low cardiac output, increased SVR and reduced oxygen consumption are predictors of poor outcome after major surgery.[155–157] These predictors are more accurate than observations such as pulse rate, CVP and urine output.[158] 'Survivor values' of cardiac index >4.5 L/min per m^2, DO_2 >600 mL/min per m^2 and VO_2 >170 mL/min per m^2 have been suggested as goals for all critically ill patients, regardless of the need for surgery,[159] and form the basis of goal-directed resuscitation.

A meta-analysis suggested that when expected mortality was greater than 10%, goal-directed therapy was associated with reduced mortality. However, when anticipated mortality was less than 10%, goal-directed therapy was not effective. There was no survival benefit when goal-directed therapy was instituted after sepsis developed.[160]

Similar studies have been performed in patients who were already showing signs of severe sepsis. Subgroup analysis implied that mortality from septic shock was significantly reduced when the cardiac index was 4.5 L/min per m^2,[161] although a subsequent trial suggested the contrary.[162] Most studies analysed had combined fluid replacement with inotropic support and it was impossible to determine whether both were important; some patients may have benefited from fluid replacement alone.

Patients who underwent major abdominal surgery were randomised to receive standard perioperative care or aggressive goal-directed treatment with pulmonary artery catheterisation, fluid loading and either adrenaline or dopexamine.[163] Significantly lower mortalities were found in the groups receiving inotropes compared with the patients receiving standard care. However, an intervention group receiving fluids alone was not included and the groups receiving inotropes also received an average of 1500 mL more fluid before surgery. In addition, only the intervention patients were treated on an ICU or HDU before and after surgery, whereas the 'control' patients came to theatre from general wards and 35% returned directly to those wards after operation.

A randomised controlled trial investigated the value of early goal-directed therapy started in the emergency department in adults with SIRS and hypoperfusion who required ICU admission.[164] Early intervention comprised goal-oriented optimisation of preload, afterload and myocardial contractility. Both standard therapy and early intervention patients received similar fluid volumes, but the latter were resuscitated faster. The early intervention group had improved acid–base status and central venous oxygenation as well as lower APACHE II scores and in-hospital mortality.

For patients with limited reserve, blinkered treatment to predetermined parameters may be detrimental. In individuals unresponsive to volume alone, high doses of inotropes may be harmful.[162] Oxygen handling in the immediate postoperative period correlates with outcome[165] and survivors of sepsis seem better able to increase oxygen delivery and utilisation when their circulatory physiology is optimised.[166] Failure to respond in this way may indicate mitochondrial dysfunction and could be a prognostic indicator. Indeed, meta-analysis demonstrated a survival benefit only when oxygen delivery was enhanced before the onset of tissue hypoperfusion or organ dysfunction.[160]

National reports in the UK have repeatedly stressed the importance of adequate preoperative resuscitation[167] but goal-directed therapy is not without risk; it may cause substantial fluid overload,[168] pulmonary oedema and impaired gastrointestinal function.[169] Further trials are required to determine the most influential elements of goal-directed therapy, not least because of resource implications.

Renal support

Ninety per cent of patients with acute renal failure (ARF) requiring replacement therapy should survive; however, survival is reduced substantially when ARF and respiratory failure coexist (50%) and catastrophically in the presence of obstructive jaundice (25%)[170] or MODS (10%).[171] While assessment of plasma urea and creatinine is essential, these variables do not deteriorate before substantial renal function is lost. Similarly, oliguria develops relatively late, but loss of renal concentrating power provides earlier evidence of impaired function.

PATHOGENESIS OF ARF IN CRITICAL ILLNESS

In health a countercurrent circulation renders the outer renal medulla relatively hypoxic compared with the whole kidney. Moreover, the outer medulla has intense metabolic activity because of active tubular transport.[172] The microcirculatory changes and increased metabolic activity associated with sepsis, together with hypovolaemia, may lead to critical hypoxia in this vulnerable area. Inflammatory mediators may cause direct renal damage, and tubular apoptosis causes plugging of nephrons by casts, worsening renal dysfunction. Pre-existing renal impairment, jaundice, hepatic failure and rhabdomyolysis predispose to ARF. Many drugs including non-steroidal anti-inflammatory agents, aminoglycosides, β-blockers, angiotensin-converting enzyme inhibitors, cyclosporin and cytotoxic agents are potentially nephrotoxic. Intravenous radiological contrast media may precipitate ARF, particularly in the presence of hypotension, and adequate fluid resuscitation before investigation is essential.[173]

MANAGEMENT OF RENAL DYSFUNCTION

Renal perfusion pressure must be maintained with correction of hypovolaemia and optimisation of cardiac output. Acute hyperkalaemia, acidosis and fluid overload should be treated appropriately, and the underlying cause for renal dysfunction addressed. Urinary outflow obstruction is excluded by bladder catheterisation; absolute anuria in a catheterised patient suggests catheter malposition or blockage. Various measures have been suggested to restore urine output in early renal dysfunction after correction of hypovolaemia. Low-dose (<3 mg/kg per min) dopamine or dopexamine have their advocates. Others recommend a loop diuretic such as furosemide (frusemide) 250 mg or bumetanide 1 mg. A placebo-controlled, randomised, prospective study of low- and high-dose dopamine in ARF showed no difference in mortality or dialysis requirement between the three groups.[174] The α-adrenergic effects of dopamine are unpredictable and there is no evidence that dopexamine influences outcome in ARF.[175] Loop diuretics have been recommended because they inhibit active solute transport in the outer medulla and possibly prevent critical hypoxia,[176] but it is uncertain whether they improve outcome. Most pharmacological studies have been conducted in patients with established ARF, and the ideal drug for restoring urine output before ARF develops is not known. Volume overload is the principal cause of morbidity in established ARF. Meticulous fluid balance, with daily weighing when possible, is essential. Plasma potassium and pH must be closely monitored, and an opinion from a nephrologist is advisable.

ARTIFICIAL RENAL SUPPORT

Indications for artificial renal support include correction of fluid overload, hyperkalaemia, persistent acidosis and rapidly climbing plasma creatinine concentration (>500 mmol/L). The threshold for intervention varies and will be lower in patients at risk of MODS than in those with isolated ARF. In critical illness, it is not unusual for the volume of essential infusions to exceed that which the patient can tolerate. This is particularly common when intravenous nutrition is required, and artificial renal support may be required to 'make space'.

Haemodialysis

During haemodialysis, blood and dialysate are pumped in opposite directions, separated by a semipermeable membrane. Solute is removed by countercurrent diffusion and solvent by ultrafiltration across a pressure gradient. Acute access is usually veno-venous in order to avoid complications of arterial cannulation, but patients requiring chronic dialysis will have surgically created shunts. When these patients present as surgical emergencies, every effort must be made to preserve the shunt; it must not be used for routine vascular access. Anticoagulation with heparin or prostacyclin is required to prevent filter coagulation. Haemodialysis enables rapid removal of large fluid volumes but may cause significant hypotension. It is indicated for uncomplicated ARF but is tolerated poorly by patients with severe sepsis or MODS. Haemodialysis may be the treatment of choice for rapid correction of life-threatening hyperkalaemia.

Continuous veno-venous haemofiltration

In continuous veno-venous haemofiltration (CVVH), anticoagulated blood is pumped through a filter and the ultrafiltrate, which is similar to the aqueous components of plasma, is discarded. Fluid is removed continuously at a slower rate than during haemodialysis, and hence CVVH causes less haemodynamic disturbance. If CVVH is performed for reasons other than fluid overload, the filtered fluid is replaced. Haemofiltration can improve outcome in animal models of sepsis by removing proinflammatory mediators,[177] although there is no convincing evidence of efficacy in humans.

When adult ICU patients who required haemofiltration were randomised to ultrafiltration rates of 20, 35 or 45 mL/hour, survival was significantly reduced in the group which had the lowest filtration rate.[178] No difference was observed between the other two groups. Most patients had a surgical cause for renal failure, but the incidence of sepsis was relatively low in each group. It was acknowledged that higher filtration rates may be difficult to achieve in patients with low blood flows.

Peritoneal dialysis

Peritoneal dialysis has little role in the management of ARF in critical illness and is contraindicated by peritoneal contamination. In patients with pre-existing renal failure already managed by peritoneal dialysis, peritoneal infection may be a subtle cause of sepsis. When a patient receiving peritoneal dialysis requires laparotomy, every effort should be made to preserve the peritoneal catheter, and prior discussion with the managing renal team is recommended.

The abdomen and gastrointestinal tract in critical illness

ABDOMINAL COMPARTMENT SYNDROME

Major abdominal trauma, surgery for leaking abdominal aortic aneurysm and massive transfusion may lead to intestinal dilatation and retroperitoneal oedema, which increase the pressure in the closed abdomen. As a consequence, ventilation pressures increase and hypoxia ensues. Cardiac output may fall and oliguria/anuria may also occur. Abdominal decompression with temporary closure is often necessary[179] (see also Chapter 13).

INFLUENCE OF THE GASTROINTESTINAL TRACT ON SEPSIS

Primary gastrointestinal disease may cause SIRS, sepsis and MODS outright. However, the gut may contribute to the patient's deterioration even when the initial insult involves other systems. The gut may be the source of the 'second hit' that precipitates progression to MODS; indeed some have labelled it the 'motor of multiple organ failure'.[180] Exposure to endotoxin or splanchnic reperfusion injury may increase mucosal permeability[181] and bacterial translocation[182] to reticuloendothelial tissue, where previously primed macrophages and Kupffer cells are activated. This hypothesis may explain why enteric bacteraemia is observed in MODS even when there is no obvious septic focus.[183]

GASTROINTESTINAL CONDITIONS THAT MAY COMPLICATE MAJOR ILLNESS

Abdominal problems may complicate, as well as cause, serious illness. Signs may be subtle, particularly in ventilated patients, and a high index of clinical suspicion is necessary. For example, an unexplained metabolic acidosis may have an abdominal cause.

Gastrointestinal motility abnormalities

Acute gastric dilatation Acute massive gastric dilatation predisposes to aspiration[184] and can limit diaphragmatic excursion and impair ventilation. If untreated, massive dilatation may progress to emphysematous gastric necrosis. Immediate treatment comprises support of breathing and nasogastric intubation.

Delayed gastric emptying Delayed gastric emptying is associated with diabetic autonomic neuropathy, subtotal gastrectomy, or gastroenterostomy performed for obstruction. Distal intestinal motility is usually normal but nasogastric intubation is required to prevent aspiration and facilitate fluid and electrolyte management. Intravenous erythromycin 1 mg/kg four times daily[185] may hasten resolution, but recovery often takes several weeks during which nutritional support will be required.

Ileus and obstruction Postoperative small bowel ileus usually resolves within days, regardless of the extent of bowel handling.[186] Drugs or electrolyte abnormalities may delay resolution, but failure to progress often indicates ongoing retroperitoneal or abdominal pathology. Ileus may be difficult to distinguish from adhesive obstruction, and contrast studies may clarify the situation. Adhesive obstruction frequently resolves but refractory cases require laparotomy. A rare form of obstruction is seen in thin bed-bound patients in which the superior mesenteric artery occludes the duodenum.[187] Surgery is seldom necessary, but nasogastric aspiration and nutritional support are required until mobilisation is possible.

Colonic pseudo-obstruction Colonic pseudo-obstruction (see also Chapter 10) is associated with immobility, electrolyte abnormalities and fractures of the spine, pelvis and lower limbs.[188] Distension may be dramatic but tenderness is uncommon. If massive colonic dilatation or peritonism develops, urgent exclusion of organic obstruction by contrast enema or endoscopy is necessary. Decompression may be achieved by rigid sigmoidoscopy or colonoscopy.

Peptic ulceration

Severe illness, mechanical ventilation and coagulopathy predispose to peptic ulceration. Significant haemorrhage may occur and carries considerable mortality.[189] The ideal prophylaxis is controversial. Reduced gastric acidity possibly predisposes to stomach colonisation by pathogenic bacteria that may subsequently cause pneumonia.

A meta-analysis suggested that sucralfate was preferable to H_2 receptor antagonists for peptic ulcer prophylaxis in the critically ill. Sucralfate was associated with reduced odds of pneumonia and possibly lower mortality.[190]

The same authors conducted a randomised controlled trial to test their conclusions. Paradoxically, this study suggested that ranitidine significantly reduced the risk of clinically important haemorrhage compared with sucralfate and that it did not predispose to pneumonia.[191]

The outcome from stress-related mucosal disease is worse than that for peptic ulceration due to other causes.[192] Prompt diagnosis is essential and early surgery should be considered for haemorrhage in this group because hypovolaemia is poorly tolerated. It is possible that proton pump inhibitors will prove superior to H_2 receptor antagonists but current data are limited.[193]

Pancreatobiliary disease

Acute acalculous cholecystitis may lead to biliary peritonitis. Non-specific derangement of liver biochemistry is common but not universal. Ultrasound may reveal gallbladder thickening, and demonstration of intramural gas is particularly concerning. The treatment is urgent cholecystectomy (see also Chapter 8).[194] Pancreatitis may present late after trauma and can complicate upper abdominal surgery, cardiopulmonary bypass and investigations such as endoscopic retrograde cholangiopancreatography (ERCP) and percutaneous transhepatic cholangiography. Diagnosis is confirmed by hyperamylasaemia, and management is usually supportive. Patients should be stratified for prognosis using biochemical criteria[195] and those with severe disease should undergo dynamic axial CT. Some advocate broad-spectrum antibiotics for severe disease[196] but opinions differ.[197] When severe pancreatitis is caused by common bile duct calculi, urgent ERCP may be beneficial,[198] and debridement is recommended for infected pancreatic necrosis.[199]

Liver dysfunction

Sepsis and intravenous nutrition can produce non-specific derangements of liver biochemistry.[200] Abnormal liver tests may also reflect infective hepatitis, liver abscesses, or drug or transfusion reactions. Imaging is indicated to exclude biliary obstruction and may also reveal occult collections, which might contribute to hepatic dysfunction. Urgent biliary decompression is required for extra-hepatic obstruction, particularly in the presence of cholangitis. In most other circumstances, treatment of liver dysfunction is supportive until resolution occurs. Cholestatic medication should be stopped, but intravenous nutrition can be continued unless liver function deteriorates. Encephalopathy, hypoglycaemia, acidosis or coagulopathy may indicate hepatic decompensation and the need for specialist care.[201] Chronic liver disease, or recent hepatic resection, predispose to liver failure, and the link between hepatic and renal failure must not be ignored. Adequate hydration is essential and sodium overload must be avoided.

Intestinal ischaemia

Small bowel ischaemia can occur secondary to low cardiac output, embolisation or venous sludging. Vasopressors and digoxin can precipitate non-occlusive ischaemia, which has high mortality.[202]

Early diagnosis is notoriously difficult but bloody diarrhoea or pain out of proportion to abdominal signs are ominous. Recent work suggests that elevated glutathione S-transferase may be a marker of bowel ischaemia.[203] In the severely ill, the treatment is resection with exteriorisation. Large bowel ischaemia is usually left-sided and is associated with low cardiac output and aortic surgery. Often only the mucosa is affected and treatment is conservative,[204] but systemic upset or peritonitis are indications for resection with exteriorisation.

Colitis

Pseudomembranous colitis, secondary to infection with *Clostridium difficile*, is associated with antibiotic exposure. The diagnosis is based on detection of toxin in the faeces. Mucosal sloughing seen on sigmoidoscopy is not universal. Most patients settle with treatment with enteral metronidazole or vancomycin. However, subtotal colectomy with exteriorisation may be necessary in severe disease. Neutropenic colitis is associated with chemotherapy for haematological malignancy. The right colon is usually affected, and plain radiography may show dilatation and oedema. Initial supportive management with broad-spectrum antibiotics is recommended. Resection is reserved for peritonitis or failure to progress.[205]

Nutrition in critical illness

Nutritional support will be required by many critically ill patients (see Chapter 17). Enteral feeding is preferred because it is relatively safe, efficacious and economical; furthermore, it may preserve the gut mucosal barrier. Enteral nutrition is contraindicated by small bowel ileus or when there is inadequate mucosa available for absorption. In such circumstances parenteral nutrition is required. Jejunostomy catheters or nasojejunal tubes may allow enteral feeding, even when there is a proximal anastomosis or delayed gastric emptying, provided distal motility is adequate. Recent studies indicate that enteral feeding is safe immediately after surgery[206] and in acute pancreatitis.[207] Neither ventilation nor absent bowel sounds are contraindications to enteral feeding provided that gastric emptying is normal.[208]

NUTRITION AS THERAPY

Starvation and parenteral nutrition are associated with compromised gut mucosal barrier function and bacterial translocation in animals[209] but similar events may not occur in humans. Nevertheless, nutritional therapy has been proposed as a means to reduce the incidence of sepsis.

 Early enteral nutrition was associated with a reduction in infective complications after blunt trauma;[210] these findings were supported by a meta-analysis of eight randomised prospective studies.[211]

Several nutrients have been ascribed specific pharmacological properties in addition to their role as energy or nitrogen sources. Enteral feeds containing arginine, ω-3 polyunsaturated fatty acids and ribonucleic acids may be beneficial for septic patients[212] but further studies are required. In animals, glutamine appears essential to maintain mucosal integrity, and intravenous replacement reverses the changes associated with starvation or parenteral nutrition.[213] However, evidence that glutamine-supplemented parenteral nutrition alters clinical outcome is lacking (see Chapter 17).[214]

Ethical considerations in critical care

Intensive care may be distressing, undignified and unjustified in insurmountable illness.[215] Similarly, surgeons should not attempt technical tours de force on patients who have no prospect of surviving them.[216] Withdrawal of treatment is ethically justified when there is no reasonable chance of benefit to the patient.[215] There is no moral or legal difference between withholding and withdrawal of treatment.[217] Complications are frequently inevitable in the critically ill and, when they occur, should be explained to patient and family. An honest approach is likely to reduce anxiety and, possibly, litigation. When bad news must be conveyed, the doctor should ensure that it is done in sympathetic surroundings with sufficient time available to answer all likely questions. It may be beneficial to arrange for a briefed counsellor to follow up the discussion. Medical staff must always act in the patient's best interest. If a doctor has a personal conscientious objection to treatment that could benefit the patient, then that patient's care should be handed over to a colleague.[215] In the UK, doctors, but not relatives, have the legal right to make decisions for the patient. When medical staff and families disagree over treatment issues, the intervention of the patient's representative or a second medical opinion is advisable.

Key points

- Sepsis is common among UK hospital patients and has a high mortality.
- Development of sepsis is associated with complex interactions between inflammatory mediators.
- A systematic approach, based on a sound understanding of pathophysiology, is essential to successful sepsis management.
- Therapeutic modulation of inflammatory mediator activity and the associated metabolic consequences may improve outcome in sepsis.
- Maintenance of tissue oxygenation is crucial and may require airway, ventilatory and circulatory support, with which the surgeon should be familiar.
- While abdominal pathology may precipitate sepsis, critical illness may also predispose to further abdominal complications.

REFERENCES

1. Friedman G, Silva E, Vincent JL. Has the mortality of septic shock changed with time. Crit Care Med 1998; 26:2078–86.

2. Crowe M, Ispahani P, Humphreys H et al. Bacteraemia in the adult intensive care unit of a teaching hospital in Nottingham, UK, 1985–1996. Eur J Clin Microbiol Infect Dis 1998; 17:377–84.

3. Angus DC, Linde-Zwirble WT, Lidicker J et al. Epidemiology of severe sepsis in the United States: analysis of incidence, outcome, and associated costs of care. Crit Care Med 2001; 29:1303–10.

4 Alberti C, Brun-Buisson, Buchardi H et al. Epidemiology of sepsis and infection in ICU patients from an international multicentre cohort study. Intensive Care Med 2002; 28:108–21.

5. Simpson JA, Weiner ESC (eds) Oxford English Dictionary, 2nd edn. Oxford: Oxford University Press, 1993.

6. Baue AE. Multiple and progressive sequential systems failure, a syndrome of the 1970s. Arch Surg 1975; 110:779–81.

7. Goris RJ, Beokhorst PA, Nuytinck KS. Multiple organ failure: generalized autodestructive inflammation. Arch Surg 1985; 120:1109–15.

8. Norton LW. Does drainage of intra-abdominal pus reverse multiple organ failure. Am J Surg 1985; 149:347–51.

9. American College of Chest Physicians/Society of Critical Care Medicine Consensus Conference. Definitions for sepsis and organ failure and guidelines for the use of innovative therapies in sepsis. Crit Care Med 1992; 20:864–74.

10. Rangel-Frausto MS, Pittet D, Costigan M et al. The natural history of the systemic inflammatory response syndrome (SIRS). A prospective study. JAMA 1995; 273:117–23.

11. Pittet D, Rangel-Frausto S, Li N et al. Systemic inflammatory response syndrome, sepsis, severe sepsis and ICU patients. Intensive Care Med 1995; 21:302–9.

12. Smail N, Messiah A, Eduoard A et al. Role of systemic inflammatory response syndrome and infection in the occurrence of early multiple organ dysfunction syndrome following severe trauma. Intensive Care Med 1995; 21:813–16.

13. Pinskey MR, Vincent JL, Deviere J et al. Serum cytokine levels in human septic shock. Relation to multiple-system organ failure and mortality. Chest 1993; 103:565–75.

14. Fry DE, Pearlstein L, Fulton RL et al. Multiple system organ failure: the role of uncontrolled infection. Arch Surg 1980; 115:136–40.

15. Zimmerman JE, Knauss WA, Wagner DP et al. A comparison of risks and outcomes for patients with organ system failure: 1982–90. Crit Care Med 1996; 24:1633–41.

16. Segal AW, Peters TJ. Characterisation of the enzyme defect in chronic granulomatous disease. Lancet 1976; i:1363–5.

17. Kuijpers TW, Van-Lier RA, Hamann D et al. Leukocyte adhesion deficiency type 1 (LAD-1)/variant. A novel immunodeficiency syndrome characterised by dysfunctional beta2 integrins. J Clin Invest 1997; 100:1725–33.

18. Bone RC. Toward a theory regarding the pathogenesis of the systemic inflammatory response syndrome: what we do and do not know about cytokine regulation. Crit Care Med 1996; 24:163–72.

19. Hunt BJ. Endothelial cell activation. Br Med J 1998; 316:1328–9.

20. Watters JM, Bessey PQ, Dinarello CA et al. Both inflammatory and endocrine mediators simulate host response to sepsis. Arch Surg 1986; 121:179–90.

21. Starnes HF, Warren RS, Jeevanandam M et al. Tumour necrosis factor and the acute metabolic response to stress in man. J Clin Invest 1988; 82:1321–5.

22. Revhaug A, Mitchie HR, Manson JM et al. Inhibition of cyclo-oxygenase attenuates the metabolic to endotoxin in humans. Arch Surg 1988; 123:162–70.

23. Goldie AS, Fearon KCH, Ross JA et al. Natural cytokine antagonists and endogenous anti-endotoxin core antibodies in sepsis syndrome. JAMA 1995; 274:172–7.

24. Deitch EA. Multiple organ failure. Pathophysiology and potential future failure. Ann Surg 1992; 216:117–34.

25. Cochrane CG. The enhancement of inflammatory injury. Am Rev Respir Dis 1987; 136:1–3.

26. Cerra FB. Hypermetabolism, organ failure, and metabolic support. Surgery 1987; 101:1–14.

27. O'Keefe SJD, Dicker J. Is plasma albumin concentration useful in the assessment of nutritional status of hospital patients? Eur J Clin Nutr 1988; 42:41–5.

28. McCluskey A, Thomas AN, Bowles BJ et al. The prognostic value of serial measurements of serum albumin concentration in patients admitted to an intensive care unit. Anaesthesia 1996; 51:724–7.

29. Whicher JT, Evans SW. Acute phase proteins. Hosp Update 1990; 16:899–905.

30. van den Burghe G, Wouters P, Weekers F et al. Intensive insulin therapy in critically ill patients. N Engl J Med 2001; 345:1359–67.

> Strict blood sugar control is associated with lower mortality in the critically ill.

31. Bernard GR, Artigas A, Brigham KL et al. Report of the American–European consensus conference on ARDS: definitions, mechanisms, relevant outcomes and clinical trial coordination. Intensive Care Med 1994; 20:225–32.

32. Anderson ID. Assessing the critically ill surgical patient. In: Anderson ID (ed.) Care of the critically ill surgical patient. London: Arnold, 1999; pp. 7–15.

33. American College of Surgeons Committee on Trauma. Shock. In: Advanced trauma life support (ATLS) for doctors, instructor course manual. Chicago: American College of Surgeons, 1997; pp. 97–122.

34. Hiramatsu K, Aritaka N, Hanaki H et al. Dissemination in Japanese hospitals of strains of *Staphylococcus aureus* resistant to vancomycin. Lancet 1997; 350:1670–3.

35. Vandenbrouke-Grauls C. Management of methicillin-resistant *Staphylococcus aureus* in the Netherlands. Rev Med Microbiol 1998; 9:109–16.

36. Standing Medical Advisory Committee Subgroup on Microbial Resistance. The path of least resistance. London: Department of Health, 1998.

37. Durack DT, Lukes AS, Bright DK et al. New criteria for diagnosis of infective endocarditis: utilization of specific echocardiographic findings. Am J Med 1994; 96:200–9.

38. Merrick MV. Blood, infection and inflammation. In: Essentials of nuclear medicine, 2nd edn. London: Springer, 1998; pp. 203–19.

39. Datz FL. Indium-111-labelled leukocytes for imaging infection: current status. Semin Nucl Med 1994; 24:92–109.

40. Anderson ID, Fearon KCH, Grant IS. Laparotomy for abdominal sepsis in the critically ill. Br J Surg 1996; 83:535–9.

41. Hinsdale JG, Jaffe BM. Re-operation for intra-abdominal sepsis: indications and results in a modern critical care setting. Ann Surg 1984; 199:31–6.

42. Zeigler EJ, Fisher CJ, Sprung C et al. Treatment of Gram-negative bacteraemia and septic shock with HA-1A human monoclonal antibody against endotoxin. A randomised double-blind, placebo-controlled trial. N Engl J Med 1991; 324:429–36.

43. Reinhart K, Karzai W. Anti-tumour necrosis factor therapy in sepsis: update on clinical trials and lessons learned. Crit Care Med 2001; 29(Suppl.):S121–S125.

44. Fisher CJ, Dhainault JF, Opal SM et al. Recombinant human interleukin 1 receptor antagonist in the treatment of patients with sepsis syndrome. Results from a randomized, double-blind, placebo-controlled trial. JAMA 1994; 271:1836–44.

45. Dhainault JF, Tenaillon A, Le Tulzo Y et al. Platelet-activating factor receptor antagonist BN52021 in the treatment of severe sepsis: a phase III randomized, double-blind, placebo-controlled, multicentre clinical trial. Crit Care Med 1994; 22:1720–8.

46. Zeni F, Freeman B, Natanson C. Anti-inflammatory therapies to treat sepsis and septic shock: a reassessment. Crit Care Med 1997; 25:1095–100.

47. Fong Y, Moldawer LL, Shires GT et al. The biological characteristics of cytokines and their implications in surgical injury. Surg Gynecol Obstet 1990; 170:363–78.

48. Tracey KJ. Tumour necrosis factor (cachectin) in the biology of septic shock syndrome. Circ Shock 1991; 35:123–8.

49. Arai K, Lee F, Miyajima A et al. Cytokines: co-ordinators of immune and inflammatory responses. Annu Rev Biochem 1990; 59:783–836.

50. Bone RC. Sir Isaac Newton, sepsis, SIRS, and CARS. Crit Care Med 1996; 24:1125–8.

51. Levi M, ten Cate H. Disseminated intravascular coagulation. N Engl J Med 1999; 341:586–92.

52. Bernard GR, Vincent J-L, Laterre P-F et al. Efficacy and safety of recombinant human activated protein C for severe sepsis. N Engl J Med 2001; 344:699–709.

> Administration of activated protein C reduces sepsis-related mortality in the critically ill.

53. Warren BL, Eid A, Singer P et al. High dose anti-thrombin III in severe sepsis: a randomized controlled trial. JAMA 2001; 286:1869–78.

54. DePaulo V, Kessler C, Opal SM. Success or failure in phase III sepsis trials: comparisons between the Drotrecogin Alfa (activated) and Antithrombin III clinical trials. Adv Sepsis 2001; 1:114–24.

55. Annane D, Sebille V, Troche G et al. A 3-level prognostic classification in septic shock based on

cortisol levels and cortisol response to corticotrophin. JAMA 2000; 283:1038–45.

56. Findling JW, Waters VO, Raff H. The dissociation of renin and aldosterone during critical illness. J Clin Endocrinol Metab 1987; 64:592–5.

57. Annane D, Bellissant E, Sebile V et al. Impaired pressor sensitivity to noradrenaline in septic shock patients with and without adrenal function reserve. Br J Clin Pharmacol 1998; 46:589–97.

58. Lefering R, Neugebauer EA. Steroid controversy in sepsis and septic shock: a meta-analysis. Crit Care Med 1995; 23:1294–303.

59. Cronin L, Cook DJ, Carlet J et al. Corticosteroid treatment for sepsis: a critical appraisal and meta-analysis of the literature. Crit Care Med 1995; 23:1430–9.

60. Annane D, Sebille V, Charpentier C et al. Effect of treatment with low doses of hydrocortisone and fludrocortisone on mortality in patients with septic shock. JAMA 2002; 288:862–71.

Physiological-dose steroid replacement improves outcome in severe sepsis.

61. Cooper MS, Stewart PM. Corticosteroid insufficiency in acutely ill patients. N Engl J Med 2003; 348:727–34.

62. Department of Health guidelines on admission to and discharge from intensive care and high dependency units. London: Department of Health, 1996.

63. Singer M, Little R. ABC of intensive care: cutting edge. Br Med J 1999; 319:501–4.

64. McQuillan P, Pilkington S, Allan A et al. Confidential enquiry into quality of care before admission to intensive care. Br Med J 1998; 316:1853–8.

65. McGloin H, Adam S, Singer M. The quality of pre-ICU care influences outcome of patients admitted from the ward. Clin Intensive Care 1997; 8:104.

66. Smith GJ, Nielsen N. ABC of intensive care. Criteria for admission. Br Med J 1999; 318:1544–7.

67. Knaus WA, Draper EA, Wagner DP et al. APACHE II: a severity of disease classification system. Crit Care Med 1985; 13:818–29.

68. Copeland GP, Jones D, Walters M. POSSUM: a scoring system for surgical audit. Br J Surg 1991; 78:355–60.

69. Champion HR, Sacco WJ, Copes WS et al. A revision of the Trauma Score. J Trauma 1989; 29:623–9.

70. Franklin CM, Rackow EC, Mamdani B et al. Decreases in mortality on a large urban medical service by facilitating access to critical care. Arch Intern Med 1988; 148:1403–5.

71. Rowan KM, Kerr JH, Major E et al. Intensive Care Society's APACHE II study in Britain and Ireland II: outcome comparisons in intensive care units after adjustment for case mix by the American APACHE II method. Br Med J 1993; 307:977–81.

72. Shapiro BJ. Blood gas analysis. In: Webb AR, Shapiro MJ, Singer M et al. (eds) Oxford textbook of critical care. Oxford: Oxford University Press, 1999; pp. 1119–23.

73. Schlichtig R. Base excess is a powerful tool in the ICU. Critical care symposium. Soc Crit Care Med 1996; 1:1–30.

74. Whitman ED. Complications associated with the use of central venous access devices. Curr Probl Surg 1996; 33:309–88.

75. Nyström B, Oleson Larsen S, Dankert J et al. Bacteraemia in surgical patients with intravenous devices: a European multicentre incidence study. J Hosp Infect 1983; 4:338–49.

76. Webb AR. Fluid management in intensive care: avoiding hypovolaemia. Br J Intensive Care 1997; 7:59–64.

77. Mythen M, Clutton-Brock T. The oxygen trail: measurement. Br Med Bull 1999; 55:109–24.

78. Elliot CG, Zimmerman GA, Clemmer TP. Complications of pulmonary artery catheterization in the care of critically ill patients. Chest 1979; 76:647–52.

79. Groenveld ABJ. Pulmonary artery catheterisation. In: Webb AR, Shapiro MJ, Singer M et al. (eds) Oxford textbook of critical care. Oxford: Oxford University Press, 1999; pp. 1094–8.

80. Connors AF, Speroff T, Dawson NV et al. The effectiveness of right heart catheterization in the initial care of the critically ill. JAMA 1996; 276:889–97.

81. Soni N. Swan song for the Swan–Ganz catheter? Br Med J 1996; 313:763–4.

82. Gnaegi A, Fiehl F, Perret C. Intensive care physicians' insufficient knowledge of right heart catheterization at the bedside. Time to act. Crit Care Med 1997; 25:213–20.

83. Espersen K. Comparison of cardiac output measurement techniques: thermodilution, Doppler, CO_2-rebreathing and the direct Fick method. Acta Anaesthesiol Scand 1995; 39:245–51.

84. Singer M, Clarke J, Bennet ED. Continuous haemodynamic assessment by esophageal Doppler. Crit Care Med 1989; 17:447–52.

85. Zhao X, Mashikian J, Panzica P et al. Comparison of thermodilution bolus cardiac output and Doppler cardiac output in the early post-cardiopulmonary bypass period. J Cardiothorac Vasc Anesth 2003; 17:193–8.

86. Jonas MM, Tanser SJ. Lithium dilution measurement of cardiac output and arterial pulse waveform analysis: an indicator dilution calibrated beat-by-beat system for continuous estimation of cardiac output. Curr Opin Crit Care 2002; 8:257–61.

87. Hamilton TT, Huber LM, Jessen ME. Pulse CO: a less invasive method to monitor cardiac output from arterial pressure after cardiac surgery. Ann Thorac Surg 2002; 74:1408–12.

88. Guttierrez G, Palizas F, Doglio G et al. Gastric intramucosal pH as a therapeutic index of tissue oxygenation in critically ill patients. Lancet 1992; 339:195–9.

89. Ivatury RR, Simon RJ, Havriliak D et al. Gastric mucosal pH and oxygen delivery and oxygen consumption indices in the assessment of adequacy of resuscitation after trauma: a prospective randomised study. J Trauma 1995; 39:128–36.

90. Hamilton MA, Mythen MG. Gastric tonometry: where do we stand? Curr Opin Crit Care 2001; 7:122–7.

91. Wagner PD, Dueck R, Clausen JL et al. Ventilation–perfusion inequality in chronic obstructive pulmonary disease. J Clin Invest 1977; 59:203–16.

92. Schlichtig R, Pinsky MR. Flow distribution during progressive haemorrhage is a determinant of critical O_2 delivery. J Appl Physiol 1991; 70:169–78.

93. Duncan AW, Oh TE, Hillman DR. PEEP and CPAP. Anaesth Intensive Care 1986; 14:236–50.

94. Hormann C, Baum M, Putenen C et al. Biphasic positive airway pressure (BiPAP): a new mode of ventilatory support. Eur J Anaesthesiol 1994; 11:37–42.

95. Antonelli M, Conti G, Rocco M et al. A comparison of non-invasive positive pressure ventilation and conventional mechanical ventilation in patients with acute respiratory failure. N Engl J Med 1998; 339:429–35.

96. Meduri GU. Non-invasive positive-pressure ventilation in patients with acute respiratory failure. Clin Chest Med 1996; 17:513–53.

97. McKibben A, Ravenscroft SA. Pressure-controlled and volume-cycled mechanical ventilation. Clin Chest Med 1996; 17:395–410.

98. Shanholz C, Brower R. Should inverse ratio ventilation be used in adult respiratory distress syndrome? Am J Respir Crit Care Med 1994; 149:1354–8.

99. Brochard L, Harf A, Lorino H et al. Inspiratory pressure support prevents diaphragmatic fatigue during weaning from mechanical ventilation. Am Rev Respir Dis 1989; 139:513–21.

100. Rouby JJ, Lherme T, de Lassale EM et al. Histologic aspects of pulmonary barotrauma in critically ill patients with acute respiratory failure. Intensive Care Med 1993; 19:383–9.

101. Ito Y, Veldhuizen RAW, Yao L et al. Ventilation strategies affect surfactant aggregate conversion in acute lung injury. Am J Respir Crit Care Med 1997; 155:493–9.

102. von Bethmann AN, Brausch F, Nusing R et al. Hyperventilation induces release of cytokines from perfused mouse lung. Am J Respir Crit Care Med 1998; 157:263–72.

103. Farge D, de la Coussaye JE, Beloucif S et al. Interactions between hemodynamic and hormonal modifications during PEEP induced antidiuresis and antinatriuresis. Chest 1995; 107:1095–100.

104. Gattinoni L, Pesenti A, Bombino M et al. Relationships between lung computed tomographic density, gas exchange, and PEEP in acute respiratory failure. Anesthesiology 1988; 68:824–32.

105. Douglas WW, Rehder K, Beynen FM et al. Improved oxygenation in patients with acute respiratory failure: the prone position. Am Rev Respir Dis 1977; 115:559–66.

106. Brimouille S, Rocmans P, de Rood et al. High-frequency jet ventilation in the management of tracheal laceration. Crit Care Med 1990; 18:338–9.

107. Gluck E, Heard S, Patel C. Use of ultrahigh frequency ventilation in patients with ARDS. A preliminary report. Chest 1993; 103:1413–20.

108. Frostell CG, Blomqvist H, Hedenstierna G et al. Inhaled nitric oxide selectively reverses human hypoxic pulmonary vasoconstriction without causing systemic vasodilatation. Anesthesiology 1993; 78:427–35.

109. Gerlach H, Rossaint R, Pappert D et al. Time-course and dose–response of nitric oxide inhalation for systemic oxygenation and pulmonary hypertension in patients with adult respiratory distress syndrome. Eur J Clin Invest 1993; 23:49–52.

110. Rossaint R, Falke KJ, Lopez F et al. Inhaled nitric oxide for the adult respiratory distress syndrome. N Engl J Med 1993; 328:399–405.

111. Barbera JA, Roger N, Roca J et al. Worsening of pulmonary gas exchange with nitric oxide inhalation in chronic obstructive pulmonary disease. Lancet 1996; 347:436–40.

112. Sokol J, Jacobs SE, Bohn D. Inhaled nitric oxide for acute hypoxemic respiratory failure in adults and children. Cochrane Database of Systematic Reviews 2003; 1:CD002787.

113. UK Collaborative ECMO Trial Group. UK collaborative randomised trial of neonatal extracorporeal membrane oxygenation. Lancet 1996; 348:75–82.

114. Zapol WM, Snider MT, Hill JD et al. Extracorporeal membrane oxygenation in severe acute respiratory failure. JAMA 1979; 242:2193–6.

115. Leonard RC. Liquid ventilation. Anaesth Intensive Care 1998; 26:11–21.

116. Hirschl RB, Pranikoff T, Wise C et al. Initial experience with partial liquid ventilation in adult patients with adult respiratory distress syndrome. JAMA 1996; 275:383–9.

117. Evans TW, Smithies M. ABC of intensive care: organ dysfunction. Br Med J 1999; 318:1606–9.

118. Meduri GU, Headley AS, Golden E et al. Effect of prolonged methylprednisolone therapy in unresolving acute respiratory distress syndrome: a randomised controlled trial. JAMA 1998; 280:159–65.

119. Gattinoni L, Pelosi P, Suter PM et al. Acute respiratory distress syndrome caused by pulmonary and extrapulmonary disease: different syndromes? Am J Respir Crit Care Med 1998; 158:3–11.

120. Malbrain ML. Abdominal pressure in the critically ill: measurement and clinical relevance. Intensive Care Med 1999; 25:1453–8.

121. Gattinoni L, Vagginelli F, Chiumello D et al. Physiological rationale for ventilator setting in acute lung injury/acute respiratory distress syndrome patients. Crit Care Med 2003; 31:S300–S304.

122. Acute Respiratory Distress Syndrome Network. Ventilation with lower tidal volumes as compared with traditional tidal volumes for acute lung injury and the acute respiratory distress syndrome. N Engl J Med 2000; 342:1301–8.

123. Brower RG, Rubenfeld GD. Lung-protective ventilation strategies in acute lung injury. Crit Care Med 2003; 31:S312–S316.

Volume- and pressure-limited ventilation improves outcome in acute lung injury.

124. Keogh BF, Ranieri VM. Ventilatory support in the acute respiratory distress syndrome. Br Med Bull 1998; 55:140–64.

125. Association of Anaesthetists of Great Britain and Ireland. Suspected anaphylactic reactions associated with anaesthesia. London: Association of Anaesthetists of Great Britain and Ireland, 2003.

126. Forrester JS, Diamond GA, Swann HJC. Correlative classification of clinical and haemodynamic function after acute myocardial infarction. Am J Cardiol 1977; 39:137–45.

127. Schierhout G, Roberts I. Fluid resuscitation with colloid or crystalloid solutions in critically ill patients: a systematic review of randomised trials. Br Med J 1998; 316:961–4.

128. Cochrane Injuries Group Albumin Reviewers. Human albumin administration in critically ill patients: systematic review of randomised trials. Br Med J 1998; 317:235–40.

129. Choi P T-L, Yip G, Quionnez LG et al. Crystalloids vs. colloids in fluid resuscitation: a systematic review. Crit Care Med 1998; 27:200–10.

130. Grootendorst AF, van Wigenburg MGM, de Laat PHJM et al. Albumin abuse in intensive care medicine. Intensive Care Med 1988; 14:554–7.

131. Moon MR, Lucas CE, Ledgerwood AM et al. Free water clearance after supplemental albumin replacement for shock. Circ Shock 1989; 28:1–8.

132. Mallick A, Bodenham AR. Present and future prospects of haemoglobin solutions in resuscitation and intensive care. Br J Intensive Care 1999; 9:87–97.

133. Hebert PC, Wells G, Tweeddale M et al. Does transfusion practice affect mortality in critically ill patients? Am J Respir Crit Care Med 1997; 155:1618–23.

134. Hebert PC, Wells G, Blajchman MA et al. A multicenter, randomized, controlled clinical trial of transfusion requirements in critical care. N Engl J Med 1999; 340:409–17.

Liberal transfusion of non-leucocyte-depleted blood may be detrimental in normovolaemic critical care patients.

135. Nelson DP, Samsel RW, Wood LD et al. Pathologic supply dependence of systemic and intestinal O_2 uptake during endotoxaemia. J Appl Physiol 1988; 64:2410–19.

136. Dahn MS, Lange P, Lobdell K et al. Hepatic blood flow and splanchnic oxygen consumption measurements in clinical sepsis. Surgery 1989; 107:295–301.

137. Bennet ED. Dopexamine: much more than a vasoactive agent. Crit Care Med 1998; 26:1621–2.

138. Vincent JL, van der Linden P, Domb M et al. Dopamine compared with dobutamine in experimental septic shock: relevance to fluid administration. Anesth Analg 1987; 66:565–71.

139. Bersten AD, Hersch M, Cheung H et al. The effect of various sympathomimetics on the regional circulations in hyperdynamic sepsis. Surgery 1992; 112:549–61.

140. Hesselvik JF, Brodin B. Low dose norepinephrine in patients with septic shock and oliguria: effects on afterload, urine flow, and oxygen transport. Crit Care Med 1989; 17:179–80.

141. Bollaert PE, Bauer PH, Audibert G et al. Effects of epinephrine on haemodynamics and oxygen metabolism in dopamine-resistant septic shock. Chest 1990; 98:949–53.

142. Meier-Hellman A, Hannemann L, Specht M et al. The relationship between mixed venous and hepatic venous O_2 saturation in patients with septic shock. Adv Exp Med Biol 1994; 345:701–7.

143. Vincent JL. Preiser JC. Inotropic agents. New Horiz 1993; 1:137–44.

144. Shoemaker WC, Appel PL, Kram HB et al. Oxygen transport measurements to evaluate tissue perfusion and titrate therapy: dobutamine and dopamine effects. Crit Care Med 1991; 19:672–88.

145. Marik PE, Mohedin M. The contrasting effects of dopamine and norepinephrine on systemic and splanchnic oxygen utilization in hyperdynamic sepses. JAMA 1994; 272:1354–7.

146. Tan LB, Littler A, Murray RG. Beneficial haemodynamic effects of intravenous dopamine in patients with low-output cardiac failure. J Cardiovasc Pharmacol 1987; 10:280–6.

147. Maynard N, Bihari DJ, Dalton RN et al. Increasing splanchnic blood flow in the critically ill. Chest 1995; 108:1648–54.

148. Ralph CJ, Tanser SJ, Macnaughton PD et al. A randomised controlled trial investigating the effects of dopexamine on gastrointestinal function and

organ dysfunction in the critically ill. Intensive Care Med 2002; 28:884–90.

149. Chatterjee K. Enoximone in heart failure: mechanisms of action. Br J Clin Pract 1988; 64:19–25.

150. Gage J, Rutman H, Lucido D et al. Additive effects of dobutamine and amrinone on myocardial contractility and ventricular performance in patients with severe heart failure. Circulation 1986; 74:367–73.

151. Boldt J, Brosch C, Suttner S et al. Prophylactic use of phosphodiesterase III inhibitor enoximone in elderly cardiac surgery patients: effect on hemodynamics, inflammation, and markers of organ function. Intensive Care Med 2002; 28:1462–9.

152. Kikura M, Sato S. The efficacy of preemptive milrinone or amrinone therapy in patients undergoing coronary artery bypass grafting. Anesth Analg 2002; 94:22–30.

153. Weber KT, Janicki JS. Intraaortic balloon counterpulsation. A review of physiologic principles, clinical results, and device safety. Ann Thorac Surg 1974; 17:602–36.

154. Solomon SM, Kirby DF. The refeeding syndrome: a review. J Parenteral Enteral Nutr 1990; 14:90–7.

155. Shoemaker WC. Cardiorespiratory patterns of surviving and non-surviving surgical patients. Surg Gynecol Obstet 1972; 134:810–14.

156. Shoemaker WC, Montgomery ES, Kaplan E et al. Physiologic patterns in surviving and non-surviving shock patients. Use of sequential cardiorespiratory parameters in defining criteria for therapeutic goals and early warning of death. Arch Surg 1973; 106:630–6.

157. Shoemaker WC, Chang PC, Czer LSC et al. Cardiorespiratory monitoring in postoperative patients. 1. Prediction of outcome and severity of illness. Crit Care Med 1979; 7:237–42.

158. Shoemaker WC, Chang PC, Czer LSC et al. Evaluation of the biologic importance of various haemodynamic and oxygen transport variables. Crit Care Med 1979; 7:424–9.

159. Bland RD, Shoemaker WC, Shabot MM. Physiologic monitoring goals for the critically ill patient. Surg Gynecol Obstet 1978; 147:833–41.

160. Boyd O, Bennet ED. Enhanced perioperative tissue perfusion as a therapeutic strategy. New Horiz 1996; 4:453–65.

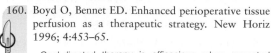

   Goal-directed therapy is efficacious when expected mortality is high.

161. Tuchschmidt J, Fried J, Astiz M et al. Supranormal oxygen delivery improves mortality in septic shock patients. Crit Care Med 1991; 19:S66.

162. Hayes MA, Timmins AC, Yau AH et al. Elevation of systemic oxygen delivery in the treatment of critically ill patients. N Engl J Med 1994; 330:1717–22.

163. Wilson J, Woods I, Fawcett J et al. Reducing the risk of major elective surgery: randomised controlled trial of preoperative optimisation of oxygen delivery. Br Med J 1999; 318:1099–103.

   Aggressive optimisation before surgery is associated with reduced mortality.

164. Rivers E, Nguyen B, Havstad S et al. Early goal-directed therapy in the treatment of severe sepsis and septic shock. N Engl J Med 2001; 345:1368–77.

   Early institution of goal-directed therapy is associated with improved outcome.

165. Kusano C, Baba M, Takao S et al. Oxygen delivery as a factor in the development of post-operative complications after oesophagectomy. Br J Surg 1997; 84:252–7.

166. Vallet B, Chopin C, Curtis SE et al. Prognostic value of the dobutamine test in patients with sepsis syndrome and normal lactate values: a prospective multicenter study. Crit Care Med 1993; 21:1868–75.

167. Buck N, Devlin HB, Lunn JN. The report of a confidential enquiry into perioperative deaths. London: Kings' Fund Publishing Office, 1987.

168. Lobo DN, Bjarnason K, Field J et al. Changes in weight, fluid balance and serum albumin in patients referred for nutritional support. Clin Nutr 1999; 18:197–201.

169. McRay PM, Barden RP, Randin IS. Nutritional oedema: effect on the gastric emptying time before and after gastric operations. Surgery 1937; 1:53–64.

170. Wait RB, Kahng KU. Renal failure complicating obstructive jaundice. Am J Surg 1989; 157:256–63.

171. Standards and audit. In: Galley HF (ed.) Critical care focus I: renal failure. London: BMJ Books, 1999.

172. Brezis M, Rosen S. Mechanisms of disease: hypoxia of the renal medulla: implications for disease. N Engl J Med 1995; 332:647–55.

173. Solomon R, Werner C, Mann D et al. Effects of saline, mannitol and furosemide to prevent acute decreases in renal function induced by radiocontrast agents. N Engl J Med 1994; 331:1416–20.

174. Chertow GM, Sayegh MH, Allgren RL et al. Is administration of dopamine associated with adverse or favourable outcomes in renal failure. Am J Med 1996; 101:49–53.

175. Woolfson RG. Dopamine and dopexamine in the prevention of renal failure. In: Galley HF (ed.) Critical care focus I: renal failure. London: BMJ Books, 1999; pp. 35–44.

176. Brezis M, Agmon Y, Epstein FH. Determinants of intrarenal oxygen I. Effects of diuretics. Am J Physiol 1994; 267:F1059–F1062.

177. Lee PA, Matson JR, Pryor RW et al. Continuous arteriovenous haemofiltration therapy for *Staphylococcus aureus*-induced septicaemia in immature swine. Crit Care Med 1993; 21:914–24.

178. Ronco C, Bellomo R, Homel P et al. Effects of different doses in continuous veno-venous haemofiltration on outcomes of acute renal failure: a prospective randomised trial. Lancet 2000; 355:26–30.

   Improved outcome associated with higher ultrafiltration rates.

179. Ivatury RR, Diebel L, Porter JM et al. Intra-abdominal hypertension and the abdominal compartment syndrome. Surg Clin North Am 1997; 4:783–800.

180. Meakins JL, Marshall JC. The gut: the 'motor' of MOF. Arch Surg 1986; 121:197–201.

181. O'Dwyer ST, Michie HR, Zeigler TR et al. A single dose of endotoxin increases intestinal permeability in healthy humans. Arch Surg 1988; 123:1459–64.

182. Deitch EA, Berg R, Specian R. Endotoxin promotes the translocation of bacteria from the gut. Arch Surg 1987; 122:185–90.

183. Border JR, Hasset JM, LaDuca J et al. Gut origin in septic states in blunt multiple trauma (ISS-40) in the ICU. Ann Surg 1987; 206:427–48.

184. Barr H. Gastric volvulus and acute gastric dilatation. In: Morris PJ, Malt RA (eds) Oxford textbook of surgery. Oxford: Oxford University Press, 1994; vol. I, pp. 953–5.

185. Summers GE, Hocking MP. Preoperative and post-operative motility disorders of the stomach. Surg Clin North Am 1992; 72:467–86.

186. Condon RE, Cowles VE, Schulte WJ et al. Resolution of post-operative ileus in humans. Ann Surg 1986; 203:574–81.

187. Ahmed AR, Taylor I. Superior mesenteric artery syndrome. Postgrad Med J 1997; 73:776–8.

188. Doradi S, Berry AR, Kettlewell MGW. Acute colonic pseudo-obstruction. Br J Surg 1992; 79:99–103.

189. Cook DJ, Fuller H, Guyatt GH. Risk factors for gastrointestinal bleeding in the critically ill. N Engl J Med 1994; 330:377–81.

190. Cook DJ, Reeve BK, Guyatt GH et al. Stress ulcer prophylaxis in critically ill patients: resolving discordant meta-analyses. JAMA 1996; 275:308–14.

191. Cook DJ, Guyatt G, Marshall J et al. A comparison of sucralfate and ranitidine for the prevention of upper gastrointestinal bleeding in patients requiring mechanical ventilation: Canadian Critical Care Trials Group. N Engl J Med 1998; 338:791–7.

   Ranitidine is effective and safe prophylaxis.

192. Peura DA, Johnson LF. Cimetidine for prevention and treatment of gastroduodenal mucosal lesions in patients in an intensive care unit. Ann Intern Med 1985; 103:173–7.

193. Steinberg KP. Stress-related mucosal disease in the critically ill patient: risk factors and strategies to prevent stress-related bleeding in the intensive care unit. Crit Care Med 2002; 30(Suppl.):S362–S364.

194. Barie PS, Fisher E. Acute acalculous cholecystitis. J Am Coll Surg 1995; 180:232–4.

195. Imrie CW, Benjamin IS, Ferguson JC et al. A single-centre double-blind trial of Trasylol therapy in acute pancreatitis. Br J Surg 1978; 65:337–41.

196. Powell JJ, Miles R, Siriwardena AK. Antibiotic prophylaxis in the initial management of severe acute pancreatitis. Br J Surg 1998; 85:582–7.

197. Barie PS. A critical review of antibiotic prophylaxis in severe acute pancreatitis. Am J Surg 1996; 172(Suppl. 6A):38S–43S.

198. Neoptolemos JP, Carr-Locke DL, London NJM et al. Controlled trial of urgent endoscopic retrograde cholangiopancreatography and endoscopic sphincterotomy versus conservative treatment in patients with acute pancreatitis due to gallstones. Lancet 1988; ii:979–83.

199. Bradley EL. Necrotizing pancreatitis. Br J Surg 1999; 86:147–8.

200. Fisher RL. Hepatobiliary abnormalities associated with total parenteral nutrition. Gastroenterol Clin North Am 1989; 18:645–66.

201. Stanley AJ, Lee A, Hayes PC. Management of acute liver failure. Aetiology, complications and management. Br J Intensive Care 1995; 5:8–16.

202. Bassiouny HS. Non occlusive mesenteric ischaemia. Surg Clin North Am 1997; 77:319–26.

203. Delaney CP, O'Neill S, Manning F et al. Plasma concentrations of glutathione S-transferase isoenzyme are raised in patients with intestinal ischaemia. Br J Surg 1999; 86:1349–54.

204. Robert JH, Mentha G, Rohner A. Ischaemic colitis: two distinct patterns of severity. Gut 1993; 34:4–6.

205. Willams NS, Scott ADN. Neutropenic colitis. Br J Surg 1997; 84:1200–5.

206. Carr CS, Lang KDE, Boulos P et al. Randomised trial of safety and efficacy of immediate postoperative enteral feeding in patients undergoing gastro-intestinal resection. Br Med J 1996; 312:869–71.

207. Kalfarentzos F, Kehagias N, Mead N et al. Enteral versus parenteral nutrition in acute pancreatitis. Br J Surg 1997; 84:1665–9.

208. Columb MO, Shah MV, Sproat LJ et al. Assessment of gastric dysfunction. Current techniques for the measurement of gastric emptying. Br J Intensive Care 1992; 2:75–80.

209. Alverdy JC, Aoys E, Moss GS. Total parenteral nutrition promotes bacterial translocation from the gut. Surgery 1988; 104:185–90.

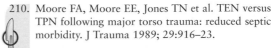

210. Moore FA, Moore EE, Jones TN et al. TEN versus TPN following major torso trauma: reduced septic morbidity. J Trauma 1989; 29:916–23.

211. Moore FA, Feliciano DV, Andrassy RJ et al. Early enteral feeding compared with parenteral reduces postoperative septic complications: the results of a meta-analysis. Ann Surg 1992; 216:172–83.

   Early enteral nutrition is associated with improved outcome after blunt abdominal trauma.

212. Bower RH, Cerra FB, Berdashadsky B et al. Early enteral administration of a formula (Impact®) supplemented with arginine, nucleotides and fish oil in intensive care patients: results of a multicentre, prospective, randomised, clinical trial. Crit Care Med 1995; 25:436–9.

213. O'Dwyer ST et al. Maintenance of small bowel mucosa with glutamine-enriched parenteral nutrition. J Parenteral Enteral Nutr 1989; 13:579–85.

214. Powell-Tuck J, Jamieson CP, Bettany GEA et al. A double blind, randomised, controlled trial of glutamine supplementation in parenteral nutrition. Gut 1999; 45:82–8.

215. British Medical Association. Withdrawing and withholding life-prolonging medical treatment: guidance for decision making. London: BMJ Books, 1999.

216. Hoyle RW. In: Gray AJG, Hoyle RW, Ingram GS et al. (eds) National confidential enquiry into perioperative death 1996–1997. London: National Confidential Enquiry into Perioperative Death, 1998.

217. *Airdale NHS Trust* v. *Bland* [1993] 1 All ER 821.

Index

Notes
Page numbers followed by 'f' indicate figures, those followed by 't' indicate tables or boxes.
vs. indicates a comparison or differential diagnosis.

inguinal hernias (*cont.*)
 complications, 68, 233f
 infants/neonates, 62–63, 233
 laparoscopic repair, 65, 67, 67t, 69–70, 70t
 open approach, 69t
 recurrence rates, 67t, 68, 68t, 69t
 recurrent hernias, 68–70
 sutured procedures, 68–69, 68t
 technique popularity, 64f
 tension-free mesh, 64–65, 65f, 66f, 69
 recurrent, 68–70
injection sclerotherapy, 125, 126–127
inotropes, critical care, 343
insulin, trauma effects, 310, 311t
insulin resistance, trauma, 310
insurance, 296
integrated care pathways (ICPs), 12
intensive care databases, 301
intensive-care unit (ICU)
 abdominal trauma, 247
 cardiovascular support, 341–344
 colonic emergencies, 183
 ethical considerations, 348
 goal-directed therapy, 344–345
 nutrition, 348
 nutritional support teams, 321
 physiological variables, 338t
 renal support, 345–346
 respiratory support, 339–341
 sepsis management, 337–348
 indications for, 335–336, 336, 336t
 tissue oxygenation/perfusion, 337–339
intermittent positive-pressure ventilation (IPPV), 340
internal validity, 3
Internet, as source of evidence, 4–5
intersphincteric anorectal abscess, 216
 management, 220f
interview, 297
intestine
 developmental abnormalities
 anorectal, 231
 duplications, 232
 malrotation, 231–232
 intussusception, 170, 234–235, 235f
 ischaemia, 85, 172, 347
 large *see* large bowel
 obstruction
 critical illness, 347–348
 large bowel *see* large bowel obstruction
 neonatal *see* neonatal intestinal obstruction
 small bowel *see* small bowel obstruction
 small *see* small bowel
intraabdominal pressure (IAP), 247
 measurement, 249
 raised, 247–250
 diagnosis, 248
 pathophysiology, 248–249

treatment, 249–250
intra-aortic balloon counterpulsation, 343–344
intracranial pressure (ICP), 249
intraperitoneal hernia repair, 67
intravaginal torsion, 236
intravenous urography, abdominal trauma, 241
intrinsic coagulation cascade, 265f
intussusception
 infants, 234–235, 235f
 small bowel obstruction, 170
invasive arterial blood pressure, 337
investigations, day surgery, 43
ischaemia–reperfusion injury, inflammation, 331
'ischaemic colitis', 172, 196
ischiorectal abscess, 216
 management, 220f

jejunostomy, 169, 317
 critical care, 348
Journal of the American Medical Association (JAMA), 4
journals, as sources of evidence, 4
judgement, professional, 291

kidney
 abdominal compartment syndrome, 248
 acute renal failure, 345–346
 ventilation-induced problems, 340
 see also entries beginning renal
Kocher's manoeuvre, 129, 245, 254
KyberSept trial, 335

Lactobacillus plantarum, 155
Laparoscopic Groin and Hernia Trial Group, 2–3
laparoscopic surgery
 appendicectomy, 176
 cholecystectomy
 angiography during, 141, 142f
 day case, controversy, 47–48
 early, advantages, 143
 colonic bleeding, 199
 evidence-based medicine, 2–3
 hernia repair
 adult inguinal hernias, 65, 67
 femoral hernias, 71
 incisional hernias, 75
 open repair *vs.* 75, 75t
 recurrence rates, 67t
 recurrent inguinal hernias, 69–70, 70t
 perforated peptic ulcer, 108–109
 small bowel obstruction, 171
laparoscopy
 diagnostic
 abdominal trauma, 242
 acalculous cholecystitis, 145
 acute abdomen, 83, 90–91
 history, 90
 minilaparoscopy, 91, 91f
 surgery *see* laparoscopic surgery

laparotomy
 abdominal trauma, 243–247
 bleeding control, 245
 damage control, 245–247
 injury assessment, 245
 physiological control, 245
 preparation, 244–245
 timing, 243–244
 complications, incisional hernia, 71–75
 investigative
 abdominal trauma, 242–243
 acute pancreatitis, 149–150
 GI bleeding, 122
 laparoscopy before, 90
 sepsis management, 333–334
large bowel
 acute conditions
 anorectal, 215–226
 colonic, 183–214
 obstruction *see* large bowel obstruction
 preparation for surgery, 183–184
 stercoral perforation, 203–204, 207
 endoscopy damage, 206, 207
 lavage, 197
 see also anus; colon; rectum
large bowel obstruction
 computed tomography, 191, 192f
 contrast radiography, 87–88, 88f, 189, 191, 191f
 functional (pseudo-obstruction) 87–88, 188–190, 207
 malignant, 190–195, 191f, 192f, 207
 hospital stay following surgery, 194
 left-sided obstruction, 193–195
 non-operative management, 191–192, 192f
 presentation, 191
 procedure choice, 195
 right-sided obstruction, 193
 surgical management, 192–195
 transverse obstruction, 193
laser photocoagulation, 123–124, 125
laser therapy, malignant large bowel obstruction, 192
lateral sphincterotomy, 221
league tables, cost-effectiveness analysis, 33–34
left-ventricular end-diastolic pressure (LVEDP), 337
leg compression, 281
leucocytosis, acute cholecystitis, 140
limb elevation, 281
lipolysis, trauma, 311
lipoma, inguinal hernia, 64
liquid ventilation, 341
literature reviews, evidence-based practice, 7–8
lithium dilution measures, 338
liver
 anatomy, 254, 255t